NURSING EDUCATION
Principles and Concepts

NURSING EDUCATION
Principles and Concepts

Second Edition

R Sudha
MSc(N) PhD
Professor and Principal
VHS—MA Chidambaram College of Nursing
(Affiliated to the Tamil Nadu Dr MGR Medical University)
Voluntary Health Services
Chennai, Tamil Nadu, India

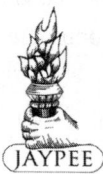

JAYPEE BROTHERS MEDICAL PUBLISHERS
The Health Sciences Publisher
New Delhi | London

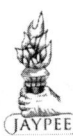

Jaypee Brothers Medical Publishers (P) Ltd

Headquarters
Jaypee Brothers Medical Publishers (P) Ltd
EMCA House, 23/23-B
Ansari Road, Daryaganj
New Delhi 110 002, India
Landline: +91-11-23272143, +91-11-23272703
+91-11-23282021, +91-11-23245672
Head Office: 011-43574357
Email: jaypee@jaypeebrothers.com: www.jaypeebrothers.com

Corporate Office
Jaypee Brothers Medical Publishers (P) Ltd
4838/24, Ansari Road, Daryaganj
New Delhi 110 002, India
Phone: +91-11-43574357
Fax: +91-11-43574314
Email: jaypee@jaypeebrothers.com

Overseas Office
J.P. Medical Ltd
83 Victoria Street, London
SW1H 0HW (UK)
Phone: +44 20 3170 8910
Fax: +44 (0)20 3008 6180
Email: info@jpmedpub.com

Website: www.jaypeebrothers.com
Website: www.jaypeedigital.com

© 2021, Jaypee Brothers Medical Publishers

The views and opinions expressed in this book are solely those of the original contributor(s)/author(s) and do not necessarily represent those of editor(s) of the book.

All rights reserved. No part of this publication may be reproduced, stored or transmitted in any form or by any means, electronic, mechanical, photocopying, recording or otherwise, without the prior permission in writing of the publishers.

All brand names and product names used in this book are trade names, service marks, trademarks or registered trademarks of their respective owners. The publisher is not associated with any product or vendor mentioned in this book.

Medical knowledge and practice change constantly. This book is designed to provide accurate, authoritative information about the subject matter in question. However, readers are advised to check the most current information available on procedures included and check information from the manufacturer of each product to be administered, to verify the recommended dose, formula, method and duration of administration, adverse effects and contraindications. It is the responsibility of the practitioner to take all appropriate safety precautions. Neither the publisher nor the author(s)/editor(s) assume any liability for any injury and/or damage to persons or property arising from or related to use of material in this book.

This book is sold on the understanding that the publisher is not engaged in providing professional medical services. If such advice or services are required, the services of a competent medical professional should be sought.

Every effort has been made where necessary to contact holders of copyright to obtain permission to reproduce copyright material. If any have been inadvertently overlooked, the publisher will be pleased to make the necessary arrangements at the first opportunity. The **CD/DVD-ROM** (if any) provided in the sealed envelope with this book is complimentary and free of cost. **Not meant for sale.**

Inquiries for bulk sales may be solicited at: jaypee@jaypeebrothers.com

Nursing Education: Principles and Concepts

First Edition: 2013
Second Edition: 2021
Reprint **2023**
ISBN: 978-93-89776-94-2
Printed at: Sterling Graphics Pvt. Ltd.

Dedicated to

My Teachers and Nursing Profession

Preface to the Second Edition

Seventh year since the first edition of this book was published, I have received numerous responses and messages from readers commenting on the book. The feedback from the postgraduate students is overwhelming and encouraging. I have been extremely grateful for the positive responses and was excited to undertake a challenge of the new edition. Beyond simply updating the concepts, this second edition provided me an opportunity to further explore the topics and give an in-depth reading.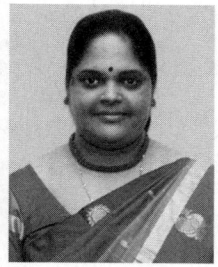

In this second edition, I have made the following changes and additions:
- The literature of all chapters is updated.
- In the first chapter, the additions are the concepts on social and economic factors influencing nursing education, technological advancements and nursing, and the National Education Policy, 2016.
- In the second chapter, revised Bloom's taxonomy and the relevant verbs with examples of specific objectives for each level are updated and the concept on Problem-based Learning is elaborated.
- The literature on Objective Structured Clinical Examination (OSCE) was revised in chapter four.
- Nursing education programs in the United Kingdom and China are added in chapter five.
- Lesson plan for the topic on cognitive and psychomotor domain learning are included in the Appendices.

Despite removing the obsolete information in all chapters, the concepts are refined and updated with the current information. Hope this book will fulfill all your expectations. Waiting to hear from you the valuable feedback as extended for the first edition.

R Sudha

Preface to the First Edition

It gives me an immense pleasure to introduce a textbook on nursing education. Indeed, I feel happy to write a textbook on nursing education. I always think and be proud of our profession where we have the opportunity to serve the humanity. Everyone accepts the demand for nurses globally. It is the responsibility of the society especially the nursing regulatory mechanisms to monitor the preparation of nurses to meet the societal and global demand. The nurse educators are accountable to this cause and ultimately held responsible for the preparation of nurses.

Nursing education as a subject has to be studied for two purposes that is to understand what nursing education is and to teach and enhance the teaching-learning process for learning other nursing subjects. A teacher who understands the concept of teaching and learning and who has the attitude to teach will automatically develop skill in teaching. A student who understands the basic concept of learning will learn quickly.

With this concept and belief, this textbook is prepared to share and communicate the principles of nursing education. This book will be of great use to undergraduate and postgraduate nursing students who can easily follow and understand the concepts as it is organized sequentially and written in a simple language. This book will also be a good reference book for the nursing teachers who have the passion to teach and educate the nursing students and the nurses.

I would appreciate the readers for their suggestions and comments for the improvement of the content of the book.

R Sudha

Acknowledgments

Gratitude is the best attitude. An individual alone cannot accomplish any task. It is the help, support and encouragement of people which helps him/her to accomplish a task.

I take immense pleasure to express my deep sense of gratitude to my parents Mr P Radhakrishnan, EE, TAHDCO (retired) and Mrs R Rajalakshmi for their selfless help and support in all my endeavors. I also thank my husband Mr C Arumugam and my daughters, AS Neya and AS Dhaya for their love, tolerance and understanding which helped me to succeed in my career.

I express my sincere thanks to Shri Jitendar P Vij (Group Chairman), Mr Ankit Vij (Managing Director), Mr MS Mani (Group President), Dr Madhu Choudhary (Publishing Head–Education), Ms Pooja Bhandari (Production Head), Ms Sunita Katla (Executive Assistant to Group Chairman and Publishing Manager), Ms Samina Khan (Executive Assistant to Publishing Head–Education), Ms Dolly Dominic (Development Editor), Ms Seema Dogra (Cover Visualizer), Mr Binay Kumar (Proofreader), Mr Dinesh Bhardwaj (Typesetter), Mr Suhel Ahmed (Graphic Designer) and the whole team of M/s Jaypee Brothers Medical Publishers (P) Ltd, New Delhi, India, for their efforts in publishing the book.

Contents

1. Introduction to Education and Nursing Education 1
- **Concepts of Education** *1* • Introduction *1* • Meaning and Definition *1* • Forms of Education *2*
- **Philosophy and Education** *3* • Meaning and Definition *3* • Main Divisions in Philosophy *3*
- Relationship between Philosophy and Education *5* • Value Theory *6*
- Significance of Philosophy of Education *7* • **Major Systems of Philosophy and its Educational Implications** *7*
- Idealism *7* • Realism *9* • Naturalism *10* • Pragmatism *11* • **Indian School of Philosophy** *12*
- The Vedanta Philosophy *12* • The Bhagvad Gita *13* • Jainism *13* • Buddhism *14*
- **Aims of Education** *15* • General Aims of Education *15* • Aims of Education in Independent India *16*
- Aims of Nursing Education *16* • Factors Determining Educational Aims *17* • **Functions of Education** *17*
- General Functions of Education *17* • Functions of Education to Individual *18*
- Functions of Education in National Life *18* • Agencies of Education *19*
- Classification of Agencies of Education *20* • Principles of Education *20*
- Impact of Social, Economical, Political and Technological Changes on Education *21*
- Economic Factors and Education *23* • Political Factors Influencing Education *26*
- Technological Factors Influencing Education *27* • **Challenges in Nursing Education** *29*
- Professional Education *33* • Trends in Development of Nursing *34* • National Policy on Education *35*

2. Teaching-Learning Process 45
- Educational Process *45* • Dimensions of Educational Process *45* • Elements of Educational Process *46*
- **Learning** *46* • Definition of Learning *46* • Characteristics of Learning *46* • Pillars of Learning *47*
- The Learning Process *47* • Learning Styles or Learning Modalities *48* • Theoretical Orientations to Learning *49*
- **Teaching** *49* • Meaning and Definition *49* • General Principles of Teaching *50*
- Effective Teaching Principles and Practices *50* • Maxims of Methodological Teaching *51*
- Phases of Teaching *52* • Variables of Teaching *52* • Stages of Teaching *52*
- Characteristics of Good Teaching *53* • Models of Teaching-Learning Process and its Application in Nursing *53*
- Relationship between Teaching and Learning *56* • Teaching Strategies *56*
- **Outcome-based Education** *57* • Meaning and Definition *57* • **Competency-based Education** *61*
- Meaning and Definition *61* • **Educational Objectives and Instructional Objectives** *62*
- Meaning and Definition *62* • Types of Educational Objectives *62* • Characteristics *62*
- Purposes of Specific Objectives *62* • Elements of Specific Objectives *63*
- Taxonomy of Educational Objectives *63* • **Lesson Plan** *66* • Points to Remember in Planning a Lesson *66*
- Prerequisites for Good Lesson Planning *67* • Types of Lesson Plan *67*
- Essential Elements of Good Lesson Plan *67* • Steps in Developing a Lesson Plan *67*
- How to Prepare a Lesson Plan *67* • Teachers' Requirements in Lesson Planning *68* • **Unit Plan** *68*
- Criteria for a Good Unit *68* • Characteristics of Unit Planning *68* • Types of Unit Planning *68*
- Essential Activities in Planning a Unit *69* • Steps in Writing a Unit Plan *69* • **Course Outline** *70*
- Meaning and Definition *70* • Classroom Management *71* • Management of Students *72*
- Managing Inappropriate Behavior *72* • Promoting Appropriate Use of Consequences *72*
- Role of Teacher in Classroom Management *72* • Role of Student in Classroom Management *73*
- Classroom Management Mistakes New Teachers Often Make *73* • **Methods of Teaching** *74*
- Introduction *74* • Classification of Methods of Teaching *74*
- Principles to Follow in Selection of Methods of Teaching *74* • Lecture Method *74* • Demonstration *78*
- Group Discussion *79* • Seminar *80* • Symposium *82* • Panel Discussion *83* • Exhibition *84*
- Field Trip *85* • Project Method *86* • Role Play *87* • Programmed Instruction *88*

- Problem-based Learning *91* • Self-directed Learning/Self-learning Packets/Individualized Learning Packet *95*
- Self-instructional Module *95* • Workshop *96* • Simulation *97* • Computer-based Simulation Programs *99*
- Microteaching *100* • Computer Assisted Learning *101* • Peer Tutoring *102* • Humor *104*
- MUDD Mapping *107* • Clinical Teaching Methods *108* • Nursing Case Study *108* • Bedside Clinic *109*
- Nursing Rounds *110* • Conference *111* • Process Recording *112*

3. Instructional Media and Methods 114

- IDefinition *114* • Senses as Gateway of Learning *114* • Where to use Audio-visual Aids *115*
- Classification of Audio-visual Aids *115* • Graphic Aids *117* • Charts *117* • Pictures *119*
- Posters *120* • Graphs *121* • Maps *123* • Cartoons *123* • Flash Cards *124*
- Pamphlets, Booklets and Leaflets *125* • Chalkboards *125* • Flannel Board *128*
- Bulletin Board *128* • Three-dimensional Models Objects, Specimens, and Models *129*
- Slides and Films *131* • Puppets *132* • Handouts *134* • Overhead Projector *135* • Radio *137*
- Tape Recorder *138* • Public Address System *139* • Television *139* • Films *140* • Computer *141*
- Camera *142* • Liquid Crystal Display Projector *143* • Powerpoint Presentation *145*
- Video Compact Disk *145* • Video Cassette Recorder *145* • Microscope *146*

4. Measurement and Evaluation 149

- Meaning and Definition *149* • Meaning of Measurement, Assessment, Evaluation and Testing *149*
- Assessment *150* • Measurement *150* • Test *150* • Evaluation *150* • Evaluation Process *150*
- Concepts of Evaluation *151* • Principles of Evaluation *151* • Purpose of Evaluation *151*
- Scope of Evaluation *152* • Common Errors in Evaluation *152* • Types of Evaluation *152*
- Criteria for Selection of Evaluation *155* • Steps of Evaluation *156* • Evaluation Methods for Different Domain *156*
- Tools and Techniques of Evaluation *156* • Multiple Choice Questions/Select the Best Answer *162*
- Checklists *165* • Item Analysis *165* • Item Difficulty and Item Discrimination *166*
- True or False Items *168* • Matching Items *168* • Observation *169* • Unstructured Techniques *170*
- Sociometry *170* • Anecdotal Records *173* • Critical Incident Records *174* • **Structured Techniques** *175*
- Checklists *175* • Rating Scale *175* • Practical Examinations *177* • Viva Voce/Oral Examination *179*
- Objective Structured Practical Examination (OSPE)/Objective Structured Clinical Examination (OSCE) *179*
- Attitude Scale *183* • Question Bank *185* • Test *188* • Grades *190* • Assigning Grades *191*
- **Standardized Tools or Tests** *193* • Meaning *193* • Classification of Psychological Tests *193*
- Design and Scoring of Standardized Tests *194* • Steps in Constructing Scales *194* • **Various Tests** *196*
- Interest Inventories *196* • Measurement of Interest *196* • Inventories of Standardized Interest *197*
- Limitation of Interest Inventories *197* • Achievement Tests *197* • Aptitude Tests *197*
- Personality Tests *199* • Intelligence Tests *200* • Socioeconomic Status Scale *200*

5. Nursing Educational Programs 202

- Nursing Education at Global Level *202* • Professional Socialization *204*
- Nursing Education in United Kingdom (UK) *205* • Nursing Education in China *205*
- Patterns of Nursing Education in India *206*

6. Continuing Education in Nursing 212

- Meaning and Definition *212* • Concept of Continuing Education *212* • Need for Continuing Education *213*
- Purposes of Continuing Nursing Education *213* • Forms of Continuing Education Programs *213*
- Philosophy of Continuing Education *214* • Planning Continuing Education Programs *214*
- Characteristics of Continuing Education *214*
- Elements Essential for Successful Implementation of Continuing Education *215*
- Relationship between Practice and Need for Continuing Education *216*
- Implications of Continuing Education *216* • Areas to be Addressed by Continuing Education *216*
- Recommendations *216* • Principles of Adult Learning *217* • Steps in CE Program Development *218*
- Steps in Conducting Continuing Education in Nursing *218* • Research in Continuing Nursing Education *220*

- *Distance Education in Nursing 221* • *Webcast 223* • *Videoconferencing 224*
- *Usage of Technology in Distance Learning—the Benefits of e-SIM 226*
- *Tutor Competencies for Online Teaching 227*

7. Curriculum Development 229
- *Meaning and Definition 229* • *Concepts of Curriculum 230* • *Three Facets of Curriculum 230*
- *Determinants of Curriculum 230* • *Approaches of Curriculum 232* • *Nature of Nursing Curriculum 232*
- *Types of Curriculum/Patterns of Curriculum Organization 232* • *Elements of Curriculum 233*
- *Forces and Issues Influencing Curriculum Development 234* • *Models of Curriculum 235*
- *Curriculum Planning 241* • *Curriculum Design 244* • *The ABC of Curriculum Organization 246*
- *Conceptual Framework for Curriculum Design 247* • *Selection of Learning Experiences 249*
- *Master Rotation Plan 251* • *Individual Rotation Plan 251* • *Curriculum Implementation 251*
- *Print-based Resources—Textbook 252* • *Curriculum Change/Innovation/Revision 253*
- *Factors Influencing Decisions about Curriculum 256* • *Curriculum Evaluation 257*

8. Teacher Preparation 263
- *Concepts of Teacher 263* • *Essential Qualities of a Teacher 264* • *Duties of a Teacher 266*
- *Broad Classification of a Teacher's Role 267* • *Teacher's Multifarious Role in Pupil Development 267*
- *Major Functions and Responsibilities of a Teacher 267* • *New Demands of the Role of Teacher 268*
- *Some Salient Attributes of an Effective Teacher 269*
- *Essential Qualities and Characteristics of Effective Teacher 271* • *The Qualities of a Good Teacher 273*
- *Teaching Skills and Teacher Competency 274* • *Teacher Education and Training 275*
- *Teacher Educator 279* • *Functions of Teacher Education Institutions 282*
- *The Twelve Roles of the Teacher 283* • *Multiple Roles of the Teacher 284*
- *Professionalization: Concepts and Characteristics 284*
- **Organizing Professional Aspects of Teacher Education 289** • *Need for Evaluation of Teachers 291*
- *Preparation of Nursing Teacher 295*

9. Guidance and Counseling 297
- *Meaning and Definition of Guidance 297* • *Significant Guidance Principles and Assumptions 297*
- *Characteristics of Guidance Program 298* • *Meaning and Definition of Counseling 298*
- *Basis of Guidance and Counseling 298* • *Need for Guidance and Counseling 299*
- *Principles of Guidance and Counseling 300* • *Organization of Counseling Services 301*
- *Types of Counseling 302* • *Approaches to Counseling 303* • *Phases of Counseling 304*
- *Tools and Techniques of Guidance and Counseling 305* • *Guidance Bureau in Colleges 305*
- *Roles of the Counseling Team Members 306* • *Qualifications of a Counselor 306*
- *Skills Required of a Counselor 306* • *Group Guidance 307* • *Problems in Guidance and Counseling 308*
- *Issues Faced by Novice Counselors 309* • *Key Dimensions of Counseling 310*
- **Disciplinary Problems and Actions 310** • *Types of Disciplinary Actions 310*
- *Ground for Disciplinary Actions 311* • *Management of Disciplinary Problems 312*
- *Procedure for Minor Misconduct 312* • *Procedure for Serious Misconduct 313* • *Preventive Strategies 313*
- *Responding to Student Misconduct 314* • *Management of Crisis and Referral Services 314*
- *Crisis Intervention 315*

10. Administration of Nursing Curriculum 317
- *Curriculum Planning 317* • *Curriculum Organization 317* • *Curriculum Evaluation 318*
- *Curriculum Development 318* • *Need Assessment 318* • *Facilitators of Curriculum Development 318*
- *Designing the Curriculum 318* • *Developing Curriculum Structure 318* • *Curriculum Enhancement 319*
- *Evaluation of Educational Programs in Nursing 321* • *Models of Evaluation 322*
- *Criteria for Evaluation of a Program 324* • *Curriculum Improvement 324* • *Curriculum Research in Nursing 325*
- *Different Models of Collaboration between Education and Service 326* • *Interfaces 329*

11. Management of Nursing Educational Institutions 331

- Management of Nursing Educational Institutions 331   • **Nursing Programs-Purpose, Requirements, Facility** 332
- Auxiliary Nurse Midwifery 332   • Diploma in General Nursing and Midwifery 333
- Bachelor of Science in Nursing [BSc(N)] 333   • Post-basic BSc(N) [PBBSc(N)] 334   • MSc(N) 335
- Nurse Practitioner in Critical Care 335   • Master of Philosophy in Nursing 335
- Doctor of Philosophy in Nursing 335   • Post-basic Diploma in Nursing 336
- Functions of Education Management Planning 336   • Institutional Planning 337   • Organizing 337
- Organization Structure 338   • Human Resource Planning 339   • Objectives 339   • Recruitment 340
- Budgeting 342   • Discipline 344   • Public Relations 346   • Meaning and Definition 346
- The Role of Public Relations for Nursing 346   • Advantages of Public Relations 346
- Disadvantages of Public Relations 347   • Objectives of Public Relations 347   • Public Relations Tools 347
- Additional PR Activities 349   • Trends in Public Relations 350   • Performance Appraisal 351
- Importance of Performance Appraisal 351   • Principles of Performance Appraisal 352
- Teaching Evaluation Model 352   • Performance Appraisal Process 352
- Components of Comprehensive Appraisal System 352   • Tool for Performance Appraisal 353
- Alternative Types of Performance Appraisal 353   • Academic Audit 354
- Format for Academic Audit to Teachers 355   • Staff Welfare Services 357   • Library 358   • Hostel 359
- Nursing Standards 360   • Purpose of Standards 361   • Characteristics of Standards 361
- Purposes of Standards in Education 361   • Classification of Standards 361   • Accreditation in Nursing 362
- National Assessment and Accreditation Council 363   • Indian Nursing Council 364
- State Nursing Council 365   • Board-CMAI 365   • University 365   • Professional Associations 366
- Benefits of Belonging to a Professional Association 366   • Deciding which Associations to Join 366
- Becoming a Productive Association 366   • Whom do Professional Associations Serve 367
- Professional Association Activities 367   • Joining and Using Professional Associations in Nursing 367
- Types of Associations 367   • List of Some Nursing Organizations (International) 367
- The Trained Nurses' Association of India 367

12. Communication and Educational Technology 372

- Definition of Educational Technology 372   • Objectives of Educational Technology 372
- Uses of Communication Technology 373   • Some Specific Educational Uses of Communication Technology 373
- Barriers of Communication Technology to Education 373   • Some of the Educational Technologies Used 374
- Online Teaching and Online Learning 378   • Virtual Campus 380   • Virtual Classroom 381
- E-learning 383   • Teleconferencing 384   • Multimedia 385   • Internet in Education 386
- Internet Services 387   • Developing an Internet Connection 387

Appendices 391

Bibliography 415

Index 417

1. Introduction to Education and Nursing Education

"Being ignorant is not so much a shame as being unwilling to learn to do things the right way".
—Benjamin Franklin

Objectives

After reading this unit, you will be able to:
- State the meaning and definition of education
- Understand the relationship between various philosophy and education
- Enumerate the aims and functions of education
- Explain the agencies of education
- Describe the principles of education
- Explain the factors influencing education
- Appreciate the trends in development of nursing education in India
- Explain the challenges in nursing education
- Understand professional education
- Explain the role of various educational commissions

Concepts of Education

"Education is not preparation for life; education is life itself".
—John Dewey

Introduction

Everybody uses the term "Education" in our day-to-day life. Different people attach different meaning to it. According to Aristotle, education means creation of sound mind in a sound body. Swami Vivekananda has said education is the manifestation of perfection already in man. Education encompasses both the teaching and learning of knowledge, proper conduct, and technical competency. Education thus is a purposive activity. It has to set forth clearly its objectives. The content is also to be developed and organized in an effective way based on the objectives. They are the goals toward which education is oriented. Methods of teaching are formulated as the intermediary between the "Why" and "What" of education. Learning is facilitated by instruction, teaching, and training. Instruction refers to the intentional facilitating of learning toward identified goals, delivered either by an instructor or other forms. Teaching refers to learning facilitated by a real-life instructor. Training refers to learning toward preparing learners with specific knowledge, skills, or abilities that can be applied immediately. Learning experiences are the means of realizing the objectives. The emphasis now is on objective-based education or instruction. Objectives are reduced to specifications in terms of the specific changes in behavior of the students which are tangible, observable, and concrete. The scheme of evaluation in education is to find out how far the objectives have been translated into practice as outcomes. This unit focuses on the essential concepts of philosophy and education, various educational commissions, and the trends in education and professional education.

Meaning and Definition

There is a great controversy in regard to the meaning and definition of the term "Education".

Etymologically education is said to have been derived from the Latin term *"Educatum"*. The alphabet "E" indicates *"from internal"* and *"Duco"* stands for *"to lead"* which mean the art of leading out. The derivation may also be from the term *"Educere"* which means the art of bringing up.

Divergent views have been expressed by scholars from Socrates and Plato up to present day. Some of the views have been tabulated below:

Scholars	Views about education
Socrates	Education means bringing out of the idea of universal validity which is latent in the mind of every man.
Froebel	Education is a process by which a child makes its internal, external.
Dewey	Education is the development of all those capacities in the individual which will enable him to control his environment and fulfill his possibilities.
Mahatma Gandhi	Education is "an all-round drawing out of the best in child and man—body, mind and spirit".

Contd...

Contd...

Scholars	Views about education
Redden and Ryan	Education as "the deliberate and systematic influence exerted by the mature person upon the immature through instruction, discipline and harmonious development of all the powers of the human being—physical, social, intellectual, esthetic and spiritual according to their essential hierarchy, by and for their individual and social uses and directed toward the union of the educand with his creator as the final end".

Education is human endeavor. It is essentially confined to "modification of human behavior". If the modification is to bring about "desirable" changes in the behavior of individuals, the word, "desirable" pertains to the philosophical question. Education is defined as influence effected by one set of individuals on another so as to enable the latter to grow properly. Education is thus equated with guidance.

Combining all the above, we can discern broadly three stand points:
1. **Education as development**: This means education acts as a process to develop the hidden potentialities of the individual.
2. **Education as acquisition**: This is an external process. Education is acquisition of knowledge from teachers.
3. **Education as transaction**: As mentioned above, education is both developmental and acquiring knowledge. This means helping the individual grow from within and from outside.

Education is thus regarded as a process of adjustment of the individual to himself and to society or environment. In other words, education is the adjustment of a physically and mentally developed individual to the intellectual, moral, and volitional environment.

Wider and Narrower Meaning of Education

In the wider sense, it is actually a process of development from cradle to grave. It includes all sorts of influence like home-life influence, the influence of friendship, recreation, hobbies, etc. This is a long process which is never ending.

In the narrower sense, "Education" is limited to some specific spheres. It is confined to school and university instruction. It is believed that education starts as soon as the child enters the school. It is over when he leaves it after completing a particular course of studies. In a narrower sense, it may be taken to mean any consciously directed effort to develop and cultivate our powers.

Forms of Education

There are various forms of education. *The table below enumerates the various forms of education and difference between them.*

Formal education	Informal education
• It has predetermined aims and methods of teaching	• It does not have predetermined aims, curricula, methods, teachers and is natural and incidental
• Definite doses of knowledge are thrust into the mind of a child at a specific place during a set duration of time by a particular individual.	• This process of imparting education goes on unconsciously
• It is rewarded invariably in the form of a certificate, diploma, or degree	• It is not rewarded with a certificate or a degree or diploma
• Agencies of formal education are school, library, museum, zoo, picture galleries, etc.	• Agencies of informal education are the family, the neighborhood, the playground, the social and religious activities, etc.
• Example: Obtaining a Degree in Nursing	• Example: Good habits, personal grooming, moral values, etc.
Direct education	**Indirect education**
• Education in which the teacher and the child are face to face, and predetermined doses of knowledge are given to the child in a specific way during a specific duration of time	• Indirect education is not a predetermined plan. It has no aims, no methods, and no fixed duration of time
• It takes place in a controlled environment, and the personality of the teacher/instructor directly influences the personality of the child/learner	• The child enjoys full freedom to structure his own experiences in a natural way according to his interests and needs
General education	**Specific education**
• General education is also called as liberal education. Here the aim of education is imparting general education for all children up to a certain stage	• Specific education has specific aim. Such education is imparted to children having special interests and aptitudes for it
• General education is imparted to sharpen the intellect of the child who is able to lead a general life successfully	• The aim of specific education is to prepare a child for a specific vocation
• Example: Primary education	• Example: Nursing and engineering education are the examples of specific education
Individual education	**Collective education**
Individual education is that education which is provided to each child separately according to his interests, inclinations, needs, and capacities	Collective education is imparted to groups or classes. This is a common pattern of education organization in our country

Philosophy and Education

"The philosophy of one century is the common sense of the next".
—Henry Ward Beecher

Meaning and Definition

The word "philosophy" is derived from the Greek words "philos" meaning loving and "sophia" meaning wisdom, and hence philosophy means "love of knowledge and wisdom". Thus etymologically the word "philosophy" means "love of wisdom". In ordinary usage it means "fundamental beliefs and convictions".

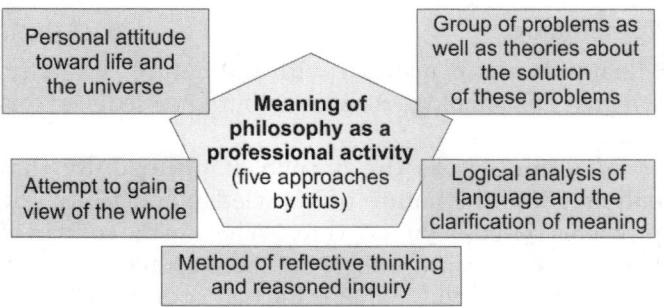

Philosophy is defined as "the persistent critical and systematic attempt to discover and consistently formulate in relation to each other the basic characteristics, meanings and values of our experience in its widest perspectives".

According to *RW Sellars*, "philosophy is a persistent attempt to give insight into the nature of the world and of ourselves by means of systematic reflection".

"Philosophy like other studies, aims primarily at knowledge," said by *Bertrand Russell*.

Main Divisions in Philosophy

The main divisions in philosophy are:
- Metaphysics
- Epistemology
- Axiology

Metaphysics

Metaphysics is the record of the explorations of the human mind into the ultimate nature of man and of the world. It is the result of an attempt to answer the question: "What is really real?" For example, one of the questions for which no one has been able to find a universally convincing answer is: "Does man possess a soul apart from his body?" Philosophers belonging to the Idealist school declare that man is essentially a soul and they accord the visible body only an insignificant status. Realists, another school of philosophers, give equal status to the body and the mind of man. Naturalists look upon the mind as a byproduct of matter and give primacy to the body. It is obvious that no specific empirical science like physiology or psychology can undertake to inquire into the matter. If they could, we would have got an unambiguous answer long ago. For these, empirical sciences investigate hypotheses on the basis of objective and impartial evidence which commands universal agreement. Unfortunately, no one has as yet been able to design an experimental method for answering in an objective way as to whether man possesses a soul apart from his body. Until such an experiment is designed, the answer given to the question will be purely speculative.

Thus, metaphysics begins where positive empirical science ends. Metaphysics is concerned with the hidden assumptions behind the scientists' work.

Metaphysics is the branch of philosophy that examines the problems of ultimate reality. It asks, "What is the nature of the universe, of life, of mind and its products, the freedom of mankind, the existence of God?"

Two major points of difference emerge in education as a consequence of metaphysical positions:
1. Man is essentially spiritual in nature; and
2. Man is a material organism that is one with nature.

Man is Essentially Spiritual in Nature

Philosophers who affirm the spiritual nature of man usually rest their case on the idea that the mind is substantially different from matter. To many philosophers, the mind is synonymous with the soul. Others agree that all of reality is reducible to mental states, and therefore they assume that the reality is basic to all; entities are immaterial.

Educational implications: This position—that man is essentially a spiritual being has numerous implications for education and educators. On the whole, philosophers supporting this position agree that education affects eternity. Further, they hold that because man is essentially spiritual, human nature is unchanging and the mind is free. Their beliefs have caused them to take rather definite positions on such matters as the aim of education, standards, the curriculum, mental discipline, higher education, academic freedom, and educational opportunity.

Aim of education: There can be only one basic educational aim. Education must aim at self-realization, self-knowledge, and self-development. The ultimate goal of education must, of course, be to develop self-knowledge, which is the beginning of wisdom.

Absolute standards: Wisdom and virtue are that part of human nature constituting the ultimate aim of a person. Educators, who hold this position, are inclined to see values as absolute and fixed, and they do not change. In teaching, the unchangeable ideals of intellectual and moral development must never be sacrificed for any reason.

Curriculum: The curriculum ought to be designed so that it liberates the mind and prepares one for his ultimate end. The fundamentals of reading, writing, and arithmetic are instrumental in the development of the individual. The subjects dealing with human values should be taught. These subjects are called as liberal or liberating arts. Philosophers of this persuasion favor a traditional and unchanging curriculum for everyone.

Mental discipline: Although the mind is spiritual in nature, it is subject to discipline and the mind can be trained in concentration, industrial alertness, observation, memory, ability, and self-discipline. Certain disciplines help to develop these desirable intellectual and moral habits. According to this position, curriculum builders should select those studies that provide the most vigorous training for the mind.

Higher education: Theorists of the spiritual persuasion have been particularly interested in higher education. In their view, the higher educational institutions must be completely free of all vested interests. The administration should be in the hands of the scholars and professionals, who are not influenced by public whims, political pressures, or monetary interests.

The curriculum must include the humanities, the arts and sciences because they believe that mathematics and science lead the individual to understand the nature and the arts to enrich their life, and the humanities are the most liberating of all and must be studied in the curriculum. Vocational skills, including teacher training, ought to be based upon a solid education in the humanities, arts, and sciences.

Academic freedom: Because of their belief that mind is spiritual, these thinkers are very much concerned about academic freedom. In their judgment, freedom in teaching and learning is essential to the free development of the individual. It must exist at every level of education.

Educational opportunity: Because they believe that it is important to train the mind as vigorously as possible, these educators insist that everyone should be provided with the opportunity to develop his potential through education. Individuals vary in their abilities. When it is evident that a student has arrived at the highest level of his ability, it is time to train him in some useful vocational skill.

Man as a Material Organism

Naturalists, materialists, experimentalists, pragmatists, and some realists believe that man is a material organism that is one with nature. They find no evidence for the existence of anything spiritual in man or nature. Man has evolved as a material part of nature; an organism that must make satisfactory adjustments in order to survive. Obviously, their beliefs about education are in many aspects different from those, which are discussed above.

To these educators, the nature of man can be understood only in the context of nature. His welfare and happiness in a changing material world are the starting point of education. One must educate pupils for a happy material existence. "Education for living" is one of the catch phrases common with this type of educator.

Epistemology

Metaphysics is concerned with the nature of reality, whereas epistemology focuses on our knowledge of this reality.

Epistemology is the branch of philosophy that enquires into the nature of knowledge and truth. The problems raised in this area are: "What are the sources of knowledge?"; "How reliable are these sources?"; "How can one know?" and "What is the nature of truth?".

The epistemologist tries to answer questions like "What is the difference between knowing and believing?", "What can we know beyond the information provided by our sense organs?", "What is the relation between the act of knowing and the object of knowledge?" and "What is the guarantee that what we know is true?" Thus the major concerns of epistemology are knowledge and truth.

Sources of Knowledge

The sources of knowledge are:
- Authority
- Common sense
- Intuition
- Reason
- Controlled experience

Authority

A great amount of our knowledge is derived from the testimony of some authority. Such knowledge is found in encyclopedias or in the best textbooks written by experts, who are usually regarded as authoritative.

In education, there are many who stress the importance of authority in learning. In their view, a student who is left to his own interests and felt problems may neglect the essential knowledge derived from the past authorities. They insist that this knowledge should be organized and presented to students by the teacher in an effective way.

Common Sense

The second source of knowledge is common sense. Common sense knowledge is bound directly to the customs and the traditions with which one is associated. One should not confuse common sense with good sense. Every system of educational philosophy agrees that the development of good sense such as clear thinking and sound judgment—as one of the most important achievements of a good teacher.

Intuition

The third source of knowledge is "intuition". Intuition is defined as the direct and immediate apprehension by knowing the subject of itself of its conscious state, of other minds, of an external world, of universe, of values, or of rational truths. It occurs on the subliminal level, beneath the "threshold of consciousness". It is connected intimately with feeling and emotion, and contrasts with the logical processes usually associated with thinking at the conscious level.

Through intuition, a person makes sudden moves and arrives at accurate conclusions about an issue/topic without having had either previous exposure to such an issue or topic or experience in the area. A belief in intuition causes many philosophical problems regarding its interpretation and usefulness. Many think that intuition is acceptable as a source of knowledge, if it is viewed as a subconscious process in a person who intuits in a field in which he is well experienced.

Reasoning

When knowledge is derived through a series of inferences that connect ideas consciously so as to arrive at judgments or conclusions, it is called reasoning. Sometimes it is called as logical thinking, even though it involves more than the form employed in the thinking process. Through reasoning universally valid judgments that are consistent with one another are derived. There are two types of reasoning such as inductive and deductive reasoning.

Controlled Experience

Science has grown rapidly. By means of critical, exact and precise analysis of sense observations, it has advanced knowledge by accumulating a body of facts in a variety of fields. Scientists employ a variety of methods consistent with the aims and limits of their respective fields of inquiry. Moreover, the success of the procedures for controlling experimentation has especially recommended for use in education. These procedures involve the following elements:
- Identify the problem
- Gather data that are relevant to the problem
- Reason, organize, analyze, and infer suitable solutions
- Formulate testable hypotheses
- Test, analyze, and classify it in a controlled design that is precise, complete, predictable, useful, and effective.

Solution arrived at must be reproducible, accurate, open, and precise.

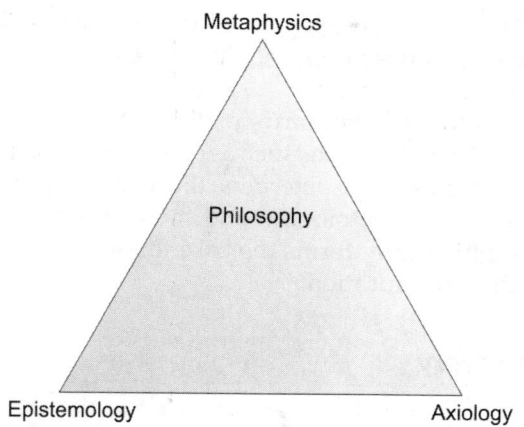

Fig. 1.1: Main divisions in philosophy.

Axiology

Axiology is the branch of philosophy concerned with the general problem of values, i.e. the nature, origin, and permanence of values. It is an attempt "to discover and recommend principles for deciding what actions and qualities are most worthwhile and why they should be so". Axiology has two major subdivisions: Ethics and Aesthetics.

Ethics, is the branch of philosophy that is concerned with morals—good and bad, right and wrong, approval and disapproval, and virtue and vice. Esthetics is the branch of science that is concerned with the problems of beauty and art.

A well-rounded system of philosophy integrates metaphysics, epistemology, and axiology (Fig. 1.1).

The tasks of philosophy are briefly formulated as follows:
- Speculation
- Description and analysis
- Prescription

Relationship between Philosophy and Education

Philosophy is a systematic and logical examination of life, so as to frame a system of general ideas, by which the sum total of human experience may be evaluated in such a manner so as to make the world more understandable. Thus, it becomes obvious that every rational person evaluates his life experiences. But the philosopher's search is systematic and determined. Conclusions must meet the rigid test of logic. The philosopher's findings provide a comprehensive interpretation of knowledge and truth of the nature of man and man's relationship with the universe and of the meaning of value, mortality, beauty, and art. These findings provide an educator with guidance in selecting goals, methods, curriculum, and the role of the educational institution in society.

John Dewey believed that philosophy is both a method of identifying problems and a source of suggestions about ways to handle these problems. This view increases the importance of philosophy to education. Generally, the relationship between philosophy and education may be approached in this way.

The values or standards of life are prescribed by philosophers in two areas such as ethics and esthetics. The theories of knowledge determine the methods of teaching or learning. The ontological and metaphysical point of view of philosophy forms the base for actual content or curriculum of education.

Value Theory

Value theory underlies every single educational activity. The content of education in any society is derived from a belief of what is good in education. The curricula, methods, and materials chosen by the educational administrators and teachers to introduce into their institutions and classes are all determined by their value outlook.

The values may be intrinsic in nature or instrumental in nature. As intrinsic, the values are absolute and permanent, and that values are arranged in an order from highest to lowest, the higher values being determined and is discovered by human reasons; and those who affirm that all values are instrumental in nature consider values as useful, constantly changing, equal and nonfactual.

Theory of Intrinsic Values

According to these theorists' viewpoints pertaining to educational aims, the curriculum, teaching-learning and the role of the institution in society are as follows:

- **Aims of education:** If values are intrinsic, they must reside in the nature of man. The aim of the school, then, should be to provide pupils with the essential knowledge that will enable them to live a successful natural and spiritual life. To meet this aim, education must give supreme priority to the development of the rational potential within each pupil. Education must stress the importance of the development of both the intellect and the will. Properly developed, it will enable one to act habitually in controlling his emotions and passions.
- **Curriculum:** Education must include those subjects that assist in the intellectual component of the pupil. The humanities are given preeminence because they contain the accumulated wisdom of civilized man.
- **Teaching-learning:** Lessons should be taught as realistically as possible. The teacher should provide as many real experiences as possible and follow the principles of the psychology of learning. The factual content must be organized systematically, proceeding from the simple to the complex. The pupil is expected individually to understand, memorize, recite, and in group drills, to explain, compare and discuss. Habits of study, concentration, and perseverance must be encouraged consistently.
- **Role of school in society:** The school should interpret and pass on to young people the accumulated knowledge, wisdom and tradition of the society. To fulfill its role, pupils must be educated to live within the values held important in their society. It must be understood that the school must remain aloof from politics. The task of the school is to educate its students. It is not the only agent of society, and it should leave other roles to the other agents.

Theory of Instrumental Values

Educators who hold this view are called as progressive educators. The Progressivists consider values in terms of their social results. To them, values are determined by an ever-changing society; therefore, values are not fixed. Ethical behavior is based upon social agreements and law, and may change as the society changes. The criteria for a society's values are the standards of the majority in that society. Behavior is evaluated in terms of the conventions of the society. There is no such thing as an absolute standard of right or wrong, or good or bad.

- **Educational aims:** From the progressivist standpoint, the major aim of the school should be to teach students how to think. Knowing "how to think" in order to make good decisions will make it possible for students to cope with life's problems and to steer themselves into the course for the good life.
- **Curriculum:** Progressivist theory tells us that the knowledge has instrumental value; that is, it is useful for the pupils to resolve problems arising as a result of their felt needs. And so, the aims of education are not ends but means to effective living. Education is life itself; therefore, the curriculum too must be life itself. It cannot be limited to the academics. A problem-centered, pupil-centered, and experience-centered curriculum featuring such approaches as shared activities, critical evaluations, pupil involvement in decision-making, community service projects, and the like is to be used. The school is a miniature society and may bring about the desired result.
- **Teaching-learning:** The heart of the progressive approach to teaching and learning is problem solving. For this method to be successful, it is essential that each pupil accepts a problem as his own. If pupils are to learn, they must have an active role in selecting, defining, working on, and evaluating their activities in resolving the problem. The teacher must never impose solutions.
- **Role of the school in society:** The school as seen by progressivists is an integral part of the society; it reflects all the social problems. The school must, therefore, emphasize social living and must assume an active role in improving the society.

Significance of Philosophy of Education

The philosophical implications on education are as follows:
- Aims of education
- Curriculum
- Methods of teaching
- Concept of freedom and discipline
- Philosophy and textbooks
- Role of the teacher.

Aims of Education

Rusk says, "Philosophy formulates what it conceives to be the end of life; education offers suggestions how this end to be achieved". Philosophy is the determining force for laying down the aims of education. A philosopher lays down ultimate values of life and these are virtually the aims of education. Different philosophical schools have prescribed different aims of education.

Curriculum

By means of curriculum, desired behavioral changes are to be achieved to attain the goal of life determined by a particular philosophy. The content of education is determined by the objectives of life. If religions circumscribe the actions in life, education in terms of religious scriptures becomes virtually the curriculum. If experiences are to be thought as goal-seeking activities, problems of modern living constitute the curriculum. If, on the other hand, child's free expressive activities are stressed, curriculum is determined in terms of direct experience provided by such areas as geography, physical sciences, and nature studies. Thus, philosophy is the force that shapes the type of curriculum.

Methods of Teaching

Method is a means by which a contact is developed between the students and the subject matter. The choice of method is governed by the philosophical ideas and values. For instance, the teacher's position as an exemplar of virtue is what we find in the idealistic philosophy. He is to expound through scholarly discourses in order to "impress" on the pupils' growth. Child-centered activities such as play techniques are favored by naturalists.

Concept of Freedom and Discipline

Philosophy determines the nature and form of discipline. Whether the school discipline should be strict and rigid or flexible and free is also a philosophical problem. Regarding freedom and discipline, while naturalism stresses free activity, idealism stresses discipline to raise the individual above "self".

Philosophy and Textbooks

To achieve aims of life and education, textbooks are of great importance and value. As curriculum is powerfully influenced by the philosophy of times, so also the textbooks are affected by the prevailing philosophy of the day. Since textbook contains the matter which reflects the ideology, ideals, and values of society, the government should keep an eye on the production of desirable books for children.

Role of the Teacher

The teacher's role and his behavior depend on the philosophical attitudes which influence him. Lofty ideals, higher values, and spiritual freedom are stressed by the school of Idealism. He should be a morally upright scholar who should be a model to be emulated. Pragmatism feels that the teacher is a consultant, coordinator, and research director stimulating the pupils in group thinking in group situations. School is regarded as a miniature society and the role expectation of teachers is in conformity with this spirit.

To conclude, philosophy remains as the foundation for education. The diverse educational theories, systems, and processes are the result of the philosophical thoughts. All great educationists are all great philosophers. Ultimately all changes, innovations, and novel experiments in educational ideas and practices are the direct or indirect results of the philosophy of education. Philosophy is a search for truth and reality. It is a search for a comprehensive view of nature, an attempt at a universal explanation of nature of things. According to Dr S Radhakrishnan, "It is a logical enquiry into the nature of reality". It must include not only the training of the intellect but also the refinement of the heart and the discipline of the spirit. Education is always guided by certain ideas, values, and standards of life.

Major Systems of Philosophy and its Educational Implications

Idealism

"All truths are easy to understand once they are discovered; the point is to discover them".
—Galileo

Idealism is the oldest system of philosophy known to man. Its origin goes back to ancient India in the East, and to Plato in the West. Its basic viewpoint stresses the human spirit as the most important element in life. The universe is viewed as essentially nonmaterial in its ultimate nature. Although, Idealist philosophers vary enormously on many specifics, they agree on the following points:

The human spirit is the most important element in life;

The universe is essentially nonmaterial in its ultimate nature.

In the philosophic sense, idealism is a system that emphasizes the preeminent importance of mind, soul, or spirit.

Basic Metaphysics of Idealism

As a philosophical doctrine, idealism recognizes ideas, feelings and ideals more important than material objects, and at the same time emphasizes that human development should be according to moral, ethical, and spiritual values so that he acquires knowledge of unity in diversity. Idealism holds that spiritual world is more important than material world. The chief reason is that material world is destructive and mortal. Hence, it is untrue and myth.

In Idealism, all of reality is reducible to one fundamental substance—spirit. Matter is not real; rather, it is a notion, an abstraction of the mind. It is only the mind that is real. Therefore, all material things that seem to be real are reducible to mind or spirit. On the universal level, finite minds live in a purposeful world produced by an infinite mind. Because man is a part of this purposeful universe, he is an intelligent and purposeful being.

Epistemology of Idealism

Idealists believe that all knowledge is independent of sense experience. The act of knowing takes place within the mind. The mind is active and contains innate capacities for organizing and synthesizing the data derived through sensations. Man can know intuitively; that is, he can apprehend immediately some truth without utilizing any of his senses. Man can also know the truth through the acts of reason by which an individual examines the logical consistency of his ideas.

Idealistic Value Theory

Idealists generally root all values either in a personal God or in an impersonal spiritual force of nature. They all agree that values are eternal. Idealists identify God with nature. Values are absolute and unchanging because they are a part of the determined order of nature.

> **Fundamental principles of idealism**
> - Idealism stresses the two forms of whole world, i.e. spiritual world and material world
> - The spiritual world is real whereas the material world is transitory and mortal
> - Ideas are more important than objects (material things)
> - Man is more important than the material nature
> - The prime aim of life is to achieve spiritual values such as Truth, Beauty and Goodness
> - Self-realization is the prime of the personality development
> - Idealism believes in unity in diversity.

Educational Implications of Modern Idealism

Aims of education: The purpose of education is to contribute to the development of the mind and self of the pupil. The school should emphasize intellectual activities, moral judgments, esthetic judgment, self-realization, individual freedom, individual responsibility and self-control in order to achieve this development. The aims of education according to idealism are:
- Self-realization
- Spiritual development
- Cultivation of truth, beauty and goodness
- Conservation, promotion and transmission of cultural heritage
- Conversion of inborn nature into spiritual nature
- Preparation for a holy life
- Development of intelligence and rationality.

Curriculum: The curriculum is based upon the idea or assumption of the spiritual nature of man. In preserving the subject matter content, which is essential for the development of the individual mind, the curriculum must include those subjects essential for the realization of mental and moral development. These subjects provide one with culture, and they should be mandated for all pupils. Moreover, the subject matter should be kept constant for all. The subjects are Literature, Language, Religion and Metaphysics, Culture, Sociology, Ethics, Arts and Music, etc.

Idealism and Teacher

Idealists have high expectations on the teacher. The teacher must be excellent, in order to serve as an example for the student, both intellectually and morally. The teacher must also exercise great creative skill in providing opportunities for the pupils' mind to discover, analyze, synthesize, and create applications of knowledge to life and behavior.

Methods of teaching: The classroom structure and atmosphere should provide the pupil with opportunities to think, and to apply the criteria of moral evaluation to concrete situations within the context of the subjects. The teaching methods must encourage the acquisition of facts, as well as skill in reflecting on these facts. It is not sufficient to teach pupils how to think. It is very important that what pupils think about being factual; otherwise, they will simply compound their ignorance.

Teaching methods should encourage pupils to enlarge their horizons; stimulate reflective thinking; encourage personal moral choices; provide skills in logical thinking; provide opportunities to apply knowledge to moral and social problems; stimulate interest in the subject content; and encourage pupils to accept the values of human civilization.

Idealism and Discipline

Idealists attach impressionistic discipline in comparison with expressionistic discipline. The teacher should impress the students by his affectionate and sympathetic behavior. They should make the child realize that self-discipline is for his own good and development.

Idealism and School

School is a place where the mental power and other spiritual ideals of the child are developed by the teachers.

Realism

"Reality does not conform to the ideal, but confirms it".
—*Gustave Flaubert*

Realism is possibly the oldest philosophy of man—older than even idealism. It was Aristotle who provided the first firm foundation for realism as a school of philosophy. In the modem period, GE Moore, Bertrand Russell and John Wild are notable exponents of realism. Among educational philosophers, Broudy (1965), Breed (1942), Bagley (1935), and Finney (1929) are realists.

Metaphysics of Realism

The world is made of real, substantial, and material entities. In material nature, there are natural laws, which determine and regulate the existence of every entity in the world of nature.

Realistic Epistemology

The mind of individual is blank on birth and in the rest of his life, a variety of sensations are impressed in his brain. It is how the man learns. Knowledge, then is derived through sense experience. However, man can capitalize on this knowledge by using reason to discover objects and relationships which he does not or cannot perceive.

Realistic Value Theory

Anything consistent with nature is valuable. Standards of value are found by means of the act of reason. However, a value judgment is never considered to be factual; it is a subjective judgment based on feeling. Acceptable individual values are values that conform to the values of the prevailing opinion of society.

Forms of Realism

a. **Humanistic realism:** Proponents of humanistic realism believed that education should be realistic. Such an education only can promote human welfare and success.
b. **Social realism:** It aims to make human life happy and successful by fulfilling the needs of the society. They opposed mere academic and bookish knowledge, and advocated that education should be useful to life and practical in nature. Education should promote work efficiency of the individuals.
c. **Sense realism:** Knowledge primarily comes through the senses, not from words. In education all sense organs should be used to the maximum. Without exercising his sense organs, no knowledge will be gained.
d. **Neorealism:** Neorealism believes that like other rules and procedures, rules and procedures of science are also changeable. They are valid only in certain conditions and circumstances. When those circumstances change, the rules also change.

> **Fundamental principles of realism**
> - Phenomenal world is true and there is no world beyond this
> - Senses are the doors or gateways of knowledge
> - God, soul and other world are merely a human imagination
> - Man is a part of material world
> - Observation and experiment are ways of finding the truth
> - The present life is real and the spirituality and spiritual values are unreal.

Characteristics of Realistic Education

- It is based on science
- It emphasizes on present life of child
- It emphasizes on experiment
- It opposes bookish knowledge
- It emphasizes training of senses
- It gives an equal importance to individual and society.

Educational Implications of Modern Realism

Aims of education: The basic purpose of education in Realist educational theory is to provide the pupil with the essential knowledge required for survival in the natural world. Such knowledge will provide the skills necessary to achieve a secure and happy life.

Curriculum: Realists believe that the curriculum is best organized according to subject matter—that is, it should be subject–centered. These subjects should be organized according to the psychological principles of learning. The subjects should proceed from the simple to the most complex. Subjects must include science, vocational studies, mathematics, humanities, and social science.

Teacher: The Realist classroom is teacher-centered. Subjects are taught by a teacher who is impersonal and objective, and who knows the subject fully. The teacher must utilize pupil's interest by relating the material to the pupil's experiences, and making the subject matter as concrete as possible. He maintains discipline by rewarding efforts and achievements, controlling the attention of the child by keeping the pupil active.

Methods of teaching: The teaching methods recommended by the Realist are authoritative. The teacher must assure that the pupil is able to recall, explain and compare facts; to interpret relationships, and to infer new meanings. Evaluation is an essential aspect of teaching. The teacher must use objective methods by evaluating and giving the type of test that lends itself to accurate measurement of the pupil's understanding. Frequent tests are highly desirable. For motivational purposes, Realists stress that it is important for the teacher to reward the success of each pupil. When the teacher reports the accomplishments of his pupils, he reinforces what has been learned.

Realism and Discipline

They advocate a synthetic form of impressionistic and emancipatory forms of discipline.

Realism and School

Realists have different views about school. Some do not feel any need of school at all. They prescribe wide traveling, tours and teaching by private tutors as the best means of education. On the contrary other realists emphasize the importance of school. They regard school as a mirror of society reflecting its true state of affairs. According to them, the school is an agency which meets the needs of the child.

Naturalism

> "We cannot command nature except by obeying her".
> —*Francis Bacon*

Rousseau, Comenius, Basedow, and Pestalozzi are prominent educationists of this naturalist movement. Naturalism is also termed as materialism. According to this philosophy, the basis of the world is matter. Mind is also a form of matter. Nature is everything. Nothing is before and beyond it. Hence, man should investigate the truth of nature.

Metaphysics of Naturalism

Naturalism believes that the ultimate reality is the nature of matter. Matter is supreme. Mind is the functioning of the brain which is made up of matter. Laws of nature are unchangeable and the whole universe is governed by them.

Epistemology of Naturalism

The naturalists subscribe to the dictum that the senses are the gateways of knowledge. They accept the validity of empirical data as a source of knowledge. The naturalists made reasoning as an instrument for understanding natural phenomena. Thus, the naturalist would accept the empirical and rational form of knowledge and between the two would give primacy to empirical knowledge.

Values of Naturalism

Since man is innately good according to naturalists, value consisted in the flowering of the innate potentialities of man.

Forms of Naturalism

- **Physical naturalism:** It studies the processes of matter and phenomena of the external world. It explains human activities and experiences in terms of material objects and natural laws. Physical naturalism lays more stress on the external material phenomena than the conscious human being.
- **Mechanical naturalism:** The universe is a lifeless huge machine which gets its form through matter and motion. Man is considered as a mere part of this huge machine and is himself a small machine. This is also set in motion by external stimuli and forces of nature.
- **Biological naturalism:** It is based on a Darwinian theory of evolution. According to this theory, man has evolved from lower animals by a gradual process of development. Man is a supreme product of this process of evolution. In this way, biological naturalism emphasizes the development of man's natural impulses, natural potentialities and inborn tendencies.

Principles of naturalism
- The universe is a huge machine and man is also a part of this machine
- All the capacities of an individual human being are delimited by his nature. Those are his innate and inherent tendencies and basic instincts
- The present life is the real life. There is no other world beyond it
- Reality is of the external nature only. All objects are born or made out by this nature and ultimately disappear in nature
- Unchanging laws of nature explain all the events and occurrences of the world
- The changes in the life of man and his physical conditions are due to scientific discoveries and inventions
- The ultimate reality is of matter. God, soul, mind, heaven and hell, moral values and prayers are all illusions.

Characteristics of Naturalistic Education

- Back to nature—the best teacher of the child is nature
- Opposition of bookish knowledge
- Education should be progressive
- Negative education—to protect from error
- Child is the center of the educational process
- Child should be given full freedom for the development
- Training of senses is mandatory.

Educational Implications of Naturalism

Aims: Self-expression or "unfolding of the self" is stressed. No control of any kind over the developing organism is allowed, and complete freedom should be given. Perfectioning of the human machine for the attainment of present and future happiness is important. The education should prepare a child for the struggle for existence and adaptation to environment.

Curriculum: This is based on the needs, interests, and abilities of the child in relation to its level of development. In fact child-centered curriculum is definite answer of the Naturalist. Individual differences are recognized. The experience of the child should form the central core of the curriculum.

Methods of teaching: Play is the natural mode of self-expression; play way is stressed. Learning by doing and learning by experience are also advocated. Learning should be through the joyous, spontaneous, and creative activity of play. The method of discovery is stressed. Excursions, fieldtrips, and practical experiments are highly commended.

Teacher: The teacher should remain in the background. The child's natural development should be stimulated. In fact the teacher should remove himself from the scene, since nature is the best educator.

Discipline: Freedom is a means to discipline. The child should be controlled only by his own learning and experiences. Discipline by natural consequences is what they believe in. Nature will punish the child if he contravenes the law of nature. Self-government by the students is advocated.

Naturalism and the School

The school environment should be completely free, flexible, and without any rigidity. Nature will do all the planning and processing for the natural development of the child.

Pragmatism

> "Good judgment comes from experience, and often experience comes from bad judgment".
> —Rita Mae Brown

Etymologically the word pragmatism is derived from the Greek word "Pragma" which means activity or work done. Pragmatism gives importance to change, processes, and relativity. It is essentially the practical approach. It has been expounded by the American philosophers like William James and John Dewey.

Metaphysics and Pragmatism

Uniformly, all Pragmatists reject metaphysics as a legitimate area of philosophical inquiry. Reality, they argue, is determined by an individual's sense experience. Man can know nothing beyond his experience. Therefore, questions pertaining to the ultimate nature of man and the universe simply cannot be answered. Attempts to answer metaphysical questions are little more than guessing games, in their opinion.

Epistemology in Pragmatism

The Pragmatists reject the dualism that separates the perceiver from the object that is perceived. Man is both in the world of his perception and of the world of his perception. All that can be known is dependent upon experience. This experiencing of phenomena determines knowledge. Because the phenomena are constantly changing, it follows that knowledge and truth must similarly be changing. Truth is something that happens to an idea. Whatever is considered true today must also be considered as possibly changing tomorrow.

Value Theory in Pragmatism

In Pragmatist theory, values are derived from the human condition. Because man is a part of his society, the consequences of his actions are either good or bad, according to their results. If the consequences prove worthwhile socially, then the value of the action is proven to be good. Thus, value in ethics and esthetics depends upon the relative circumstances of the situation as it arises.

Forms of Pragmatism

- **Humanistic pragmatism:** According to this ideology, only those things or principles are true which satisfy the needs, requirements, aspirations, and objectives of human being.
- **Experimental pragmatism:** Any thing or principle is true which can be verified as true by experiment.
- **Biological pragmatism:** The power or capacity of human being is valuable and important, which enables him to adjust with the environment or which makes him to change his environment according to his needs and requirements.

Principles of pragmatism
- Change is the essence of this universe. Nothing is permanent or final
- Reality is what one experiences. There is no absolute reality
- There is no absolute truth. Truth always changes according to time, place, and person
- Problems form the motivation for the search of truth
- Action must precede knowledge. True experience is knowledge, and it is functional. Action is more important than knowledge or thought
- Man is a biological organism getting a social stimulation. Human personality can be developed only in a social context

- The present is stressed, neither the past nor the future
- There are no absolute values or universal moral principles. Man creates his own values. Man is the measure of all things
- What is good is what works; what works for all
- Means are more important than ends. They are closely related. The ends once realized become means for realization of further ends
- Mind is dynamic. The growth of personality is the interaction of the individual with the environment
- Critical intelligence is of great value. Democracy is a way of life promoting a permissive atmosphere.

Educational Implications of Pragmatism

Aims of education: There is no final aim as there is no finality about life. Education becomes the laboratory of life. Education is a continuous reconstruction of experience. It must be a social process. Education has only a functional value in helping the children realize their potentialities. Problem solving is the attitude to be developed both as ends and means. This should result in an adaptable mind which is both resourceful and enterprising in all situations.

Curriculum: Pragmatism believes in life-centered curriculum. There is only one subject—the Art of Modern Living. School curriculum must be built around the particular problems of life which are meaningful and purposeful for the students. Generally, subject-matter of social experience and social studies would receive greater emphasis and cultural activities will receive a comparatively low priority.

Methods of teaching: The pupils should learn by doing and problem-solving. Cooperative group work should be encouraged. Project method is the method of the pragmatism. The pupils should be made to think and act for themselves, to do rather than to know, to originate rather than to repeat.

Role of the teacher: The teacher is a Research Project Director. The student is an active participant in the business of learning, investigating, enquiring, reading, thinking, testing, etc. The teacher has to set the proper environment and guide them in planning, executing and evaluating the whole activity or project. The teacher works as a friend, philosopher and guide to the children.

Discipline: Discipline should grow out of purposeful group activity. It is self-discipline that has to be cultivated in the pupils and this is developed through involving the students in the moral dimensions of the classroom. "Learning by Living" is the formula here. The predominant condition for moral training is community life of the school. The school is a "miniature society".

Pragmatism and School

As already mentioned, the school is a miniature society where a child gets a real experience to act and behave according to his interests, aptitudes and capacities.

Indian School of Philosophy

The Vedanta Philosophy

The term "Vedanta" means that which comes at the end of the *Vedas*. The term "*Veda*" means knowledge and it has two aspects:
1. Mantras or hymns or *Samhitas* like the four "*Vedas*"—*Rig*, *Yajur*, *Sama*, and *Atharvana*.
2. The Brahmans.

The appendage to the "Brahmans" is called the *Aranyakas* where philosophical speculation has its beginning. The concluding portions of the *Aranyakas* are called the *Upanishads*. The *Upanishads* are the cream of the Vedic philosophy. The *Mantras* and the *Brahmans* are the *Karma Kanda* (action) and the *Aranyakas* and the *Upanishads* are the *Gnanakanda* (knowledge). The *Upanishads* are also known as "The Vedanta" as it comes at the end of the *Vedas*.

The Upanishads have two terms for Ultimate Reality—the "*Brahman*" and the "*Atman*" which are two pillars on which the edifice of Indian philosophy rests. The *Brahman* is the ultimate source of the outer world and the *Atman* the inner self of man. *Atman* is the soul; *Brahman* is the single source of the visible universe. *Brahman* and *Atman* are complementary. The subjective side is the *Atman* and the objective side is "*Brahman*".

In the scholarly discourses, discussion was promoted. There was no question of any dogmatic acceptance and faithful adherence to the views of Guru. The disciples can raise questions (*Prasna*) and put supplementaries (*Anuprasna*), *Anathu Prasna* (intercepting of irrelevant questions for arguments), *Vyakarna* (explaining), and *Dristanta* (illustration and analogy).

Educational Implications of the Vedanta Philosophy

- The spiritual personality of the individual is the central core of the Vedanta Philosophy. In education it is, therefore, "respect the individual personality" as the object of transformation.
- There was mutual esteem between the teacher and the pupil. The pupil is accepted by the teacher only after a "Probationary period of a year or so, obviously to find out the fitness of the individual for education".
- Cultivation of the detachment of the self or the removal of *Ahamkara* (Egoism) or *Vairagya* is the attitude toward the world in a selfless approach. The four *ashrams* in life or the disciplinary stages are the stages of:

- Religious student (*Brahmacharya*)
- The house-holder (*Grahastha*)
- Anchorite (*Vanaprastha*) and
- The sage (*Sanyasi*).

- Acquisition of knowledge is through detachment. The methods are *Sravana* or Hearing, *Manana* or Reflection, *Nididhyasana* or Meditation.
- The *Upanishads* prescribe several *upasanas* or meditative exercises. Powers of concentration are cultivated through *upasanas*.
- The four-fold ideals of life are "*Artha*", "*Kama*", "*Dharma*" and "*Moksha*", i.e. acquisition of wealth, enjoyment of earthly pleasures, practice of righteousness and the attainment of God realization.

The Bhagvad Gita

This literally means, The Lord's song. It is called the "Gospel of Humanity". It deals with metaphysics, religious outlook, and ethical codes. But essentially the central point is the philosophy of action. The *Gita* is a philosophy of *Karma* (action) based on *Jnana* (knowledge) and supported by *Bhakti* (devotion) "to fight against the evil is the duty of man". Thus, the *Gita* represents a unique synthesis of Action, Devotion, and Knowledge. Disinterested, dispassionate, and detached devotion to duty may be called the quintessence of the *Bhagvad Gita*. "*Nishkamya karma*" or selfless devotion to duty is advocated for everybody. Detached action is what is prescribed.

Secular studies are also emphasized in connection with one's spiritual duties. A number of disciplines like mathematics, astronomy medicine, politics, and sculpture also received attention during the *grahastha* period. Practical knowledge was given relevant importance. The disciple was required to fetch fuel, kindle the fire, beg and render household duties along with Vedic studies.

Educational Implications of Bhagvad Gita

- Self-effort is the key note for success. Be manly, Be self-reliant, Be bold and cheerful. Do not be despondent.
- Do your duty with a sense of devotion.
- Develop a Balanced Mind. Humility, uprightness, purity, and self-control are the qualities to be inculcated, and qualities such as egoism, laziness, prejudice, fear, and brooding should be eschewed.
- Follow the Golden Mean. Do not follow the extremes of renunciation and attachment to worldly things.
- Be of service to others.
- Be a Jnani—you have to merge all desires in the supreme desire. There are four kinds of devotees of God: (a) the sufferer (*Artha*), (b) the seeker (*Jignasu*), (c) the self-interested (*Artharthi*), and (d) the Wise (*Jnani*). The last one is the one who sees the Lord in everything and everything in the Lord.

- The three qualities in men are *Sattva*, *Rajas* and *Tamas*. Greed and unrest arise when *Rajas* is dominant. Darkness, inertness and wrong understanding arise when Tamas is predominant. One who is calm, intelligent and dispassionate has *Sattva* predominant in him.

Jainism

Jainism derives its name from the word "*Jina*" which means one who has conquered his passions and achieved mastery over his self. Jainism is said to have its origin in prehistoric times.

Jainism believes in the premise and possibility of liberation. It has been characterized as realistic, pluralistic and relativistic. It is realistic because it believes in the reality of the external objective world. It is pluralistic because it believes that the souls are many in number and they continue to be so forever. Jainism is relativistic because it maintains that our judgments about the world are relative to our time and place.

The following are the essential features of the Jaina philosophy:

- The Universe is brought under two categories—Jiva and *Ajiva*—the conscious and the unconscious spirit. The *Jiva* is capable of expansion and contraction. It resembles a lamp which illumines the whole of the space enclosed in a small room. The category of *Ajiva* is divided into: *Kala*, *Akasa*, *Dharma*, *Adharma* (space), and *Pudgala* (motto).
- The metaphysics is the doctrine of manyness of reality (*Anekantavada*). It is thus realistic and pluristic. The Jaina says that he, who knows all the qualities of one thing, knows all the qualities of all things. Human knowledge is relative and limited.
- Reality is unity in difference and difference in unity. Jainism emphasizes the partial views of accepting performance and change. It is called *Anekantavada*.
- Ignorance is the cause of bondage. Right knowledge is the act of liberation. Right faith, Right knowledge, and Right conduct are the three jewels of Jainism. So it is primarily ethical.
- Discipline is enforced strictly. There are five vows—Ahimsa, Astega, Nonstealing, Celibacy, and Renunciation. The last two are not for the laymen.
- The final aim is the development of personality. Individual and social aspects of personality are equally emphasized.
- Jainism is a religion of self-help. It denies God. But every liberated soul is God.

Metaphysics

The basic category of Jaina metaphysics is dravya or substance. Every substance is the locus of two characters—essential and accidental. The essential characters of a substance persist as long as the substance endures. The accidental characters of a substance may come and go. For example, consciousness is an essential character of a soul. Desires, volitions, pleasure, and pain are accidental characters. It is through accidental characters that a substance undergoes modification. They are, therefore, also described as modes. According to the Jains, both changes and modifications are real.

Next to *dravya* or substance, there are two main categories in Jains metaphysics. They are *jiva* (Soul) and *ajiva* (non-soul). Consciousness is the essential character of Soul; non-consciousness that of the non-soul. Non-soul in turn consists of the following five sub-categories—*Kala* (time), *Akasa* (space), *Dharma* (medium of motion), *Adharma* (medium of rest), and *Pudgala* (matter).

Epistemology

The Jainas admit perception (pratyaksha), inference (anumana), and testimony (sabda) as valid sources of knowledge. Testimony, of course, means in their case the testimony of the omniscient liberated saints (Jinas) and not Vedic testimony. In terms of their own classification there are five different forms of knowledge. They are:
1. Mati jnana (perceptual knowledge)
2. Srut jnana (scriptural knowledge)
3. Avadhi jnana (clair-voyance)
4. Manaparyaya jnana (telepathy)
5. Kevala jnana (perfect knowledge).

The first two belong to the category of mediate knowledge and the rest to immediate knowledge. The Jains admit that individuals differ in the kinds of knowledge, they attain and the degrees to which they attain them. These individual differences are determined by one's past Karma.

The Jainas argue that the knowledge of reality formed by imperfect beings is always relative. According to them, only the liberated who has attained Kevala jnana can obtain an immediate and total knowledge of the various aspects of reality. This theory of the relativity of our judgment about reality is called *Syadvada*. It is a distinct feature of Jains through which he has influenced its metaphysics. *Syadvada* is a hedge against dogmatism.

Values

Liberation from bondage is the goal of life in the Jaina scheme of values. Tri-ratna or 'three-gems' is the means for liberation. It consists of *samyag-darsana* (right faith), *samyag-jnana* (right knowledge), and *samyak charita* (right conduct). Of the three, knowledge is central.

Right faith and right knowledge constitute the foundation for right conduct (*samyak charita*). Right conduct is what helps the soul to get rid of the *karmas* that lead to bondage. For the arrest of the influx of new *karmas* and the eradication of the existing ones the following steps are prescribed:

- Take the five great vows (Pancha mahavrata).
- Practice extreme carefulness (Samiti) in everyday speech and movements so as to avoid harming any living being.
- Practice restraint of thought, speech, and bodily movements.
- Practice dharma of 10 different kinds namely forgiveness, humility, straight forwardness, truthfulness, cleanliness, self-restraint, austerity (internal and external), sacrifice, nonattachment, and celibacy.
- Mediate on the cardinal truths taught regarding the self and the world.
- Conquer through fortitude all pains and discomforts that arise on account of the body, and
- Attain equanimity, purity, absolute needfulness, and perfect conduct.

The five great vows are *ahimsa* (abstinence from all injury to life), *satyam* (abstinence from falsehood which means not merely speaking what is true but speaking good and pleasant as well), *arteyam* (abstinence from stealing), *brahmacharayam* (abstinence from self-indulgence and not merely sexual celibacy), and *aparigraha* (abstinence from all attachment).

Educational Implications of Jainism

Development of the personality of the student is the educational aim. Jainism does not have any predetermined absolute goals. It believes in the development of the self.

Knowledge is relative. By knowing the different parts, we may hope to get all about one relatively.

The moral aspect of the individual's growth in terms of right conduct was emphasized.

There was strong emphasis on memory. The spiritual aspect was stressed. Curriculum was based on three Ratnas—Right faith, Right knowledge, Right conduct. The mother tongue was the medium of instruction. Debate and discussion were used as methods of instruction. Residential life of the pupil was stressed.

Buddhism

Siddhartha or Gautama Buddha is the founder of Buddhism who lived in the sixth century BC.

Metaphysics

Buddhism recognizes the distinction between the Soul and its material environment. Thus, Buddhism is, in a sense, dualistic and realistic. Buddhism views the world as mere process. There is neither being nor nonbeing in the cosmos, but it is a ceaseless process of becoming.

Epistemology

Buddhism recognizes only pramanas as valid. They are pratyakas (perception) and anumana (inference).

The Buddha was pragmatic in its conception of truth whatever was useful in overcoming evil and suffering that the Buddha considered to be true. Buddhism explicitly emphasizes reasoning and excludes whatever is not positively, i.e. perceptually known. Accordingly, the Buddha rejected the authority of Vedic tradition, especially as regards to ritual.

Ethics

Buddhism accepts the inexorable law of *Karma*. The teaching of Buddha was threefold:
1. **The four noble truths:** There is suffering; there is a cause of suffering; there is cessation of suffering; there is a way leading to cessation of suffering (Nirvana).
2. **The eightfold path to nirvana:** They are Right faith, Right resolve, Right speech, Right action, Right living, Right effort, Right thought, and Right concentration.
3. **Dependent origination:** All phenomenal things hang between reality and nothingness. Every object of reality is relative. Ignorance is bondage; knowledge is liberation. According to the theory of Momentariness (Kshana Bangavada), everything is conditional, dependent and relative. Everything is merely a link in its chain, a spoke in the wheel, a transitory phase in the senses.

Educational Implications of Buddhism

- Buddhist philosophy admits the possibility of attaining peace here and now, though it starts with a pessimistic note. Teachers, therefore, need not be despair.
- Buddhistic philosophy is positivistic and has a careful logical systematization of ideas.
- It is pragmatic. Everything is in a state of flux as it is only momentary. Change is the rule of the universe. It does not believe in absolutism.
- It believes in the integration of personality by developing the various aspects of the individual which are interlinked.
- It is ethical. The eightfold path to *Nirvana* makes a universal appeal.
- It is democratic as it believed in the freedom of enquiry.
- Its belief in *Karma* lays stress on the necessity to be constantly on vigil to maintain one's conduct in the present life. Buddhist Viharas or monasteries have their methods of initiation and training of the apprentices. The preceptor must give his disciples, possible intellectual and spiritual help and guidance.
- The Buddha Bhikku (Monk) took the vows of chastity and of poverty. Character was the basis of moral discipline.
- Training of manual skills like spinning and weaving was emphasized to enable men to earn for their living.
- The method of instruction was oral. Preaching, repetition, exposition, discussion, and debates were all used. The Buddhistic Council organized seminars to scholars to discuss the major issues at length.

Aims of Education

"The only true wisdom is in knowing you know nothing".
—Socrates

Education is mostly a planned and purposeful activity. It must have clear aims and objectives. An aim is a predetermined goal which inspires the individual to attain it through appropriate activities. Educational aims are necessary in giving direction to educational activity.

General Aims of Education

> *Mnemonic for General aims of education –*
> **VLCC CHIKS**
> **V**ocational, **L**eisure, **C**ultural development, **C**omplete living, **C**itizenship, **H**armonious development, **I**ndividual and social, **K**nowledge, **S**elf-realization

- **Vocational:** Education should help a person to become self-sufficient and economically and socially sound.
- **Knowledge:** Knowledge is power and strength. It is an asset which no one can destroy. Knowledge is the source of all activities of a person. It is must for growth of a person and modification of behavior. So attainment of knowledge is the aim of education.
- **Complete living:** It means living a meaningful life which includes activities such as bearing and rearing children, self-development and preservation, attainment of self-esteem and self-actualization and fulfilling one's duties and responsibilities toward family and society.
- **Harmonious development:** It means the harmonious cultivation of the physical, intellectual, esthetic and moral aspects of human nature. The aim of education is to produce a well-balanced personality. Mahatma Gandhi emphasized this aim of education very much when he said, "By education I mean an all-round drawing out of the best in child and man—body, mind and spirit". Education directs a person to develop sound mind in a sound body. It enables a person to become emotionally mature and mentally healthy person. It also cultivates moral values and virtues such as truthfulness, goodness, honesty, purity, reverence and courage. By developing moral values, one can develop good and desirable characters. So the aim of education is harmonious development of physical, mental, emotional, moral, and character development.
- **Self-realization:** Education helps a person to realize his or her maximum potentials. It helps him to assess

his strengths and shortcomings and plan for what he wants to achieve.
- **Cultural development:** Every individual has to become cultured and civilized through education. Cultural development if attained truly gives refinement, esthetic sense and a concern and respect for others and others' culture.
- **Citizenship:** The child has to be educated to become a good citizen of his country. Education should enable him to cultivate such qualities that are beneficial to the society. In a democratic set-up, being a member of society, a person should have knowledge about his duties, functions, and obligations toward society.
- **Individual and social aim:** Education is essential for optimum growth and development of the individual as well as social development of an individual. Individual and society are inseparable. Social contacts and relationships are essential for individual development whereas individual development is essential for social development. There should be a balance between the individual and social aims of education and they should complement each other.
- **Education for leisure:** Leisure is the time which is used for enjoyment and recreation. Leisure is also a part of human life. Leisure time should be utilized in such activities that are beneficial to the individual as well as the society.

Aims of Education in Independent India

The secondary education commission of *1952 (Mudaliar Commission)* suggested the following aims of education in free India.
- **Democratic citizenship:** Education should prepare people for democratic citizenship. It means to train persons with capacity for clear thinking, receptivity to new ideas, clarity in speech as well as in writing and true patriotism.
- **Development of personality:** All-round development of personality is an important aim of education. Education should develop the liberty, artistic, esthetic and cultural interests of students for this purpose. Subjects like art, dance and craft, etc. should be included in the curriculum.
- **Development of leadership:** If democracy is to function successfully, there should be people to assure leadership in the social, political, industrial, and cultural fields. Education should train the youth to assume such responsibilities.
- **Vocational efficiency:** For improving the poor economic situation of the country, the commission emphasized the need for increasing productivity through vocational and technical efficiency. One of the aims of education should be to develop vocational efficiency of the youth. Education should help to create a new attitude toward work and dignity of labor.
- **Initiating students to the art of living:** Through education the child should learn the art of harmonious living. Education should enable a person to acquire the necessary interpersonal skills and adjustment abilities for successful and happy living together in society.

The *Kothari Education Commission* of 1964–1966, proposed some more aims of education in India. They are as follows.
- **Education for increased productivity:** Increased productivity is an essential need of our country. Education should help us to satisfy this need through the production of manpower that is people who are equipped with advanced scientific knowledge, complex technical ability, and efficient work experience.
- **Social and national integration:** Education should inculcate the feeling of oneness and belongingness. This is a very important aim of education of our country which has the tendency to divide on the basis of language, culture, caste, religion and so on. This aim should be accomplished through some kind of public educational system and some form of obligatory national service.
- **Education for modernization:** The world is moving very fast with all kinds of scientific and technological advancements. India also should keep pace with the advancements of the modern world. Our education should aim at producing people who are able to think and judge independently and effectively. Intellectually efficient and technically competent persons must be prepared.
- **Education for social, moral and spiritual values:** Another important aim of education is to integrate social, moral and spiritual values in the minds of children and young people. The curriculum should include instruction in these subjects. All religions should be given equal importance.

The National Educational Policy of 1986 has set the following educational aims of our country which are still in force. They are:
- All-round material and spiritual development of all people
- Cultural orientation and development of interest in Indian culture
- Scientific temper
- National cohesion
- Independence of mind and spirit
- Furthering the goals of socialism, secularism, and democracy
- Manpower development for different level of economy
- Fostering research in all areas of development
- Education for equality.

Aims of Nursing Education

Nursing education is the professional education for the preparation of nurses to enable them to render professional nursing care to people of all ages, in all phases of health and illness, in a variety of settings. Need for nursing care is universal.

The purpose of nursing education is to meet the nursing needs of the country which ultimately requires knowledge of nursing.

It (the knowledge of nursing) is recognized as the knowledge which everyone ought to have distinct from medical knowledge, which only a profession can have. (Nightingale, 1860).

The aims of nursing education are:
- Nursing manpower development
- Knowledge aim
- Leadership aim
- Professional development
- Personality development
- Nursing research
- Democratic citizenship.

Factors Determining Educational Aims

There are certain factors determining educational aims. They are:
- Philosophy of life
- Elements of human nature
- Religion
- Political ideologies
- Socioeconomic factors
- Emerging problems of the nation
- Cultural factors
- Exploration of knowledge and technology.

Functions of Education

"The sole meaning of life is to serve humanity".
—Tolstoy

Education to be true must fit in with the capacity of the individuals, quite in keeping with the needs of the larger whole, namely the country. The only way of changing the psychology and social and personal habits of the people and to prepare them for the new task of democracy and freedom, is to educate them —Dr RS Mani.

General Functions of Education

Progressive Development of Innate Powers

Each child is endowed with some inherent tendencies as love, affection, curiosity, reasoning, imagination, and selfrespect, etc. The function of education is to develop these inborn capacities. According to pestalozzi, "Education is a natural, harmonious and progressive development of man's innate powers".

All-round Development of Personality

The total development of personality includes the physical, mental, emotional, and social development. The individual may not be fully equipped when any of these aspects remain undeveloped.

Control, Redirection and Sublimation of Instincts

An infant is born with some basic instincts. These instincts direct and mold his activities. The function of education is to control, redirect and sublimate the animal instincts into desirable patterns of behavior conducive to the good of the individual and welfare of society by pursuing higher goals of life.

Character Formation and Moral Development

Basically the instincts are neither good nor bad. Goodness or badness results from their proper or improper sublimation and modification. Education helps to build a strong moral character of the child by molding and sublimating the basic instincts. According to Herbert also, "The one and the whole work of education may be summed up in the concept—Morality".

Preparation for Adult Life

The child of today is a citizen of tomorrow. Education develops such abilities and capacities in the child that as he grows older, he is able to confront the problem of life courageously and solve them successfully.

Inculcation of Social Feelings

The school environment and social activities in the school develop social feeling and spirit of social service in children. Other social qualities such as love, fellow feeling, kindness, cooperation, tolerance, sympathy, and sacrifice are also inculcated in children by education and education alone.

Creation of Good Citizenship

For a good and great country, its citizens need to be good and dynamic. Good citizenship qualities are the sense of responsibility, fellow-feeling, cooperation, love, service, sense of duty, and qualities of leadership. Education prepares and develops these qualities in good citizens.

Preservation of Culture and Civilization

Each society has its own traditions, customs, morality concepts, and religious ideals. Prosperity promotes standards of civilization. Each nation is proud of its own culture and civilization. It is the function of the education to preserve and transmit this cultural heritage from one generation to another generation.

Social Reform

Education helps to remove blind beliefs, useless traditions, and evil customs which mar the progress and development of the society. Education shows the new ways of improvement for reform and development.

National Security

Education develops such necessary qualities in the individuals so that they are eager to sacrifice everything including lives for the security and honor of the nation. Education gives us the necessary training and inculcates the noble qualities such as patriotism, nationalism, and sacrifice.

Functions of Education to Individual

Adaptation to Environment

It is natural that everybody should struggle for existence. Adaptation leads to life and maladjustment leads to decay and destruction. Education teaches this adaptation so essential for life and existence.

Modification of Environment

Education inculcates good habits and values. By this he is able to modify his environment according to his needs and requirements. Thus, education not only helps him to adapt to his environment but helps him to modify the environment according to the changing situations and circumstances.

Making the Man Civilized

Education is a process to reform and culture the child. At birth, the child is like an animal with all basic instincts. The education makes him and directs him to behave like a civilized and cultured human being.

Satisfaction of Needs

Every individual human being has his physical, emotional, educational, and social needs. All these needs can be fulfilled by education.

Vocational Efficiency

Education helps the individual to achieve more and more vocational efficiency and professional competency.

Dr Radhakrishnan said, "To help the students to earn a living is one of the functions of education".

Achievement of Self-sufficiency

Education makes an individual to be self-reliant and self-supporting. It also promotes the sense of self-sufficiency and independence of others.

Development of Character

The main function of education is to develop the character of an individual. A man of character is devoted to high ideals of life. He is a man of virtue and nobility, and sincerely pursues the highest ideals of Truth, Beauty, and Goodness.

Development of Personality

Education develops moral qualities and social attitudes in the individual. It also inculcates the spirit of service and sacrifice, and stimulates a sense of responsibility and duty. Not only this, the latent capacities are stimulated and developed, and this leads to the development of wholesome personality.

Preparation for Life

Education develops and promotes preparation for the present as well as future life of an individual. It may be noted that life is a continuous struggle and an individual faces various problems from time to time in his life. Education develops his capacities and powers to the full, so that he is able to solve problems with self-confidence and lead a successful life.

Reorganization and Reconstruction of Experiences

A man undergoes various experiences in relation to his environment and through contact with other fellow beings. He classifies and consolidates those experiences which are conducive to his good and progress. Through this continued reconstruction and reorganization of experiences, the individual goes on developing himself to higher and higher levels of progress.

Creation of Good Citizens

Education creates good citizens. India is a secular democratic state. Hence, each and every citizen of this state should be dynamic, enterprising and resourceful. He should be fully conscious of his duties and responsibilities toward society and the nation to which he belongs.

Practical Knowledge of Spheres of Work

Education provides to the individual knowledge about various spheres of human thoughts and activities. But this knowledge should not be mere theoretical and merely academic. Citizens need practical efficiency in work.

Functions of Education in National Life

Training for Leadership

Success of democracy is possible only with efficient public leadership. The able leaders guide national programs of development in political, social, cultural, and economic fields.

Education provides this training for leadership at all levels. It inculcates the required values in the people who develop the needed qualities of effective and efficient leadership.

National Development

Education is the foundation stone of national development. Hence, all citizens should be provided with minimum standard of education, and after that various types of education should be made available to those who have a need, aptitude and zest for any other types.

National Integration

For national development, national unity is must. Our's is a country of diversities of language, religions, castes and modes of living. Our education should achieve unity in diversity. It should inculcate a feeling of oneness in all people irrespective of all types of differences.

Emotional Integration

National integration can be achieved through emotional integration. India is a country of diversities and differences in almost all spheres of national life. Narrow feelings develop hatred, enmity, jealousy, and rivalry. These feelings of citizens have to be molded and sublimated into desirable feelings of tolerance, fellow-feeling, cooperation, and adjustment. These desirable feelings and emotions will bring about emotional integration and promote discipline, unity, and national integration. Education can only inculcate such feelings.

National Discipline

Education promotes national discipline which is essential for the growth and development of a country. Our educational system should be shaped in such a way that desirable feelings and healthy emotions promoting national discipline at all levels are inculcated in all the citizens of State.

Inculcation of Civil and Social Duties

It is essential that all the citizens perform their duties and obligations toward the nation and all individuals discharge their responsibilities toward the society of which they are integral parts. Education is the only means to develop these social and moral qualities in individuals.

Training in Morality

Morality is the valuable treasure of every nation. Without a high sense of morality, national character does not develop. Even individual character is not formed without the inculcation of moral and spiritual values. Education is the only means to develop these moral values in individuals.

Supply of Skilled Manpower

Today is the age of materialism, where the eminence and greatness of a nation is evaluated in terms of its material prosperity and effluence. Only a trained and skilled manpower force can achieve material prosperity and industrial advancement.

Priority to National Interests

To promote national progress, it is essential that all citizens of the country give priority to national good over their own interests. The past history of our nation is a record of sacrifice for the freedom, integrity, security, and honor of the nation. Such qualities of sacrifice, service, patriotism, and nationalism should be developed in our children who are the citizens of tomorrow. Education alone can do it through its various activities and programs.

Promotion of Social Efficiency

Education can produce socially efficient person who is self-reliant and does not depend upon the income of others. Such a person helps to promote social welfare.

The functions of education are in nutshell represented in the table below.

Functions of education

For Family	For an Individual
• Growth of the family	• Self-understanding
• Economic stability and sustainability	• Physical development
	• Mental development
• Status symbol	• Moral development
• Preservation and transmission of culture	• Social development
	• Personality development
	• Vocational development
	• Increased productivity
	• Preparation for adult life
	• Satisfaction of needs
	• Achievement of material prosperity
	• Achievement of self-sufficiency

For Society	For Nation
• Supply of skilled manpower	• National integration
• Promotion of social efficiency	• National development
	• Emotional integration
• Increased employment opportunities	• National discipline
• Better understanding among people of varied caste, creed and religion	• Inculcation of civil and social duties
	• Peace
	• Improved status among other nations

Agencies of Education

It is generally believed that children are educated in schools and colleges. But the truth is that a child receives his education from various sources besides schools and colleges. The family, the school, the community, the church, the state, the library, the newspaper, etc. are all the means which provide diverse opportunities for the child to learn something or the other and bring about a modification in his behavior. All these means are the sources of education. Precisely, these means or sources of education are called as "agencies of education".

BD Bhatia has rightly remarked, "Society has developed a number of specialized institutions to carry out these functions of education. These institutions are known as agencies of education".

Classification of Agencies of Education

The agencies of education can be broadly classified as given below:

Classification	Types	Meaning	Examples
First	Formal	Agencies which impart formal education	School, religious institutions, library, museum, zoo, art galleries, organized games, educational programs
	Informal	Agencies which prepare the child for general as well as various types of education	Family, general games, state, community or society
Second	Commercial	These agencies give various kinds of knowledge, discoveries, inventions, and achievements of human race. Through these agencies, the child develops social attitudes and receives all kinds of social education and experiences	Radio, TV, cinema, clubs, theaters, newspapers, press
	Noncommercial	Noncommercial agencies came into being for social good. They are not linked with any commercial motive. Noncommercial agencies of education create the sense of dynamic citizenship and social service	Sports club, social welfare centers, dramatic clubs, scouting and guiding, youth welfare clubs, adult education centers
Third	Active	Active agencies of education act and react upon the growing child. Here, the child is active and can influence the working of the agencies	Family, school, community, religion, state, social clubs, organized games, entertainment programs, etc.
	Passive	Passive agencies act in one way only. The child is not in a position to influence them at all and remains a passive recipient only	Cinema, TV, radio, newspapers, magazines and market places, etc.

Principles of Education

Education is Pervasive

It involves everybody. It is invasive and it is not just learning and forgetting. A true learning involves the application of whatever learned whenever and wherever necessary.

Education is Goal Oriented

Everybody learns to achieve certain goal. The goal may be differing based on the individual needs. The needs might vary according to their life goal, philosophy, opportunities available, etc.

Education is a Continuous Process

There is no limit for education. Education starts in womb and ends in tomb. We learn something every day and every moment. It is a lifelong process.

Education is the Modification of Behavior

The aim of education is to bring desirable changes in the behavior of the educand and remove the unwanted behavior from the child.

Education is Flexible

Any education cannot be rigid. It is based on many factors especially the learner. Individuals are unique and differently endowed with various capacities and abilities. The educators should consider the individual difference and adopt a suitable method.

Education is for All Age Groups

We have variety of educational systems called preprimary, primary, secondary, higher secondary, collegiate education, distance education, and a system of Open University. Because of this, now opportunities are available for all age group people to undergo educational process.

Education is a Group Activity

In order to learn something at least two people are necessary. Education is the interaction between the teacher and the student.

Education is a Social Process

It is a social process because the close cooperation of all the members is essential. It is the interaction between the teacher and the student. The aim of education is to prepare a human being to lead a happy life in the society.

Education is Dynamic

Education is an active process, where the learner is actively involved in the process of learning. The aim of education is to bring the desirable changes in the behavior. Education is mostly a planned, purposeful and dynamic activity.

Education is a Science and Art

Education is a body of systematized knowledge and hence a science. It includes the principles of psychology, sociology, philosophy, humanities, etc. It is an art in the sense that it includes the art of teaching, learning, and imparting knowledge.

Education is Multidisciplinary

It draws its knowledge from many disciplines such as sociology, psychology, anthropology, philosophy, humanities, etc. Hence it is multidisciplinary.

Impact of Social, Economical, Political and Technological Changes on Education

Social Factors Influencing Education

"Culture" means refinement of feelings and "education" means knowledge of literature. Education is a means and culture is the end.

Each generation of a society passes on its social heritage and cultural tradition to the next generation which is known as the transmission of culture. The teachers prepare the students to face the challenges of career and life by inculcating in them values of the culture and developing in them a positive attitude; values and the right attitude helped their own progress and the progress of their society.

Earlier, in the man making education, the head saw the meaning of information, the heart saw its righteousness and its use within the boundaries or morality and the hands put it into action. But modern higher education has ignored the heart; it has ignored the fact that students are a subject matter of immense significance both for the present and the future of their country. Higher education in science and technology, which majority of the students opt tries to equip them for materialistic development, which is mistaken for "progresses". The engineers, doctors, scientists, economists, and men of commerce change very much in the name of civilization and they advance materialistically. Change and materialistic development do not signify human progress and the progress of society.

The present day youth stretch themselves beyond the limits to the extent of disturbing their mental poise and affecting the psychological well-being due to which values are forsaken and the interpersonal relationship break down. The youth have become the victims of over-vaulting materialistic ambition and unknowingly have accelerated the pace of their life. The result is gastric neurosis, mental disorder, and behavioral problems.

Unfortunately, the meaning of higher education generally these days is teaching the youth to live by machines and gadgets and not by the universal human values like truth, nonviolence, love, and compassion. The young men want to be always busy with their business and industry, which can multiply their money. Leisure and social get together are generally neglected.

The present way of thinking, behavior and life is changing so adversely that there is now an urgency to make value education an integral part of higher education. Machines like computer and internet have become so advanced that we cannot wait any longer for natural proofs to redeem the youth from the commercialized way of functioning and artificial way of living. Life has become so artificial and materialistic that young men and women have begun to think whether they need any value system at all that will guide them to the right way of living. If this doubt becomes a conviction, life will not be human and our society cannot be called a human society.

Education was the key to the alleviation of all social ills. Society engages itself in many activities. Education is one of the manifold activities of society. The type of education given will be largely determined by the type of skills required in carrying out the various activities of society.

Education is a powerful and pervasive agent for all-round development and individual and social transformation. This alone can sustain culture and civilization. Sarvapalli Dr Radhakrishnan said: "The three things—vital dynamism, intellectual efficiency and spiritual direction together constitute the proper aim of education". Moral and spiritual training is an essential part of education. A balanced development of mind and body in harmony with the spirit is the key to the enrichment of human personality.

UNESCO Report on Education, Culture and Values

A UNESCO report on education for the 21st century entitled "Learning: The Treasure Within" also pleads for an education which is "rooted to culture and committed to progress". Developing a harmonious and integrated personality would just not be possible, if the system does not inculcate values of culture, heritage and traditions. Indian heritage, culture, and values need to be thoroughly studied, analyzed and incorporated comprehensively in the educational system right from the initial stage to higher dimensions of education. It also lays emphasis on the challenge of improving quality of life. It suggests that educational process needs to be restructured to draw out the hidden talents in students. It has also identified four icons namely, learning to know, learning to do, learning to live together, and learning to be. It is the responsibility of the educational managers to ensure that the four special features are included in all their education programs.

It is in this context that UNESCO identified the decade (2001–2010) as the International Decade for a Culture of Peace and non-violence for the Children of the World. A culture of peace will be achieved when citizens of the world understand global problems, have the skill to resolve conflicts and struggle for justice, nonviolence and live by international standards of human rights and equity.

Culture of peace is a set of values, attitudes, traditions and modes of behavior and ways of life based on:
- Respect for life, ending of violence and promotion and practice of nonviolence through education, dialogue and cooperation;
- Full respect for the principles of sovereignty, territorial integrity, and political independence of states;
- Full respect for and promotion of all human rights and fundamental freedom;
- Commitment to peaceful settlement of conflicts;
- Efforts to meet the developmental and environmental needs of present and future generations;
- Respect for and promotion of the equal rights of and opportunities for women and men;
- Respect for and promotion of the rights of everyone to freedom of expression, opinion and information;
- Adherence to the principles of freedom, justice, democracy, tolerance, solidarity, cooperation, pluralism, cultural diversity, dialogue and understanding at all levels of society and among nations; and fostered by an enabling national and international environment conducive to peace.

The National Council of Educational Research and Training (NCERT), the National Open School, Universities and the University Grants Commission (UGC) are now engaged in the development modules and instructional packages in the area of value education to incorporate in the school and higher education curriculum.

Teacher Preparation

The role of teachers in changing society may be summarized in the following points:
- The teachers should be above to create and sustain an academic environment
- The teachers should not be restricted to teaching only but should take part in extension activities
- The teachers should be conscious of their roles in terms of teaching, training, consultancy, and research
- Teachers should be active researchers and lifelong learners
- The teachers have to encourage student to be willing partners in the learning process
- The teachers are expected to dedicate their efforts and energy toward the development of the institution they are working for and in the process of developing themselves as professionals.
- The teachers should practice superior standards of *morality*
- The teachers have to be accountable to both their employers and the students.

Social Factors and Nursing Education

The general aim of nursing education is to prepare nurses to serve the human beings in the society to promote optimum health and prevent illnesses and nursing revolves around the care of individual and the society. Dr Dennis Raphael developed the Social Determinants of Health model which looks at non-medical factors and its influence on someone's health and their healthcare needs. These sociopolitical factors are issues outside of someone's individual control; they are imposed by society or life circumstances. Knowledge on these factors and its influence on health of people are important for nurses to promote health and well-being of the individual and the society.

According to Dr Raphael the 14 determinants are:
1. Income and income distribution
2. Education
3. Unemployment and job security
4. Employment and working conditions
5. Early childhood development
6. Food insecurity
7. Housing
8. Social exclusion
9. Social safety network
10. Health services
11. Aboriginal status
12. Gender
13. Race, and
14. Disability

The Sustainable Development Goals (SDGs), otherwise known as the Global Goals, are a universal call to action to end poverty, protect the planet, and ensure that all people enjoy peace and prosperity. The SDGs came into effect in January 2016, and they will continue to guide United Nations Development Programme (UNDP) policy and funding until 2030. There are 17 SDGs. The third goal is "Good Health and Well-being" which is directly related to Nursing and Nursing Education. The UNDP data state that at least 400 million people have no basic health services and 40% of the world's people lack social protection. In every 2 seconds someone aged 30–70 years dies prematurely from noncommunicable diseases—cardiovascular disease, chronic respiratory disease, diabetes or cancer.

The 2030 agenda reflects and responds to the increasing complexity and interconnectedness of health and development, including widening economic and social inequalities, rapid urbanization, threats to the climate and the environment, the continuing burden of HIV and other infectious diseases and emerging health challenges such as noncommunicable diseases. Universal health coverage, based on the principles of equity, access and quality, will be integral to achieving SDG-3, ending poverty and reducing inequalities.

By 2030, there are targets fixed to achieve in the areas such as global maternal mortality, preventable deaths of newborns and children under 5 years of age, ending the epidemics of AIDS, tuberculosis, malaria and neglected tropical diseases and combat hepatitis, water-borne diseases and other communicable diseases, reduction by one-third premature mortality from noncommunicable diseases through prevention and treatment and promotion of mental health and well-being, reduction of global deaths and injuries from road traffic accidents, ensuring universal access to sexual and reproductive healthcare services, including family planning, information and education, and the integration of reproductive health into national strategies and programs, achieving universal health coverage, etc.

The goals such as 1: No poverty; 2: Zero hunger; 3: Quality education; 4: Gender equality; 5: Clean water and sanitation, etc. are interrelated and concerning health and well-being of the people. All these goals are interconnected and the progress in one area will influence positively on the other. The nursing education should focus on these areas to address the challenges in achieving these goals and the role of nurses. The curriculum restructuring and revision need to be done to incorporate the content and strategies to face emerging problems of the people and attain the SDGs.

Economic Factors and Education

Economic conditions, economic policies, and the economic system are important external factors that constitute educational environment in a country. Income of the people and their purchasing power influences the demand for education. In countries where investment and income are steadily and rapidly increasing, educational prospects are generally bright. The economic policies of the government influence education environment in a country. Education tie up of collaboration with foreign universities, exchange of students and faculty members from one country to another country also influences education environment. Economic conditions of a country determine infrastructure for schools, colleges and universities and other educational oriented development activities.

There may be a positive correlation between economic conditions of a country and growth of educational sector. A substantial growth in education can be seen in developed countries and students of developing countries prefer to do their higher studies in developed countries.

Indian educational institutions are governed by the economic policies and economic systems of the Government of India. Trends in domestic trade, export, inflation, money supply, foreign exchange reserved growth of industry, agriculture and services sector determine status of education and its prospects. Reducing interest rate influences educational environment. Students pursuing higher studies come forward to get educational loan from public sector banks to meet their expenditure on education. Loans are also provided to educational institutions for constructing required infrastructure.

Government also frequently interferes to fix various types of fees to be collected from students of professional education. Curriculum improvement is one of the factors contributing to increase in the cost of education. Modern infrastructure in educational institutions increases cost of education to students. Modern teaching methods and technologies increase the cost of diversified courses offered by educational institutions and the need to increase the students' competitive skills also increase the cost of education.

Universal Declaration of Human Rights establishes that higher education shall be accessible to all on the basis of merit. No discrimination can be accepted, no one can be excluded from higher education or its study fields, degree levels and types of institutions on ground of race, gender, language, religion or age because of any economic or social distinctions or physical disabilities.

Funding for Education

The University Grants Commission (UGC) has no funds of its own. It receives both plan and nonplan grants from the central government, through the Ministry of Human Resource Development to carry out the responsibilities assigned to it by law. The UGC also has a variety of programs under which financial assistance is available for promoting career advancement and research.

Investment in Education

Investment in education is of vital significance especially in the developing countries for enriching the quality of human life which in turn can promote economic development.

The funding from the government sources is drying up in the context of new economic and industrial policies which call for privatization and a decreasing role for the government in higher education. Hence, there is a need to look for more funding from other sources and devising innovative strategies for attracting these funds. The universities and technical institutions have to be prepared to market and offer their strengths to earn the enhanced funding.

Strategies for Resources Mobilization

There are essentially two strategies for resource management, namely, increasing avenues and reducing costs.

Universities can succeed in increasing revenues by offering some of the following services to industries:
- Consultancy
- Research and development services
- Short-term specialized courses
- Technology transfer
- Running continuing education courses on commercial basis
- Developing workshops as training cum production centers
- Corpus fund, and
- Utilization of available resources by industries.

In addition to raising resources, there is a need to look at the internal efficiency and effectiveness in these universities. The Punnayya Committee has suggested certain areas for improving internal efficiency of the universities such as: Development of appropriate Management Information System, cost analysis, approaches to budgeting, comparative studies of costs and expenditures, strategic planning, and several incentives and structures.

However, the higher education institutions can think of introducing reforms with regard to:
- Better utilization of teaching materials and facilities
- Better management of physical resources
- Equipment management
- Management of resources, and
- Use of new techniques.

Education is an economically and socially productive investment. In many developing countries, education is financed and provided predominantly by the state. It is widely accepted that the state of higher education is an indicator of future progress and prosperity of the country. Higher technical and professional education has the power to produce change agents for moving the country along the development continuum.

Technical and professional education in India has witnessed a rapid expansion in terms of the stock of technical manpower, number of institutions/enrollment and the out turn of degree and diploma holders. The attraction of earning higher salaries, western lifestyle, liking for upgrading living standards, charm of going abroad, parental pressures, all these inspire our youth to get skilled with professional education. Professional and technical education supplies qualified manpower. Hopes for the better future inspire the students to invest money in professional education; availability of money through educational loans has become an easy task. The social benefits include mainly economic growth, income distribution, etc. The demand for these courses has been growing faster than the institution's capacity to absorb them.

Privatization in Higher Education

There is a problem in providing adequate funds by the central and state government for the higher and professional education and in opening new professional colleges to meet the growing demands of the increasing number of aspirant boys and girls. The only alternative available before the government was to allow the entry of private trusts, corporate houses, and individuals to set-up "Self-financing institutions" to provide education as also qualified manpower. The decision by the Government of India to allow entry of private enterprises to set up self-financing institutions helped the central and state government to share the burden of ever-growing demand for admission into colleges and professional courses.

The higher education in India continues to be in a financial crisis, with escalating cost and increasing needs of the system, on the one hand, and declining resources, on the other, despite large investments made on higher education.

The Gnanam Committee stated as follows:
"It will not be possible for the state government to fund adequate resources, to create endowment funds for each university. Universities, however, should make efforts to raise own resources but must be ensured that there are no conditions attached like preference in admission, etc. Rising of resources should not affect academic standards and universities should lay down guidelines for the same."

Issues Related to Privatization of Higher Education

Admission based on capitation fee lead to commercialization of education. Thus, self-financing higher education institutions have become a place where money power replaced the merit of the students. This has violated the basic concept of equity as has been enshrined in the Indian Constitution.

Another important issue is related to the quality of these self-financed or private institutions. But there is a contradiction in the opinion of different people regarding the concept of quality. There are few who believe that increased fees will lead to better quality because when the people pay for educations, they ask for quality. Institutions also feel accountable to satisfy the aspirations of parents regarding better quality education.

Privatization of higher education will have its adverse effects upon future employment opportunities. The people who are spending thousands and lakhs of rupees to get a degree of a particular profession will definitely exercise their influence on money in securing employment. It is happening now and will continue in future too due to deterioration of values of life.

Tilak (1991) defines privatization of higher education on the basis of funding that "Private universities may generate large amount of resources from private sources". He classified privatization of higher education into four categories.

An extreme version of privatization implies total privatization of higher education, colleges and universities being managed and funded by the private sector, with little government intervention. Therefore, the pure or unaided institutions do provide financial relief to the government in providing higher education, but at huge long-term economic and noneconomic cost to the society.

There is strong privatization concept, which means recovery of full costs of public higher education from users, students, their employers or both. Due to externalities associated with higher education, privatization of this type may not be desirable and empirically feasible.

A moderate form of privatization implies public provision of higher education but with reasonable level of financing from nongovernment sources. Since higher education is a quasi-public good, 100% public financing of education can be seen as economically unjustified. Since private individuals also benefit, it is reasonable that they share a portion of the costs.

Pseudo-privatization, which cannot be really called privatization, higher education under this category is private but government-aided. Private bodies originally created them, but receive nearly the whole of their expenditure from governments. Thus, these institutions are privately managed but publicly funded. Hence, strictly from the financial point of view such private colleges do not play any significant role.

Curriculum improvement is one of the factors contributing to increase in cost of education. Modern infrastructure in educational institutions increase cost of education to students. Modern teaching methods and using educational gadgets also increase cost of education.

Despite the recent expansion of higher education, levels of participation and chances of academic success are still lowest among young people from deprived neighborhoods. This report identifies what affects the experiences of the minority or disadvantaged young people who do enter higher education.

Although there has been an increase in the numbers of university entrants from more disadvantaged backgrounds in recent years, such young people have been enjoying less success within higher education. The research by Alasdair Forsyth and Andy Furlong of the University of Glasgow, details the barriers to success within higher education faced by students from disadvantaged backgrounds. The researchers found that:

Students from disadvantaged backgrounds were more likely to prematurely reduce their level of participation within higher education, by dropping out of courses or by foregoing the opportunity to progress to more advanced courses. They were also more likely to follow complicated paths within higher education, including deferred enrollment, gap-years and switching, repeating or restarting their courses for nonacademic reasons. A number of factors seem to lie behind these difficulties:

- A lack of familiarity with higher education, which often resulted in such young people enrolling in inappropriate courses or at unsuitable institutions;
- A lack of funds, which limited their choices of course or institution and also the length of time which the young person was willing to remain within higher education;
- A fear of debt, which could exert a much greater deterrent effect on disadvantaged students' continued participation than could actual debt, especially when this fear was coupled with a lack of confidence, about both their chances of academic success and their chances of finding a job at the end of it, all to pay off this debt;
- Feelings of cultural isolation, particularly at the more prestigious institutions, which could compromise the disadvantaged students' identity and lower morale, and lessen their commitment to continued study.

As might be expected, many of the disadvantaged students in this research felt that the length of their student career would be limited by their finances rather than by their academic ability. To overcome their financial problems, various sources of income, particularly paid work and debt, were budgeted against hardship and study time. Interestingly, it was often the fear of debt rather than actual amount of debt which led to reduced participation.

Financing Higher Education

The National Policy on Education of 1986 and its modified version (1992) stressed the need of financing higher education through such avenues:

- Enticement of fees coupled with provision of soft loans to the needy students
- Consistency
- Testing
- Sponsored projects
- Community contribution
- Institutional chairs
- Raising donations for infrastructural development with a provision for tax exemptions
- Establishment of industrial foundations
- Charging fees for specific facilities such as laboratories, libraries, games, and magazines, etc.

Private institutions tap the untapped resources available in the society and generate the much needed resources for the development of higher professional education.

Economic Factors and Nursing Education

There is a common belief that upon completion of a course in nursing, there will be a job opportunity and it is true. The scope for nursing is good in the current scenario. At any point of time, the demand for healthcare will not decline, even at the time of recession. This reminds that the hospital should be staffed adequately at all times. Because of the gender advantage in the profession of nursing, female nurses add income to the family.

Despite the scope in nursing, there is a greater disparity in the salaries paid to the nurses working in the private and government sectors. The nursing workforce staged a chain strike for their pay hike in the private sectors. The need for nursing and nurses is global and there begins the opportunity to work in any part of the world and nurses serve as a vital part of global health work force.

Nurses nowadays aim for higher education and are motivated to pursue higher studies in nursing. The number of students pursuing higher education such as PBBSc(N), MSc(N), and PhD in nursing is increasing. Affordability, cost of education, availability of courses, and career advancement are the factors attributed to enrollment of candidates for higher education in nursing.

Political Factors Influencing Education

Political environment consists of the political system (i.e. democracy, autocracy, etc.), the political institutions (the national and regional parties, their structure and their style of functioning, etc.), the political ideologies of the parties, political stability (continuance of same party in power, continuance of same policies pursued by the party in power, etc.), and strength of opposition and political culture of parties. As long as there is no absolute majority for the ruling party in the parliament, support of the opposition and supporting political parties becomes essential for introducing any new policies or enacting any new laws relating to any subject matter.

Government policies in education are based on the prevailing environment. Dual degree course, job oriented courses, vocational course, short-term courses relating to information technology, specific courses/studies needed to get employment opportunities abroad are planned based on the government policies in education. Uniform curriculum in all educational institutions and uniformity in conducting examinations and publishing results are also the outcome of government policies in education. Education to all is the primary objective of education policies of the government. Government provides financial support and other infrastructural facilities for organizing training programs to improve teaching skills to the teachers. Teacher education program is given priority. Refresher and orientation course are conducted to the teachers of higher education in order to refresh them with multi-faceted developments in various disciplines of education.

Two major governmental policies which have impacted the growth and dissemination of education are discussed briefly as below:

Sarva Shiksha Abhiyan

Sarva Shiksha Abhiyan (SSA) is Government of India's flagship program for achievement of Universalization of Elementary Education (UEE) in a time-bound manner, as mandated by 86th amendment to the Constitution of India making free and compulsory education to the children of 6–14 years age group, a Fundamental Right.

SSA is being implemented in partnership with State Governments to cover the entire country. The program seeks to open new schools in those habitations which do not have schooling facilities and strengthen existing school infrastructure through provision of additional classrooms, toilets, drinking water, maintenance grant, and school improvement grants.

Existing schools with inadequate teacher strength are provided with additional teachers, while the capacity of existing teachers is being strengthened by extensive training, grants for developing teaching-learning materials and strengthening of the academic support structure at a cluster, block and district level.

SSA seeks to provide quality elementary education including life skills. SSA has a special focus on girl's education and children with special needs. SSA also seeks to provide computer education.

Samagra Shiksha

The Union Budget, 2018–19, has proposed to treat school education holistically without segmentation from prenursery to Class 12. Samagra Shiksha—an overarching program for the school education sector extending from preschool to class 12 has been, therefore, prepared with the broader goal of improving school effectiveness measured in terms of equal opportunities for schooling and equitable learning outcomes. It subsumes the three schemes of Sarva Shiksha Abhiyan (SSA), Rashtriya Madhyamik Shiksha Abhiyan (RMSA), and Teacher Education (TE).

The Goal SDG-4.1 states that "By 2030, ensure that all boys and girls complete free, equitable and quality primary and secondary education leading to relevant and effective learning outcomes." Further the SDG-4.5 states that "By 2030, eliminate gender disparities in education and ensure equal access to all levels of Education and vocational training for the vulnerable, including persons with disabilities, indigenous peoples and children in vulnerable situations."

The scheme envisages the "school" as a continuum from preschool, primary, upper primary, secondary to senior secondary levels. The vision of the scheme is to ensure inclusive and equitable quality education from preschool to senior secondary stage in accordance with the SDG for education.

The major objectives of the scheme are Provision of quality education and enhancing learning outcomes of students; bridging Social and Gender Gaps in School Education; ensuring equity and inclusion at all levels of school education; ensuring minimum standards in schooling provisions; promoting vocationalization of education; support States in implementation of the Right of Children to Free and Compulsory Education (RTE) Act, 2009; and strengthening and upgradation of SCERTs/ State Institutes of Education and DIET as nodal agencies for teacher training.

The scheme will be implemented as a Centrally Sponsored Scheme by the Department through a single State Implementation Society (SIS) at the State/UT level.

This scheme is introduced in selected schools in India. The primary objective of this program is to provide required infrastructure in schools for providing basic education to the children. Increasing enrollment rates and reducing dropout rates for school children are the objectives of this program. Noon-meal scheme to the school children also motivates and encourages school-going children. Government encourages community participation in education institutions in order to make the community to actively involve for the progress of educational institutions.

National Policy on Education

National Policy on Education is a basic document for taking steps and planning programs for upliftment of education sector in India. Budgetary allocation for education is also based on government policies. Renowned and reputed institutes of higher education and professional education are given deemed university status. Colleges are given autonomous status. They design their courses and curriculum based on the ever-changing environment related to industry, agriculture, and services. Streamlining higher secondary education, common entrance test for professional education, and centralized admission for professional education are also monitored by the policies of the government. Medium of instruction in educational institutions is also based on the education and language policies of the government. Reservation policy to be followed in educational institutions is decided by the government and based on the policy, student admission process is completed. Some of the programs at elementary education stage are District Primary Education Program, Mid-day Meal Scheme, Pradhan Mantri Gramodaya Yojana, etc.

The government policies on education will influence education environment. Government will frame policies relating to students admission, teacher selection, and administration of educational institutions. Policies relating to above should be followed strictly. Economic policies and systems will support as well as monitor educational institutions. There may be a perfect positive correlation between economic conditions of a country and growth of education sector.

After privatizing education sector, government frequently interferes to fix various types of fees to be collected from students of professional education. In some cases judicial body also interferes for fixing fees to be collected from the students of professional education.

Technological Factors Influencing Education

Growing influence of telecommunication and advances in information technology has significantly influenced the daily lives, as making the concept of global village a reality. Higher education system has to accept this changing environment and adopt new technologies to break its traditional boundaries. Similarly other scientific revolutions have influenced increasingly the areas of research and teaching with greater emphasis on biomedical environment with the ultimate aim to improve the quality of life.

Academic autonomy warrants special efforts of the institution to provide appropriate teaching and learning experiences to the students. The institutions and the faculty have to introduce teaching aids and use of technology to make system learner-centered.

We have arrived at a global village concept with all virtual realities on the desktops. But still teacher education has largely remained unaffected by this. An explosive growth in technology, on the other hand, is providing a new wave of teaching tools, computer aided video instruction, hypermedia, multimedia, CD-ROMs, LANS, Internet connections, and collaborative software environment. Video conferencing and Internet allow people to communicate more effectively for pleasure, business, and learning. Accessed through the World Wide Web, the Internet brings people a range and quantity of information that would be impossible to find through any other source. The educational paradigm is changing due to educational technology (Table 1.1).

Teaching and Learning

It is important that student-teachers, teachers at colleges and university departments of education to be enabled to achieve the following IT qualifications through teacher training or in-service and further training.

Teachers must have a basic qualification including IT related topics, from the viewpoint of their professional pedagogic and didactic considerations. They must be able to communicate, in much easier and effective way, the knowledge about the social information and communication technology. If this goal is to be achieved, it will require that teachers have the following qualification:
- A general knowledge of how it helps education.
- Knowledge of methods and concepts in IT-based technology supported learning, teaching and education.

Table 1.1: Changing educational paradigm.

Traditional model	Emerging model	Technological aspects
• Information delivery	• Individual initiative and self-exploration	• CD-ROMs, networked computers with access to online databases
• Classroom lectures passive/absorption	• Learning by doing or apprenticeship	• Requires simulations for skill development
• Emphasis on individualism	• Emphasis on collaboration and team learning	• Requires collaborative tools and e-mail
• Teacher knows all	• Teacher as a guide	• Provide access to experts over network and USENET
• Stable content	• Rapidly changing content tools	• Requires access to real time news and publishing

- Basic knowledge and skill in the use of information and communication technology as an instrument in the daily preparation and teaching activities.
- The experience of various methods for evaluating the quality and utility of IT-based and technology supported learning, teaching and education.
- Insight and experience of, the development of methods to evaluate IT-based and technology supported learning, teaching and education.

In the technology environment, the human interaction is reduced in the learning process, thereby leading to partial loss of effective skills learned through personal contact and modeling other's behavior. In a world, which is gradually becoming more impersonal, the retention of large amounts of human interchange in learning seems important, both for socialization purposes and to enhance the quality of life.

Online Education

Online instruction is the most recent form of what is generically termed distance education, which includes satellite courses, computer-based programs, video instruction, educational television, correspondence or home study courses. The emphasis is to provide opportunities to students who are unable to attend classes at the traditional, centralized classrooms because of schedule or physical problems or unavailability of desired course. It makes use of available media. Online education thus represents a learning domain which is distinct from other technology based delivery systems. It offers a unique learning mode which is place- and time-independent, and provides for many to many communications.

The online education will not only change the way courses are taught and the way students learn, but also fundamentally change the institutions and individuals involved in universities, colleges, schools, publishers, and authors.

Virtual University

A virtual university imparts education through virtual classes sometimes augmented with video, and supplemented with a couple of face-to-face meetings. The distinguishing features of a virtual university in contrast to a physical university can be summarized as follows:
- It is a university in abstract with global coverage, whereas a physical university has to be located at a city
- It imparts education asynchronously in multiple modes of delivery
- Its education process flows from a course ware (not from course book) that can be media-rich in its presentation
- Its education process is learner centric as against faculty centric of the face-to-face classes
- It provides better attention to each individual student
- It provides better collaborative learning environments
- It decomposes the multiple roles of a traditional faculty, facilitating multiple professionals to participate in a coordinated way in conducting a course.

Technological Advancements and Nursing

No area is left untouched by Information Technology, and nursing is no exception. Nurses make up the most significant number of healthcare professionals and technology has changed the way nurses practice from the bedside to nursing education.

Medical and technological advancements in the field of healthcare have largely influenced nursing practice and nursing education. Medical technology has improved patient outcomes by allowing faster diagnosis, more precise therapies, and more hands-on patient care. Nurses use tablets to access information and portable computers which are at the bedside. Charts are continuously updated in real time which improves patient outcomes and the delivery of appropriate and timely care. Mobile apps are developed and utilized for health promotion of the patients. Today cell phone apps are quick references for useful information and are vital to the speedy delivery of excellent care. Information processing speed has grown exponentially. Digital technology advancements in telehealth and telemedicine bring providers and patients together from worlds apart.

The use of electronic gadgets and monitors is inevitable in patient care which facilitates the delivery of nursing care. Whatever was once done manually, now has been replaced with technology. Advances in simulation make clinical learning effective and the use of high fidelity simulators is the need of the hour in nursing education. Instructors can program the mannequins to mimic scenarios nurses might see in clinical practice. It is a safe environment where students can practice their critical thinking and decision-making skills. Health informatics is an evolving specialization that links information technology, communication and healthcare to improve the quality and safety of patient care. The nursing curriculum must incorporate the technological changes and its influence on health and nursing so as to equip the students to cope with the reality.

Challenges in Nursing Education

"Nothing is more purifying on earth than knowledge"
—*Bhagvad Gita*

According to Tagore, the widest road leading to the solution of all our problems is education. Education may be compared to a Kalpavriksha as it fulfills human desires. Nursing education provides the learners with the opportunity to acquire, integrate, apply, and synthesize knowledge in the delivery of nursing care.

The challenges can be discussed under the following headings. They are:
- Students
- Teachers
- Education environment
- Political environment
- Controlling bodies
- Healthcare problems
- Healthcare industry
- Environment
- Globalization
- Modern technology
- Research.

Students

Geographical Variation

Today's classrooms are very different from those in the past. There is greater diversity in the student body. For education, students from different parts of the country travel to different places. By using the strength and originality of diverse students, the final classroom product can be much stronger than the product of assimilated one. There is a cultural interaction, exchange of communication, language, etc. in addition to learning.

Diverse Intelligence, Learning Styles and Personality

Not only the geographical variation, there is also a variation in the forms of learners in terms of intelligence (Box 1.1),

---

Box 1.1: Seven Forms of Intelligence —*by Gardner*

1. *Linguistic*: It is related to written and spoken words and language.
2. *Musical/Rhythmic*: Based on sensitivity to rhythm and beat, recognition of total patterns and pitch and appreciation of musical expression.
3. *Logical/Mathematical*: Related to inductive and deductive reasoning, abstractions and discernment of numerical patterns.
4. *Visual/Spatial*: Ability to visualize an object or to create internal (mental) images, thus able to transform or recreate.
5. *Bodily kinesthetic*: The taking in and procession of knowledge through use of bodily sensations. Learning is accomplished through physical movement or use of body language.
6. *Interpersonal*: Emphasis communication and interpersonal relationships, recognition of mood, temperament and other behaviors.
7. *Intrapersonal*: Inner thought processes, such as reflection and metacognition, include spiritual awareness and self-knowledge.

Box 1.2: Four Learning Styles —*by Kolb*

1. *Convergers*: Prefer abstract conceptualization and achieve experimentation. These individuals are more detached and work better with objects than people. They are problem solvers and apply ideas in a practical manner.
2. *Divergers*: Prefer connect experience and reflective observation. Individuals with this tendency are good at generating ideas and displaying emotionalism and interest in others. Divergers are imaginative and can see the big picture.
3. *Assimilators*: Prefer abstract conceptualization and reflective observation. Assimilators easily bring together diverse items into an integrated entity, sometimes overlooking practical aspects or input from others. Theoreticians are likely assimilators.
4. *Accommodators*: Prefer correct experience and active experimentation. These individuals, while intuitive are risk takers and engage in trial and error and ever problem solving. Accommodators are willing to carry out plans and they like and adapt to new circumstances.

---

learning styles (Box 1.2) and personality, etc. Students with different forms of intelligence and learning styles also join nursing. To cater to the needs of these students is a challenge.

Economic Status

Students from different economic status join nursing profession. Their school education and attitude toward nursing is influenced by economic status.

Teachers

Adaptive Personality

Personality of the teacher influences nursing education. Teachers' willingness to accept changes and also to incorporate it in nursing is a challenge. Professional pride and growth is influenced by the attitude of the teacher toward nursing education.

Updated Knowledge

All faculty members are pushed to develop curricula responsive to the needs of today's healthcare delivery system, which demands greater efficiency, an ability to work in a highly technical environment, knowledge of new protocols, community experiences, and greater responsibility and accountability. A knowledge explosion and the emphasis on evidence-based practice challenges nurse educators to be aware of the current newer developments and flexible when it comes to change.

Meeting Increased Demands of Education

Members of the nursing faculty are pushed to meet the increasing demands of education, clinical excellence, tenure and possibly vocational certification or research. The workload and the time invested in performance of professional responsibilities often are greater than the same for instructors in other disciplines, even though they are considered colleagues in the educational setting.

Technological Skill Upgradation

Another challenge is skill in usage of technology. We all pass through three defined stages before we become more or less comfortable with using the new technology. These three stages are classic in the adoption of computing and information technology.
1. *Replacement:* The first stage is called replacement. In this stage, we are replacing a function that we have done manually by this new tool, the computer.
2. *Innovation:* We move from replacement into what is called the innovation stage. We have gone beyond what we could originally do manually to doing things with the computer we could not do before. The new technology begins to be diffused throughout our profession. Computer systems become common place in large scale hospital information systems, as they have in radiology and clinical laboratories.
3. *Transformation:* In the healthcare profession, the one area that has entered into this third stage is radiology, e.g. CAT scan. When we look into nursing profession and its practices, it is very exciting to realize that we are going through these phases and are involved in this process. Most of us are still in the replacement stage, moving into innovation. Over the next 5 or 6 years, there will be a revolution—not even an evolution—a revolution into a transformed profession.

In today's scenario, many colleges find it difficult to appoint a qualified and experienced teacher. Due to mushrooming of colleges, it is not an easy job to find adequate number of suitable faculty members to employ in the institution which is also a challenge.

Education Environment

Feasibility

All colleges preparing graduates for practice must meet the criteria established by the council. Adequate financial support is a major concern. All nursing programs are relatively expensive to operate in comparison with other forms of education provided in colleges and universities.

Finding Appropriate Learning Experiences

Most programs find themselves competing with other institutions for learning experiences in clinical agencies.

The increase in the number and size of colleges in urban areas create a high demand for clinical facilities.

Changes in the Attitudes of the Consumer and the Agency

The concept of teaching hospital is not as viable as it once was. Consumers paying for the high cost of care wanted that the care must be provided by the qualified nurses rather than by students who are still learning.

Constructing and Teaching the Curricula

Educators in all types of nursing programs struggle to construct and teach curricula that will prepare the graduate for entry into a profession who practices in a much larger arena, with much more technical equipment and requiring greater critical thinking skills than ever before.

Self financing Institutions in Higher Education

There is a problem in providing adequate funds by the central and state government for the higher and professional education and in opening new professional colleges to meet the growing demands of the increasing number of aspirant boys and girls. The only alternative available before the government was to allow the entry of private trusts, corporate houses and individuals to set up "Self-financing Institutions" to provide education as also qualified manpower. The decision by the Government of India to allow entry of private enterprises to set up self-financing institutions helped the central and state government to share the burden of ever-growing demand for admission into colleges and professional courses.

Political Environment

It is the government who develops policies related to education and reservation for various categories. It is the commitment of the government to allocate money for the development of medical and paramedical education and healthcare services. The National Education Policy reflects the changes to be incorporated based on the current need and future demand for professionals and professional education.

Controlling Bodies

State Nursing Council, Indian Nursing Council, University and Professional Association establish standard for nursing education. The Indian Nursing Council will revise syllabus when required, verify the provisions and facilities of the nursing colleges by periodically conducting inspections. Legal concerns are demanding more time and attention. Programs are caught up in more legal concerns than in the past, because applicants and students are seeking their "rights as individuals" and challenging admission, progression and dismissal policies. The National Student Nursing Association had formulated student bill of rights and responsibilities is widely accepted by schools of nursing in the United States. It sets forth the students' basic rights and establishes grievance procedures if a student believes that these rights have been violated.

Healthcare Problems

Emergence of newer diseases, development of drug resistance and societal trend leads to many other chronic health problems which present a challenge for nursing education. Because of increased mobility of people from one place to another, the diseases are easily spread in other parts of the world. It is imperative that the nursing curriculum should provide knowledge on global health problems.

Healthcare Industry

Computerized Healthcare Delivery System

Today's healthcare settings could not operate without computers and computerized equipment. Computers are used for business operations, medical records, and collection of clinical data. Computers may be used for writing nursing care plans, for communication from the physicians' office to nursing stations, for regulating the administration of medications, and for many other facets of operation and patient care. Most of the equipment used in today's modern hospital is computerized. New graduates move into a highly technical world when they seek their first nursing positions. The education they receive to prepare them for these positions also must include the skills necessary to work in this highly computerized environment.

Increased Community-based Practice Experiences

Another significant change in nursing practice is the trend toward community-based practice. Nurses are expected to provide care in client's homes, the workplace, schools, nursing homes, community health agencies, clinics, shelters, and community gathering places. As the arena in which nursing is practiced begins to shift, nursing educators are challenged to define what part of the nursing curriculum should be taught in a community setting. Often this requires different clinical teaching strategies and approaches.

Healthcare delivery system is differing in developing and developed countries. Sub-specialization in nursing also depends upon the healthcare delivery system. Nurses have to be prepared for the use of advanced technology, which is used in the healthcare delivery system. The trends affecting healthcare delivery system are demographic trend, social trend, economic trend, health workforce trend, and technological trends.

Environment

Managing victims of natural disasters like Tsunami, Earthquake, and man-made disasters like pollution, war and violence are a challenge for nurses. The topic disaster management is given much importance nowadays.

Globalization

Higher Education under Globalization

The process of globalization and internationalization are increasing at alarming rates. Their combined impact on higher education along with other factors is of great concern to the educators and also to policy makers which may be summarized as follows:
- The perceived importance of knowledge for the economic, social, and cultural welfare of society world wide.
- Ongoing integration and application of information communication technologies to the process of teaching, learning, and research.
- Increasing pressures and demands for higher education institutions to prepare graduates for life and work in an international content.
- Mobility for highly qualified human resources creating a competitive and international labor market for academic scientific workers.
- Stagnating public funding for higher education in most countries around the world, without a respective decline in demand for access to higher education.
- Increased pressure on higher education institutions to diversify funding sources in order to meet demands which in many respects leads to commercialization or commodification of education.
- The advent of new providers and innovations in the delivery of higher education as well as in the overall knowledge production system.

The General Agreement on Trade in Services (GATS), which came into force in 1996, is a multilateral agreement that is based on the promise that progressive liberalization of trade in commercial services will promote economic growth in the World Trade Organization (WTO) member countries. It provides legal rights to trade in all services except those (like defense) provided entirely by the government.

Under GATS, member nations have obligations of two types—general and conditional. General obligations are those that apply automatically to all member countries regardless of existence of commitments. Mode for any sector relates to Most Favored Nation (MFN) treatment, transparency, and establishment of administrative reviews, procedures, and disciplines under conditional obligations. Each country has to identify if it so wishes, sectors, sub-sector, and modes of supply under which it is willing to make commitments (with limitations if it so desired) relating to member access and national treatment.

Education tie-up of collaboration with foreign universities will contribute to increase in quality in the entire education spectrum. Exchange of students/research scholars from one country to another country also influences education environment. These types of exchange program is encouraged and funded by the UGC and many other private institutions and deemed universities. Economic conditions of a country determines infrastructure for colleges and universities and other development oriented activities.

Foreign universities may enter into India to provide their educational services to Indian students. This is the outcome of globalization of education market. Reducing interest rate influences education environment. Students pursuing higher education services come forward to get educational loan from public sector banks to meet their expenditure on education. Public sector banks also encourage educational loan. Loans are also provided to educational institutions for constructing required infrastructure.

Despite the above, the World Bank document puts forward the argument that the developing countries should not invest their scarce resources in higher education. The argument is supported by setting up of primary education against higher education.

WTO and Education

In these changed circumstances, "knowledge products" are freely traded in the international market place. The World Trade Organization (WTO) would help to guarantee that academic institutions or other education providers could set up branches in any country, export degree programs, award degrees and certificates with minimal restriction, invest in overseas educational institution, employ instructors for their foreign ventures, set up educational and training programs through distance technologies without controls, and so on.

Once India makes commitments for trade in higher education under WTO policy regime and allows market access, the commercial presence mode will be further strengthened. Thus, India must realize the impending threats of trade in education and try to convert these into opportunities.

Modes of Trades

- *Cross border supply:* The Indian Universities have, in recent years, commenced offering degree and diploma programs, through the distance education mode, in countries having a large Indian Diaspora. The Indira Gandhi National Open University has formulated a policy in this regard and is offering programs in both liberal arts and professional areas like computer application.
- *Consumption abroad:* For more than a century now, Indian students are going to the Western countries, mainly UK and USA for higher education and research. In contrast, we have only limited number of international students in India, mainly from the developing countries of East Africa and South Asia but number is slowly increasing.
- *Commercial presence:* An encouraging aspect from the Indian viewpoint is that the deemed universities are now permitted to open institutions/campuses abroad. The institutions that have taken the advantage of this liberalization are the Birla Institute of Technology and Science, Pilani and Birla Institute of Technology, Ranchi. The Manipal Education and Medical Group have set up campuses in Nepal and Manipal.
- *Movement of natural persons:* Faculty members from universities and researchers have been moving to developed countries for temporary period, or for permanent employment, or on individual initiatives. The number is, however, not large. Flow in the opposite direction is still lesser.
- *Distance education in India*: The NPE, 1986, recognizes that educational opportunities in India are both inadequate and unequal. It emphasizes that a cost-effective alternative to the present conventional system of higher education can be seen in distance education.

The modular structure and flexible delivery system makes distance education program ideal to meet the desired higher educational needs of a wide class of learners.

Distance education has emerged as a viable and an effective option to a large section of youth having no access to the conventional universities. It also helps in upgrading and updating knowledge of the working people. The distance learning system provides flexibility in terms of combination of courses, age of entry, pace of learning, and methods of evaluation.

Modern Technology

As technology advances, nursing and nursing education remain responsive to the changes that occur. It is imperative that nursing education undergoes modification. In the healthcare setting, computers are used for patient records, business functions and increasingly as a support to effective decision making. Computer and its usage in the field of nursing education are imperative. Computer Assisted Classroom Instruction, Internet, Web-based courses and instruction, online courses, and virtual university are newly emerging technologies in the field of education.

Telemedicine and Tele Nursing

It refers to the provision of healthcare services by health professionals where distance is a critical factor. One can use information and communication technologies for the exchange of valid information of diagnosis, treatment, prevention of disease and injuries and for continuing education of healthcare providers as well as research and evaluation aiming at advancing the health of the individuals and communities. It is one of the recent advancements in the field of medicine and from which emerges tele nursing which can be used by nursing faculty members and students in the field of nursing education.

Research

Research is seen as a requirement to be fulfilled rather than an enquiry conducted to advance the frontiers of science as far as many private institutions are concerned. As the nursing profession continues to grow, one of the areas receiving more emphasis is nursing theory and research. This emphasis will undoubtedly continue. As nursing education keeps pace with the advancement of nursing knowledge, there is a push to envelop curricular patterns that respond to the work of nursing theorists.

We require many researches conducted in all areas of nursing in order to improve specific body of knowledge for nursing. Evidence-based approach is another aspect in which nurses seek evidence from the research findings and apply it in the day-to-day practice for the clinical problems.

Professional Education

Profession and Professional Education

Any man or woman who has prepared for exacting service by thorough and disciplined scholarship and training, and who lives and works in the spirit of professional standard, may well be recognized as a member of a profession. Professional education is the process by which men and women prepare for exacting responsible service in the professional spirit. The term may be restricted to preparation for fields requiring well informed and disciplined insight and skill of a high order. Less exacting preparation may be designated as vocational or technical education.

The Responsibilities of Professional Education

The professional man has the responsibility to contribute toward the welfare of the society in which he lives. He must devote his moral energies and intellectual powers to solve current and long-range problems. The professional education should bring intelligence and patriotism thus helps to promote peace and order in the society. A professional man should have purpose and philosophy for his work and life. If a person lacks in such purpose and philosophy, the total effect may be great internal stress and even social deterioration.

Fundamentals of Professional Education

The foundation of professional education should be not only technical skill, but also a sense of social responsibility, an appreciation of social and human values and relationships, and disciplined power to see realities without prejudice or blind commitment. While professional men largely set the pattern of national life, that pattern is much influenced by their earlier intellectual and moral experiences, especially their professional training. The standards and motives of professional practice in the coming years are largely being made in the professional schools of today. An increased sense of social responsibility in the professions cannot be brought about in the man by trying to re-educate mature professional men. It requires a changing of professional education in method and spirit, so that young men entering the professions shall be living and working in the spirit of the new, democratic India.

One of the primary needs is that the professional man shall see the whole problem with which he deals, not merely its technical phases. All technical education should transmit technical understanding, skill and method, not as an isolated discipline, but in its total human and social setting. Failure to do that is largely responsible for failure of modern civilization to produce social peace and harmony.

The problem of professional teaching is one of content as well as of method. If the professional student has acquired widely selected basic knowledge and the professional way of thinking and working with representative increments of particular knowledge, then he can himself acquire the particular knowledge, he especially needs from time to time. Every practitioner of professional stature knows that human and social problems are inherent, in all major professional questions and must be dealt with if such questions are to be handled on a professional level.

The professional man faces problems in the practice of his profession in everyday life. To find a solution for his professional problems, he must ask himself, what all things which are truly considered as professional, should be done? Only then can a professional man accept moral responsibility for his own professional conduct, and determine for himself what values his technical competence will serve, instead of leaving this to be determined by others. General human motive and purpose need to be so much a part of professional training that to the student they will be one and inseparable.

Professional development plays an essential role in successful education reform. Professional development serves as the bridge between where prospective and experienced educators are now and where they will need to meet the new challenges of guiding all students in achieving to higher standards of learning and development.

High-quality professional development as envisioned here refers to rigorous and relevant content, strategies, and organizational supports that ensure the preparation and long career development of teachers and others whose competence, expectations and actions influence the teaching and learning environment. Both pre- and in-service professional development require partnerships among schools, higher education institutions, and other appropriate entities to promote inclusive learning communities of everyone who impacts students and their learning. Those within and outside schools need to work together to bring to bear the ideas, commitment and other resources that will be necessary to address important and complex educational issues in a variety of settings and for a diverse student body.

Equitable access for all educators to such professional development opportunities is imperative. Moreover, professional development works best when it is part of a system wide effort to improve and integrate the recruitment, selection, preparation, initial licensing, induction, ongoing development and support, and advanced certification of educators.

High-quality professional development should incorporate all of the principles stated below. Adequately addressing each of these principles is necessary for a full realization of the potential of individuals, school communities, and institutions to improve and excel.

The mission of professional development is to prepare and support educators to help all students to achieve high standards of learning and development.

Professional Development

- Focuses on teachers as central to student learning, yet includes all other members of the school community;
- Focuses on individual, collegial, and organizational improvement;
- Respects and nurtures the intellectual and leadership capacity of teachers, principals, and others in the school community;
- Reflects best available research and practice in teaching, learning, and leadership;
- Enables teachers to develop further expertise in subject content, teaching strategies, uses of technologies, and other essential elements in teaching to high standards;
- Promotes continuous inquiry and improvement embedded in the daily life of schools;
- Is planned collaboratively by those who will participate in and facilitate that development;
- Requires substantial time and other resources;
- Is driven by a coherent long-term plan;
- Is evaluated ultimately on the basis of its impact on teacher effectiveness and student learning; and this assessment guides subsequent professional development efforts.

Trends in Development of Nursing Education in India

Before independence, the progress of nursing and nursing education was not good. The factors like caste system among Hindus, poor and low status of women, the notion that nursing is done by low people and it is servant's work failed to attract public toward nursing.

In 1664, the East India Company helped to start a hospital for soldiers at Fort ST George, Madras (now the Tamil Nadu Secretariat is functioning). Later a civilian hospital was built and the medical staff appointed by the East India Company, served in these hospitals. In 1797 a lying in hospital was built and in 1854 a training school for midwives was started. In 1871 in the Government General Hospital, Madras, a training course for nurses was started. Simultaneously, in Mumbai, there were some development in the field of nursing education. The Jamshedjee Jeejeebhoy Group has opened the earliest hospital in Mumbai in the year 1843. In 1886, another hospital called Pestanji Hormusji Cama Hospital for women and children opened. During this period, people did not come forward to do nursing. There were only few Anglo-Indian and Christian girls from India did nursing. The sisters of all saints from England who were called by then ruling British Government in India started training for nurses in these hospitals in India. The training was initially for 2 years and later it was changed to 3 years. Ms TK Adranvala was one of the outstanding students of this JJ Group of hospitals and she served as a ward sister to nursing superintendent of the hospitals. Later she worked as a nursing advisor to the Government of India.

Until the late 19th century, there were insufficient care provided for the women and children since there were no women doctors. Upon hearing this, Queen Victoria instructed Lady Dufferin who was coming to India with her husband who was on British Government Service to look into this issue. Lady Dufferin collected funds for providing medical aid which was later known as Dufferin fund. In 1885, Lady Dufferin was responsible for starting the "National Association for Supplying Medical Aid by Women to Women of India" which not only provided medical services for women and children but also started training doctors, nurses and midwives to render care for women and children.

Between 1890 and 1900 many schools were started either by the government or missionaries under the head of English or American people. There was no uniformity in training and the courses were offered according to the belief of the heads of the institution.

In 1909, the Bombay Presidency Nursing Association was started. During 1907–1910 the North India United Board of Examiners for Mission Hospitals was organized and set up rules for admissions and standards of training. In 1909, the Indian Medical Mission Association granted the nursing diploma after examining student by Central Board for Nurses' training schools in South India. After few years, the Mid India and the South India Boards of Nurse examiners were similarly set up. Later the name of the South India Board was changed to the Board of Nursing Education, Nurses' League of Christian Medical Association of India.

The first degree program in nursing was started in the year 1946 in Tamil Nadu, India in the Christian Medical College Hospital, Vellore. Then the Rajkumari Amrit Kaur College of Nursing, New Delhi was established in 1946 by the Union Ministry of Health and Family Welfare, Government of India, with the objective of developing and demonstrating model programs in Nursing Education. In 1959, the two years Master of Nursing programme was started and M Phil, in Nursing was started in 1986 as a foundation course for undertaking doctoral work and in the year 1992, Doctoral programme in nursing was started under Department of Nursing, University of Delhi. In the meanwhile, private sectors have been permitted to start Colleges of Nursing and Schools of Nursing by the respective State Government.

There are five levels of nursing education in India today.
1. Auxiliary Nurse and Midwife
2. General Nursing and Midwifery (GNM)
3. BSc Nursing and PBBSc(N)
4. MSc Nursing
5. MPhil and PhD.

The ANM and GNM are conducted in schools of nursing. The last three are university level courses and the respective universities conduct examinations. Besides there are several certificate and diploma courses in specialties.

National Policy on Education

The National Policy on Education (NPE) is a policy formulated by the Government of India to promote education amongst India's people. The policy covers elementary education to colleges in both rural and urban India. The first NPE was promulgated in 1968 by the former Prime Minister Indira Gandhi, and the second by Prime Minister Rajiv Gandhi in 1986.

Based on the report and recommendations of the Education Commission (1964–1966), the former Prime Minister Indira Gandhi announced the first NPE in 1968, which called for a "radical restructuring" and equalize educational opportunities in order to achieve national integration and greater cultural and economic development. The policy called for fulfilling compulsory education for all children up to the age of 14 years, as stipulated by the Constitution of India, and the better training and qualification of teachers.

Three Language Formula

This policy emphasizes on learning of three language formula that is the instruction of the English language, the official language of the state where the school was based, and Hindi, the national language.

Although the decision to adopt Hindi as the national language had proven controversial, the policy called for use and learning of Hindi to be encouraged uniformly to promote a common language for all Indians. The policy also encouraged the teaching of the ancient Sanskrit language, which was considered an essential part of India's culture and heritage. The NPE of 1968 called for education spending to increase to 6% of the national income.

New Education Policy, 1986

Every country develops its system of education to express and promote its unique sociocultural identity and also to meet the challenges of the times. The Government of India announced in January 1985 that a new Education Policy would be formulated for the country; the former Prime Minister Rajiv Gandhi introduced a new NPE in May, 1986. The new policy called for "special emphasis on the removal of disparities and to equalize educational opportunity", especially for Indian women, Scheduled Tribes (ST) and the Scheduled Caste (SC) communities. To achieve these, the policy called for expanding scholarships, adult education, recruiting more teachers from the SCs, incentives for poor families to send their children to school regularly, development of new institutions and providing housing and services. The NPE called for a "Child-centered approach" in primary education, and launched "Operation Blackboard" to improve primary schools nationwide. The policy expanded the Open University system with the Indira Gandhi National Open University, which had been created in 1985. The policy also called for the creation of the "rural university" model, based on the philosophy of Indian leader Mahatma Gandhi, to promote economic and social development at the grassroot level in rural India.

Modified National Education Policy

The 1986 National Policy on Education was modified in 1992 by the government by Mr PV Narasimha Rao. In 2005, Prime Minister Manmohan Singh adopted a new policy based on the "Common Minimum Program" of his United Progressive Alliance (UPA) government.

The 1968 Education Policy and After

The National Policy of 1968 marked a significant step in the history of education in post-independence India. It aimed to promote national progress, a sense of common citizenship and culture, and to strengthen national integration. It laid stress on the need for a radical reconstruction of the education system, to improve its quality at all stages, and gave much greater attention to science and technology, the cultivation of moral values and a closer relation between education and the life of the people.

Since the adoption of the 1968 policy, there has been considerable expansion in educational facilities all over the country at all levels.

A beginning was also made in restructuring of courses at the undergraduate level. Centers of Advanced Studies were set-up for postgraduate education and research.

National Policy on Education 1986 and Program of Action 1992

The National Policy of Education of 1986 is the result of the reviews which was discussed and adopted during the budget session of 1985 when Rajiv Gandhi was the prime minister of India. Again, a committee was set up under the chairmanship of Acharya Rammurti in May 1990 to review NPE and to make recommendations for its modifications. The Central Advisory Board of Education, a committee set up in July 1991 under the chairmanship of Shri N Janardhana Reddy, Chief Minister of Andhra Pradesh, considered some modifications in NPE taking into considerations the report of the Ramamurti Committee and other relevant development having a bearing on the policy. This Committee submitted its report in January 1992, which is known as National Program of Action of 1992. This policy aimed to promote national progress, a sense of common citizenship and culture, and to strengthen national integration. It laid stress on the need for a radical reconstruction of the education system, to improve its quality at all stages, and therefore gave much greater attention to science and technology, the cultivation of moral values and a closer relation between education and the life of the people. The salient features of 1986 and 1992 policies are as follows:

> In our national perception, education is essentially for all. This is fundamental to our all-round development, material and spiritual.
>
> Education has an acculturating role. It refines sensitivities and perceptions that contribute to national cohesion, a scientific temper and independence of mind and spirit, thus furthering the goals of socialism, secularism and democracy enshrined in our constitution.
>
> Education develops manpower for different levels of the economy. It is also the substrate on which research and development flourish, being the ultimate guarantee of national self-reliance.

Common Educational Structure

It envisages a common educational structure, i.e. 10 + 2 + 3 which was recommended by Kothari Commission (1964–66). This structure has now been accepted in all parts of the country. Regarding the further break-up of first 10 years efforts will be made to move toward an elementary system comprising 5 years of primary education and 3 years of upper primary followed by 2 years of High School.

The policy has emphasized on the minimum levels of learning and lifelong learning. The NPE-86 recommended for the strengthening of the institutions like University Grants Commission (UGC), the All India Council of Technical Education (AICTE), the Indian Council of Agricultural Research (ICAR), and the Indian Medical Council (IMC). Integrated planning will be instituted among all these bodies so as to establish functional linkages and reinforce programs of research and postgraduate education. These, together with the National Council of Educational Research and Training (NCERT), the National Institute of Educational Planning and Administration (NIEPA), and the International Institute of Science and Technology Education (IISTE) will be involved in implementing the education policy.

It laid stress on the education for equality including women equality, Education of Scheduled Castes and Scheduled Tribes, other backward sections, minority people and other challenged people. It stressed on Early Childhood Care and Education (ECCE), ICDS program, and elementary education. The new thrust in elementary education emphasized two aspects. Universal enrollment and universal retention of children up to 14 years of age and a substantial improvement in the quality of education. It recommended for the exclusion of corporal punishment from the educational system and adjustment of school timings as well as vacations to the convenience of the children. The features of nonformal education, secondary education, higher education, the concept of Open University and distance learning, rural university, science education, value education, sports and physical education, teacher education were also included.

National Education Policy, 2016

The National Education Policy (NEP), 2016, provides a framework for the development of education in India over the coming few years. It seeks to address both the agenda relating to the goals and targets set in the previous national policies on education and the current and emerging national development and education sector-related challenges.

The National Education Policy, 2016, envisions a credible and high-performing education system capable of ensuring inclusive quality education and lifelong learning opportunities for all and producing students/graduates equipped with the knowledge, skills, attitudes, and values that are required to lead a productive life, participate in the country's development process, respond to the requirements of the fast-changing, ever-globalizing, knowledge-based economy, and society. This vision recognizes the central role of education in India's social, economic, political, and cultural development. The vision also implies that good quality education will help amalgamate globalization with localization, enabling India's children and youth to become global citizens, with their roots deeply embedded in Indian culture and traditions.

The policy framework covers recommendations and policy initiatives with respect to Pre-school Education, Protection of Rights of the Child and Adolescent Education, Learning Outcomes in School Education, Curriculum Renewal and Examination Reforms, Inclusive Education and Student Support, Literacy and Lifelong Learning, Skills in Education and Employability, Use of ICT in Education, Teacher Development and Management, Language and Culture in Education, Self-development through Comprehensive Education, School Assessment and Governance, Governance Reforms in Higher Education, Regulation in Higher Education, Quality Assurance in Higher Education, Open and Distance Learning and MOOCs (Massive Open Online Courses), Internationalization of Education, Faculty Development in Higher Education, Research, Innovation and New Knowledge and Financing Education.

The National Education Policy, 2016, has charted out many new directions and it is imperative to note that the Center and the States have to work together in a spirit of cooperative federalism to translate the intended goals and actionable strategies into realities that can result in the transformation of the education landscape.

Some of the policy initiatives planned are as follows:
- Implementation of program for preschool education for children in the age group of 4–5 years in coordination with the Ministry of Women and Child Development
- Developing a framework and guidelines for ensuring school safety and security of children and will be made a part of the eligibility conditions for a school education institution for recognition and registration
- Development of norms for learning outcomes and uniform application to both private and government schools in elementary education
- Laying down of minimum standards for provision of facilities and student outcomes across all levels in school education
- Expansion of open schooling facilities to enable dropouts and working children to pursue education without attending full time formal schools.

Curriculum Renewal and Examination Reforms

- It is stated in the draft policy, 2016, that National Council of Educational Research and Training (NCERT) will undergo a re-orientation to address issues of deteriorating quality of school education and periodic renewal of curricula and pedagogy to move from rote learning to facilitate understanding and encourage a spirit of enquiry. For science, mathematics and english subjects, a common national curriculum will be designed. For other subjects, such as social sciences, a part of the curricula will be common across the country and the rest will be at the discretion of the states. For teaching of science subjects, practical components will be introduced gradually from class VI onwards.
- Curriculum and textbook development agencies should ensure that the textbooks should promote harmony and do not contain any discriminating issues/events/examples in the context of gender, disability, caste, religion, etc. Citizenship education, peace education, character building, legal and constitutional literacy, financial literacy, environmental sustainability and other common core should be promoted through all the subject areas.
- Adoption of a zero tolerance approach on gender discrimination and violence. The State will endeavor to enhance induction, retention, and substantive presence of women in the higher education sector through various kinds of affirmative action. For this, greater efforts will be made to ensure the placement and recruitment of women in the higher echelons of university administration.
- To promote skill development in children, a detailed plan for the creation of skill schools for improving employment opportunities for secondary school students in special focus districts will be prepared. Joint certificates by the Sector Skill Council and the School/College authorities will be issued to help students take up wage-employment or start their own enterprise.
- *Use of ICT in education:* Online maintenance of all records of a child from the time of admission till the time of leaving the school will be made mandatory. IT-based applications will be used for monitoring teacher and student attendance, performance evaluation of teachers and school administrators, performance of

students and also for administrative functions like maintenance of records and accounts.
- To promote learning in mother tongue, all states and UTs, if they so desire, may provide education in schools, up to class V, in mother tongue, local or regional language as the medium of instruction.
- *School assessment and governance:* Principals/head teachers will be held accountable for the academic performance of the schools and its improvement. The education department will fix the minimum tenure of principals/head teachers.
- *Governance reforms in higher education:* An Education Commission comprising of academic experts will be set up, every 5 years to assist the Ministry of Human Resource Development (HRD) in identifying new knowledge areas/disciplines/domains as well as pedagogic, curricular and assessment reforms at the global level, which will help to keep up with the change in global scenario and national aspirations. Efforts will be made to move toward a university system integrating UG, PG and doctoral studies, with faculty concurrently teaching both at UG and PG levels which will help improve synergies between teaching and research. Universities will be multi-disciplinary in nature and not single discipline specific.
- *Regulation in higher education:* State Councils of Higher Education will be mandated to monitor periodically the academic standards of universities and colleges in consultation with approved accrediting agencies. Every higher education institution will have a dedicated website for more transparency disclosing standard information of admissions, fees, faculty, programs, examination results, placements, governance, finance, business tie-ups, management, and a report on academic and co-scholastic activities, as well as other relevant information relating to the institution.
- *Quality assurance in higher education:* It is stated that several problems including inadequate infrastructure and facilities, large vacancies of faculty positions, poor quality of faculty, outdated teaching methods, declining research standards, etc. are faced by the universities and colleges. In addition, there is widespread geographical, gender and social imbalances within the sector. These problems are also a reflection of the poor quality of higher education. As a part of quality assurance, it is now mandatory for institutions to get accredited by NAAC or NBA. It is a matter of concern that very few higher education institutions find a place in the global ranking of universities. The global ranking of universities is based on an assessment of the institutional performance in the areas of research and teaching, reputation of faculty members, reputation among employers, resource availability, share of international students and activities, etc. Recently, MHRD has launched the National Institute Ranking Framework (NIRF) for ranking of our higher education institutions covering engineering, management, pharmacy, and architecture, universities and colleges. The following policy initiatives will be taken:
- An expert committee will be constituted to study the systems of accreditation in place internationally. It will draw from the experiences of some of the best practices followed by countries having well performing systems and will suggest restructuring of NAAC and NBA as well as redefining methodologies, parameters, and criteria.
- Evaluation/Accreditation details of each institution will be available to the general public through a dedicated website, to enable students and other stakeholders to make informed choices.
- The government will take steps for reaching the long pending goal of raising the investment in education sector to at least 6% of GDP as a priority.

Educational Commissions

In India various educational commissions were appointed from time to time to look into the matters of education. Though the major objective of each committee was to improve the education and the system, each one was appointed with the specific purpose.

Educational Commissions

Name of the Committees/Commissions	Recommendations

1. Overseas Scholarship Committee, 1947
Chairman: DR BC Roy
	To consider whether the award of Government Scholarship is serving the purpose for which it was established and the number of scholars to be sent abroad in 1948 and in subsequent years should be increased or reduced and whether the range of subjects should be enlarged. If so, to what extent;
	    To consider what modifications, if any, may be desirable in the existing arrangements for inviting applications selecting candidates, placing them in training institutions abroad, and generally supervising their welfare while overseas;
	    To consider what arrangement should be made in this country to ensure that scholars who have successfully completed their courses abroad are absorbed without delay into suitable employment on their return;
	    To consider what steps should be taken to coordinate the Overseas Scholarship Scheme with any existing arrangements by other Government Departments or by any University for sending persons abroad for advanced training.

Contd...

Contd...

2.	Committee on Secondary Education in India, 1948 Chairman: Dr Tara chand	To examine the aims and objectives of secondary education as defined in the report of the Central Advisory Board of Education on (CABE) Post-War Education; • To determine the period of and gradations in secondary education; • To consider the place of the national language and english in secondary education; • To consider the procedure to be adopted for selecting pupils for secondary education; • To consider the relation of secondary education to basic education and university education; • To consider the nature of the examination to be held at the end of the secondary stage and how it could be utilized for administration to universities; • To consider the steps to be taken for training an adequate number of teachers with the qualifications necessary and the conditions of their service; • To consider the financial implications of the proposed system of secondary education. **Summary of recommendations** • Admission to the degree course should be preceded by a course of primary and secondary education for at least 12 years. • Of the above 12 years, 5 years should be spent at the junior basic stage, 3 years at the senior basic or presecondary and 4 years at the secondary stage. • The Federal language should become a compulsory subject at the secondary stage when English ceases to be the medium of instruction in the universities. • There should be one public examination at the end of the secondary stage; the universities may, for admission purposes, lay down such conditions as they deem fit. • The pay and conditions of service of teachers should be the same as recommended by the CABE. Trained graduates can take charge of the teaching in the first 2 years of the secondary stage. • Education should be one of the subjects in the university course of studies. • Provincial boards should be set up to advice provincial educational authorities on problems connected with secondary education. There should be All India Council at the center to act as a coordinate body for the proposed provincial boards. • Youth Movements, Scout Movements, etc. should be encouraged in all schools. • A number of public schools may be established to foster the growth of leadership among pupils. Admission to such schools should be governed by merit alone. There should also be provision for scholarships and free places up to 50% of available seats in such schools.
2.	Committee on the Ways and Means of Financing Education Development in India, 1948 Chairman: Shri BG Kher	To consider in the light of present conditions, the finance (recurring and nonrecurring) required for the different stages of a comprehensive system of education in India; To consider the ways and means of raising the necessary finances. **Summary of recommendations** • The state must undertake the responsibility of providing at least junior basic education for everybody without, however, detriment to existing facilities for secondary and higher education. Special attention should be given to the provision of such higher studies as it will be necessary for increasing the industrial and agricultural potential of the country. • The provinces should aim at introducing universal compulsory education for the children of 6–11 age-group within a period of 10 years but if financial conditions compel, the program may be extended over a larger period but in no circumstances should it be given up. • In view of the present emergency, the committee, with great reluctance, agrees that only for 5 years, the teacher-pupil ratio may be 1:40 instead of 1:30, though from the educational point of view, this change would be most undesirable. The ratio of 1:30 should be restored earlier, if possible, but in any case the position must be reviewed at the end of 5 years. • In urban areas, where conditions justify, the same school buildings should be used for two shifts provided different teachers are employed in each shift. • Voluntary efforts should be encouraged for meeting the capital and recurring cost of education and voluntary organizations should be induced to run educational institutions with such assistance from the government as may be feasible. • Wherever conditions permit, loans should be raised for meeting the capital cost or such part thereof as may be necessary. • About 70% of the expenditure on education should be borne by the local bodies and provinces, and the remaining 30% by the center. • All contributions for education approved by the provincial or central government should be exempted from income tax.

Contd...

Contd...

3. Indian University Education Commission, 1948 Chairman: Dr S Radhakrishnan	To consider and make recommendations in regard to: • The aims and objectives of university education and research in India; • The changes considered necessary and desirable in the constitution, control, functions and jurisdiction of universities in India and their relations with governments, central and provincial; the finance of universities; • The maintenance of the highest standards of teaching and examination in the universities and colleges under their control; • The course of study in the universities with special reference to the maintenance of a sound balance between the Humanities and Sciences and between Pure Science and Technological Training and the duration of such courses; • The standards of admission to university and the avoidance of unfair discriminations which militate against Fundamental Rights. The medium of instruction in the universities; • The provisions for advanced study in Indian Culture, History, Literature, Languages, Philosophy and Fine Arts; • The need for more universities on a regional or other basis; • Religious instruction in the universities; • The qualifications, conditions of service, salaries, privileges and functions of teachers and the encouragement of original research by teachers; • The discipline of students, hostels and the organization of tutorial work and any other matter which is germane and essential to a complete and comprehensive enquiry into all aspects of university education and advanced research in India. **Summary of recommendations** • The ordinary amenities and decencies of life should be provided for women in colleges and there should be no curtailment in educational opportunities for women, but rather a great increase. • There should be intelligent educational guidance, by qualified men and women, to help women, to get a clearer view of their real educational interest, to the end that they shall not try to imitate men, but shall desire as good an education as men get. Women's and men's education should have many elements in common, but should not in general be identical in all respects, as is usually the case today. • That women students in general should be helped to see their normal places in a normal society, both as citizens and as women and to prepare for it, and college programs should be so designed that it will be possible for them to do so. • That where new colleges are established to serve both men and women students, they should be truly coeducational institutions, with as much thought and consideration given to the life needs of women as to those of men. That women teacher should be paid the same salaries as men teachers for equal work. • Separate schools between the age of 13 and 18 years. The University Education Commission was of the view that there seems to be a definite preponderance of opinion that from the 13th or 14th year of age until about the 18th, separate schools for boys and girls are desirable. **Coeducation at the college level** As the age of entry to degree colleges would, on the recommendation, be approximately 18, college education may be coeducational. Separate institutions at this level would demand an unjustified increase in expense. To maintain separate institutions for men and women side by side, duplicating equipment, even when it is very inadequate, would be an undue tax upon limited financial resources. The University Education Commission recommended: • The importance of a teacher and his responsibility be recognized. • There should be four classes of Teachers-Professors, Readers, Lecturers and Instructors. • The promotions from one category to another should be solely on grounds of merit. • Each university should have some research fellows. • Care must be taken for the selection of proper teachers. • That the age of retirement be ordinarily 60 years but extension can be allowed up to 64 in the case of a professor. • That conditions regarding provident fund, leave and hours of work be definitely laid down. **Finance** The commission recommended: • The state should recognize its responsibility for the financing of higher education. • The steps should be taken to amend income-tax laws to encourage donations for educational purposes. • That additional grants be made to colleges and universities in order to enable them to give effect to the recommendations. • That the University Grants Commission be setup for allocating grants.

Contd...

Contd...

4.	Kothari Commission (1964–66) Chairman: PS Kothari	Kothari Commission was appointed by the Government of India in 1964. The commission began its work on 2nd October, 1964.
		
		Need for appointment of commission:
		• Need for a comprehensive policy of education in spite number of education committees after independence, satisfactory progress would not be achieved.
		• Need for detailed study even though a good deal of expansion of education facilities took place; it was at the expanse of quality.
		• Need to emphasize role of people in national development. To make people aware that they have a share in the national development along with the government.
		• Need for overview of educational development. To create more integration between various parts and consider it as a whole not as fragments.
		• Need for positive approach to the status of teacher. The teacher community had been neglected suffering many hardships requiring a positive approach to the problem.
		
		Facts of educational resolution
		• Internal transformation to relate to the life needs and the aspirations of the people.
		• Qualitative improvement so that the standards achieved are adequate, kept continually raising and become internationally comparable.
		• Expansion of educational facilities broadly or the basis of manpower needs with an accent on equalization of educational opportunities.
		
		Goals of education
		• Education for increasing productivity:
		  – Make science a basic component of education and culture
		  – Vocationalization of education to meet the needs of the industry of agriculture
		  – Improving scientific and technological research and education at university level.
		• Education for an accelerating process of modernization:
		  – Adopting new methods of teaching
		  – Proper development of instructional attitudes and values and building essential skills
		  – Educating people of all strata of society
		  – Emphasizing teaching of vocational subjects and science
		  – Establishing universities of excellence in the country.
		• Educating for promoting social and national integration:
		  – Introducing common school system of public education
		  – Developing all modern Indian language
		  – Taking steps to enrich Hindi as quickly as possible
		  – Encouraging and enabling students to participate in community living.
		• Education for inculcation of national values:
		  – Introducing moral, social and spiritual values
		  – Providing syllabus giving information about religions of the world
		  – Encouraging students to meet in groups for silent meditation
		  – Presenting before students high ideas of social justice and social service.

5.	CABE Committee on Gnanam Committee. Dr Sudhir Ray	The Minister of Human Resource Development, in his capacity as Chairman of the Central Advisory Board of Education (CABE), has nominated Dr Sudhir Ray, Member of Parliament (Lok Sabha) and Member, CABE, as a member of the CABE Committee on Gnanam Committee constituted vide this Ministry's Order of even number dated on 9th December, 1991. **General** Universities are the centers of excellence as also of regional/national development. The objective of the universities and their modes of funding should be reviewed and redefined accordingly. The students-teachers, administrators, and the society's representatives must be involved in setting the new goals and objectives of the universities. In deciding the management pattern of universities it should be recognized that the academic administration is very different from that in vogue in the governmental or in the corporate system and it should be based on the principle of participation, decentralization, autonomy, and accountability. The managerial patterns of a university system must necessarily have an in-built flexibility to adapt itself quickly to the changing needs of the country and the region it serves and to carry out innovations and experiments. Any effort, therefore, to bring the structures of all universities within the framework of a single pattern of University Act will prove to be an impediment in this process.

Contd...

Contd...

Legislations, therefore, should, while laying down the broad pattern of university management, leave the details to be framed by each university through statutes and ordinances.

University autonomy should be considered as an essential prerequisite for ensuring academic excellence and development. The Acts of the universities should be so designed as to strengthen the autonomous character and particularly in academic and administrative matters and prevent external interference.

Universities should have accountability in financial matters since they are not raising their own resources.

Elections to various university bodies should be kept at a bare minimum and the selection of principal should be based on seniority and nomination-based on seniority.

Representation of teachers on various university authorities/bodies should normally be on rotation or on the basis of criteria lay down by the university concerned.

The nomination of student representatives to university representatives on the senate should be based on their excellence in academic excellence for curricular, cocurricular and hostel/sports and other coextracurricular activities.

More women should be inducted in the planning and management bodies of the departments/faculties/university.

More women should be involved in the planning and management bodies of the departments/faculties/university by having substantial representation.

Ministers or Members of Legislatures or office bearers of political parties should not hold any office in the university system.

Members of the staff (teaching as well as nonteaching) of the university or office bearers in holding a college should not be permitted to contest election system.

The political parties should work out for themselves and adhere to a Code of Conduct ensuring that the student community is left completely free to engage.

6. **High Power Committee 1990**
   Chairperson: Mrs Sarojini Vardappan

This committee after being set-up by the central government did an extensive survey into the nursing profession and the nursing conditions and submitted a report to the central government, which was released at the end of March 1990. The summary of the report is as follows:

Strength of the nursing staff to be increased in all fields of work before a nursing service of even modest standards can be reached.

Expansion of nursing education programs has not been as per requirement from time to time with the result that at that time of appointment of commission only one nurse was available for 100 patients at night in many hospitals.

Practice of using student labor continued. Nursing education at the 20th century remains only curative and hospital-based in spite of the country's commitment to the goal of "Health For All by 2000 AD".

Steps by the INC to reorient nursing have not been implemented mainly because of shortage of nurses in the hospitals where the training of GNM and ANM is conducted.

Schools have no budget for nursing education, shortage of teachers, lack of library facilities and absence of modern methods of teaching add up to the misery of education of nurses.

Overcrowded and poorly furnished hostels and classrooms, delays in admission and examinations, low salary and poor status, long working hours, poor salary, inadequate work place, improper accommodations, lack of supplies and equipments, forced performance of non-nursing duties hampered or poor progress of quality nursing education and nursing services are due to the concepts of role of nurses as a medical technician or someone to carry out orders. Independent practice by nursing personnel is not being recognized. Retarded development of nursing is due to the fact that no serious thought has been given to this discipline by the government for years. Nurses or nursing personnel are excluded generally from governmental bodies.

Most decision concerning nursing care and nurses are made by other people usually physicians, without the benefit of professional input by the nurses.

Recommendations
1. Working conditions of nursing personnel.
   - Employment
     - Uniformity in employment procedure to be made
     - Similar recruitment rules for all categories of nursing personnel
   - Job description
     - For all categories to be prepared by the central government to provide guidelines.
   - Working hours
     - Should be reduced to 40 hrs per week
     - Extra working hours to be compensated either by leave or extra pay

Contd...

Contd...

- To be given all the weekly day offs and government holidays
- In no case the weekly day off be reduced.
- Work load/Working facilities
    - Nursing norms for patient care and community care to be adopted as recommended by the committee
    - Polices for breakage, loss to be developed and nurses not to be made responsible for breakage and losses.
- Pay and Allowances
    - Uniformity of pay scales for all categories of nurses is not possible but special allowances for nursing personnel throughout the country should be for uniform.
- Promotional opportunities
    - For promotion to the post of ward sister post Basic-BSc nursing to be made compulsory
    - Each nurse must have three promotions during her work period. Promotions are based on merit cum seniority.
    - Promotion to senior most administrative or teaching post to be made only by open selection.
- Career development
    - Provision of deputation for higher studies after 5 years of regular service is made by all states
    - Every nursing personnel must have on opportunity to attend at least one refresher course every 2 years.
- Accommodation
    - As far as possible nursing staff should be considered for priority allotment of accommodation near work place.
- Transport
    - During odd hours, calamities, etc. arrangement for transport must be made for safety and security of nursing personnel.
- Special incentives
    - Scheme of special incentives in terms of awards, increment (special) for meritorious work for nurse working in each state/district/city, etc. to be worked out.
- Occupational hazards
    - Medical facilities as provided by the central government be extended by state governments to nursing personnel. Till such time as medical services are provided free to all the nursing personnel
    - Risk allowance to be paid to nursing personnel working in rural and urban areas.
- Other welfare measures
    - Hospitals should provide other welfare measures like crèche facilities for children of working staff
    - Children's educational allowance as granted to other employees be paid to nursing personnel.

Additional facilities for nurses working in rural areas.
- Family accommodation at subcenter is a must for safety and security of ANM's/LHV's
- Woman attendant, selected from the village must accompany the ANM for visits to other villages.
    - The District Public Health Nurse be provided with a vehicle for field supervision.
    - Fixed travel allowance with provision of enhancement from time to time.
    - Rural allowance as granted to other employees be paid to nursing personnel.

Nursing education:
- Nursing education to be filled into national stream of education to bring about uniformity, recognition and standards of nursing education. The committee recommends that:
    - There should be two levels of nursing personnel viz, professional nurse, auxiliary nurse/vocational nurse.
    - Admission to professional nursing should be with 12 years schooling with science.
    - Admission to vocational/auxiliary nursing should be with 10 years of schooling.
    - Duration of course should be 2 years in health related vocational stream.
- All schools attached to medical college hospitals be upgraded to degree level in a phased manner.
- All ANM schools and schools of nursing attached to district hospitals be affiliated with Senior Secondary Board.
- Post certificate BSc-nursing degree to be continued to give opportunity to the existing diploma nurses to obtain higher education.

Contd...

Contd...

- Masters in nursing program to be increased and strengthened over the period of time.
- Doctoral program in nursing to be started in selected universities.
- Central assistance to be provided for all levels of nursing education in terms of budget.
- Nursing personnel should have complete say in matters of selection of students.
- All schools to have adequate budget for libraries and teaching equipment.
- All schools to have independent teaching block called as School of Nursing with adequate classroom facilities.
- Adequate living accommodations to be provided to students.
- Students should learn under supervision in wards.
- Community nursing experience should be as per requirements of the INC.
- Indian Nursing Council requirements for staffing the schools and meeting the minimum requirements should be followed by all the schools as these are statutory requirements.
- Specialty courses at postgraduation level to be developed at certain special centers of excellence.
- Institutes like National Institute of Health and Family Welfare, RAK College of Nursing and several others may develop courses on Nursing Administration for several senior nurses leading to doctorate level.
- Provision of higher training abroad and exchange program be made.

Source: Indian Nursing Year Book;1988–89.pp.3-7.

Each committee recommendation was taken into consideration by the Government from time to time for the betterment of education. Budgetary allocations and special programs were devised to implement the recommendations given by these committees. Educational infrastructure and the scheme of study and examinations were strengthened.

Summary

- Education means creation of sound mind in a sound body. It is imparted by means of different agencies of education. Many scholars namely Soccrates, Froebel, dewey, Redden and Ryan have explained the meaning of education. A number of factors determine the educational aims for e.g. philosophy of life, elements of human nature, religion, political ideologies, socioeconomic factors, emerging problems of the nation, cultural factors and exploration of knowledge and technology.
- Philosophy on the other hand, is a persistent attempt to give insight into the nature of the world and of ourselves by means of systematic reflection. It has three main divisions namely Metaphysics, Epistemology, and Axiology and has varied implications on education.
- The major systems of philosophy of education are Idealism, Pragmatism, Naturalism and Realism.
- The Indian schools of philosophy are the Vedanta philosophy, Jaina philosophy, and Buddha philosophy.
- Professional education is the process by which men and women prepare for exacting, responsible service in the professional spirit. Nursing as a profession evolves from five levels of nursing education in India today. They are:
  1. Auxiliary Nurse and Midwife,
  2. General Nursing and Midwifery (GNM),
  3. BSc Nursing and PBBSc(N),
  4. MSc Nursing,
  5. MPhil and PhD.

Government initiatives in the form of policies and committees, plays an important role in promoting and propagating education to one and all.

2. Teaching-Learning Process

"Tell me and I forget. Show me and I remember. Involve me and I understand".
—*Chinese Proverb*

Objectives
After reading this unit, you will be able to:
- Explain the educational process
- Understand the concepts of learning
- Explain the concepts of teaching
- Explain the educational objectives
- Understand and prepare the lesson plan, unit plan and course plan
- Describe the techniques of classroom management
- Explain the various methods of teaching.

Introduction

Teaching-learning process is a means whereby society trains its young ones in a selected environment as quickly as possible to adjust themselves to the world in which they live. Education is modification of behavior. Teaching-learning process enhances education. Teaching is one of the instruments of education and its special function is to impart understanding and skill. Teaching is a relationship which is established between three focal points in education—the teacher, the child and the subject. Teaching is the process by which the teacher brings the child and the subject together. The teacher and the taught are active, the former in teaching and the latter in learning.

Educational Process

Education is a process, the chief goal of which is to bring about desirable changes in the behavior of the learner in the form of acquisition of knowledge, proficiency in skills, and development of attitudes. The three main components of the educational process are development of educational objectives, organization of the teaching-learning activities, and evaluation. This is called the educational spiral (Fig. 2.1).

The two-way arrows indicate that there is a mutual feedback and influence of one component on the other; for instance, if it is not possible to give an adequate T-L experience for a particular objective, then that objective needs rethinking.

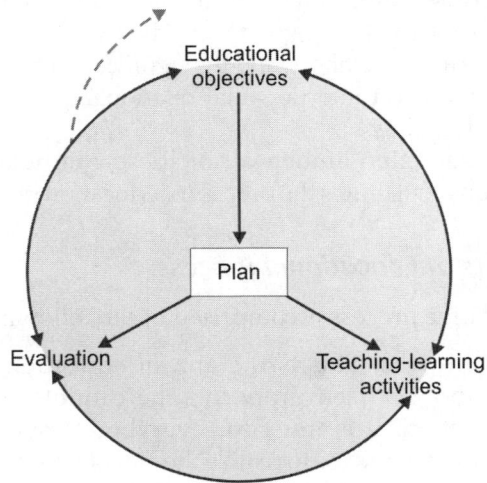

Fig. 2.1: Educational spiral.

The relationship between the three components is best depicted as a spiral and not a closed circle to show that there is a constant scope for improvement and revising of old objectives and development of new objectives depending on the requirements of the process and the feedback obtained from earlier cycles.

Dimensions of Educational Process

The four dimensions identified in the educative process are:
1. Substantive dimension
2. Procedural dimension
3. Environmental dimension
4. Human relations dimension.

Substantive dimension: It pertains to what is taught and what is learned. This is the knowledge, attitude, and skill learned from education. This is what is known as curriculum. It is the content of the teaching and learning activities planned for a specific group of students in order to achieve an objective.

Procedural dimension: It refers to the way in which the teacher helps the students to learn. It deals with the techniques and methods, the teacher uses to impart knowledge and enhance learning. It includes the learner(s), teacher, and methods and procedures of teaching and learning.

Environmental dimension: It refers to an environment where the teaching and learning occur. It includes the classroom, laboratory, hospital, etc. and also includes the climate prevailing in that environment.

Human relations dimension: It refers to the interpersonal relationship existing among the members in the educative process. Usually, the members are the teacher, students, healthcare team members, and the significant others. There should be a good interpersonal relationship in order to promote learning.

The interaction among all of these components or dimensions constitutes the process of education in nursing.

Elements of Educational Process

An educative process is comprised of the following:

Why to educate: This is the aim of education. If the aims are not realized properly, one cannot go in the right direction. It is must for everybody involved in the educational process to realize the aim of education and such aim should be achievable, practical and based on the current needs of the learner and the society.

Whom to educate: It is the learner in the educational process. In nursing, it refers to the student nurses. While choosing students for nursing, the administrators should choose the candidates who have the right attitude and being willing to take nursing as their profession.

Who is to educate: It refers to the teacher. The teacher must be dedicated and should not teach for the sake of teaching. She should possess all the essential qualities required of a good teacher.

What to educate: This is the content of the curriculum. Usually, it is devised by the respective professional organization such as the Indian Nursing Council (INC). Same thing can be adopted by the university and the institution offering the nursing education.

Where to educate: The students are educated in the Schools or Colleges of Nursing. The environment, especially the physical environment, should be conducive with all facilities to promote learning.

How to educate: It refers to the methods and techniques of teaching and learning activities. The teacher uses various techniques, methods, and strategies to facilitate learning in various set-ups such as classroom, hospital, community, laboratory, etc.

Learning

"Teachers open the door. You enter by yourself".
—*Chinese Proverb*

Definition of Learning

"It is any relatively permanent change or modification of behavior that results as a result of practice or experience."
—*Murthy, Gates and others.*

Webster's Dictionary defines learning as "the act or experience of one that learns"; "knowledge or skill acquired by instruction or study"; "modification of a behavioral tendency by experience".

Learning is often defined as a change in behavior (Birkenholz, 1999), which is demonstrated by people implementing knowledge, skills, or practices derived from education.

It is a process by which behavior is originated or changed by practice or training.

Learning is the process of growth and development whereby the learner acquires a body of knowledge, develops ideas which she makes a part of herself and develops the ability to use her knowledge in the pursuit of her ideals. Learning is a part of education and brings modification of behavior.

Characteristics of Learning

Learning is Unitary

The learner responds as a "whole person" in a unified way to the whole situation or total pattern. She responds intellectually, emotionally, physically and spiritually, and these occur simultaneously. All these dimensions are coordinated and integrated toward achievement of goals.

Learning is Individual

Learner differs from one another. Therefore, the teaching-learning situation is approached differently by each learner and with different goals with the result that each learner responds differently.

Learning is Social

Learning takes place in response to the environment in which there are other individuals as well as physical things.

Learning is Self-active

Learning is a personal process. An individual can learn only through her own reactions to situations.

Learning is Purposive

Learning is directed toward the goal. Goals are determined directly by motives and indirectly by incentives. Motives are conditions, physical and psychological, within the persons that dispose him to act in certain ways.

Motives take in different variety of forms, e.g. needs, desires, tensions, attitudes, interest, and so on. Motives energize behavior by releasing energy and arousing activity, by selecting or determining the activities in which the individual will engage. Goal setting comprises both momentary and long-term goals.

Learning is Creative

Human learning is both selective and creative. In learning, the learner is the primary force, and the teacher is the secondary force. Learner decides and chooses to learn. The learner has the power to vary her responses at will and thus creates new forms of response.

Learning is Transferable

Transfer means whatever is learned in one context or situation will apply or affect another context or situation. Transfer depends on understanding; it depends on the discovery of essential relationship applied deliberately to the situation of a practical problem.

Learning is Growth

Learning leads to the growth of the individual by integrating past and present learning. Learning is the process of growth and development whereby the learner acquires a body of knowledge, develops ideas which she makes a part of herself and develops the ability to use her knowledge in the pursuit of her ideals.

Learning is Adjustment

Learning leads the individual to make adjustment in day-to-day life for the betterment of an individual.

Learning is Organizing Experience

Learning occurs through sensory experiences. Mere presence of experience will not lead to learning. In order to learn effectively, the experiences need to be organized in such a manner that it leads to maximum learning.

Learning is Intelligent

Certain level of intelligence is required to learn. Learning style depends upon the intelligence. There are different types of intelligence possessed by the learners. They are verbal and linguistic, logical and mathematical, musical, kinesthetic, visual and spatial, interpersonal and intrapersonal.

Learning Affects the Conduct of the Learner

Learning brings the desirable changes in behavior of the person. Learning makes a person to make effective adjustment in his environment. Each and every activity of the learner is influenced by learning.

Learning Takes Place through Trial and Error

We learn out of our own mistakes. Such learning is lifelong and permanent because a person is actively involved in the process of learning.

Learning Depends upon Insight

Learning is basically a process of understanding and critically analyzing. Learning out of rote memory is only temporary. Permanent learning is the one which a person can integrate and reproduce at any time.

Pillars of Learning

- The first pillar of learning is the "Learning to know".
- The second pillar of learning is "Learning to do".
- The third pillar which, in some way, is the most important is "Learning to live together".
- The fourth pillar is "Learning to be".

The Learning Process

Certain elements must be presented for learning to take place.

Elements of Learning Process

- Goal
- Stimulus
- Perception
- Response
- Consequence
- Integration.

Types of Learning

According to Arthur Melton, the categories of learning are:
- Conditioning
- Role learning
- Problems learning
- Skill learning
- Problem-solving.

Eight Kinds of Learning

Gagne proposes eight kinds of learning:
1. Sign learning
2. Stimulus response learning
3. Changing
4. Verbal association learning

5. Multiple discrimination learning
6. Concept learning
7. Principle learning
8. Problem-solving.

Factors Influencing Learning
- Learning experiences and behavioral objectives
- Teaching-learning environment
- Motivation toward objectives
- Individual differences
- Association of concepts
- Active participation and practice
- The learning preparation
- Sequencing or ordering of subject content.

Learning Styles or Learning Modalities

Auditory, Visual, and Kinesthetic Learners

Differing aptitudes, abilities, and experiences have caused individuals to develop a preference for sending and receiving information through one sense over another. A preference for one type of learning over another may be seen in the following ways:

Visual learners prefer, enjoy or require graphical illustrations such as bar graphs or cross tables to explain data; color codes to highlight salient information; maps to find their way on the subway or while driving in a new city; written material to study new concepts; wall charts that display points to be remembered; written outlines; drawings or designs to illustrate overhead presentations; sitting "up close" in a presentation in order to see the presenter's face, gestures or visuals; taking notes during a lecture; instructors to repeat verbal directions.

Auditory learners prefer, enjoy or require a verbal presentation of new information, such as a lecture; group discussions to hear other points of view or practices; fast-paced verbal exchanges of ideas; a good joke or story that they can repeat for others; verbal cues or pneumonic devices to help them remember information; music at the beginning or during transitions in a training setting; words to accompany a cartoon; oral reports of working groups.

Kinesthetic learners prefer, enjoy, or require movement, such as rocking or shaking a leg during a lecture; hands-on experience to learn a task; gestures while making a point; role play exercises over discussion groups; shaking hands when meeting or greeting people; trying new things without a lengthy explanation of the activity; frequent breaks; regular opportunities to change seating or room arrangement; "just doing it" rather than talking about it.

While it is thought that people have developed a preference for or have greater skill in processing one type of input over others, most people simultaneously process information through multiple senses. In fact, the retention of learned material is enhanced if the learner is asked to process information using more than one sense. Presentations that are multi-sensory (using visual and auditory components) in combination with interactive activities will increase learning and retention for most adults.

Gardner proposes seven broader dimensions of learner possesses intelligence in various areas such as:
1. *Verbal and linguistic*: Ability to deal with words and language, both written and spoken.
2. *Logical and mathematical*: Ability to do inductive and deductive thinking, ability to use numbers, abstract patterns, and reasoning ability.
3. *Musical*: Ability to recognize tonal patterns, pitch, melody, rhythms, and tone.
4. *Kinesthetic*: Ability to use the body skillfully.
5. *Visual and spatial*: Ability to observe and process visual stimuli and visualize or create visual images.
6. *Interpersonal*: Ability to develop and maintain relationships and understand, communicate, and work with other people.
7. *Intrapersonal*: Understanding of self and one's own feelings, values and purpose.

Many instructors have found applications for this new way of defining intelligence or aptitude. In general, the instructors have utilized this theory to support the notion that instruction should entail for more than a verbal/linguistic presentation of ideas, and include experiential opportunities that enable people with varying types of "intelligence" to be successful.

Kolb (1976) describes learners as:

Divergers—have the ability to synthesize diverse opinions and observation. They are creative, intuitive, imaginative, and are people oriented. The same attributes sometimes obscure their ability to make decisions.

Assimilators—are systematic, focused learners who use logic and inductive reasoning to organize new information. They may feel uncomfortable in situations of ambiguity and when the practical relevance of the information is not clear.

Accommodators—grasp new information through their feelings and are highly action oriented. They enjoy taking risks and exploring new ideas and environments. They tend to use trial and error method to solve problems. They may disregard well established procedures and theory in the process.

Convergers—tend to be logical, highly pragmatic, and are able to transform information to new ideas or solutions to problems. Their range of interests tends to be narrow and they are often accused of being close-minded and unimaginative.

Adult preferences regarding a learning environment:

Physical factors	Emotional factors	Learning factors
Learning setting: • Noise level • Lighting • Temperature • Structure • Time of day	**Social needs:** • Learn alone • Learn with others • Motivation: – Extrinsic – Intrinsic	**Learning styles:** • Auditory • Visual • Kinesthetic

An instructor must recognize that learners' preferences in these areas may affect their responsiveness in the session. Efforts should be made to accommodate differences by providing a variety of learning activities in which participants may feel comfortable. The able educator delivers instruction in a stimulating, rich and diverse environment through a variety of instructional methods to appeal to adult participants' learning styles and preferences. (Please refer to the factors influencing learning environment in the table given above.)

Theoretical Orientations to Learning

Four different orientations to learning were explained in relation to the view of the learning process, locus of learning, purpose of education, educator's role and manifestations in adult learning is a Table 2.1 in given:
- Behaviorist orientation to learning
- Cognitivist orientation to learning
- Humanist orientation to learning
- Social/situational orientation to learning.

Teaching

"Teaching = helping someone learn".

—L dee Fink

Meaning and Definition

Education encompasses both the teaching and learning of knowledge, proper conduct and technical competency. Formal education consists of systematic instruction, teaching and training by professional teachers. It thus focuses on the cultivation of skills, trades or professions, as well as mental, moral and esthetic development. Teaching is the action of teachers. The passing of knowledge from generation to generation allows students to grow into useful members of society. Good teachers can translate information, good judgment, experience and wisdom into relevant knowledge that a student can understand, retain and pass to others. Teaching is a process which facilitates learning by encouraging learners to think, feel and do.

Teaching is a system of directed and deliberate actions that are intended to induce learning through a series of directed activities designed to induce learning (Heidgerken, 1953).

Bevis (1989) defined teaching as an art and science in which the content is structured and the processes used enable student learning.

Teaching is the stimulation, guidance, direction and encouragement of learning.—Burton.

"Teaching is an arrangement and manipulation of a situation in which there are gaps and obstructions which an individual will seek to overcome and from which he will learn in the course of doing so."—John Brubacher.

Table 2.1: Four orientations to learning.

Aspect	Behaviorist	Cognitivist	Humanist	Social and situational
Learning theorists	Thorndike, Pavlov, Watson, Guthrie, Hull, Tolman, Skinner	Koffka, Kohler, Lewin, Piaget, Ausubel, Bruner, Gagne	Maslow, Rogers	Bandura, Lave and Wenger, Salomon
View of the learning process	It is the change in behavior of the learners	It is the internal mental process, which includes insight, information processing, memory, perception, etc.	It is a personal act to fulfill potential	It is an interaction/observation in social contexts
Locus of learning	Stimuli in external environment	Internal cognitive structuring	Affective and cognitive needs	Learning is a relationship between the people and environment
Purpose of education	To produce behavioral change in desired direction	To develop capacity and skills to learn better	To become self-actualized and autonomous	To promote full participation in community activities and utilization of resources
Educator's role	Arranging the environment to elicit desired response	Structuring the content of learning activity	Facilitating the development of the whole person	Working to establish and maintain activities of community in which conversation and participation can occur
Manifestations in adult learning	• Behavioral objectives • Competency based education • Skill development and training	• Cognitive development • Intelligence, learning, critical thinking creativity and use of memory, etc.	Andragogy self-directed learning	• Socialization • Social participation Associationalism • Conversation

General Principles of Teaching

- The principle of aim: There should be a definite aim for every lesson. It is a goal for the teacher.
- The principle of activity or learning by doing.
- The principle of linking with actual life and other subjects.
- The principle of planning.
- The principle of interest or motivation.
- The principle of flexibility and cooperation.
- The principle of diagnostic and remedial teaching.
- The principle of creativity.

Principle of Individual Differences

Teaching must take into consideration the individual differences of children in various aspects.

Principle of Motivation

Teaching must be based on various techniques which appeal to the motives of students.

Principle of Stimulations

Best learning takes place when the teacher is successful in arousing the interest of the student.

Principle of Goal Setting

A definite goal should be set before each child according to the standard expected of him. Immediate goals should be set before small children and distant goals for older ones. It must be remembered that the goals should be very clear and the children must understand these goals.

Principle of Association

Thorndike points out that thing which we want to do together should be put together. Many different things should be brought together as a part of one process.

Principle of Emotional Development

Children should be praised when they show good results. This will give them encouragement to show all the more better results and they develop confidence, hope, self-reliance and self-respect. Sympathetic attitude on the part of the teachers gives stimulus and a sense of security to the students.

Principle of Law of Readiness

The law is indicative of learners' state to participate in the learning process. According to Thorndike readiness is preparation for action.

Principle of Law of Effect

It states that a response is strengthened, if it is followed by pleasure and weakened if it is followed by displeasure.

Law of Principle of Exercise or Repetition

The learning is better and concrete when the concepts are repeated often. Exercising a particular skill very often helps in skill learning.

Law of Use and Law of Disuse

Anything which is used, remembered and learned well than which is not used or less used. The learner tends to forget the concept or skill which is not used.

Principle of Attitude

The learner performs the task well if he has his attitude set in the task.

Principle of Law of Similarity

This law states that "other things being equal" the stimuli that are more similar to one another will have greater tendency to be grouped. This learning of similar things is easier than learning dissimilar things.

Principle of Law of Proximity

According to this law "perceptual groups are favored according to the nearness of parts". This means that we perceive all closely situated or located things as groups. The maxims of teaching aim at quickening the interest of the students. They make learning inspirational, interesting, effective and meaningful. They keep the students attentive to the teaching-learning process. They make the students active participants in the work.

Effective Teaching Principles and Practices

The Teacher

Principle 1: Sets clear goals and intellectual challenges for student learning.

Exemplary practices:

- Demonstrates and shares a clear vision of intellectual goals and learning outcomes for the class
- Identifies key concepts or ideas in the field, and helps students to understand and apply them
- Integrates current research and conceptual approaches into learning activities
- Identifies key steps in achieving learning goals
- Actively helps students to accomplish goals and meet challenges as defined in the course outline
- Sets high, yet reasonable, expectations of students' learning.

Principle 2: Employs appropriate teaching methods and strategies that actively involve learners.

Exemplary practices:

- Shows awareness in teaching activities, that learning is a process which transforms and changes learners

- Encourages appropriate student participation
- Organizes effective learning experiences to meet intellectual goals and learning outcomes, both in the classroom and (as possible) beyond
- Evaluates and assesses learning in a manner consistent with established goals and learning outcomes
- Integrates appropriate teaching methods and technologies, tailored to course goals and learning outcomes
- Integrates appropriate teaching methods and technologies, tailored to course goals and learning outcomes, and facilitates student participation
- Encourages and assists students to participate in self-directed learning activities.

Principle 3: Communicates and interacts effectively with students.
Exemplary practices:
- Expresses goals, intended outcomes, and expectations clearly and effectively and discusses these with students
- Balances collaborative and individual student learning to reflect the course aims and outcomes
- Attends to classroom dynamics that enhance or inhibit learning
- Engenders enthusiasm and interest in subject matter
- Uses fair and reasonable methods of evaluating learning.

Principle 4: Attends to intellectual growth of students.
Exemplary practices:
- Provides and discusses with students, explicit criteria for assessing learning
- Acquires regular and varied feedback on students' intellectual accomplishments
- Reviews students' progress in achieving intellectual goals and learning outcomes
- Provides advanced learning opportunities for those students who seek them.

Principle 5: Respects diverse talents and learning styles of students.
Exemplary practices:
- Promotes a stimulating learning environment
- Recognizes and accommodates different learning styles
- Demonstrates sensitivity to intellectual and cultural issues.

Principle 6: Incorporates learning beyond the classroom.
Exemplary practices:
- Encourages appropriate student-faculty interaction
- Helps students connect their learning experience to the world outside the classroom (both within and outside of the university)
- Helps students to apply their learning in a variety of ways.

Principle 7: Reflects on monitors and improves teaching practices.
Exemplary practices:
- Seeks regular student feedback on teaching effectiveness
- Reflects on teaching practice through creation of a teaching dossier or other self-reflection activity
- Seeks peer feedback to enhance teaching
- Regularly revises and updates course content, format, teaching strategies and assignments
- Takes advantage of opportunities to enhance teaching by attending professional development activities.

Source: From the "Report of the Ad Hoc Senate Committee on Teaching Quality, Effectiveness and Evaluation, May 1999".

Maxims of Methodological Teaching

- Known to unknown
- Easy to difficult
- Simple to complex
- Concrete to abstract
- Particular to general
- Analysis to synthesis
- Whole to part
- Empirical to rational
- Psychological to logical
- Actual to representative.

Maxims of Teaching

From known to unknown: This means that the teacher should arouse interest by putting questions on the subject matter already known to the pupils. The teacher has to proceed step by step to connect the new matter to the old one.

Proceed from easy to difficult: Lessons must be graded in order of difficulty to suit the pupil standards. This will help in sustaining the interest of the students. In determining what is easy and what is difficult, teachers have to take into account the psychological make-up of the child. Logically viewed, one skill may be easy but psychologically it may be difficult. There are many things which look easy to teachers but are in fact difficult for children. The interest of the child has also to be taken into account.

Proceed from simple to complex: Teachers should not curb the initiative and interest of the pupils by presenting them complex problems before the simpler ones are presented.

Proceed from concrete to abstract: Small children learn first from things they can handle and see.

Proceed from indefinite to definite: Early ideas of children are very vague, indefinite and incoherent.

These ideas have to be made precise, clear, definite, and systematic.

Proceed from particular to general: The study of general rules should be undertaken with the help of the particular examples. Particular is more defined to the child than the general.

Proceed from empirical to rational: Empirical knowledge is based only on observation or experience and for which any reasonable account cannot be given. Rational knowledge is that for which we have scientific explanation. Sometimes teachers have to start from less general to more general laws. To reach the rational type of knowledge, empirical observations have to be collected, analyzed and rationalized.

Proceed from psychological to logical: Logical approach is concerned with the systematic exposition of the subject matter. It is concerned with the arrangement of the subject matter. The psychological approach looks at the child's interests, needs, reactions, and mental make-up.

Proceed from main operation to exceptions: To avoid confusion and doubt, teachers should teach main operations and draw attention of the students to exceptions later on.

Phases of Teaching

Preactive Phase

This phase involves planning and preparation for teaching. The teacher prepares the lesson plan, decides on teaching methods, and prepares the teaching materials.

Interactive Phase

It is the phase of implementation where the teacher teaches the students. She adopts appropriate teaching methods and uses audio-visual aids planned earlier. In this stage, more interaction occurs between the teacher and the students.

Postactive Phase

It is mainly of testing the effectiveness of teaching-learning process. The teacher uses various methods of evaluation in assessing the success of her teaching and learning by the students.

Variables of Teaching

It comprises three variables which operate in the process of teaching-learning conditions or situations.

Teacher as Independent Variable

The teacher does the planning, organizing, leading and controlling of teaching. He/She is free to perform various activities to provide a learning experience to the learners.

Student as Dependent Variable

The student is required to act according to the planning and organization of the teacher. The teaching activities of the teacher influence the learning of the students.

Content and the Strategy of Presentation as Intervening Variables

The intervening variables lead to an interaction between the teachers and the students. The content determines the mode of presentation—telling, showing, and doing.

The variables perform three functions:
1. **Diagnostic function**: The teacher as an independent variable is more active and diagnoses the following:
   – Entering behavior of the students
   – Teaching problems
   – Individual variations
   – Content analysis in view of learning conditions.
   The student as a dependent variable diagnoses on the basis of his perception for his activities and responses. In the process of interaction both teacher and the student diagnose for initiations and responses.
2. **Prescriptive function**: The main objective of this function is to bring desirable changes in the behavior of the learner. The teacher makes efforts to organize the intervening variables in such a way so as to select teaching techniques and feedbacks that help in the realization of the objectives. The student helps the teacher by actively participating in teaching-learning process.
3. **Evaluative functions**: This aims at examining the effectiveness of the prescriptive function. The evaluative function has two main activities:
   – Construction of criterion test.
   – Evaluation of change of behavior.

Stages of Teaching

One of the analyses of teaching describes the whole process as comprising of three different stages:

Preteaching + Teaching-learning process + Post-teaching

Preteaching

Preteaching consists essentially of the planning of a lesson. The planning of lesson needs to be seen in broader terms, not merely the designing of a lesson plan. Planning includes identifying the objectives to be achieved in terms of students learning, the strategies and methods to be adopted, use of teaching aids and so on.

Teaching-Learning Process

The second stage includes the execution of the plan, where learning experiences are provided to students through suitable modes and evaluation of students learning is done.

Post-teaching

Post-teaching includes the performance evaluation of students, the extent of students' achievements and problems, reflecting on the performance of self and also on deciding on changes in the way of proceeding with the entire process of teaching-learning if required.

As it is obvious from the above analysis, the roles that teacher has to play at different stages are different ranging from a designer, to a participant, to a decision maker, etc. Instruction is the complex process by which learners are provided with a deliberately designed environment to interact with, keeping in focus prespecified objective of bringing about specific desirable changes. Whether instruction goes in a classroom, laboratory, outdoors or library, this environment is specifically designed by a teacher so that students interact with certain specific environmental stimuli, like natural components (outdoor), information from books, certain equipment (laboratory), etc. Learning is directed in predetermined directions to achieve certain prespecific goals. The predetermined environment will ensure learning of what the teacher has decided as instructional objectives to take place. The variety of experiences that students go through with a teacher, among themselves provides learning opportunities.

Characteristics of Good Teaching

Palmer's (1998) Thoughts on Good Teacher

Good teachers possess a capacity for connectedness. They are to weave a complex web of connections among themselves, their subjects, and their students so that students can learn to weave a world for themselves.... The connections made by good teachers are held not in their methods but in their hearts—meaning heart in ancient sense, as the place where intellect and emotion and spirit and will converge in the human life.

- Good teaching is as much about passion. It is about not only motivating students to learn, but teaching them how to learn, and doing so in a manner that is relevant, meaningful, and memorable.
- Good teaching is treating students as consumers of knowledge. It is about doing the best to keep on top of the field, reading sources, inside and outside the areas of expertise, and being at the leading edge as often as possible. Good teaching is also about bridging the gap between theory and practice.
- Good teaching is about listening, questioning, being responsive, and remembering that each student and class is different. It is about eliciting responses and developing the oral communication skills of the quiet students. It is about pushing students to excel; and being professional at all times.
- Good teaching is about not always having a fixed agenda and being rigid, but being flexible, fluid, experimenting, and having the confidence to react and adjust to changing circumstances. Good teaching is about the creative balance between being an authoritarian dictator on the one hand and a pushover on the other.
- Good teaching is also about style. Effective teaching is not about being locked with both hands glued to a podium or having the eyes fixated on a slide projector. Good teachers realize that they are the conductors and the class is the orchestra. All students play different instruments and at varying proficiencies.
- This is very important—good teaching is about humor. It is about being self-deprecating and not taking oneself too seriously. It is often about making innocuous jokes so that the ice breaks and students learn in a more relaxed atmosphere.
- Good teaching is about caring, nurturing, and developing minds and talents. It is about devoting time, often invisible, to every student.
- Good teaching is supported by strong and visionary leadership, and very tangible institutional support—resources, personnel, and funds.
- Good teaching is about mentoring between senior and junior faculty, teamwork, and being recognized and promoted by one's peers. Effective teaching should also be rewarded, and poor teaching needs to be remediated through training and development programs.
- At the end of the day, good teaching is about having fun, experiencing pleasure and intrinsic rewards. Good teachers practice their craft not for the money or because they have to, but because they truly enjoy it and because they want to. Good teachers could not imagine doing anything else.

Models of Teaching-learning Process and its Application in Nursing

Learning is the process of growth and development whereby the learner acquires a body of knowledge, develops ideas which one makes a part of oneself, and develops the ability to use such knowledge in the pursuit of chosen ideals. Learning is a part of education, which brings modification of behavior. Teaching is a process which facilitates learning by encouraging learners to think, feel and do. Teaching is a system of directed and deliberate actions that are intended to induce learning through a series of activities designed to induce learning (Heidgerken, 1953). Both teaching and learning involve series of actions and activities. A model tries to explain the concepts involved and its interrelationship. It is a visual aid or a picture which highlights the main ideas and variables in a process or a system. Many researchers have tried to put together classroom or school-based models that describe the teaching-learning process. The main models discussed and compared are by Carroll (1963), Proctor (1984), Cruickshank (1985), Gage and Berliner (1992) and Huitt (1995). This aims at explaining the various models of teaching-learning process and their application in nursing.

John Carroll's Model

It is basically related to school learning. However, it can be applicable to nursing. Carroll states that time is the most important variable in school learning. A simple equation for Carroll's model is:

School learning = f(Time spent/Time needed)

Time spent is the function of opportunity and perseverance. Opportunity is determined by the classroom teacher; the specific measure is called allotted or allocated time (that is allocated for learning by classroom teacher). Perseverance is the students' involvement with academic content during that allocated time. Carroll proposed that perseverance be measured as the percentage of the allocated time during which students are actually involved in the learning process, and was labeled as engagement rate. Allocated time multiplied by engagement rate produced the variable which Carroll proposed as a measure of time spent, which came to be called engaged time or time on task.

Application in Nursing

Learning = f (Time spent/Time needed)

Time spent = Opportunity + Perseverance.

Opportunity: It depends upon the allocated time for theory and practical for each subject by the Indian Nursing Council, the university, the institution, faculty planning, faculty commitment, and the ability to provide comprehensive teaching-learning experience.

Perseverance is the nursing students' involvement with the academic content during that allocated time. It includes the number of days/hours attended, leave taken, quality teaching and learning, motivation, aptitude, attitude, intelligence, memory, immediate need, etc.

Engagement rate = Time spent in teaching-learning/Time allocated for teaching and learning.

Time on task = Engagement rate × Time allocated for teaching and learning.

Students can learn if:

They are given enough time to learn the concept and information taught in school and are provided quality instruction. By quality instruction it is meant that the teacher should:
- Organize subject matter into manageable learning units.
- Develop specific learning objectives for each unit.
- Develop appropriate formative and summative evaluation measures with sufficient time allocations.
- Plan and implement group teaching strategies with sufficient time allocations, practice opportunities, and corrective instructions for all students to reach the desired level of mastery.

Proctors' Model

This model emphasizes the importance of schools' social climate in the teaching-learning process. The school climate is influenced by a number of factors. The two important factors are student characteristics and the interaction among the individuals involved in the schooling process.

Application in Nursing

Student learning ∝ School climate

Student learning or achievement is directly proportional to school climate.

School climate = Student characteristics + Interaction among the individuals

Student characteristics include race, gender, economic level and past academic performance, attitudes, norms, beliefs and prejudices.

Interaction includes the input of administrators, teachers and students.

The outcome of learning and student's achievement will go up when the institution has good qualified faculty members, adequate infrastructural facilities, committed students, quality instructions, corrective feedback, and good communication among students, parents, and educators. On the other hand, adverse or negative attitudes on the part of the instructors and administrators will erode student's self-esteem and consequently lower the achievement level. It is hypothesized that there is a cyclical relationship among the variables and changes can be made at any point along the way. These changes will affect the institutional achievement, which will continue to affect the social climate of the school.

Cruickshank's Model

It is based on the classroom and teacher. He has taken the concept of Mitzel and Biddle and incorporated it in his model. Mitzel classified variables as Product, Process, and Presage. Biddle classified variables such as school and community contents, formative experiences, classroom situations, teacher properties, teacher behaviors—intermediate and long-term consequences.

Application in Nursing

Product <—> Process <—> Presage

Product is the outcome of learning on the part of the students. It is the gain in knowledge, changes in attitude and skill attainment in nursing students. Process involves interaction between student and teacher in various contexts such as classroom, hospital, and community set-up. Presage is the teacher's intelligence, experience and success, and other teacher characteristics such as personality, attitude, aptitude, experience, motivation, commitment and sincerity, etc. Presage is supposed to affect the process and then, of course, process will affect the product.

Biddle variables include the following:

School and community contents: It includes the philosophy, aims and objectives, climate of the school and environment, facilities available in the institution and in the environment.

Formative experiences: It is the experience gained from the past events by the teachers, administrators, students, etc.

Classroom situations: The climate, physical facilities, furniture, control of external noise, adequate lighting, ventilation, seating facilities, etc.

Teacher properties: Teacher's personality, attitude, knowledge, experience, communication, and assertive skills.

Teacher's behavior and intermediate and long-term effects: Ability to handle the students of various personalities, problematic students, way of disciplining the students, techniques used to correct the wrong behaviors of the students, being impartial to all students, maintaining good interpersonal relationship with the students, etc.

Gage and Berliner's Model

This model is classroom and teacher-based and centers on the question, "What does a teacher do?" A teacher begins with an objective and ends with an evaluation. Instruction connects objectives and evaluations and is based on the teacher's knowledge of the student's characteristics and how best to motivate them. If the evaluations do not demonstrate that the desired results have been achieved, the teacher re-teaches the material and starts the process all over again. Classroom management is subsumed under the rubric of motivating students. Gage and Berliner suggest that the teacher should use research and principles from educational psychology to develop proper teaching procedures to obtain optimal results.

Application in Nursing

Objectives ←—Instruction—→ Evaluation

The teacher starts teaching with the formation of specific learning objectives and based on this, she instructs the students. After the instruction, she evaluates the students. So instruction connects the objectives to evaluation. Evaluation in turn helps them to revise or modify the specific learning objectives and prepare for further instruction or remedial instruction.

Huitt's Model

This model is not only classroom, teacher and student-based, but includes additional contextual influences as well. This adds variables related to context, and student and teacher characteristics. Huitt advocates that the important context variables must be considered because our society is changing rapidly. From this perspective, children are members of a multifaceted society, which influences and modifies the way they process learning as well as defines the knowledge and skills that must be acquired to succeed in society.

His model shows a relationship among the categories of context (family, school, home and community environment), input (what students and teachers bring to the classroom process), classroom processes (what is going on in the classroom), and output (measures of learning done outside the classroom).

Application in Nursing

Input—> Classroom process—> Output

Input: It is the beginning of teaching-learning process. Input variables include:
- Teacher characteristics such as values, beliefs, knowledge of student, teaching-learning process, communication skills, personality, etc.
- Student characteristics such as study habits, learning style, age, sex, gender, race, ethnicity, motivation, moral, socio-emotional, cognitive, character development and aptitude, etc.

Output: It is the end of the teaching-learning process. Educators must identify or propose an end result or outcome of teaching and learning. Until the outcome objectives are known, nothing else can be considered. Output measures are gain in knowledge, learning new concepts, reading, language, mathematics, etc.

Classroom processes include teacher's behavior, student's behavior and other variables such as classroom climate, student leadership roles, etc.
- Teacher's behavior includes planning (getting ready for classroom interaction), management (getting the class under control) and instruction (guiding the learning process). Planning activities have a little predictable relationship with student achievement. The other two are moderately related to student achievement. Lack of a strong relationship may be due to teacher inconsistency, which depends on change of the time

of day or the characteristics of a particular group of students. The three variables such as correct feedback by the teacher, reinforcement and level of student teacher interaction are the classroom predictors of student's success.
- Student's behavior includes planning, preparation for the class, learning readiness, need, preference for learning and learning styles, study habits, age, sex, gender, race, ethnicity, motivation, moral, socio-emotional, cognitive, character development and aptitude, etc.

Context variables include mother's education, family expectation, technology at home, facilities in the institution, institutional climate, specific needs of the community, prevailing health problems, demand, etc.

Intermediate outcome: Academic Learning Timer (ALT) is the best classroom process predictor of student achievement. ALT is defined as the amount of time students are successfully involved during the learning of content that will be tested. Huitt proposes that ALT should be considered as the "vital signs" of a classroom. It is influenced by:
- *School year*: The number of days available for going to school.
- *Attendance year*: The number of days the student actually attends school.
- *School days*: The number of hours the student attends school each day can influence ALT.

Teaching and learning is the fundamental concept of nursing education. The aim of nursing education is to prepare the nurses with head, heart and hand. The knowledge of nursing is enhanced by teaching and learning. The above mentioned models and concepts can be understood and applied in nursing education to facilitate teaching and learning.

Relationship between Teaching and Learning

Teaching is a system of action intended to induce learning. Learning is modification of behavior. Teaching action includes provision of learning experiences and guidance that facilitates learning in formal situations such as classrooms and informal situations as clinics, wards, etc.

Teaching action: Preparing and planning materials, evaluation, observation, lecture, question answer, discussion, discovery and assignments, etc.

Teaching Strategies

Objective	Teaching	Learning type
1. Cognitive	Lecturing	Knowing
2. Affective	Dramatization	Feeling
3. Psychomotor	Experimentation	Doing

> Chickering and Gamson (2004) describe seven principles at the core of "good practice in undergraduate education".
> 1. Encouragement of contact between students and faculty
> 2. Development of reciprocity and cooperation among students
> 3. Encouragement of active learning
> 4. Transmission of prompt feedback
> 5. Emphasis on time "on task"
> 6. Communications of high expectations
> 7. Respect for diverse talents and ways of learning.

What is Taught and What is Learned

It is a simple point that what is taught is not the same as what the students learn, but it does have a number of implications.

A teacher designs teaching to induce learning but every student is not able to learn. Thus no learning is possible without teaching and all teaching may not result in learning. In Figure 2.2, it is clear that some of what we teach is wasted effort: but the diagram is a representation of only one learner's learning. It may be that within a class as a whole, everything we teach is learned, by someone. The shape representing the teaching is smaller than that for learning because students are also learning from other sources, including colleagues and the sheer experience of being in the educational system, as well as from more conventional other resources such as books.

Teaching BIASes

Pratt and associates, across a wide range of people, disciplines, and contexts they found that teachers vary on four dimensions that are called teaching BIASes:

B: Beliefs about learners, about the process of learning, about the content or skills to be learned, and about the role and responsibilities of a teacher.

I: Intentions as to what learners are to learn or what the person teaching them is trying to accomplish.

A: Actions or ways in which the teacher enacts the role of teacher using techniques and methods in particular ways to help people learn.

S: Strategies or ways in which a teacher combines beliefs, intentions, and actions into strategic thinking and decision-making.

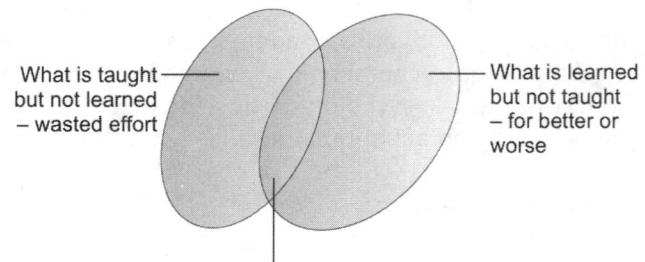

Fig. 2.2: What is taught and what is learned.

> *Stevens and Cassidy* (1999) defined evidence-based teaching as "the conscientious, explicit and judicious use of current best evidence in making decisions about the education of profession nurses".

What is Student-Centered Teaching

It is an approach to teaching that contrasts with the traditional content-centered and teacher-centered approaches that most of us experienced as students. *Content-centered teaching* focuses on mastery of specific material designated by the curriculum that is implemented by the instructor. In such teaching, there is little or no flexibility to shape the content to the needs of the learners or to the styles of the teachers or learners. In a *teacher-centered teaching*, the instructor is the expert on the content and delivery method. Here the teacher determines what will be taught with students as a passive recipient of information. The students are empty vessels to fill on blank slates upon which the teacher writes his or her knowledge. By contrast, in student-centered teaching, the shift moves away from the content and teacher to the learner. The teacher must meet everyone's needs; rather, the boundaries of the content and modes of teaching expand to better accommodate learners (Piccinin, 1997).

> **Why student-centered teaching in nursing?**
> In nursing, a shift to a student-centered approach to teaching not only provides nurse educators with a new vision for teaching, but also parallels a paradigm shift in nursing practice from nurse-centered to client-centered nursing practice. Nurse educators who embrace student-centered teaching not only prepare student nurses with the substantive knowledge necessary for competent practice, but also create an environment in which students learn to think critically, practice reflectively, work effectively in groups, and access and use new information to support practice.

Teaching Strategies to Create Empowering Learning Environments

Siu HM, Spence Laschinger HK and Vingilis E (2005) mentioned certain teaching strategies to create empowering learning environments. They are:
- Strategies to increase students' formal and informal power
  - Instill a shared governance approach to education with students
  - Encourage students to set goals and agendas for class sessions
  - Encourage students to decide educational content to explore in class
  - Facilitate the educational use of small-group projects or assignments
  - Encourage students to facilitate the learning of their peers and nursing faculty
- Strategies to increase students' access to opportunity
  - Encourage students to be self-directed and autonomous in their learning
  - Encourage students to conduct self-assessments of their learning needs
  - Help students develop their own individualized learning plans
  - Explore with students creative learning opportunities, such as attending nursing conferences, conducting an educational in-service, or developing an educational pamphlet.
- Strategies to increase students' access to resources
  - Allow adequate class time for students to accomplish their learning objectives and to share their knowledge development with their peers
  - Be available to help students with their learning needs
  - Direct students to use other resources, such as the library, nursing experts, allied health care professionals, professional associations, and community agencies.
- Strategies to increase students' access to information
  - Share with students the teaching and learning values
  - Discuss with students what is expected of them
  - Offer students one's nursing expertise and knowledge
  - Provide students with verbal and written feedback about their learning progress and performance
  - Encourage students to provide each other with verbal and written feedback about their learning progress
  - Challenge students to critique the effectiveness of their learning resources.
- Strategies to increase students' access to support
  - Foster an open-door philosophy
  - Take time to listen to students' learning needs and ideas
  - Recognize students' learning skills and accomplishments
  - Encourage students to assume roles and engage in learning activities that showcase their strengths
  - Encourage students to pursue their individualized learning needs.

Outcome-based Education

"People differ not only in their ability to do but also in their will to do".
—Paul Hersey

Meaning and Definition

Outcome-based education is a method of teaching that focuses on what students can actually do after they are taught. All curriculum and teaching decisions are made based on how best to facilitate the desired outcome.

Outcome-based education (OBE) is a student centered learning philosophy that focuses on empirically measuring student performance, which is called outcomes. OBE contrasts with traditional education, which primarily focuses on the resources that are available to the student, which are called inputs.

Outcome-based education is a model of education that rejects the traditional focus on what the school provides to students, in favor of making students demonstrate that they "know and are able to do" whatever, the required outcomes are.

Outcome-based education is a method of curriculum design and teaching that focuses on what students can actually do after they are taught. OBE addresses the key questions as:
1. What do you want the students to learn?
2. Why do you want them to learn it?
3. How can you best help students learn it?
4. How will you know what they have learnt?

Thus, the OBE's instructional planning process is a reverse of that associated with traditional educational planning. The desired outcome is selected first and the curriculum, instructional materials and assessments are created to support the intended outcome (Spady 1988; 1993). All curriculum and teaching decisions are made based on how best to facilitate the desired final outcome.

Towers (1996) listed four points to the OBE system that are necessary to make it work:
- What the student is to learn must be clearly identified.
- The student's progress is based on demonstrated achievement.
- Multiple instructional and assessment strategies need to be available to meet the needs of each student.
- Adequate time and assistance need to be provided so that each student can reach the maximum potential.

Meaning of Outcomes

The term "outcomes," "standards", and "goals" frequently are used interchangeably. These terms are also used to refer to different types of results, including content outcomes, students' performance outcomes, and college performance standards.
- **Content outcome:** It describes what students should know and be able to do in particular subject areas.
- **Student performance outcomes:** It describes how and at what level students must demonstrate such knowledge and skills.
- **College performance standards:** It defines the quality of education an educational institution must provide in order for students to meet content and/or performance outcomes.

An educational institution can specify its own outcomes and its own methods of measuring student achievement according to those outcomes. The results of these measurements can be used for different purposes. For example, one institution may use the information to determine how well the overall education system is performing, and another may use its assessments to determine whether an individual student has learned required material. Under the OBE model, education agencies may specify any outcome (skills and knowledge), but not inputs (field trips, arrangement of the school day, teaching styles).

The emphasis in an OBE education system is on measured outcomes rather than "inputs," such as how many hours students spend in class, or what textbooks are provided. Outcomes may include a range of skills and knowledge. Generally, outcomes are expected to be concretely measurable, that is, student can draw the heart in less than one minute instead of "student enjoys anatomy class".

An important byproduct of this approach is that students are assessed against external, absolute objectives, instead of reporting the students' relative achievements. The traditional model of grading on a curve (top student gets the best grade, worst student always fails (even if they know all the material), everyone else is evenly distributed in the middle) is never accepted in OBE or standards-based education. Instead, a student's performance is related in absolute terms: "Mary answered 80% of questions correctly" instead of "Mary answered more questions correctly than Mala".

The arguments developed by the proponents of OBE are:
- OBE is able to measure, "What the students are capable of doing"—something which the traditional education system often fails to do. For example, assessment methods in a conventional education system often grade students based on their ability to choose a correct answer from a group of four or five possible answers. OBE requires the students to understand the contents by "extending the meaning of competence far beyond that of narrow skills and the ability to execute structured tasks in a particular subject area and classroom" (Spady, 1995).
- OBE goes beyond "structured tasks" (e.g. memorization) by demanding that students demonstrate his/her skills through more challenging tasks like writing project proposals and completing the projects, analyzing case studies and giving case presentations, etc. Such exercises require students to practice and demonstrate their ability to think, question, research, make decisions, and give presentations.

Approaches to Grading, Reporting and Promoting

Under OBE, teachers can use any objective grading system they choose, including letter grades. For the purposes of graduation, advancement, and retention, a fully developed OBE system is generally useful. Instead of giving a single overall grade for a subject, information about several specific outcomes within that subject helps the teacher, student and the parents about the students' performance in different areas. For example, rather than just getting a passing grade for pediatric nursing, a student might be assessed as level 4 for pediatric history collection, level 5 for growth and development assessment and physical examination, level 3 for communication skills, etc. This approach is valuable to colleges and parents by specifically identifying a student's strengths and weaknesses.

In one alternate grading approach, a student can be awarded "levels" instead of letter grades. From 1st year to the 4th year till a student completes his or her course in nursing, he may have to pass through many fixed levels for example level 1 to 6. A student completing a level one by fulfilling certain requirements, he may have to go to level two. In the simplest implementation, earning a "level" indicates that the teacher believes that a student has learned enough of the current material to be able to succeed in the next level of work. A student technically cannot flunk in this system as a student who needs to review the current material will simply not achieve the next level at the same time as most of his same-age peers. This acknowledges differential growth at different stages, and focuses the teacher on the individual needs of the students.

OBE-oriented teachers think about the individual needs of each student and give opportunities for each student to achieve at a variety of levels. Thus, in theory, weaker students are given work within their grasp and exceptionally strong students are extended. In practice, managing independent study programs for thirty or more individuals is difficult.

The Basic Principles of OBE

- OBE has significant, culminating exit outcomes as the focus
- Let the students know what they are aiming for
- Design curriculum backward by using the major outcomes as the focus and linking all planning, teaching and assessment decisions directly to these outcomes
- Set the expectation that OBE is for all learners
- Expect students to succeed by providing them encouragement to engage deeply with the issues they are learning and to achieve the high challenging standard set (Spady, 1994)
- Develop curriculum to give scope to every learner to learn in his/her own pace
- Cater for individual needs and differences, for example, expansion of available time and resources so that all students succeed in reaching the exit outcomes
- Use outcomes to guide instructional planning.

Instructional Planning Under OBE System

Four major steps of planning under OBE system are as follows:

1. **Deciding on the outcomes:** It is very important to define the outcomes of a program in specific and precise manner. Spady and Marshall (1994) wrote:

   Outcomes are clear, observable demonstrations of student learning that occur after a significant set of learning experiences. Typically, these demonstrations, or performances, reflect three things:
   i. What the student knows
   ii. What the student can actually do with what he or she knows
   iii. The student's confidence and motivation in carrying out the demonstration. A well-defined outcome will have clearly defined content or concepts and be demonstrated through a well-defined process beginning with a directive or request such as "explain," "organize" or "produce".

   Thus most outcomes and standards should be described in terms of three dimensions:
   i. Content—simple to complex
   ii. Context—simple to complex
   iii. Competence—low to high

2. **Demonstrating outcomes:** Expected demonstrations will be defined by setting "benchmarks" for each level of the program. Each benchmark is a skill that must be demonstrated by the student. Unlike the outcomes, the list of benchmarks is different in every level of study. Benchmarks should address and define specifically the goals of the curriculum and determine ways to assess whether students have reached these goals at that level of study.

3. **Deciding on contents and teaching strategies:** One of the most common questions among teachers is "what experiences will I need to provide?" At the beginning of any class, the teachers will delineate expectations and outcomes to make the students feel like participants in classroom decisions. When this is done the students tend to be more supportive of activities and leaning processes taken in all aspects of the class.

   There are two general approaches to implementing outcome-based models:
   i. "Whole-class" models which seek to bring all learners in a classroom up to high levels of learning before proceeding further, and
   ii. "Flexible" models which use flexible grouping, continuous progress, technological approaches and instructional management.

   The latter model requires the instructor to make a sincere attempt to meet each student at his/her level of competency and build upon the "strengths already there" throughout the course. After the first few days of the course, students must have clearly understood the objectives of the program.

4. **Assessments in OBE:** The entire curriculum in OBE is driven by assessments that focus on well-defined learning outcomes and not primarily by factors such as what is taught, how long the student takes to achieve the outcomes or which path the student takes to achieve their target. The learning outcomes are set out on a gradation of increasing complexity that students are expected to master these outcomes sequentially. Willis and Kissane (1995) suggested two techniques for assessing students' learning outcomes i.e. "Standard-referenced assessment" (similar to criterion-referenced assessment but with a clearer description of expected performance), and student portfolios documenting their progress.

Differences with Traditional Education Methods

In a traditional system, students are given grades and rankings compared to each other. Content and performance expectations are based primarily on what was taught in the past to students of a given age. The highest-performing students are given the highest grades and test scores, and the lowest-performing students are given low grades. Schools used norm referenced tests, such as inexpensive, multiple choice computer-scored questions with single correct answers, to quickly rank students on ability. These tests do not give criterion-based judgments as to whether students have met a single standard of what every student is expected to know and do: they merely rank the students in comparison with each other. In this system, grade-level expectations are defined as the performance of the median student, a level at which half the students score better and half the students score worse.

Claims in Favor of OBE

Outcome-based education proponents believe that all students can learn, regardless of ability, race, ethnicity, socioeconomic status, and gender. The adoption of measurable standards is seen as a means of ensuring that the content and skills covered by the standards will be a high priority in the education of students. While recognizing that some students will learn certain material faster than others, the standards movement rejects the idea that only a few can succeed. All students are capable of continuous improvement.

The opportunities that were previously afforded to those at the top of a bell curve are opened up to the diversity of all students, in a democratic vision, sometimes connected to social justice.

The movement presents the following positions and viewpoints on OBE:

- All students will complete rigorous academic coursework
- All students, including those who live in poverty, will meet district, state, and national standards
- Staff will maintain high expectations and standards, believing all students will succeed if kept to high expectations
- Students should be measured against a fixed yardstick, or "against the mountain" rather than against other students
- Students should demonstrate that they have met standards, not just put in seat time to advance to the next level.

Criticism of OBE Falls into a Few Major Groups

Opposition to Standardized Testing

Standards can be set too low: Most fear that the focus on achievement by all students will result in "dumbing down" the definition of academic competence to a level which is achievable by even the weakest students. Critics are unhappy with having all students meet a minimum standard, instead of most students meeting a somewhat higher standard.

Standards can be set too high: Others object that the standards are too high. OBE models do not approve of social promotion, so nondisabled students who perform significantly below the stated standard may be held back or required to take additional instruction. Especially, when the standards are relatively new, and the schools are just beginning to adjust to the new standards, a majority of students struggle with at least some of the requirements.

Criticism of Inappropriate Outcomes—Dislike of Specific Outcomes

Finally, many complaints are directed against the nature of certain standards. Controversial standards are opposed because of their content, not simply because they are standards. OBE models always leave the choice of the exact standards to the educational authority, so that families can influence the choice of standards according to their community's preferences.

Additional Work for Teachers

- Teachers sometimes oppose OBE because of the amount of paperwork that often accompanies it. Rather than issuing a single letter or number to summarize an entire term's achievements, an OBE system may require that the teacher track and report dozens of separate outcomes. Some critics have objected to additional resources being spent on struggling students while some teachers find their marking workload significantly increases.

Outcome-based education promises high level of learning for all students as it facilitates the achievement of the outcomes, characterized by its appropriateness to each learner's development level and active and experience-based learning. Moreover, knowing that this system is going to be used would also give students the freedom to study the content of the course in a way that helps them learn it. OBE must involve administrators, educators, parents, teachers and students for successful implementation. Outcome-based education reforms emphasize setting clear standards for observable, measurable outcomes.

The key features which may be used to judge if a system has implemented an outcomes-based education systems are:
- Creation of a curriculum framework that outlines specific, measurable outcomes.
- A commitment not only to provide an opportunity of education, but to require learning outcomes for advancement. Promotion to the next grade, a diploma, or other reward is granted upon achievement of the standards, while extra classes, repeating the year or other consequences entail upon those who do not meet the standards.
- Standards-based assessments that determine whether students have achieved the stated standard.
- A commitment that all students of all groups will ultimately reach the same minimum standards. Colleges or schools may not "give up" on unsuccessful students.

Competency-based Education

"Eighty percent of success is related to attitude rather than competency".

Meaning and Definition

Competency-based education (CBE) is an institutional process that moves education from focusing on what academics believe graduates need to know (teacher-focused) to what students need to know and be able to do in varying and complex situations (student and/or work place focused).

Competency-based education is focused on outcomes (competencies) that are linked to workforce needs, as defined by employers and the profession. CBE's outcomes are increasingly complex in nature, rather than deriving from the addition of multiple low level objectives.

Competency-based education often necessitates more complex assessment, involving experiential learning assessment in field experience, demonstration in varying contexts, role play, use of standardized patients or clients, etc.

Competencies

Large skill sets are broken down into competencies, which may have sequential levels of mastery. Competencies reinforce one another from basic to advance as learning progresses; the impact of increasing competencies is synergistic, and the whole is greater than the sum of the parts.

Competencies within different contexts may require different bundles of skills, knowledge and attitudes. The challenge is to determine which competencies can be bundled together to provide the optimal grouping for performing tasks. Another challenge is designing-learning experiences that support students as they practice using and applying these competencies in different contexts. Continual refinement of defined competencies is necessary so that enhanced performance in a variety of contexts can be assessed. In essence, CBE is a process, not a product. In addition to clarifying educational outcomes as they relate to workforce needs and expectations, competencies are critical to linking course learning objectives to the instructional objectives.

Measurable objectives specify the minimum acceptable performance in terms of quality, quantity or time. These objectives are used by the institution to evaluate progress in meeting its basic educational mission and may be expanded as appropriate to encompass the complex nature or special focus of each institution.

All objectives and competencies, regardless of the level for which they are intended, should be specific, measurable and written in behavioral terms. Each should specify an observable learning outcome, and all objectives have two parts—an action verb and a content area.

Important Considerations

- Each set of competencies should be made available to school or program constituents, especially students. Competencies are equivalent to a "contract" between the student and the school or program. They state specifically what the student should expect to learn and be able to do upon completion of the program of study.

  This allows students to monitor their own progress and identify any gaps in skill attainment. Additionally, if an institution intends to assess student achievement and learning based on the identified competencies, it is imperative that they are shared with students.
- Competencies should be reviewed regularly and redefined to reflect the changing needs of public health practice.
- Finally, while course learning objectives are most appropriately developed by the course instructor (as part of a collaborative curriculum development process), instructional objectives and competencies should be developed through a process of consensus-building. Ideally, all affected parties should be involved

in their development, faculty in particular, but also students and representatives from the public health practice community and workforce quality assurance processes. The process of obtaining consensus will inevitably take longer than it would if the chair of the curriculum committee or the program director simply writes the competencies, but in the end will produce a sense of ownership.

Educational Objectives and Instructional Objectives

"Goals are not only absolutely necessary to motivate us. They are essential to really keep us alive".
—Robert H Schuller

Meaning and Definition

Educational objectives tell us what the learner should be able to do after undertaking an educational program. It is a statement which explains what the learner would be able to do after successful completion of an educational program that he/she was unable to do or could not do so well before. Educational objectives are the statements of those changes in behavior which are desired as a result of specific learner and teacher activity, which is a two-way process. It is usually derived from the aims of an educational program. It is stated as teacher centered, learner centered or behavior centered or subject centered (Fig. 2.3).

Types of Educational Objectives

Central Objective

It is otherwise known as the institutional objective. It corresponds to the aim of a particular educational program. A course objective may be a central objective. It is usually broad, comprehensive and clear. It refers to the capabilities of the individual trained by the institution. For example, after successful completion of the BSc nursing degree course, the student would be able to provide preventive and curative care to the individual and the community in health and in sickness.

Intermediate Objectives

It is arrived at by breaking down the professional functions into components or activities which together indicate the nature of the function. It is otherwise known as departmental objectives. It is derived from the institutional objectives. One institutional objective may give rise to several departmental objectives. For example, after completion of the course in child health nursing, the students would be able to provide preventive and curative care to the children and their family in health and in sickness.

Specific Instructional Objectives

Instructional objectives are statements which tell us, what the student should be able to do at the end of a learning period that he would not beforehand. Educational process aims at evaluation of the learner and not the teacher. It is advantageous to have objectives written in terms of learner behavior. It is specific and pertains to a particular learning activity. All specific learning activities are derived from the departmental objectives. It corresponds to or derived from precise professional tasks, whose results are observable and measurable against given criteria.

For example, the student would be able to draw 2 mL of blood sample from a child in not more than two attempts. A specific educational objective should be:
- Relevant
- Logical
- Unequivocal
- Achievable
- Feasible
- Measurable
- Observable.

Characteristics

The objectives should state what the learner must do under what circumstances with what degree of skill:
- It should be written in behavioral terms
- It should reflect the standard and the condition
- It must be reasonable in number
- It must be consistent with one another
- Each one should be distinctive but not completely independent
- It should be descriptive.

Purposes of Specific Objectives

For teachers:
- It serves as a guide for selection of content for teaching
- It describes behavior in terms of students performance
- It serves as a basis for evaluation.

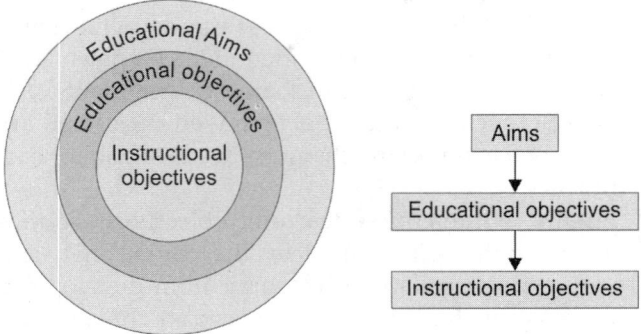

Fig. 2.3: Relationship between educational objectives and instructional objectives.

For students:
- Students can understand what they are supposed to learn or master at the end of the program
- Gives direction to the students toward in-depth study.

Elements of Specific Objectives

The four elements are:
1. **Condition**: It is the condition under which the learner should display the desired behavior. For example, after attending the class on hypothesis, the students will be able to formulate the hypothesis.
2. **Activity or behavior**: It denotes the behavior or action the learner is expected to perform after attending a class. For example, the learner will be able to calculate the drug dosage or administer injection or list out the causes of obesity.
3. **Standard**: It is otherwise known as criterion. It states the norms or acceptable level of performance expected from the student. For example, the learner will be able to start IV line with a single attempt. The learner will be able to list four causes of anemia. Here, the single attempt or four causes are the standard.
4. **Content**: It describes the subject, object or theme in relation to which the activity is performed.

An instructional objective should consist of all the above mentioned four criteria. A few examples have been illustrated below.

Example 1: At the end of the class on instructional objectives, the students will be able to name the four criteria of an instructional objective.

At the end of the class on instructional	- Condition
Name	- Behavior
Four criteria	- Standard
Instructional objective	- Content

Example 2: At the end of class on health, the students will be able to define health by WHO correctly.

At the end of the class on health	- Condition
Define	- Behavior
Correct WHO definition of health	- Standard
Health	- Content

Example 3: At the end of the class on anatomy of heart, the students will be able to draw the structure of heart within five minutes.

At the end of class on anatomy of heart	- Condition
Draw	- Behavior
Within five minutes	- Standard
Anatomy of the heart	- Content

Taxonomy of Educational Objectives

The Taxonomy of Educational Objectives, often called Bloom's taxonomy, is a classification of the different objectives and skills that educators set for students (learning

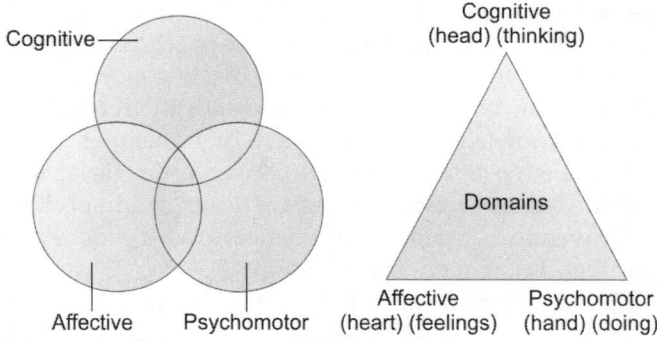

Fig. 2.4: Bloom's taxonomy.

objectives). The taxonomy was proposed in 1956 by Benjamin Bloom, an educational psychologist at the University of Chicago. Bloom's Taxonomy divides educational objectives into three "domains": Cognitive, Affective and Psychomotor (Fig. 2.4). Like other taxonomies, Bloom's is hierarchical, meaning that learning at the higher levels is dependent on having attained prerequisite knowledge and skills at lower levels (Orlich et al. 2004). A goal of Bloom's taxonomy is to motivate educators to focus on all three domains, creating a more holistic form of education.

A group of cognitive psychologists, curriculum theorists and instructional researchers, and testing and assessment specialists published in 2001 a revision of Bloom's taxonomy with the title "A Taxonomy for Teaching, Learning and Assessment". This title draws attention away from the somewhat static notion of "educational objectives" (in Bloom's original title) and points to a more dynamic conception of classification.

The authors of the revised taxonomy underscore this dynamism, using verbs and gerunds to label their categories and subcategories (rather than the nouns of the original taxonomy). These "action words" describe the cognitive processes by which thinkers encounter and work with knowledge. A statement of a learning objective contains a verb (an action) and an object (usually a noun). The verb generally refers to (actions associated with) the intended cognitive process. The object generally describes the knowledge students are expected to acquire or construct (Anderson and Krathwohl, 2001).

Cognitive Domain

According to Bloom, cognitive domain is concerned mainly with description of learning designed to acquire, recall or recognize knowledge and the development of intellectual abilities and skills of the students. This is also referred to as the "domain of intellectual skills". There are six levels in the taxonomy, moving through the lowest order processes to the highest. The cognitive process dimension represents a continuum of increasing cognitive complexity—from remember to create.

Remembering: It refers to recall of previously learned information. It is exhibiting memory of previously learned material by recalling facts, terms, basic concepts, and answers. The cognitive process includes the retrieval of relevant knowledge from the memory. It includes the:
- Knowledge of specifics: Terminology, specific facts
- Knowledge of ways and means of dealing with specifics: Conventions, trends and sequences, classifications and categories, criteria, methodology
- Knowledge of the universals and abstractions in a field: Principles and generalizations, theories and structures.

Example: The students will be able to state the names of medication.

Understanding: Demonstrate understanding of facts and ideas by organizing, comparing, translating, interpreting, giving descriptions, and stating main ideas. It requires remembering.

Example: The students will be able to interpret the type of anemia based on Hb values.

Applying: Using new knowledge, solve problems arising in new situations by applying acquired knowledge, facts, techniques and rules in a different way. It requires remembering and understanding.

Example: The students will be able to modify the nursing action when she observes a side effect of a particular medicine

Analyzing: Examine and break information into parts by identifying motives or causes. Make inferences and find evidence to support generalizations. It requires remembering, understanding and applying. It includes the following:
- Analysis of elements
- Analysis of relationships
- Analysis of organizational principles.

Example: The students will be able to compare the merits of hot and cold application.

Evaluating: Present and defend opinions by making judgments about information, validity of ideas or quality of work based on a set of criteria. It requires remembering, understanding, applying and analyzing. It includes the following:
- Judgments in terms of internal evidence
- Judgments in terms of external criteria.

Example: The students will be able to evaluate the effectiveness of treatment given.

Creating: Compile information together in a different way by combining elements in a new pattern or proposing alternative solutions. It requires remembering, understanding, applying, analyzing, evaluating. It includes the following:
- Production of a unique communication
- Production of a plan, or proposed set of operations
- Derivation of a set of abstract relations.

Example: The students will be able to prepare an individualized dietary plan for a woman with anemia considering all factors.

The table below gives a comprehensive picture of cognitive domain levels and verbs.

Level	Verbs
Remembering	Define, describe, identify, know, label, list, match, name, outline, recall, recognize, reproduce, select, state
Understanding	Classify, compare, contrast, demonstrate, explain, extend, illustrate, infer, interpret, outline, relate, rephrase, show, summarize, translate, comprehend, distinguish, estimate, explain, extend, generalize, paraphrase
Applying	Apply, build, choose, construct, develop, experiment, identify, interview, plan, select, solve, utilize, compute, demonstrate, modify, operate, predict, prepare, relate, change
Analyzing	Analyze, categorize, classify, compare, contrast, distinguish, differentiate, discriminate, examine, infer, identify, illustrate, outline, relate, select, separate
Evaluating	Appraise, assess, compare, conclude, criticize, determine, estimate, evaluate, explain, interpret, justify, describe, discriminate, relate, summarize
Creating	Combine, compile, compose, create, devise, design, explain, generate, modify, organize, plan, rearrange, reconstruct, relate, reorganize, revise, rewrite, summarize, formulate.

Affective Domain

This domain deals with description of learning tasks concerning changes in interests, attitudes, values, and the development of appreciations and adequate adjustments. Skills in the affective domain describe the way people react emotionally and their ability to feel another living thing's pain or joy. Affective objectives typically target the awareness and growth in attitudes, emotion, and feelings.

There are five levels in the affective domain moving through the lowest order processes to the highest.

1. **Receiving**
   It means becoming aware of an idea and of being willing to receive it and give some attention. It is the lowest level. Without this level no learning can occur.
   Example: The students will be able to identify the anxiety of a patient waiting for admission.

2. **Responding**
   It implies being willing to accept an idea, to respond to it.
   It requires receiving.
   Example: The students will be able to answer the doubts of the anxious patient waiting for a diagnostic procedure.

3. **Valuing:** It is accepting an idea or behavior as worthy, exhibiting preference for it over others and develops

sufficient commitment to promote it. It requires receiving and responding.
Example: The students will be able to explain the ward routines to the patient who is newly admitted.
The students will be able to demonstrate concern over the patients with anxiety.

4. **Organizing:** It means conceptualizing a value. It requires receiving, responding and valuing.
Example: The students will be able to organize a counseling session for a patient experiencing anxiety.

5. **Characterizing:** It implies integration of the value into a total philosophy in such a way that it becomes a consistent and predictable behavioral characteristic. It requires receiving, responding, valuing and organizing.
Example: The students will be able to perform assessment for anxiety for all patients.

The learner has held a particular value or belief that now exerts influence on his/her behavior so that it becomes a characteristic.

The below table gives the comprehensive picture of affective domains and the verbs

Level	Verbs
Receiving	Follow, select, rely, choose, point to, ask, hold, give, locate, attend
Responding	Read, confirm, help, answer, practice, present, report, greet, tell, perform, assist, recite
Valuing	Initiate, ask, invite, share, join, follow, purpose, read, study, work, accept, argue
Organization	Defend, alter, integrate, synthesize, listen, influence, adhere, modify, relate, combine
Characterization	Adhere, relate, act, serve, use, verify, question, confirm, propose, solve, influence

Psychomotor Domain

This domain deals with acquisition of physical abilities, motor or muscular skills, and manipulation of objects or acts requiring a neuromuscular coordination. Skills in the psychomotor domain describe the ability to physically manipulate a tool or instrument like a hand or a hammer.

Psychomotor objectives usually focus on change and/or development in behavior and/or skills.

Bloom and his colleagues never created subcategories for skills in the psychomotor domain, but since then other educators have created their own psychomotor taxonomies.

Simpson's Categorization

Perception

Becoming aware of objects, qualities and relations through sensory input, recognizing cues and relating to potential actions.

Example: The students will be able to identify the need for performing personal hygiene.

Set

The mental, physical and emotional readiness to initiate some kind of action.

Example: The students will be able to proceed to set the articles for performing the procedure.

Guided Response

An overt action that follows selection of an appropriate response and one that may represent imitation or trial and error.

Example: The students will be able to reproduce the steps of procedure as demonstrated.

Mechanism

Action has become part of a repertoire and can be employed with confidence under most circumstances.

Example: The students will be able to display basic skills in performing the procedure.

Complex Overt Response

Action performed without hesitation and with a high degree of skill.

Example: The students will be able to display coordination, speed and accuracy in performing the procedure.

Adaptation

Actions and skills are modified to fit special requirements or to meet a problem situation.

Example: The students will be able to reorganize the steps according to the patient needs.

Origination

Creation of new pattern to fit a particular situation of specific problem—emphasis is on creativity based upon highly developed skills.

Example: The students will be able to create new steps/techniques of doing the procedure at different settings.

The below table gives a comprehensive picture of psychomotor domain levels and verbs.

Level	Verbs
Perception	Choose, describe, detect, differentiate, distinguish, identify, isolate, relate, select
Set	Begin, display, explain, move, proceed, react, show, state, volunteer
Guided response	Copy, trace, follow, react, reproduce, respond
Mechanism	Assemble, calibrate, construct, dismantle, display, fix, grind, heat, manipulate, measure, mend, mix, organize, sketch

Contd...

Contd...

Complex overt response	The keywords are the same as mechanism, but will have adverbs or adjectives that indicate that the performance is quicker, better, more accurate, etc.
Adaptation	Adapt, alter, change, rearrange, reorganize, revise, vary
Origination	Arrange, build, combine, compose, construct, create, design, initiate, make, originate

Harrow (1972) Jewett and Mullan (1977) presented a four level taxonomy for psychomotor domain which can be seen as follows:

Fundamental Movement

They are those that form the basic building blocks for the higher level movement. For example, the students will be able to hold the syringe properly.

Generic Movement

It refers to the ability to carry out the basic rudiments of a skill when given directions under supervision. At this level, efficient motor patterns, timing and coordination are being developed and refined. However, the total act is not performed with skill. For example, the students will be able to perform hot application under supervision.

Ordinate Movement

It makes the competence in performing a skill ably and independently. The entire skill has been organized and can be performed in sequence. Conscious effort is no longer needed. The skill is mastered and there is precision of performance. For example, the students will be able to measure the blood pressure accurately.

Creative Movement

The individual will be able to invent unique motor option or improvise originality into a movement or invent a new motor pattern.

Level	Student actions
Fundamental movement	Track, crawl, hear, react, move, grasp, walk, climb, jump, stand, and run
Generic movement	Drill, construct, dismantle, change, clean, manipulate, follow, use, march, and hop
Ordinate movement	Play, connect, fasten, weigh, wrap, manipulate, play, repair, write
Creative movement	Create, invent, construct, manipulate, play, build, perform, make.

Lesson Plan

"A man who does not plan long ahead will find trouble right at his door".
—Confucius

A lesson plan is actually a plan of action. A lesson plan reveals the knowledge and philosophy of the teacher, her understanding of students, objectives of education, the content to be taught and teaching ability to utilize appropriate method of teaching. —*LB Sands*

Lesson plan is the title given to a statement of achievement to be realized and the specific means by which these are to be attained as a result of the activities engaged in during the period. —*NL Bossing*

Purposes
- It guides the teacher in presentation of subject matter and activities involved
- It provides definite objective for each day's work
- It helps to achieve definite goals and objectives
- It makes teaching economical, systematic and orderly
- It tends to prevent wandering from the subject
- It helps to maintain sequence of content presentation
- It aids in time management
- It keeps the teacher on the track, ensure steady progress and a definite outcome of teaching and learning
- It is essential for effective teaching
- It helps to enhance learning process
- It prevents waste of time
- It helps the teacher to delimit the teaching field
- It is useful to select proper learning and best technique
- It helps to avoid repetition
- Planning encourages the teacher to consider the need and level of understanding of students
- It gives the teacher greater confidence and greater freedom in teaching
- It helps the teacher to overcome the feeling of nervousness and insecurity
- It aids in deciding in advance of the AV aids and techniques of teaching
- It helps in teaching and learning outcomes
- It facilitates self and peer assessment of teaching and future improvement of lessons
- It provides guideline to the student teacher.

Points to Remember in Planning a Lesson

- It should contain only main points or ideas or concepts. It is not necessary to write down every word the teacher is going to say.
- The teacher can use her own subject notes which are different from the lesson plan.
- The teacher should not become over dependent on the lesson plan. The plan must be flexible, not rigid and adjusted according to the situation arising in the classroom.
- Fresh plan should be prepared every time a teacher prepares.
- Design for sequencing the subject matter (main heading, subheading, etc.)
- Planning must be done keeping in mind the level of understanding of the students and their previous experiences.

- The method of teaching plan should be based on the objectives to be attained (cognitive, affective, and psychomotor)
- Psychological factors related to learning should also be remembered
- Motivation to maintain interest and attention of the class is important
- Each lesson is planned in such a way that the objective of each lesson lead to the statement of unit objective then course objective and finally the objective of the curriculum.

Prerequisites for Good Lesson Planning

- The teacher should clearly state objectives
- The content should be linked with the previous knowledge of the students
- The teacher must have adequate mastery
- She should understand the students' interest and background
- She must be fully conversant with new methods and techniques of teaching
- The teacher must have a good understanding of psychology of learning, philosophy of education, etc.
- She must ensure active learner participation during a class and maintain interest and motivation of the student
- There should be variety and novelty in type of presentation
- It should not be too detailed and exhaustive
- It is preferably being written
- It should be flexible
- It should be relevant, clear, and feasible
- The teacher prepares lesson plan in such a manner that it should provide full justification to all students of varied abilities
- The lesson plan should include the methods of self-evaluation and self-criticism of the teacher
- It also should include the summary and reference materials.

Types of Lesson Plan

Lesson plan can be prepared for acquiring knowledge that is called knowledge lesson plan (cognitive domain), and it also can be prepared for affective domain and psychomotor domain.

Essential Elements of Good Lesson Plan

- Front page data such as subject, topic, class, duration, etc.
- General learning objectives/central objectives
- Specific learning objectives/behavioral objectives
- Evaluation of previous knowledge
- Set induction
- Selection and organization of subject matter—the content
- Organizing centers includes learning activities and teaching activities
- Types of illustrative material—AV aids
- Assignments
- Evaluation
- Follow-up action.

Steps in Developing a Lesson Plan

Preparation

It is a stage in which the teacher decides on the objectives, teaching learning methods and materials and she prepares it. At the end, she is ready with the write up plan and is ready to proceed for teaching.

Presentation

In this phase, she actually presents the content. She adopts various techniques and methods of teaching as planned earlier. She uses various audio-visual aids to facilitate teaching and learning. The way she communicates the information is very important. She should possess communication skills, interpersonal skills, etc. She compares and associates various concepts. Questioning, discussions, and appropriate examples from real life situations should be used to make the presentation interesting and to motivate the students to learn. While presenting the content, she compares or makes association of facts and principles. She also uses the principles of generalization and application.

Summarization/Recapitulation

After presentation, the teacher summarizes the whole content and stresses the important points and concepts. It helps the student to recall whatever she has learned. It is useful for the teacher too to recall whatever has been taught and identify any omissions so that the teacher can explain at this stage.

Evaluation and Feedback

The teacher evaluates the effectiveness of teaching and learning by various methods. Questioning is one of the effective methods used in evaluation. The teacher should follow the techniques and principles of questioning. She also can evaluate by conducting tests and giving assignments. Based on the evaluation, she has to take remedial measures for those who have not learned the concept effectively.

How to Prepare a Lesson Plan

- Topics for lesson plans are derived from the institutional and departmental objectives and course outline.

- The topic is broken down into subtopics pertaining to different domains.
- The topic and subtopics are converted into learning objectives (general and specific).
- Objectives should be stated in clear terms and specific objectives should be measurable and observable.
- Lesson time should be appropriately divided among different objectives.
- An effective set inducer that could arouse the interest of the learners has to be planned. This calls for creativity and innovation.
- To prop up learner attention, an interaction should be incorporated after about 20 minutes.
- Some follow-up activity should be arranged to strengthen and extend the message of the lesson.

Teachers' Requirements in Lesson Planning

- Mastery over the content
- Efficiency of content analysis and identifying learner's objectives in terms of taxonomic categories
- Ability to state the objectives in behavioral terms
- Skill in choosing appropriate teaching learning methods and AV aids
- Competency in using various evaluation techniques
- Ability in planning, organizing, reinforcing the students activities, and controlling their behavior
- Ability in acknowledging the individual differences of students.

Unit Plan

"A good plan is like a road map: it shows the final destination and usually the best way to get there".
— *H Stanley Judd*

Unit may be defined as a large subdivision of the subject matter. Planning the unit is known as unit planning.

Criteria for a Good Unit

- Principle of learning by whole
- Principle of simple to complex
- Principle of concrete to abstract
- Principle of integration
- Principle of relatedness
- Principle of specification
- Principle of sequence
- A good unit includes the scope for variety of learning experiences in relation to the subject matter learned
- A good unit places all the relevant topics together
- It helps us to plan for time specification to complete the unit, scheme of evaluation, etc.

Characteristics of Unit Planning

Unit planning recognizes that:
- Learning takes place most effectively in terms of whole rather than fractions
- Learning is developmental and, therefore, provides for vertical and horizontal organization of learning experiences
- Learning is maximum when there is an understanding and acceptance of goals to be achieved
- Learning needs differ in accordance with individual difference and learning interest
- Learning leads to self-directed behaviors
- Unit planning provides sound basis for evaluation.

Types of Unit Planning

Subject Matter Units

This again can be classified as:
- Topical units
- Generalization units, and
- Units based on significant aspects of environment and culture.

Subject matter units are used more widely by teachers for its easy organization. The primary emphasis of the subject matter unit is on materials to be learned. The arrangement of the subject matter and the learning activities will be shaped in accordance with the objective. Unless what is learned is understood by the learner, learning the subject matter will be of no use to the learner. In this, subject matter is given primary consideration over the learner.

Experience Unit

This is again classified as units based on center of interest, student purpose, and student needs.

Experience units on the other hand is planned by organizing the learning around or bound together by a central theme of interest. It can be used in clinical nursing studies of nursing students as taking a case study of patient otherwise the formal or theoretical part of nursing curriculum will benefit very little from this type of organization.

Teaching-learning Unit

The term "teaching-learning unit" is used by Heidgerken to describe unit planning for nursing courses. The term embodies the concept of useful learning experiences which involve comprehensive problems or projects focused on stated objectives. It permits the inclusion of knowledge components and a series of selected and organized teaching-learning activities to provide learning outcomes specified by the objectives.

Process Units

It is based on the thought process, for example, problem-solving. It is further subdivided into unit of discovery, normative units (norms and values), and unit of criticism.

Resource Units

It is compendium of suggested activities and materials, accompanied by statement of objectives, scope, educational resource materials and suggestions for everything used by teachers in their preparation for teacher-student unit planning. It serves as a guide for teacher and is constructed by a group of faculty members.

Essential Activities in Planning a Unit

There are certain common activities which are involved while planning and developing teaching-learning units. These include:
- **Selection and statement of objectives:** The teacher must select and state the objectives in behavioral terms for each unit.
- **Selection of unit plan:** The type of unit selected will be influenced by various factors. It will also depend on the ability and the experience of the teacher. Each teacher will have to select and plan the unit according to her teaching ability and mastery of the subject matter.
- **Selection of the learning situation:** The teacher has to decide the learning situations in which the unit is taught such as classroom, laboratory, and the community where students get rich learning experiences. The students should be given the right type of situations at the right time and under supervision and guidance of experienced faculty members. The learning outcomes in each situation should be evaluated.
- **Selection of content:** The knowledge or the content component of the unit plan refers to all the knowledge in the form of facts, concepts, and principles, etc. which are required to attain the objectives of the unit.

The subject matter can be from the textbook or body of materials composed of facts, information, principles, and generalizations which are organized into the fields of knowledge. Subject matter is experience and so a teaching-learning unit is drawn upon many sources for its knowledge component, i.e. textbooks, reference books, periodicals, etc.

It also includes the study of a patient or client at a hospital, home or clinic or any other life situation which may serve as an educational source. The content and learning experience for a unit vary according to the:
- Type of unit
- Objectives
- The field of study.

- **Distribution of time** and the allotment of time for the course is also another important factor influencing type and the content of unit.
- **Organization of the content of unit:** The content should be organized so as to produce a cumulative effect, reinforced in a manner to create a broader and deeper understanding of knowledge base as well as to develop, refine, and strengthen the skills already acquired.
- **Selection of teaching and learning activities:** The selection should be made keeping in mind the curriculum, administrative pattern and policies, available educational resources and flexibility, providing opportunities for students to practice the behavior they are expected to develop as a result of participation in these activities. There should be continuity, sequence and integration in organizing these activities so that they become meaningful and motivating experiences for the learner.
- **Teacher's expertise:** The teacher should have the knowledge of the subject, of the learners for whom she is planning the course, the unit, etc.
- **Selection of methods of evaluation:** The selection of adequate methods of evaluation and their use are very important in teaching and learning which should be included in unit planning.
- **Selection of reference:** The teacher should give the references to the students for their self-study according to their needs and levels. The teachers should also use the library regularly for keeping themselves updated.

Steps in Writing a Unit Plan

- Read the subject matter related to the topic in detail
- Discuss with experts on the subject and also refer to university syllabus
- Include students and develop the unit cooperatively by the teacher and student
- Write down the details such as the title of the unit, number of hour required to teach and the practical experience, placement in the curriculum, etc.
- Formulate the central objectives and contributory objectives
- Identify the content area and the methods of teaching
- Plan the teaching-learning activities to attain the objectives
- Select the instructional aides to be used
- Plan the experiences—clinical, laboratory and visits, etc.
- Decide on the approximate number of hours to be given to classroom and clinical learning
- Plan appropriate methods of evaluation and select the tools or construct test for evaluation
- Provide a list of books, journals, etc. for reference.

Course Outline

"Men never plan to be failures; they simply fail to plan to be successful".
—William Arthur Ward

Meaning and Definition

A course may be defined as a complete series of studies leading to graduation or a degree. It could also mean any of the separate units of instruction in a subject made of lectures and classes. For example, as in the case of BSc (N) degree course, a student has to complete several short courses such as a course in Anatomy, Physiology, Psychology, Fundamentals of Nursing, etc. in order to obtain BSc (N) degree. Each of these separate subjects is also called as a course. Year plan refers to planning the courses of instruction for a year. The subject content and learning experiences need to be organized so that they serve the educational objectives. All the relevant subject matters are organized under one course heading. It refers to planning course of instruction.

Principles of Course Outline Planning

- State the objectives for each course in behavioral terms which are to be achieved
- **Establish sequence:** arrange the content according to the learning experiences from simple to complex, known to unknown, whole to part
- Ensure logical and psychological continuity
- Organize the content focusing on the students rather than subject matter
- It should allow for individual differences and according to the level of students
- There should be a logic in organizing units and also should allow for problem solving
- Promote cumulative learning: Provide for reinforcement and recalling of already learned concept. The course should be organized in such a way that there is an integration of old and new concepts and encourage cumulative learning.
- **Integration:** The teachers have to plan for horizontal coordination of subjects by relating all the relevant subjects together. It aids in transfer of knowledge from one area to the other area very easily.
- **Avoid repetition:** The common topics can be combined in order to reduce the bulk of content and avoid repetition of the subjects or topics.
- It should be acceptable by all teachers.
- The course should provide variety in modes of learning. The course should include different methods of learning such as role playing, group discussions and problem solving approach, etc.

Content for a Course Plan

- State the objectives to be achieved or outcomes to be attained through the given course. For example, pediatric nursing.
- Specify the level of learners (I, II, III, IV years)
- Give a brief course description
- Mention the placement of the course within the curriculum. For example, a course in Nursing Foundation is placed in the I year of nursing curriculum
- Organize the content in topicwise and unitwise
- Describe the resource materials and methods of teaching in various set-up
- Give the plan of learning activities for students
- Describe the scheme of evaluation such as concurrent and terminal evaluation
- Give references for teachers and students
- Include a separate plan for practical learning.

Levels of Course Planning

Courses are planned at university level, institutional level and instructional level. The teacher will plan the course-based on the broad outline given by the university syllabus/INC syllabus. Each college/institution plans the course curriculum for implementation at the institutional level. The teacher, who is responsible for teaching a course, makes a detailed plan including objectives, content, teaching methods, resources, AV aids and selects learning experiences required to achieve the objectives and selects appropriate methods of evaluation.

Purpose

Teachers plan the units of work and the lesson for each course, linking it to previous learning of the students as well as related to the needs of students. Without planning, there will be little unity and cohesion in what is being learnt. It could be just a collection of unrelated facts. Students' participation in course planning is important to achieve the objectives. It also should be done based on sound educational and psychological principles.

Structure of the Course Plan

In planning courses two distinct areas of planning are involved.
1. Identifying the kinds of elements around which specific learnings are to be organized. This refers to the area of human experiences—the knowledge, the understanding, etc.
2. Selection of specific organizing centers on which the learners' interest and needs are focused.

Elements of Course Planning

A course plan should contain:

Objectives

These may be general for the entire course. These may be the central objectives of all units in the course which lead to the attainment of general objectives for the course.

Specification for a Level of Learner

The stated objectives should be according to the level of the learners. This will include the information regarding the levels of the students (1st year, 2nd year and so on), prerequisites for the course (subjects to be learnt before starting the new course) and the experiences the student should have had prior to the starting of the course.

Placement in the Curriculum

It is also decided in advance the placement of the course in the curriculum such as placement in the 1st year or 2nd year and so on.

Resource Material Needed for the Course

The resource materials such as books, magazines, audio-visual aids, etc. should be decided in planning the course.

Unit Plans

The course can be divided into appropriate units, each unit specifies its objectives and teaching-learning activities.

Evaluation Measures

Course plan should include the evaluation measures to be used to assess learning of students and to measure the learning outcomes. More than one type of evaluation methods should be used such as written test, practical examination, class examination and quiz, etc.

Bibliography

Course plan must provide a list of books for reference for teachers and students. The students can do some reading on their own from the list of books provided for reference.

Classroom Management

"Every truth has four corners: as a teacher I give you one corner and it is for you to find the other three".
—*Confucius*

Classroom management and management of student conduct are skills that teachers acquire over time. These skills will be developed only after a minimum of few years of teaching experience. To be sure, effective teaching requires considerable skill in managing the myriad of tasks and situations that occur in the classroom each day. Skills such as effective classroom management are central to teaching and require "common sense", consistency, a sense of fairness, and courage. These skills also require that teachers understand in more than one way the psychological and developmental levels of their students. The skills associated with effective classroom management are only acquired with practice, feedback, and a willingness to learn from mistakes. Sadly, this is often easier said than done. As previously mentioned, personal experience and research indicate that many beginning teachers have difficulty ineffectively managing their classrooms. While there is no one best solution for every problem or classroom setting, the following principles, drawn from a number of sources, might help. Teachers with many years of experience have contributed to an understanding of what works and what does not work in managing classrooms and the behavior of students. The following information represents some of the things that good teachers do to maintain an atmosphere that enhances learning.

An Effective Classroom Management Context

These four things are fundamental for teachers:
1. Know what you want and what you do not want.
2. Show and tell your students what you want.
3. When you get what you want, acknowledge (not praise) it.
4. When you get something else, act quickly and appropriately.

Management of Physical Environment

Room arrangement:
- While good room arrangement is not a guarantee of good behavior, poor planning in this area can create conditions that lead to problems
- The teacher must be able to observe all students at all times and to monitor work and behavior. The teacher should also be able to see the door from his or her desk
- Frequently used areas of the room and traffic lanes should be unobstructed and easily accessible
- Students should be able to see the teacher and presentation area without undue turning or movement
- Commonly used classroom materials, e.g. books, attendance, pads, and student reference materials should be readily available
- Some degree of decoration will help add to the attractiveness of the room
- The space should be adequate for the students for easy movement and it should not be too congested
- Natural lighting and ventilation can be enhanced by having adequate windows. Also there should be provisions for artificial lighting and ventilation for

use in case if the natural lighting and ventilation is inadequate
- Classrooms are constructed in such a manner that the noises are contained
- Furniture for students and teachers are designed for comfort, utility and enhance learning.

Management of Students

Setting expectations for behavior:
- Teachers should identify expectations for student behavior and communicate those expectations to students periodically.
- Rules and procedures are the most common explicit expectations. A small number of general rules that emphasize appropriate behavior may be helpful. Rules should be posted in the classroom. Compliance with the rules should be monitored constantly.
- Regulations particularly safety procedures should be explained carefully.
- Because desirable student behavior may vary depending on the activity, explicit expectations for the following procedures are helpful in creating a smoothly functioning classroom:
    - Beginning and ending the period, including attendance procedures and what students may or may not do during these times
    - Use of materials and equipment such as the pencil sharpener, storage areas, supplies, and special equipment
    - Teacher-led instruction
    - Seatwork
    - How students are to answer the questions, e.g. no student's answer will be recognized unless he raises his hand and is called upon to answer by the teacher
    - Independent group work such as laboratory activities or smaller group projects
    - Good discipline is much more likely to occur if the classroom setting and activities are structured or arranged to enhance cooperative behavior
    - Managing student academic work.
- Effective teacher-led instruction is free of:
    - Ambiguous and vague terms
    - Unclear sequencing
    - Interruptions.
- Students must be held accountable for their work.
- The focus is on academic tasks and learning as the central purpose of student effort, rather than on good behavior for its own sake.

Managing Inappropriate Behavior

- Address instruction and assignments to challenge academic achievement while continuing to assure individual student success.
- Most inappropriate behavior in classrooms that is not seriously disruptive and can be managed by relatively simple procedures that prevent escalation.

    Monitor students carefully and frequently so that misbehavior is detected early before it involves many students or becomes a serious disruption.
- Act to stop inappropriate behavior so as not to interrupt the instructional activity or to call excessive attention to the student by practicing the following unobstructive strategies.

    Moving close to the offending student or students, making eye contact and giving a nonverbal signal to stop the offensive behavior.

    Calling a student's name or giving a short verbal instruction to stop behavior.

    Redirecting the student to appropriate behavior by stating what the student should be doing; citing the applicable procedure or rule.

    Example: "Please, look at the overhead projector and read the first line with me, I need to see everyone's eyes looking here."

    More serious, disruptive behaviors such as fighting, continuous interruption of lessons and stealing require direct action according to college regulation.

Promoting Appropriate Use of Consequences

In classrooms, the most prevalent positive consequences are intrinsic student satisfaction resulting from success, accomplishment, good grades, social approval and recognition.
- Students must be aware of the connection between tasks and grades
- Frequent use of punishment is associated with poor classroom management and generally should be avoided.
- When used, negative consequences or punishment should be related logically to the misbehavior
- Milder punishments are often as effective as more intense forms and do not arouse as much negative emotion
- Misbehavior is less likely to recur if a student makes a commitment to avoid the action and to engage in more desirable alternative behaviors
- Consistency in the application of consequences is the key factor in classroom management.

Role of Teacher in Classroom Management

The teacher has to take special interest in the classroom management. She should check daily for any problem in the classroom. It is also her prime responsibility to inform the concerned members for any problems like broken furniture, repair of electrical items and non-functioning of any objects in the classroom and get it repaired as early as possible. She should instruct the students regarding the

Table 2.2: Guidelines for effective and ineffective praise.

Effective praise	Ineffective praise
• Is delivered contingently upon student performance of desirable behaviors or genuine accomplishment.	• Is delivered randomly and indiscriminately without specific attention to genuine accomplishment.
• Specifies the praiseworthy aspects of the student's accomplishments.	• Is general or global, not specifying the success.
• Is expressed sincerely, showing spontaneity, variety and other nonverbal signs of credibility.	• Is expressed blandly without feeling or animation, and relying on stock, perfunctory phrases.
• Is given for genuine effort, progress or accomplishments which are judged according to standards appropriate to individuals.	• Is given based on comparisons with others and without regard to the effort expended or significance of the accomplishment of an individual.
• Provides information to students about their competence or the value of their accomplishments.	• Provides no meaningful information to the students about their accomplishments.
• Helps students to better appreciate their thinking, problem-solving and performance.	• Orients students toward comparing themselves with others.
• Attributes student success to effort and ability, implying that similar successes can be expected in the future.	• Attributes student success to ability alone or to external factors such as luck or easy task.
• Encourages students to appreciate their accomplishments for the effort they expend and their personal gratification.	• Encourages students to succeed for external reasons—to please the teacher, win a competition or reward, etc.

proper and effective use of furniture and other goods and also give appropriate punishment for any misuse. Refer Table 2.2 for guidelines for effective and ineffective praise.

Role of Student in Classroom Management

The effective classroom management lies in the hands of students too. They should develop the sense of discipline and accept the responsibility for their actions in the classroom. They should cultivate the habit of maintaining cleanliness, proper use of furniture and electrical goods. They should appreciate the value of each item in the classroom. Students should cooperate with the teachers in the classroom management.

Classroom Management Mistakes New Teachers Often Make

New teachers often:
- Overpraise students for doing what is expected
- Do not know the difference between praise and acknowledgment and when each is appropriate
- Fail to do effective long-range and daily planning
- Spend too much time with one student or one group and not monitoring the entire class
- Begin a new activity before gaining the students' attention
- Talk too fast and are sometimes shrill. Use a voice level that is always either too loud or too soft.
- Stand too long in one place
- Sit too long while teaching
- Overemphasize the negative
- Do not require students to raise hands and be acknowledged before responding
- Always too serious and not much fun
- Always too much fun and not serious
- Fall into a rut by using the same teaching strategy or combination of strategies day after day
- Ineffectively use silence (wait time) after asking a content question
- Are ineffective when they use facial expressions and body language
- Tend to talk to and interact with only half the class (usually their favorites, and usually on the right)
- Collect and return student papers before assigning students something to do.
- Interrupt students while they are on task.
- Use "SHHHH" as a means of quieting students (one of the most annoying and ineffective behaviors)
- Overuse verbal efforts to stop inappropriate student behavior—talk alone accomplishes little
- Settle for less rather than demand more
- Use threats to control the class (short-term, produces results; long-term, backfires)
- Use global praise inappropriately
- Verbally reprimand students across the classroom (get close and personal if possible)
- Interact with only a "chosen few" students rather than spreading interactions around to all students
- Do not intervene quickly enough during inappropriate student behavior
- Do not learn and use student names in an effective way
- Read student papers only for correct answers and not for process and student thinking
- Ask global questions that nobody likely will answer
- Fail to do appropriate comprehension checks to see if students understand the content as it is taught
- Use poorly worded, ambiguous questions
- Try to talk over student noise (never ever do this, because when you do, you lose and they win)
- Are consistently inconsistent
- Will do anything to be liked by students
- Permit students to be inattentive to an educationally useful media presentation (this happens a lot)
- Introduce too many topics simultaneously (usually the result of poor planning)
- Sound egocentric

- Take too much time to give verbal directions for an activity (an inability to focus and explain effectively)
- Take too much time for an activity (usually the result of poor planning)
- Are nervous, uptight, and anxious
- Overuse punishment for classroom misbehavior—going to an extreme when other consequences work better.

> **Examples of student misconduct in the classroom:**
> - Sleeping in class
> - Talking in class
> - Discourteous
> - Uncooperative
> - Late to class
> - Poor hygiene
> - Eating, drinking
> - Cell phones
> - Early exits
> - Dishonesty
> - Disorderly conduct
> - Physical/verbal abuse
> - Cheating
> - Threats of violence against self or others

Methods of Teaching

"The job of an educator is to teach students to see the vitality in themselves".
—Joseph Campbell

Introduction

Teaching methods are the stimulation, guidance, direction and encouragement for learning and also the means to achieve the desired educational objectives. Systematic attention to methods and materials of teaching as well as mastery of the subject matter are essential to promote positive learning. Selection of right method of teaching is important to impart knowledge in an efficient manner, and it also inculcates desirable values and proper attitudes and habits of work among the students.

A teaching-learning method will help the teacher to conduct teaching in an agreeable, student-friendly and successful manner by initiating and maintaining link between the subject matter and the student.

Teachers need to build their practice, increase their knowledge base and skills and adopt pedagogy in order to realize and maintain critical roles that teachers play between learner aspirations and learner achievements. The teacher should be innovative in using the various teaching methods to achieve the educational objectives.

Classification of Methods of Teaching

- Inspirational methods: Simulation and microteaching
- Expository methods: Lecture method
- Individualized methods: Programed instruction, self-study, case method, self-instructional module and computer assisted instruction, etc.
- Encounter methods: Role play, simulation
- Natural learning method: Field trips
- Discovery methods: Problem-based learning
- Group methods: Project method, socialized classroom method.

Based on the degree of dominance enjoyed by the teacher or learner, in the teaching-learning process, teaching methods can be classified into:
- Teacher centered methods
- Learner centered methods.

In the former, teacher plays an active role and the student's role is minimized to a passive listener. In the latter, learners actively participate in the teaching-learning process. Depending upon the quantity of audience a particular method can cater to, the methods of teaching can be divided into large group methods—small group methods and individual methods.

Principles to Follow in Selection of Methods of Teaching

The following should be kept in mind while selecting the methods of teaching:
- The educational and instructional objectives
- The content of the course
- The capacity and level of students
- In accordance with the psychological principles of learning
- In accordance with the teacher's capability and style
- The extent to which it can be used creatively
- The extent to which it stimulates creativity in the students
- Availability of resources.

Lecture Method

"A good lecture is a textbook plus personality".
— Flexner

> Be sure that your brain is loaded before you shoot off your mouth. On the other hand, because your brain is loaded, you do not have to empty it into your student.

Lecture is a "formal talk" given by a trained or experienced teacher to a large group of students that definitely includes clarification or the explanation of facts principles or relationships between various concepts that are directly related to the educational objectives.

The term "lecturing" is used by most of the people synonymously with lesson and teaching. It is a particular type of educational encounter in which a teacher transmits information to a number of students, with the teacher doing most of the talking and the students mainly listening or writing.

It is a careful presentation of facts with organized thoughts and ideas by a qualified person. For many reasons, among which tradition, necessity, convenience and choice are perhaps most important, the lecture continues to be the most common teaching method. Talking by teachers alone is a less effective one way communication. It can be made more effective by changing into a two-way communication by talking with students, where questions and answers and discussions become the major activity. Most of the times, it is the appropriate method of teaching available for the teacher.

Purposes of the Lecture Method

- To motivate, sensitize, and stimulate students in their pursuit of learning objectives
- To introduce a new topic or subject as this method aids in close and personal contact with the students
- To economically use staff time
- To provide structured knowledge about a determined concept
- To motivate and guide in hunting knowledge
- To arouse the students' interest in a particular subject
- To clarify difficult concepts and stress on main points
- To assist in preparing students for a discussion
- To promote critical thinking
- To influence students
- To facilitate good human relationship.

Factors Influencing Planning Lecture

Learner Factors

- Educational background of the student
- Previous knowledge
- Class size
- Learning styles
- Personality and intelligence.

Subject Matter Factors

- Domain of the objective
- Content to be learned
- Nature of the content, simple or complex.

Environmental Factors

- Audio-video aids
- Lighting and ventilation
- Noise and climate
- Infrastructure facilities
- Furniture
- Seating arrangements.

Psychological Factors

- Emotion
- Mood
- Memory
- Abstract thinking
- Concept formation.

According to Walters and Marks (1981), there are three kinds of lecture. They are the "ideal" or "pure", the "classical" and the "experiential".

The ideal lecture: The participants attend the lecture of their own willing and this implies commitment on their part. The role of the lecture is to persuade the audience by virtue of the beliefs and values that are shared by both parties. Lectures given by the politicians are the example of the ideal lecture.

The classical lecture: In our education system, attendance at lectures is seen as being largely compulsory, in contrast to the ideal lecture. The students attend the lecture with the focus of getting good grades and marks and this is more specific in its subject matter.

The experiential lecture: This form of lecture is used prior to experiential learning and is given to participants to explain the basic concepts and explanations about the issue in question.

> Tell them what you are going to say, then say it clearly and then tell them what you have said.

Strategies to Deliver an Effective Lecture

The lecture has to be well-organized so that the learners can follow throughout the lecture. In order to deliver an effective lecture it is essential that the lecture is planned, implemented and then evaluated effectively.

Planning for a lecture should include the following:

- **Preparation**:
  - Set the objectives. Teacher, while lecturing, should keep the educational objectives clearly in her mind.
  - Find out if there is a better teaching-learning method to attain the objectives.
- **Sequencing the lecture:** Identify the main points that need to be stressed. Teacher, while lecturing, should keep a central concept of the lecture in mind and its relativity to the educational objectives. The concept is to be completed in one delivery.
- **Organizing the material**:
  - Subdivide the lecture under headings. Each concept has to be broken into simple pieces of information and the sequence of these pieces has to be maintained
  - Select appropriate AV aids
  - Plan student preparation and follow-up activities
  - Allow group discussion/buzz session to solve problems and to gain arousal feedback
  - Have a written teaching plan.

Implementing a lecture involves:
- **Delivering the lecture**:
  - Begin the lecture by arousing interest
  - Present aims and objectives of the lecture in the beginning
  - Recognize limitation of time; avoid too much of material.
  - Do not speak fast; 100 words per minute are ideal
  - Vary the pace and loudness to avoid monotony
  - Use illustrative anecdotes to teach abstract and complex ideas; aim at concept learning by all the students
  - Appear confident, look at the learners, have eye contact and establish nonverbal contact
  - Assess learner response and react accordingly
  - Give 2–3 minutes break between main parts
  - Do not dictate notes; use handouts or chalkboard to convey the outlines of the lecture
  - Present a summary at the end.
- **Steps to improve active participation by learner**: The following steps may help to activate and hold learner attention.
  - Open the lecture with a series of questions that the learners should be able to answer at the end of the lecture
  - Have wider eye coverage of the student
  - Club the lecture with discussion
  - Allow time near the end of the lecture for students to write a summary of the main presentation or answer a few questions-based on the lecture
  - Follow the principles and techniques of questioning.

Evaluation of the Effectiveness of the Lecture

- Informal feedback in the class could be sought by noticing student behavior
- Formal student evaluation helps in assessing the effectiveness of the lecture
- Peer evaluation: Opinion of colleagues or supervisors is also obtained to assess the lecture
- Feedback is also obtained by analyzing the video or audio recording of the lecture.

Note-taking during lecture: Note-taking results in loss of time for reflection and discussion. Listening without note-taking is the best method, if the learnt material had immediate use. Duplicating summary (handouts) is the best method, if the learnt content had to be used at a later period. Writing down full notes or outline during the lecture is of little use.

Strategies for Delivering a Good Lecture

In nutshell, a good method of delivering an effective lecture is to ensure that the lecture content is not read out in a monotonous voice and preparing oneself emotionally to be able to present before the class. However, a lecture may be rendered ineffective if effective strategies are not implemented. Table 2.3 explains the characteristics of effective and ineffective lecture.

Table 2.3: Characteristics of effective and ineffective lecture.

Effective lecture	Ineffective lecture
Teacher-student interaction	Teacher dominating the lecture, little or no interaction
Two-way communication	One way communication
Shared responsibility	Both have not realized the objectives
Small group and problem solving activities are used. Sharing of information facilitates learning	No such activities. Depends only on teacher
Variety of supporting media	No supporting media
Limited note-taking required	Extensive note-taking required
Humorous and good interpersonal relationship	Monotonous and less interpersonal relationship
Obtains regular feedback	Very less or no feedback

Enlisted below are some of the effective strategies for delivering a good lecture.

Opening a Lecture

- Avoiding a "cold start"
- Minimizing nervousness
- Grabbing students' attention with interesting opening
- Varying the opening
- Announcing the objectives for the class
- Establishing rapport with the students.

Capturing Students' Interest

- During class, think about and watch the audience the students
- Vary the content delivery to keep students' attention
- Make the organization of the lecture explicit
- Convey one's own enthusiasm for the material
- Be conversational
- Use concrete, simple, colorful language
- Incorporate anecdotes and stories into the lecture
- Do not talk into one's notes
- Maintain eye contact with the class
- Use movements to hold students' attention
- Use movements to emphasize an important point or to lead into a new topic
- Use facial expressions to convey emotions
- Laugh at self when one makes a mistake
- Keep track of time
- Be humorous
- Use AV aids to stimulate the students.

Mastering Delivering Techniques

- Vary the pace at which one speaks
- Project one's voice or use a microphone
- Vary one's voice
- Pause. Watch out for vocalized pauses
- Adopt a natural speaking stance
- Breathe normally.

Learner's Criteria of a Good Lecture:
- Concentrates on concept-teaching; inculcates the main concept of the lecture into the mind of the learner
- Presents material clearly and logically
- Clearly audible, writes legibly and concisely
- Has mastery of the content and is an expert of the subject
- Maintains appropriate pace in lecture
- Uses constructive criticism while giving feedback to the students
- Stimulates critical thinking on the part of the learners
- Presents the material using the principles of learning
- Facilitates easy learning by moving from known to unknown and from simple to complex
- Appears confident and at ease
- Avoids excess of factual details
- Possesses good sense of humor
- Illustrates practical applications related to the subject matter
- Utilizes instructional aids judiciously
- Avoids personal mannerisms
- Appreciates learner's accomplishments
- Does not ridicule wrong answers
- Is democratic and friendly
- Invites questions and listens to answers
- Enjoys teaching and loves the subject
- Maintains eye-contact with the students, and do not teach the blackboard
- Maintains conducive and nonthreatening environment
- Above all, maintains good interpersonal relationship with the students.

Advantages of Lecture Method

Lecture, being the oldest method, has its own merits and demerits both for the teacher and the learner.

Though many creative and innovative methods of teaching have come into practice, lecture method remains to be the most prime method of teaching. No one can deny the importance and vitality of this technique. We cannot prevent any teacher from using this method as it is very natural and spontaneous for a real teacher.

Lecturalgia—"Painful lecture"
Causes:
- Lecture objectives were unclear
- Lecture was disorganized
- Lecturer did not relate to students
- Lecturer did not respond to students
- Lecture was boring.

Disadvantages of Lecture Method

The fact that "All teachers are not good lecturers" envisages that however vital, if not presented properly, the lecture method may become the most boring one and may not serve the purpose.

- Lecturing makes the learner more passive in the learning process. Most of the time, the students do not participate in the learning process, remaining dormant
- Attention span of the students decreases considerably after 20 minutes with a reduction of information assimilated
- As readymade information is being fed to the students, there is no place for any practical activity, observation, experimentation or demonstration

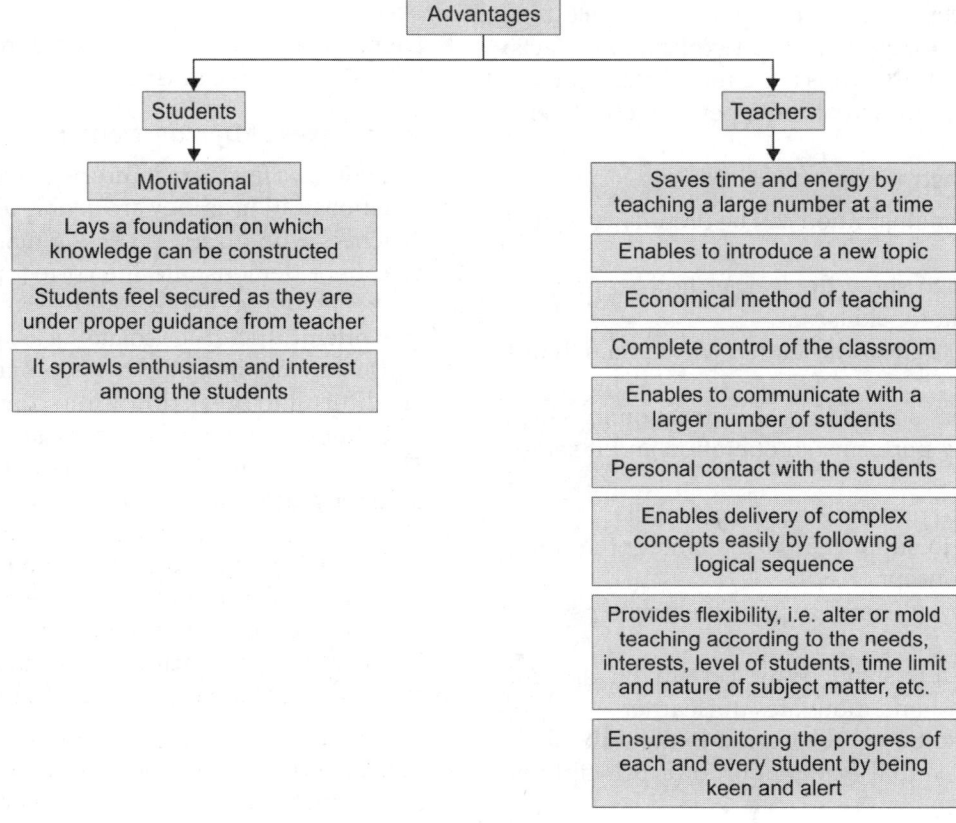

- This method pays little attention to needs, interests and abilities of individual students
- It may leave gaps in understanding, if the teacher is not having very good communication skills
- A very monotonous presentation may not be successful in attracting the students' attention
- Pace of lecture does not suit all students.

All these demerits are the drawbacks of the lecturer, not the lecture method. Hence, all these a teacher could overcome easily and this method could be used more successfully and productively.

Morning lectures seem superior to afternoon lectures for the recall on information, but this may not apply to the "evening type" of learner, whose maximum physiological alertness occurs between 1500 hours and midnight.

Demonstration

"Visualized explanation of facts, concepts and procedures".

Learning is more valued only when the knowledge acquired is combined with skill. Lectures, discussions and many other techniques are incomplete as they do not provide a combination of knowledge and skill. This flaw is always rectified by demonstrations. Demonstrations show the learners, how something works and what procedures to be followed in doing a particular job. Demonstration of the skills is often required in order for the learner to fully comprehend as well as apply the new knowledge, competencies, skills, concepts and or truth.

Demonstrations can be defined as an accurate portrayal of a procedure, techniques or operation (Laird 1986).

It can also be defined as "Visualized explanation of facts, concepts and procedures". It is a method which requires special skills and abilities in order to perform effectively.

Purpose of Demonstrations

The purposes of demonstration can be broadly classified into the following:
- Those designed to show the learner how to perform certain psychomotor skills.
- Those designed to show the learner why certain things occur.

A demonstration is a method of instruction in which the teacher actually performs an operation and it serves the following purposes:
- It may be used to provide a model of a skill
- It may be used to support an explanation of an idea, theory, belief, concept or skill
- It shows the learner "how" to perform certain psychomotor skill
- It also helps to understand "Why" certain things occur
- It arouses interest and motivates the learner
- It directs the attention of the learner to the skill
- It supports the verbal explanation of a principle or physical process
- It provides a visual image that contributes to encoding of information
- Demonstration provides a means to illustrate, clarify an approach and skill
- It is a method where a teacher involves many learners at one time, thereby aiding for an economical use of time, materials and equipment
- It shows a process in action.

Advantages of Demonstration

Demonstrations are an excellent way to illustrate points which enable the learner to comprehend complex and difficult material in a short period of time.
- When properly prepared, several minutes of demonstrations may accomplish more than hours of lecture.
- Demonstrations reduce the gap between theory and practice. The teacher can provide practical examples which reflect actual practice.
- Complex models and processes become real by way of demonstration.
- Demonstration activates more than one sense, which enhances learning. It involves visual, aural and kinesthetic sense of individuals that improves recall and transferability of the knowledge and skill learnt.
- Demonstration provides variety to the learning situations, thereby reducing boredom. Exchange of learning becomes more relaxed and joyful.
- Demonstration allows the learner, to see the exact manner in which a skill or behavior is to be performed.
- Demonstration trains the learner in the art of careful observation.
- Demonstration stimulates the interest of the learners by use of concrete illustration.

Disadvantages of Demonstration

- Sometimes, a few learners are negatively motivated after a demonstration as they are unable to perform the skill.
- Teachers who do not possess a mastery level of skill or cannot demonstrate the correct procedure and or her behavior may confuse and discourage the learners.
- It is often difficult to isolate tasks, skills, procedures and behaviors in a step-by-step manner. Some skills are difficult to break down into components and may be better understood from a holistic perspective.
- They may be time consuming, as they require more time for practice and review.
- Demonstrations are usually best with small groups.
- Even the most skilled and talented teacher may find it difficult to provide timely detailed feedback on performance to each individual in a group.

For the demonstration to be more effective, the demonstrator should possess certain skills and qualities.

According to Laird (1986) good demonstrators:
- Rehearse the presentation prior to delivery to make certain that information is correct and clear.

- Explain the goals of the demonstration at the beginning, in a two-way discussion with the learner.
- Present the operation one step at a time and explain each step as the demonstration proceeds.
- Allow the earliest possible tryout of the demonstrated skill, procedure or behavior.
- Reinforce everything learners do correctly in their practice session.

Role of the Demonstrator before the Procedure:
- Should have a clear understanding of the learning objectives.
- Formulate behavioral objectives for the particular demonstrative session.
- Perform a skill analysis of self and students.
- Possess mastery of skill and confidence in demonstrating.
- Analyze the process completely and break it into sequential steps.
- Have all material in place.
- Check the operation of all equipment before the demonstration.
- Assess the entry behavior of the students and determine prerequisites.
- Give an overview of the procedure to the students before demonstrating.

During the procedure:
- Conduct demonstration at a normal pace.
- Make sure everyone can see each step of the procedure.
- Proceed in a step-by-step fashion without carrying or overlapping steps.
- Motivate them by explaining why the skill is important.
- Demonstrate the total skill at normal speed.
- Follow sequence in demonstration.
- Ensure that a particular step is clear to the learners before proceeding to next step.
- Intersperse demonstration with lecture, discussion and questioning.
- Communicate clearly and directly.
- Avoid use of negative examples and variations in technique.

After the procedure:
- Get feedback from all learners.
- Arrange for return demonstration by the student.
- Provide immediate supervised practice, with adequate time allowance.
- Provide verbal, rather than physical guidance.
- Remember that initial interest may wane, so provide motivation and encouragement.
- Replace all articles and equipment.
- Ensure whether the learning objectives are attained or not.

Group Discussion

"Cooperative, problem-solving activity".

Discussion is an interchange of opinions and reactions, sharing of ideas and information regarding the solution of a problem or issue.

Definition

Discussion may be defined as a problem-solving activity which seeks consensus of the group regarding the solution of a problem rather than a decision by the majority.

According to Aggarwal, discussion is a thoughtful consideration of relationships involved in the topic or problem under study. These relationships are analyzed, compared, and evaluated for drawing conclusions.

Group discussion, basically is a cooperative, problem-solving activity, which seeks a consensus regarding the solution of a problem rather than a decision by majority vote. It is the working together in the search for the solution of a problem of common concern rather than just talking about a topic. It is a constructive process involving listening, thinking as well as speaking in utilizing relevant facts and ideas to advance the groups understanding and action.

Discussions may be formal or informal. Formal discussion is preplanned and guided by preset rules in order to achieve predetermined goals. Informal discussion is characterized by free verbal exchanges between the participants in the absence of preset rules or predetermined goals.

Purposes of Discussion Method

The purposes of the discussion method are:
- To make the learner to be an active participant in the teaching-learning process.
- To promote cooperative decision-making.
- To develop skills in problem-solving and decision-making.
- To develop communication and verbal skills of the student.
- To increase the knowledge, intellectual abilities and skills in the students.
- To promote group dynamics.
- To develop the skills of analyzing, comparing, evaluating a problem and drawing conclusions for the same.
- To share information.
- To foster democratic values.

General Principles for Organization of Discussion
- The goals and objectives of the discussion should be clearly defined and understood by all participants.
- An appropriate topic for discussion should be chosen that would stimulate the interest of the participants and invite their attention.
- Discussion on factual materials should be avoided, as nothing can be gained by discussing facts. It is merely a waste of time.
- The physical arrangement of the environment should be done in such a way that it promotes fair discussion.
- The members of the group should come well prepared; have basic knowledge about the topic to be discussed.
- The teacher has to guide and coordinate the proceedings so that the discussion should be kept to the point.

- The group leader introduces the topic, sets the time limits for various aspects of the discussion, and asks questions pertaining to the topic periodically so that important aspects are covered.
- A recorder should be selected from among the group, to record the main points of discussion as it is going on.
- Each one in the group should feel free to participate and everyone should be encouraged to get involved in the discussion.
- The discussion should be properly closed with a report, decision, recommendations if any or summing up of the matter discussed.
- All points of view should be fairly discussed.

Advantages of Discussion Method

- Discussion method of teaching is a democratic method used for teaching a particular subject and to supplement a lecture. It is an excellent student centered method.
- Discussion helps in clarifying and sharpening the issues. Old ideas and values may be replaced by new concepts.
- It helps the students to crystallize their thinking and identify concepts needed for their study.
- Discussion helps the students in discovering what he does not know and what he has over looked.
- Discussion engenders toleration of various viewpoints.
- Discussion activates thinking along the lines of self-evaluation. It is helpful in establishing an attitude of looking forward to progress and growth.
- It promotes conversational skills, listening skills, speaking skills among the students.
- It develops the capacity of respecting the ideas of others.
- It promotes group dynamics. A group learns together and presents important information, makes suggestions, shares responsibility, shows interest, respects the opinions and ideas of others, comprehends the topic, evaluates the findings, and summarizes the results.
- Discussion enhances the self-esteem of the students, as their opinions and suggestions are accepted.
- Active participation in the discussion not only results in better learning but also promotes retention and recalling ability of students.
- It helps the students to develop problem-solving skills, critical thinking ability, self-confidence and self-expression skills.

Disadvantages of Discussion Method

- Discussion is time-consuming.
- The teacher may find it difficult to control the group and sometimes a few students, who have very good communication skills may dominate the discussion.
- Both students and teacher are to be well prepared for the session otherwise discussion may not be productive.
- Discussion may be less effective when the number of students exceeds 20.

Forms of Group Discussion

Discussion techniques for small groups:
- Individual conference
- Informal class group discussion
- Seminar
- Role playing
- Case-analysis
- Clinical conference.

Discussion techniques for large groups:
- Multiple discussion groups
- Symposium
- Panel.

Seminar

"Exchange of ideas in some particular area; guided discussion of concepts".

Seminar is an instructional technique where the teacher takes less of a leadership role as students meet under the teacher's direction to discuss topics that are generally related to a particular subject.

Seminar can be defined as an exchange of ideas in some particular area; guided discussion of concepts.

A seminar as an instructional technique involves generating a situation for a group to have guided interaction among themselves on different aspects or components of a topic, which is generally presented by one or more members.

Teaching Tips

- Student preparation time may be reduced by having students rotated as discussion facilitators. So the individual student is responsible for an in-depth preparation of only a few topics.
- The teacher is a part of the group, sometimes acting as a participant or a consultant or the leader.
- Energy, creativity and planning by the teacher and the students are required for the effective use of this strategy.
- A clear connection of the seminar discussions to the course objectives is necessary or students will be bored and perceive the seminar as a waste of time.
- Some control is needed so as a vocal person (either student or teacher) does not dominate the discussion.

Important Features of a Seminar

- Seminar combines the formality of a lecture and the work of a simple discussion session. Seminars combine the formal presentation of material on a relevant subject matter combined with any form of discussions on the

floor or in groups. A talk or the reading of a paper by one or more persons is very basic to any seminar.
- Seminar is an academic get-together in which well-prepared papers are read by one or more persons followed by discussions of a variety of kinds. Not only schools and colleges, but various organizations hold seminars as a usual practice.
- A seminar is important because of a level of independence it has as an academic procedure to handle a topic of importance and to arrive at an understanding among the participants and to arrive at a set of conclusions.

A seminar offers opportunity for:
- A presentation of a short paper
- Establishing close contacts between presenter and audience
- Inquisitive and searching questions on the part of audience
- Controlled and guided discussion on the topic covered.
- Arriving at an understanding of a problem and its possible solutions on hand.

Discussion and listener participation are intrinsic to the very nature of a seminar and because of its characteristics, it gives the seminar greater scope for handling topics that are creative, communicative and perennial by nature. Seminars thus have greater relevance to teaching. This method has been accepted as part of the college curriculum.

Creative Aspects of the Seminar Method

The seminar method is a system which consists of a large variety of components or aspects that go into its making. The teacher should view the relevance of seminars from these aspects and try to tap its resources for the classroom.

The Art of Presentation

A seminar enables students to develop the art of presenting a discourse to an audience. Presentation of a paper or a talk to an educated audience is not a matter of joke. It is a more scientific, enlightened and concentrated activity and requires training at a higher level. Presentation in this context means those elements of public speaking that are required just for reading a paper in a meaningful and acceptable manner. A seminar is an opportunity for developing this specific element and teacher needs to keep this in mind while organizing a seminar.

Meaningful Interaction with the Audience

A seminar helps students develop the ability to achieve meaningful interaction with the audience. Meaningful contacts with the listener are important. A paper is read aloud, and reading aloud is always meant for others.

Developing the Paper for the Seminar is an Aspect that Requires Care and Training

Under the guidance of the teacher, the students organizes the material for the seminar. It provides opportunity to develop and organize the paper, keeping in mind the needs of the listeners and the role of the discussion that is played later.

Reference and Gathering Information

The seminar paper should be scientific in nature of a relative level. The material to be presented should have a theoretical basis for which the student should know how to use source books and materials. The teacher should guide the students in developing this skill of gathering materials from books. Seminars contribute to the development of the skill of reference in a significant manner.

Coordination of Materials and One's Frame of Mind

Seminar paper and its presentation help the student learn how to coordinate the information that he gathers with his frame of mind with reference to the topic. The students understanding of the topic is the framework in which he will build the new information. If this coordination is achieved, the presentation of the paper at the seminar will be most effective. The teacher can enlighten him in regard to the ways of doing this.

Developing the Art of Collective Thinking

Seminars provide opportunity to the students to engage in collective thinking. This is an aspect of the seminar. When the seminar paper is developed the student foresees the problems to some degree but collective thinking and group reasoning becomes a reality when the paper is presented. The student who presents the paper may not impose his ideas on the group but is required to lead the group step-by-step in developing a discussion by means of thinking and reasoning.

Answering Questions with a Focus

Another aspect of the seminar is its potential to help students answer questions with a definite focus. The framework of theory or practice that is presented through the people enables the leader to answer the participant's questions with a definite focus.

Learning to Defend One's Points

The seminar is an academic procedure that requires the student to defend his ideas. He presents a body of information through the paper that may naturally have some or other area that is relatively controversial. The student would have made references and gathered information from certain sources and only he knows the nature of these sources and how valid these points are. On several occasions, he is expected to defend his ideas and viewpoints during the discussion. This again requires training that is slow and painstaking. Seminars thus contribute to the development of how to defend one's viewpoint without hurting others.

Learning to Revise One's Position

Just as one needs to defend one's position that has a solid foundation, one also is required to revise and change one's position at a given instance when the participants has provided arguments to the contrary. It often happens that a new insight is obtained or someone highlights a point that one has not seen before and one's stand point has to be changed. It is called as obstinacy, when a student keeps on defending himself too far even after he is proved wrong. With a true sense of sportsmanship, the student should know how to give up his viewpoint and accept the new idea.

Participant Involvement

Seminars are providing ground for student involvement and for generating high level interaction. The participants should be able to have an involvement in the discussion and follow-up work. The teacher should regard this as an important aspect of the seminar and work toward it.

Each one of these aspects seen above goes into the making of a seminar. The teacher needs to be very conscious of this systematic perspective of seminar and guide students toward the effective implementation of these aspects.

Advantages of a Seminar

The seminar method has the following advantages:
- Facilitates active student engagement with content
- Collaborative, cooperative learning, peer sharing and dialog facilitates comprehension and practical application of concepts
- Allows teachers to role model, clarify concept and problem-solving
- Improves articulation in discussion
- Improves thinking skills
- Limited preparation time for teachers, but planning is still necessary to ensure effectiveness
- Does not typically require additional supplies like handouts or audio visuals
- Student can learn group problem-solving techniques.

Disadvantages of a Seminar

- Requires that students possess adequate knowledge for active discussion and comprehension
- May require high amount of student preparation time
- May allow a student to "slip through" without sufficient knowledge or thinking skills
- Students may require instruction in how to participate in seminars.

Symposium

"Investigation of a single problem from several points by a group with a special knowledge of the subject."

A symposium is a systematic presentation of different approaches of a single problem by group of two or more persons belonging to a particular discipline with a special knowledge of the subject. The main purpose is to investigate a problem from several points. As an alternative to the lecture method, for the presentation of a new material, symposium method can be used.

The symposium can be defined as a method of group discussion in which two or more persons under the direction of a chairman, present separate speeches which give answers to several aspects of one question (Hiedgerken).

In the words of Struck, "we think of a symposium as a group of comment either spoken or written, which portrays contrasting or at least different points of view".

Shortly it is a meeting for an exchange of ideas in some area; a guided discussion of a concept.

Purpose of Symposium

The chief purpose of the symposium is to clarify thought upon controversial questions. For presentation of new and sensitive issues or a concept, symposium may be most suitable.
- The main purpose of symposium is to analyze a problem from several different points of view.
- To relieve the students from boredom of monotonous lecture method.
- To make students active and alert as opposed to lecture method in which students are more or less passive listeners.

The Symposium Technique

In the symposium process, the participants present to the audience their views about various aspects of a selected problem or topic through speeches or paper reading.

The whole discussion process could be divided into three phases.
1. Preparation phase
2. Conduction phase
3. Conclusion phase.

Preparation Phase

- The apt topic for the symposium is selected and various aspects of the topic are spelled out. Planning

is the foundation for success of any activity, hence all planning regarding the discussion should be done well ahead of time.
- A group of participants, who are good in communications, are to be selected and from among them a chairman is selected. (Sometimes, the teacher may need more control of the group; hence, she may function as the chairman.) The ideal number of pupil participants in a symposium is four or five.
- It should be kept in mind that there is a clear connection of the symposium discussion to the course objectives necessarily or else students will be bored and perceive the symposium as a waste of time.
- Each member including the chairman should know the objective of the symposium and the breadth of topic to be discussed.
- All speeches to be prepared well ahead to avoid confusion and overlapping or repetition of material.
- Date and venue are to be decided.

Conduction Phase
- Chairman opens the topic for discussion with a brief introduction and also introduces the speakers to the audience.
- He sets the time limit for presentation of papers by the speakers.
- Chairman may also invite questions from the audience and directs the discussion. He maintains the sequence of information presented.
- Each speaker may be given an opportunity to make a final statement.
- The chairman finally sums up after all the speakers have spoken and closes the session.

Conclusion Phase
- The general audience listens to the discussions and each person forms his own conclusions based on the validity or value of the viewpoints presented.
- The chairman gives brief summary of all the speeches and opens the topic for discussion to the students.
- Finally under the leadership of chairman, a consensus is reached after verifying the pros and cons of different viewpoints expressed by the speakers as well as the participants.

Advantages of Symposium
- Promotes collaborative, cooperative learning, and peer sharing.
- Facilitates comprehension and practical application of concept.
- Improves the capability of students to approach a problem through various facts.
- Improves articulation in discussion and communication.
- It does not require any additional supplies such as handouts or audio-visuals.
- Students can learn group problem solving techniques.

Disadvantages of Symposium
- Requires extensive preparation and planning on the part of students.
- Time consuming.
- Requires that students possess adequate knowledge for active discussion and comprehension.
- Inadequate opportunity to participate actively for all the students.

Panel Discussion

"Small group discussion for the benefit of a larger group".

The panel method, originated by Professor Harry A. Overstreet is a discussion in which a few persons (the panel) who are qualified to talk about the topic carry over a conversation and discuss the given problem in front of an audience. The purpose of the panel is to reproduce the features of a small group discussion for the benefit of a larger group. The panel discussion does not try to solve a problem. Solutions or conclusions are seldom reached. It is a socialized group conversation in which difficult points of view are produced.

When handled intelligently and creatively, the panel stimulates thought and discussion and clarifies thinking. Because several people engage in a free exchange of opinions, the panel usually influences the audience to an open minded attitude and respect for the opinion of others. The quick exchange of facts, opinions, and plans develop a more critical attitude and better judgment.

Technique
A panel discussion is composed of three components:
1. The members of the panel
2. The chairman
3. The audience.

The panel consists of four to eight members, all seated in a semicircle facing the audience. The members of the panel should be prepared by knowing the limits of the topic to be discussed and the regulations which are to guide the discussion.

The members should be quick thinkers and facile talkers, and represent different points of view. The chairman does not contribute any ideas or information, but merely serves as a neutral referee and controls the trend of the discussion. He should be selected carefully, as the success of the panel will depend on his leadership. He should be a person with wide mental flexibility. The chairman must keep the discussion to the subject and see that all members of the panel get an equal opportunity to express their view.

The chairman begins the discussion by exploring the whole proceeding. First the members of the panel are introduced by name and background of experience. The topic is announced and the limits of the discussion are stated. The chairman may start the discussion by making a comment or two or by directing a question to a particular person. After that he keeps the conversation to the topic, encourages expression of the difference of opinion and organizes the discussion with occasional summaries. A general summary before discussion is opened to the audience.

Uses of a Panel

- A very effective group learning technique; students are directly and actively involved
- Encourages social learning
- Aids in attaining higher cognitive and affective objectives
- Develops ability of logical thinking and analyzing
- Helps to approach a problem in different points of view.

Limitations

- The panel is limited in its usefulness as a teaching tool because it makes no attempt to arrive at a solution. Another drawback is that the panel may lead to a certain tenseness of feeling if the topic is difficult to control.
- There are chances for deviation from the topic. Some members may dominate the discussion reducing other's opportunity.

Exhibition

"Visual treat with the purpose".

Many times, in the school or college, a particular department or class puts up their work for showing it to people outside the school, and such a show is called an exhibition. The pieces of work done by the students for an exhibition are called exhibits. Preparation, display, and explanation of exhibits by students provide them an excellent learning opportunity. It is worthwhile to display the projects done by the students and invite parents and others to see them and interact with the students.

For the school or college (especially a nursing college), who wish to foster close ties with the community around them, exhibitions are the most effective means to achieve it. If the exhibition is held in a prominent part of the institution, and people are invited to see the same, it will help the community members to know about the school or college, and appreciate the good work done by them.

Requisites for an Exhibition

An exhibition provides an excellent opportunity for the students to prepare projects and other exhibits by themselves, therefore induces better learning. For an exhibition to be of a good standard, the following requisites should be met:

- The exhibition should have a central theme with a few subthemes to focus attention to a particular concept
- The exhibits should be clean and labeled properly
- The concept of contrast in color and size should be used in preparing exhibits
- The exhibits should be so placed that most visitors can see them
- As exhibitions are meant to be mainly seen, all exhibits and the whole place should be well lighted
- To capture interest and attention of visitors, both motions and sounds should be utilized. All kinds of audio-visual materials relevant to the theme must be displayed
- The exhibition should have some exhibits with operative mechanism such as switches, handles, levers to be operated by the visitors to observe some happening
- The exhibition must include a lot of demonstrations as they involve both the students and the visitors more deeply
- The exhibition should be able to relate various subject areas to provide integrated learning, e.g. existing health issues and problems to create awareness to public.

Advantages of Exhibition

Exhibitions can serve as excellent teaching aids as they are able to capture the interest of the students and impart learning in a relaxed mood. Some of the advantages of exhibitions are as follows:

- Exhibitions inspire the students to learn by doing things themselves which automatically incurs a sense of involvement in them.
- They give students a sense of accomplishment and achievement.
- They develop social skills of communication, cooperation, and coordination.
- They foster better college–community relations and make community members conscious about the institution.
- They diffuse and disseminate knowledge among students easily by developing an interesting network among them.
- They couple information with pleasure.
- They foster creativity among students.

Disadvantages of Exhibition

Though exhibitions are considered as a creative and interesting method of teaching that reduces boredom,

there are also certain constraints in conducting an exhibition. They are as follows:
- Exhibitions need intensive planning on a focused manner otherwise the objective will not be met
- Exhibitions are time consuming. Preparing exhibits and conducting the exhibition requires a longer time span.
- Exhibitions are comparatively costlier than other methods of teaching.
- Unless very careful, can easily get diverted from the central theme.
- It should be kept in mind that the exhibits should be prepared by the students themselves using readily available and low-cost materials. The school can make use of the classrooms, corridors and quadrangles for laying out the exhibits. If utilized properly, exhibitions can serve as the best and successful method of teaching.

Field Trip

"A visit for an educational purpose".

Life in the classroom can cover only a small part of our total learning, and if learning has to be complete, it has to expand beyond the walls of the school. To attain this, school authorized, teacher planned, curriculum-integrated field trips are the most concrete and most real of visual techniques.

A field trip is especially planned for its possible contribution to the objectives of the curriculum, course, project, lesson or other unit of instructions. It is one of the most realistic educational procedures and the oldest method of teaching.

Definition

A field trip, also called as an observational visit, is defined as an educational procedure, by which the students obtain first-hand information by observing places, objects, phenomena or activities and processes in their natural setting to further learning.

Organization of a Field Trip

Organization of a field trip includes the following phases:
- Preplanning
- Actual conduct of the trip
- Evaluation phase.

Preplanning

Any project may fail badly if proper preplanning is not done. The teacher has to plan the following along with the students' participation:
- Decide on the trip
- Know the resources
- Obtain administrative sanction of the school/college
- Obtain permission from the organization that is to be visited and fix the date and time of visit
- Formulate objectives for the visit and inform them to the students
- List down specific information to be obtained
- Arrange transport
- Prepare a guide sheet and formulate questions to be asked to the guide
- Divide and allot the students into groups
- Brief students the following instructions—equipment and accessories needed, date and exact time of transport, actual location and setup of place being visited, conduct and behavior expected during the visit and safety precautions to be observed.

Actual Conduct of the Trip
- Follow the schedule exactly, avoiding alterations
- Strictly follow safety precautions
- Observe and collect information needed based upon the educational objectives
- Collect source/study materials as per availability
- Teacher has to be a good supervisor and should call the attention of the students toward pertinent points
- Observe formalities and extend courtesies.

Evaluation Phase

A well-planned follow-up session after the field trip increases its educational value. It should include a group discussion about the effectiveness of the trip and extent to which the educational objectives are obtained. Any learning material collected during the field trip should be displayed for others.

> **Teacher's role**
> - Watches students closely
> - Gives specific help as and when needed
> - Avoids frequent interruption
> - Avoids loud voiced comments
> - Acts as a guide, resource person or consultant
> - Supplements learning by timely explanation
> - Gives relevant follow-up activities.

Advantages of Field Trips

- Field trips supplement and enrich curriculum experiences
- They provide first hand experiences
- They break the monotony of classroom lectures, and add spice to the teaching of various subjects
- They offer varied types of experiences to the students
- They provide accurate information about objects, processes and systems in their real settings
- They involve all senses while learning
- They develop social skills among the students
- They are more meaningful and permit easier transfer of learning

- Ideals learnt in classroom can be better fixed in mind in actual situations
- Outdoors, students are able to work with large size materials. It can be used for review and drill.

Limitations of Field Trip

A field trip can provide learning to only one part of the curriculum rather than the whole syllabus. They are expensive and require proper planning to make them effective and meaningful.

Project Method

"Modern method of teaching based on the philosophy of pragmatism".

Project method is one of the modern methods of teaching in which the students' point of view is given importance in designing the curricula and content of studies. It is one of those methods which illustrate the use of problem-solving attitude.

Project method is the direct outcome of the philosophy of pragmatism. As both teaching and learning are experimental in character, this method is the most suitable one to test or assess the outcome of each and every educational activity, as it is more scientific and practical. It can be defined as "a whole hearted purposeful activity, proceeding in a social environment" (Kilpatrick).

According to Ballard, "A project is a bit of real life that has been imported into the school".

Qualities of a Good Project

"Learning by Living" is a better description of project method, according to Ballard. The peculiar qualities of this method are:
- Spontaneity: It is the necessary quality of the project because the project grows out of the students' own purposes. They are not forced to do anything.
- Aimed at a definite attainable goal.
- Purposeful: A purpose on the part of the learner is of absolute necessity, while doing a project. The student's whole mind is set toward the achievement of that particular goal.
- Significance and interest: When there is a strong purpose, then activity takes on great significance and creates intense interest to the student. The strong desire to achieve a certain end provides intense stimulus and increases the interest of the student in what he is doing.
- Learning activity of the project should be problematic in nature.
- Whole project is directed and planned by the student.
- Practical in nature with emphasis on a single complete unit of purposeful activity, resulting in a concrete achievement.

Types of Project

Project may generally belong to two forms:
1. Individual
2. Group.

The group projects are comparatively more valuable and usually called as the "socialized activities". They are the group enterprises providing rich experience in cooperation.

Another classification of projects is according to the purposes and objectives by which the learning activities are unified and shaped. This provides the following three types:
1. Projects calling for the production of some physical or material object (making a model).
2. Learning projects, where the chief concern is the acquisition of some ability.
3. Intellectual or problem projects.

Stages of a Project Method

A typical project method comprises the following stages:

Providing a Situation

The teacher has to be alert to recognize or create situations that are suitable for a project and should help the students to select their own project. Much opportunity should be given for the students to express their own ideas and to have discussions among themselves as well as with the teacher, in the initial step.

Choosing and Purposing

The aim of the project method is to teach students to think for themselves and to have the ability to select, choose and to carry out the project. The more the children feel that the subject and choice is their own, the better will they be able to plan and carry out their own chosen project.

Planning of the Project

The students themselves should plan out the project under the guidance of the teachers. Success of the project depends on the care with which the details of the procedures have been worked out. A good plan is to have the student to draw up a detailed written outline of how she intends to proceed and critically and deliberately examine every proposed step for the accomplishment of the project.

Executing the Project

Execution is the most interesting and vital phase of the project. The teacher should provide the students, opportunity for creative expression and self-activity. Care must be taken that the student's attention and energy are centered on educational value. The project should always lead to completion.

Evaluating the Project

The student should be given the necessary standards for evaluation of the project work. The students review their work, and try to see what mistakes they have made in planning or in carrying out their purpose. They learn to criticize their own work, which is very valuable.

A project may be said to be a success if judged by the following criteria:

The quality of the experience: It gives the students a socially valuable experience.

The activities of the students: The project is successful in which the students have the maximum responsibility left in their own hands.

Useful and practicable aim: A successful project is one in which the aim is useful and practicable.

Experience must be fruitful: The experience obtained from the project must actually bear fruit, i.e. the activities must be completed, knowledge must be gained and lead to further acquisition of knowledge.

Economy: We want the best results with the least waste. The students exert many efforts and do a great many things, but at the same time they should get the best results.

Role Play

"A dramatic approach to learning".

Role playing is relatively new educational technique in which people spontaneously act out problems of human relations and analyze the enactment with the help of other role players and observers. It is a small group discussion technique that makes it possible to get maximum participation of a group through acting out an example of some problem or idea under discussion.

A role play can be defined as "A dramatic approach in which individual students assume the roles of others".

What is a role?
A role is a patterned sequence of feelings, words and actions.

Aims of role playing:
- To illustrate interpersonal problems
- To gain insight into personal attitudes, values, and behaviors
- To understand about social and psychological issues
- To understand feelings and opinions of others
- To develop interpersonal communication skill
- To enable even the shy and introverts to express their views.

The Role Play Process

Role playing is one of the techniques of simulation. The students simulate the particular role of a person or actual life-situation, to depict a particular behavior. The role, false or actual, is performed in an artificial environment. This may give the student an understanding of a situation or relationship among real life participants of a social process. She will gain some perceptions of the actions, attitudes and insight of persons or situations.

Preparation Phase

The teaching staff has to plan thoroughly for the role play. They also need to be prepared to monitor and modify the student actions and reactions as necessary.

An ideal problem, which the group is concerned with or related to, should be selected. Situations that involve conflicting emotions provide good scenarios for the role play. A small group of four or five students are selected for the role play. Usually the students participant have to assume different roles voluntarily. Only then they can place themselves in the position of the characters.

Role plays are unscripted, spontaneous interactions in a simulated setting that are observed by others for analysis and interpretation.

Organization of Role Play

Organization of role play typically involves three stages, viz.:

1. **Briefing:** After having selected the problem, the stage is set and objectives for the role play for the concerned problem are structured. These objectives are briefed to all the members along with what is being expected out of them. This is the shortest stage.
2. **Running:** This stage includes the acting out of the role play. The scenes should be played simply, spontaneously, succinctly as far as possible. This stage may take from 5 minutes to 20 minutes. The behavior of players may help the audience to analyze the problem to recognize its outcome if it continues.
3. **Debriefing:** This stage includes discussion, analysis and evaluation of the role playing experience. This is the most important stage of role play, in which students can clarify actions, decisions and alternate decisions can be explained. Observation skills can be enhanced and other interpersonal reactions can be anticipated.

Videotaping or audiotaping of the role play may aid in the debriefing stage.

The techniques work better in small groups of students and all those students who are not involved in the role play can become active observers. Students should be encouraged to respond naturally to the role play and avoid phony acting. Criticism should be directed to the behaviors exhibited in the role play and not to specific students.

To put into nutshell, the activities of the role playing are:
- Warm up the group
- Select participants
- Set the stage
- Prepare observers
- Enact
- Discuss and evaluate
- Re-enact
- Discuss and evaluate
- Share experiences and generalize.

Advantages of Role Play
- It develops skills in leadership, interviewing and social interaction
- It develops sensitivity to others feelings and generates awareness
- It develops skills in group problem-solving
- It develops ability to observe and analyze situation
- It helps them to practice selected behaviors in a real life situation without the stress of making mistake
- It helps to minimize shyness and inhibitions through role playing
- It helps the students in making adjustments
- It gives scope for free expression of feelings.

Disadvantages of Role Play
- Role play is time consuming and is effective only for small groups.
- Beyond using this as a method of learning, sometimes students may become actively involved in the role play.
- All problems cannot be role played.

Checklist for Organizing Role Play

Before the role play:
- Arrange the room to allow for free interaction
- Write out the role briefs for each actor
- Write out instructions for the participants
- Do a briefing session, outlining purpose, rules, etc
- Invite observers.

During the role play: Enact the role play.

After the role play:
- Facilitate group discussion and evaluation
- Re-enact the role play if required
- Facilitate group discussion and re-evaluation if re-enacted
- Explore the implications and applications arising out of role play
- Summarize the concepts
- Thank the actors and participants.

Possible focuses of a role playing session:
- Feelings
- Exploring one's own feelings
- Exploring others' feelings
- Acting out or releasing feelings
- Experiencing higher-status roles in order to change the perceptions of others and one's own perceptions.

Attitudes, values and perceptions:
- Identifying values of culture or subculture
- Clarifying and evaluating one's own values and value conflicts.

Problem-solving attitudes and skills:
- Openness to possible solutions
- Ability to identify a problem
- Ability to generate alternative solutions
- Ability evaluate the consequences to oneself and others of alternative solutions to problems
- Experiencing consequences and making final decisions in light of those consequences
- Analyzing criteria and assumptions behind alternatives
- Acquiring new behaviors.

Subject matter:
- Feelings of participants
- Historical realities: historical crises, dilemmas and decisions.

Programmed Instruction

"Presentation of stimuli to elicit appropriate response".

Programmed instruction is a new and modern strategy, which employs a highly individualized instructional methodology for the modification of behavior and to promote learning.

It is defined as the kind of learning experience in which a "program" takes the place of a tutor for the student and leads him through a set of frames of specified behaviors designed and sequenced to make more probable that he will behave in a desired way (Kochhar SK 1992).

According to Susan Markle, "It is a method of designing a reproducible sequence of instructional events to produce a measurable and consistent effect on behavior of each and every acceptable student."

Programed instruction implies self-instructional and self-controlled, carefully specified and skillfully arranged learning experiences. Programed learning may be defined as the arrangement of material to be learned into an orderly series of learning experiences, in each of which material is presented to the learner, a response is elicited and feedback is given.

Aim of programed learning: Usually the aim is to enable the learner to progress through a prearranged sequence of experiences to the acquisition of some kind of information or skill. Naturally the experiences are ordered in a manner to maximize the efficiency of learning.

Elements in programed learning: There are three important elements in this controlled learning process.

The learner is presented with a stimulus which gives him information, demands on his response, or does both.

There is a continual necessity for the learner to utilize his information in making some response.

After responding, he is presented with information (feedback) which enables him to ascertain the appropriateness of response.

Characteristics of Programed Instruction

- The rate and depth of learning are maximized, understanding is fostered and the motivation of the student is enhanced
- The objectives underlying the program are defined in explicit and operational terms. This makes the terminal behavior desired to be built up through the program
- The subject matter of the program is presented by breaking into small steps in a logical sequences
- Programed learning emphasizes the interaction between learner and the program
- The learner is made to respond actively
- A programed instructional sequence takes into consideration, the initial behavior of the learner with which it starts and the terminal subject matter competence which the learner is to achieve
- A programed test provides for immediate feedback information. This is based on the theory of reinforcement which emphasizes that the learner learns from the sequence of responding
- In a programed learning situation, the learner progresses at his own pace
- Programed instruction takes care of the fact that there are even differences in the rate at which an individual learner learns various kinds of subject mater
- Programed learning provides for consistent evaluation through the record of learner's responses
- Learning material in a programed instruction is presented in such a way that learning becomes an interesting game and the learner is motivated to meet the challenges set by his own capabilities
- Programs are developed by experts. They are empirically tested and modified till they are standardized. A number of students can use a single good program and thus save texts
- Since a program requires continuous response from the learner it overcomes the passivity and inertia on the part of the learner
- In programed instruction, the learner is immediately reinforced to correct his response and this reinforcement sustains the motivation of the learner.

- It permits individual student to progress at his own need.
- The introduction of programed instruction is very helpful in certain situations where human instructors are not available, e.g. small isolated schools in the hilly areas.
- The introduction of programed instruction is of great significance for developing countries which are set on the path of educating millions of masses and are short of teachers.

All these imply the following concepts of programed instructions:

- It puts forth a controlled situation, in which various kinds of intellectual, emotional and verbal experiences are provided to the learner
- It attempts to provide effective instruction without requiring the physical presence of human teacher.
- The learner can precede through the instructional material in short steps at his own pace, receiving immediate knowledge of correctness of his answers.
- The learner proceeds from known principle to unknown, through self-instruction to learn new complex principles.

The Process of Programed Instructions

The "Program" is the important thing about programed instruction. It is done in the following steps:

The subject matter to be programed is analyzed thoroughly and divided into meaningful segments of information. This segment or piece of information is called as a "frame".

At one time, only one single frame is presented to the learner, for which he is asked to make a response. After writing his response to the frame, he can compare his response with the correct response of the programer.

The items are so skillfully written and the steps are so small that the student practices mostly correct response. The sequence of items is so skillfully arranged that the student is taken from known response to the unknown response. The learner proceeds at his own pace. Thus, programing, by providing self-pacing, incorporates the principle of individual differences in the teaching learning process.

Programed Instruction Material

There are three basic types of programed instructional material, viz.:

1. *The teaching machine* is a mechanical device that presents the student, a sequential program of learning activities comprising instructional items. It requires the student to follow the instructions and make a response. It immediately provides the student the knowledge of the accuracy of his results.

2. *The programed textbook*: The whole book is divided into four or five panels and the student responds to one by one.
3. *The scrambled textbook*: In this, the student is given the material to be learnt in small logical units and is tested on each unit immediately. If the student passed the test question, he is automatically given the next unit of information and next question. If he fails, the preceding unit of information is reviewed, the nature of error is explained to him and he is retested.

Styles of Programing

Generally two types of programing are used:
1. Linear or extrinsic programing
2. Branching or intrinsic programing.

Linear or Extrinsic Programing

In this, the frames prepared are presented to the student in small steps and he actively responds to each step. Immediate knowledge of the result is given to him. Self-pacing of student is possible in this. Such sequence of a program is called linear because each learner takes the same path through the instruction. It does not provide for branching for able or slow learners. The whole program is designed by the programer extrinsically hence it is called extrinsic programing.

Branching or Intrinsic Programing

In this, the frames are not kept before the students in a numerical sequence. The student's answer determines which frame he has to see next. If he fails in a frame, he is taken back and explained why he is wrong. Depending on the answer he gives, the student may branch ahead or may branch backward. Unless he gives the correct answer, he cannot proceed to the next frame.

Steps in Program Writing

The following are the steps in program writing:

- **Preparation:** The teacher should analyze the suitability of the topic for a program and prepare a content outline. He should define objectives in behavioral terms and construct tests for entering terminal behavior expected from the students.
- **Program writing:** The whole material is presented in frames to the student and his response is confirmed and corrected.
- **Try out and revision:** When the first draft is ready, it should be tried out on several persons and re-edited. Frames are revised and final draft will be prepared.

Principles of Programed Instruction

A good programed instruction is based on the principles of learning. The fundamental principles are:

- **Principle of small steps:** The subject matter is broken into a sequence of small steps. A student can take a step at a time.
- **Principle of active responding:** Students learn best if he actively responds.
- **Principles of immediate confirmation:** After he takes a particular step, he gets the feedback or the confirmation immediately and reinforcement can be done accordingly.
- **Principle of self-pacing:** Students can work as slowly or as quickly as per his capability.
- **Principle of student testing:** A student leaves the record of his study because he has to write a response for each step on a response sheet.

Advantages of Programed Instruction

The following are the advantages of programed instruction:
- Student is kept active and alert
- Student is allowed to work at his own pace
- It is helpful for teaching complex subject matter as the complexion of material is simplified by breaking it into smaller segments
- Student can work at his own pace
- Individual attention is given to each student
- Student is provided with immediate knowledge of result
- It facilitates self-evaluation of the student
- Workload of the teacher gets reduced, so that he can concentrate on other important works like guidance, counseling, and organization activities
- It makes learning interesting
- It facilitates self-evaluation of the student
- It helps the student to develop high efficiency.

Disadvantages of Programed Instruction

- Preparation of the programed instruction material may be difficult and time consuming
- It requires special competence for the teacher to prepare the material
- Programed materials have been severely criticized as a threat to replacing the teacher
- It is also argued that there is too much emphasis in learning facts and very little emphasis on the mastery of principles and concepts.
- It is also argued that the programed instruction materials are very costly and only rich nations can afford it.

- It is stated that the development and use of programed instructional material require expert knowledge and training. An average teacher finds it very difficult to make use of this device.

Problem-Based Learning

"Learning by resolution of a problem".

Problem-Based Learning (PBL) is a teaching method in which complex real-world problems are used as a tool to promote student's learning of concepts and principles as different from direct presentation of concepts in addition to course content. It is a learning method based on the principle of using problems as a starting point for the acquisition and integration of new knowledge. PBL is an educational strategy which uses material that is as close as possible to real life as a stimulus for learning.

Definition

Problem-based learning can be explained as "the learning that results from the process of working toward the understanding or resolution of a problem".
—Barrows, 1980

Albanese and Mitchell (1993) defined PBL as an instructional method characterized by the use of patient problems as content for students to learn problem-solving skills and acquire knowledge about the basic and clinical sciences.

History of Problem-based Learning

The Faculty of Medicine at McMaster University in Canada was the first educational institute to adopt this model in 1969. Dr Howard Barrows at McMaster is the first to apply PBL to medical education. Barrow's idea came from the concepts of adult learning (Knowles 1975). From the late 1970s PBL methodology spread to several medical schools around the world and other professional courses adopted this method. Many have done so with several modifications to suit local needs and understanding. Hence, PBL method is quite heterogeneous and is continuously evolving.

> Problem-based learning is the basic human learning process that allowed primitive man to survive in his environment.
> —Barrows and Tamblyn (1980)

Characteristics of PBL

- Learning is student centered
- Learning occurs in small student groups
- Teachers serve as facilitators or guides
- Problems form the organizing focus and stimulus for learning
- Problems are a vehicle for the development of clinical problem-solving skills
- New information is acquired through self-directed learning.

Principles of PBL

PBL revolves around the following principles:
- Understanding is built through what one experiences.
- Meaning is created from the efforts to answer one's own questions and solve one's own problems.
- It appeals to students' natural instincts to investigate and create.
- It is based on real life problems.
- The student is the focus of the educational program, not the teacher, the curriculum or the curriculum contents.
- The development of his/her learning capacities is emphasized.
- The problems presented in the curriculum trigger the student's abilities to analyze, to understand and to solve. The student will memorize knowledge obtained in this way much better than by content-based learning.
- Cooperation with others and the importance of communication is emphasized.
- Working on interdisciplinary problems or projects is part of any curriculum.
- Much attention is paid to the development of practical skills, the development of analytical and creative thinking skills.
- Student-centered strategies build critical thinking and reasoning skills and further their creativity and independence.
- The development of self-directed learning ability and the integrated application of knowledge and skills within practice are encouraged.

Principles by Wood (2003)
- Based on real-life problems
- Student-centered learning
- Learning occurs in small teams of students
- Cooperative and collaborative learning
- Inquiry-based learning
- Self-directed learning
- Self-access to learning is present
- Based on the adult learning principles
- Independent responsibility for shared learning.

Goals of PBL

The common goals of PBL are to:
- Construct an extensive and flexible knowledge base
- Foster increased retention of knowledge
- Develop effective problem-solving skills

- Develop self-directed, lifelong learning skills
- Become effective collaborators
- Strengthen student's intrinsic motivation to learn
- Develop an ability to identify relevant health problems, an appreciation for the individualized nature of the physical, biological and behavioral mechanism
- Acquire the knowledge base necessary to define the health problems of the patients
- Reinforce the development of effective clinical reasoning process
- Recognize, develop and maintain the personal characteristics and attitude.

Savin-Baden (1996) listed three key reasons for PBL:
1. First reason was developing "skills" and more specifically clinical reasoning skills
2. Second reason was that learning should take place in "context" for students
3. Final reason was the promotion of self-directed learning.

Steps of Problem-based Learning (Flowchart 2.1)

1. **Presentation of the problem/case:** The teacher as the facilitator should present the problem scenario. The problem for PBL can be sourced from variety of resources, viz. paper-based clinical scenarios, a real or simulated patient, experimental/laboratory data, photos, newspaper clippings, magazines, journals, textbooks, and other multimedia sources. It requires careful preparation and is time consuming. In general, the problem statement should:
   - Be developmentally appropriate
   - Be grounded in student's experience
   - Be curriculum based
   - Should accommodate a variety of teaching and learning strategies and styles and well structured.

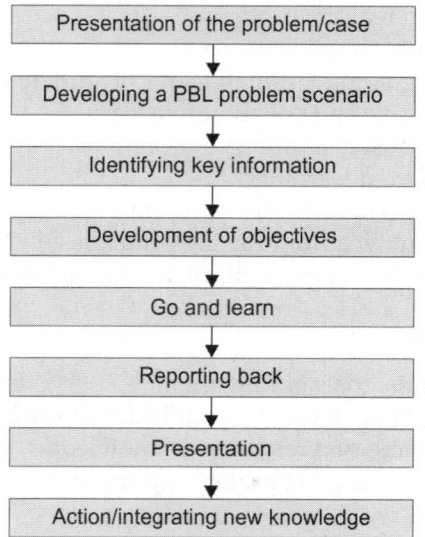

Flowchart 2.1: Steps of PBL.

2. **Developing a PBL problem scenario:** Problems are considered to be one of the three key elements of PBL. The other elements are students and instructors. Problems are to be presented in the best available format either in text or visuals or real or simulated cases. Problems should describe the situation or phenomenon set in real life contexts which require students to explain or resolve the issue. PBL is effective only if the scenario is of standard quality. The five dimensions of the problem scenario are difficulty, solution multiplicity, intrinsic interest, cooperation, and familiarity.

Criteria for PBL scenario
- The title to be of a brief content and not a hint
- Should specify core issues in clear terms
- Confined to limited topics
- Should have neutral description
- In understandable language could contain medical terms
- Should have a balance between available time and study load.

Seven principles of problem design by Dolmans et al.
i. Should simulate real life
ii. Lead to elaboration
iii. Encourage integration of knowledge
iv. Encourage self-directed learning
v. Fit in with student's prior knowledge
vi. Inspiring and interesting to the students
vii. Reflect the faculty's objectives.

Problem-based learning is characterized by students' working in small groups to increase knowledge by identifying learning objectives, engaging in self-directed work and participating in discussions. Problem-based learning environment provide students with greater access to information, support, resources, flexible approaches to learning, collaborative learning activities and opportunities for self-development and greater access to these conditions in the learning environment results in higher levels of structural environment.

Characteristics of PBL scenario
- Learning objectives likely to be defined by the students after studying the scenario should be consistent with the faculty learning objectives
- Problems should be appropriate to the stage of the curriculum and the level of the students' understanding
- Scenarios should have sufficient intrinsic interest for the students or relevance to future practice
- Basic science should be presented in the context of a clinical scenario to encourage integration of knowledge

- Scenarios should contain cues to stimulate discussion and encourage students to seek explanations for the issues presented
- The problem should be sufficiently open so that discussion is not curtailed too early in the process
- Scenarios should promote participation by the students in seeking information from various learning resources
- Each step may lead back to a previous step as well as leading to the next step.

Example of a problem: Mr Kannan, 56 years old, a bus driver who has come to the clinic. In the last month, Mr Kannan had his blood pressure checked nearby, and was found to be high. You are the nurse interviewing Mr Kannan at the clinic. He denies on any medication for high blood pressure. He is obese. He also had the complaints of headache in the last week. Mr Kannan's vital signs, on assessment, are as follows:

T: 36.8°C, BP: 170/95 mm Hg, pulse rate: 92 bpm and respiratory rate: 20 bpm.

As a nurse, how can you help him to solve the problem?

3. **Identifying key information:** In this step, students as a group understand what the problem is all about. They identify: What are the issues? What are known? What is the situation?. This involves discussing about the issues and clarifying the learning needs. The group should analyze the problem and sort out what is known and what is unknown with regard to the problem. Some guiding questions will help them to understand the key information. Brainstorming is of great help in this stage. For example, in the previous problem, his tentative diagnosis is high blood pressure. The guiding questions can be formulated as follows:
   - What is the meaning of high blood pressure?
   - What body system is involved?
   - What will be the possible physiological changes?
   - What is the meaning of obesity?
   - What kind of information do we seek for in order to understand his present situation?
   - What are the appropriate health assessment skills for this client?
   - What are the possible nursing diagnosis, goals and specific intervention for the patient?
   - What skills should one master in order to provide care to him?
   - What are the common patterns of reaction to stress?

Some areas of discussion:
   - Health history taking
   - Physical examination
   - Physiological changes
   - Body and nutritional assessment
   - Reactions to stress and coping
   - Treatment and nursing care for client with high blood pressure and headache.

Development of objectives: Once the problem is identified, the next step is the development of objectives for the learning. The group has to formulate the learning objectives in order to solve the problem. The teacher facilitates the understanding of the problem and helps in formulation of objectives and resources. Each group member identifies his role in finding the solution for the problem. The identification of gaps in knowledge helps students to define their learning objectives and these become the focus of self-directed study in the interval between tutorials. Learning objectives should be clear and specific and of appropriate scope to be addressed in the time available between tutorials (typically 2–3 days). At each tutorial, the group might identify three to five major learning objectives and perhaps an equal number of lesser objectives.

Although the PBL tutorial is student-centered, major learning objectives are identified in advance by the case writers as part of the overall curriculum design. Tutors may need to provide prompts to ensure that major objectives are identified and pursued. In PBL, as knowledge is acquired in the context of a specific clinical problem (the problem is encountered before the student has the knowledge to understand it), it is likely to be better focused and retained.

Go and learn: This step is to go and learn. Everybody in the group goes away to research all of the learning objectives by using all the resources. If all of them have understood their role in solving a problem, they will be focused in searching and learning the solution for the problem. A time limit is set by the group under the guidance of the facilitator and the time for feedback is fixed.

Reporting back: In this step, all team members come and present what they have searched and learned with regard to the problem. All learning needs identified are clarified by the members. In the follow-up tutorial, students reconvene to report on their self-directed study and share and integrate new knowledge. All students should contribute to the report-back and their unique perspectives are incorporated into the process of knowledge building. The exchange and debate of ideas promote the consolidation and elaboration of new knowledge and understanding. After each one presents about the learning they had, they have to write a report for presentation to the facilitator which is done by a member in the group who records all the points discussed. It is also used as a document for future reference.

Presentation: The group presents to the facilitator the content they have learned as per the objectives formulated and the solution to the problems. The facilitator carefully listens to them and makes suggestions/corrections if required. The final presentation makes everyone to recall, and synthesize what they have learned.

Action/integrating new knowledge: This is the last step in the PBL process where the students are expected to apply whatever they have learned in relation to the problem in real life situation.

Role of Facilitator in PBL

Integral to the success of a PBL program is the role of the tutor. The tutor performance is considered (along with the student's prior knowledge and the quality of the cases discussed) to be a prime determinant of how the tutorial group functions.

- Understand the PBL process
- Together with the team members identify and present a suitable problem
- Be familiar with the problem
- Be realistic about what the PBL team can achieve in a given time period
- Understand the big picture behind the problem
- Attend the opening meeting (and as many other meetings as is possible)
- Be enthusiastic and interested in students and their learning
- Motivate the students
- Provide positive and constructive feedback
- Ask questions and encourage reflection
- Assist in the creation of a positive atmosphere
- Be aware of group dynamics and strong and shy personalities and where there may be conflict
- Have an open door policy
- Promote an environment conducive to learning
- Guide group by asking questions, when necessary
- Ensure that the group achieves appropriate learning objectives
- Allow group adequate time to think
- Help students manage group function
- Ensure end-of-session reviews of group performance.
- Help students for their self-assessment
- Give constructive feedback to students
- Accept feedback from group nondefensively
- Help students to prioritize their learning issues
- Assist group in identifying misconceptions or learning deficiencies.

Role of Students

- Prompt and present for all sessions
- Has knowledge of the process of PBL
- Commitment to self-/student-directed learning
- Active participation in discussion and critical thinking while contributing to a friendly, nonintimidating environment
- Willingness to make constructive evaluation of self, group and tutor
- Recognize the need to continue searching for information and integrate the information into practice based on sound justifications
- Work independently and interdependently with others in the process of data collection and analysis.

Role of Group Members

Facilitator	Moderates team discussion, keeps the group on task, and distributes work.
Recorder	Takes notes, summarizing team discussions and decisions, and keeps all necessary records.
Reporter	Serves as group spokesperson to the class or instructor, summarizing the group's activities and/or conclusions.
Timekeeper	Keeps the group aware of time constraints and deadlines and makes sure meetings start on time.
Devil's advocate	Raises counter arguments and (constructive) objections, introduces alternative explanations and solutions.
Harmonizer	Strives to create a harmonious and positive team atmosphere and reach consensus (while allowing a full expression of ideas).
Prioritizer	Makes sure group focuses on most important issues and does not get caught up in details.
Explorer	Seeks to uncover new potential in situations and people (fellow team members but also clients) and explore new areas of inquiry.
Innovator	Encourages imagination and contributes new and alternative perspectives and ideas.
Checker	Checks to make sure all group members understand the concepts and the group's conclusions.
Runner	Gets needed materials and is the liaison between groups and between their group and the instructor.
Wildcard	Assumes the role of any missing member and fills in wherever needed.

Advantages of PBL

- The PBL method fosters active and cooperative learning, the ability to think critically, and clinical reasoning.
- It stimulates the students to use skills of inquiry and critical thinking, peer teaching and peer evaluation.
- It increases ability to apply knowledge in clinical situations.

- It increases student responsibility for self-directed peer learning.
- It helps in developing flexible knowledge that can be applied to different contexts.
- This learning method helps in developing lifelong learning skills.
- It encourages students to work in teams or groups, thereby facilitating group dynamics.
- Many people find it much easier to learn from examples than from abstract theory. Building up their own links and experiences helps students recall information, so PBL helps them to learn and comprehend new material more easily.
- It promotes the development of an effective and efficient clinical reasoning process and increased retention of data.
- Development of effective self-directed learning skills and increased student-faculty interaction is facilitated.
- Increased motivation for learning is the added advantage.

Disadvantages of PBL

- The PBL method involves faculty time in developing the problem situation and in learning to use the method
- Students require orientation to perform the role of a learner in PBL setting
- It is very difficult and expensive to use as a teaching technique, when the class size is large
- Evaluation is quite difficult, and sometimes may be subjective
- Resource-expensive
- Staff and students may be initially uncomfortable with PBL because they are used to subject-based learning, and they do not really understand how to proceed in PBL
- Measurement of learning outcomes is difficult.

Common Difficulties in PBL in Group

- A group member who is much quiet and not actively contributing to the group's learning is considered as a problem
- Unprepared for the tutorial
- Not given enough time by other members
- The dominating group member
- The group that keeps storming.

Professional Behaviors in PBL

- Respect
- Responsibility
- Self-awareness/self-evaluation
- Communication skills.

Approaching Group Problems in PBL

- Listen carefully to everyone
- Clarify issues with the group
- Seek underlying causes
- Facilitate group solutions
- Follow-up on decisions.

Self-directed Learning/Self-learning Packets/ Individualized Learning Packet

Definition

Information on one concept presented according to a few specific objectives in a format that allows skipping of a section if the student has previously mastered the content, typically includes self-checks (pretests, post-tests) of student learning throughout the self-contained packet. It can be used for a single class period, an entire course, enrichment or remedial learning.

Advantages

- It is good for adult learners who have busy lives and limited traditional study times
- It gives students control of when and where learning will occur
- Learning can occur without the presence of the teacher
- It is flexible according to the learner needs
- It is good for teaching psychomotor skills
- It has been found to enhance learning over combined lecture and discussion methods.

Disadvantages

- Students may procrastinate and not complete in a timely manner
- It is costly in time and money to prepare and update
- Printing costs may be high
- Students used to in-class learning may be abandoned.

Self-instructional Module

"Self-contained written material for self-learning".

Self-instructional module (SIM) is an accepted strategy for self-learning and enhancing the knowledge. It refers to self-contained written material which can be used by the students for self-learning. The purpose of SIM is to feed relevant knowledge to the students from multiple angles by providing proper quality material.

Characteristics of SIM

Self-explanatory: The content is self and is clear in concept.

Self-contained: It is self-sufficient, the student does not have to hunt for additional sources.

Self-directional: It is presented in a form of easy explanation, illustration and learning activities. It guides, instructs and regulates the learning process and performs the role of the teacher.

Self-motivating: The material arouses curiosity, raises problems and relates knowledge to familiar situation and makes learning meaningful.

Self-evaluating: It provides questions, exercise and other activities for self-evaluation and checking ones learning progress.

Self-learning: It gives directions, hints and references and motivates a person for self-learning.

The construction of self-learning materials involves three important phases that include:
1. **Preparatory phase:** This phase refers to input, concerned with collection of data regarding target groups, their characteristics, job responsibilities and learning needs. This information serves as a baseline information for construction of learning materials.
2. **Implementation phase:** This phase refers to the process comprising the program definition, preparation, production, dissemination, assessment, monitoring of activity and utilization of instructional material.
3. **Evaluation phase:** This phase is a process of arriving at judgment and decisions based on a careful appraisal of all aspects of the trained performance. This information provides concrete and precise idea of developing an SIM.

Workshop

"Series of individual sessions which render first hand knowledge and practice".

Workshop, in general, is a place where group of people work together to produce a new item or try to solve a problem in an old item. Same way, educational workshop is a type of meeting of different people to find out a solution for a problem. The regular classroom is the nucleus of all academic activities. Academic activities are carried out right from the most formal atmosphere of a lecture hall to the most informal, work-oriented and practical atmosphere of a workshop.

The success of a workshop will depend largely on the way it is planned and on the arrangements made before the opening session.

A workshop is a type of meeting that lets persons with a common interest or problem meet with specialists to receive first-hand knowledge and practice. It is a series of individual sessions.

Purposes of Workshop

- Allows a group of individuals to meet over an extended period of time, in a variety of sessions
- Gives individuals opportunity to receive help from other participants and resource people
- Provides learning situations based on interests and needs of participants
- Gives individuals in the group a chance to work out their own specific programs
- Provides group learning situations for the participants.

Attendants of the Workshop

- Participants are those for whom the workshop is planned
- Coordinator or director offers leadership or guidance throughout and plans and conducts sessions
- Resource persons present information and authoritative opinions in general sessions and or subgroups
- Staff may act alternatively as instructors, discussion leaders and or resource persons.

Organization of a Workshop

A well-planned and organized workshop will prove to be a success.

The topic for the workshop should be decided after assessment of needs and interests of those who will attend.
- Designing the workshop comprises the following steps:
  - Establishing objectives
  - Participants must be able to "learn" or "do" something
  - Relate content of workshop closely to what occurs on the job-keep it practical
  - Consider what information should be learned before, during and after the workshop
  - Determine whether practice is necessary during the workshop.
- Develop the basic plan:
  - Determine:
    i. What will be presented?
    ii. What will be discussed?
    iii. What will be practiced?
  - Consider subgroup activity and size.
  - Consider materials to be prepared for participants:
    i. Handbook
    ii. Discussion guides
    iii. Practice instructions
  - Determine what equipment will be needed:
    i. Chalkboards
    ii. Overhead visuals
    iii. Demonstration devices
    iv. Films
    v. Determine room arrangements.
- Select the best method.
- Select techniques with schedule and budget in mind.
- Determine who should do what.
- Expand outline.
- Meet with resource person as needed.

- Review with organizing committee and tasks delegated to them.
- Evaluation: Planning for methods of assessment of the workshop and its outcome.

Advantages

- Workshops are participative
- Participants identify their interests and needs and the learning situations are also based on them
- Skill sets are developed in the participants
- Workshops are flexible
- Emphasis is placed on improving individual understanding and proficiency
- Theory and practice may be combined
- Individuals are encouraged to formulate their ideas and tasks, and assistance is available.

Disadvantages

- Individuals may not perceive their own needs to be identified, either initially or in the following workshop sessions
- Much planning and organization is needed because it has limited time
- Some participants may find it more difficult to follow with this format
- Workshops may be overused
- Selection of resource person may be difficult
- Last minute changes and emergencies may affect the learners
- Sessions may not be productive or effectively inter-related.

Simulation

"Reproduction of real-life situation".

Simulation is a technique that enables adult learners to obtain skills, competencies, knowledge or behavior by becoming involved in situations that are similar to those in real-life. This method of teaching attempts to address problems of real-life conditions and to discuss them completely after the presentation is over.

Simulation is the reproduction of the essential features of a real-life situation. Although nurse educators strive to mimic reality in their practice laboratories, they find that nursing students often do not make the imaginative leap required to visualize a dummy model as a real patient. Consequently, students frequently experience difficulty making the transition from the learning laboratory to the real patient setting. To better facilitate this transition, nursing learning centers have recently begun moving from static, plastic models to costly, interactive, computerized models.

To successfully develop a simulation program, nursing faculty need a broad understanding of the tools available, the scope of their use, and the degree of their realism. With this information, faculty is better able to formulate a meaningful vision for their simulation programs.

The increased use of simulation in nursing can be attributed to:

- The nursing shortage and the need to increase, enrollment into nursing programs
- A need to supplement limited numbers of clinical sites
- Lower cost of simulation equipment
- Emphasis on evidence-based practice and competencies
- Acceptance of simulation as a useful tool
- Increasing awareness of the need to address patient safety (Institute of Medicine) IOM 2000
- The ability of simulation to enhance clinical practice.

Types of Simulation Equipment

Many types of simulation equipment are available to nurse educators. Models range from equipment that teaches a simple, single skill (e.g. inserting an intravenous access into an arm, assessing vital signs, such as heart, lung, and bowel sounds) to very advanced, realistic equipment that can simulate reality-based scenarios in a clinical setting, such as an intensive care unit. Fletcher (1995) described the term "fidelity" as the degree of accuracy depicted by the simulation, compared to the real experience. Whereas static or low fidelity models are useful for practice and testing of specific skills, high-fidelity models challenge students to make clinical decisions based on data obtained from assessments and interventions.

The word fidelity is often used in the simulation domain to describe the accuracy of the system being used. Fidelity is defined as "precision of reproduction" the extent to which an electronic device, for example, a stereo system or television, accurately reproduces sound or images.

Low-fidelity Simulators

Low-fidelity simulators are often less in detail and vitality of a living situation. In introducing and practicing psychomotor skill, they generally lack the realism. A good example of a low simulator would be a foam intramuscular injection simulator. Administering injections not only requires technology skill but also relies heavily on interpersonal skills, which are difficult to demonstrate with a foam model.

Moderate-fidelity Simulators

A moderate-fidelity simulator offers more realism than a static, low-fidelity model. They offer breath sounds, heart sounds, and pulse but may lack corresponding chest movement or functional eyes, which one would expect in a high-fidelity simulator. Moderate-fidelity simulators are useful as both introduction tools and tools for developing deeper understanding of specific, increasingly complex subject matter and competencies.

High-fidelity Simulators

High-fidelity simulators produce the most realistic simulated patient experiences. They include details that give the units personality and used to more closely identify with the unit as something they might actually encounter in real-life. High-fidelity units must not only have the outward appearance of reality (cosmetic fidelity) but also react in realistic ways to student interventions (response fidelity). These types of simulation units are the most costly.

High-fidelity models are often life-size mannequins with features such as palpable pulses, visible respirations, measurable blood pressure and pulse oximetry, vocal sounds, open orifices, and minimal movement, all programed by computer. Through interface with the computer, the data emitted from the mannequin will change based on student interventions and decisions. A faculty member can manually control the computer or small subprograms can be stored and programed into the scenario. For example, a stored subprogram may alter blood pressure and heart rate in response to administration of a specific medication. These small programs are unlimited in scope and use. Educators need to:
- Determine the content best taught through simulation
- Determine the learning objectives
- Replicate reality as closely as possible through the environment and equipment
- Use video equipment to record the activities for later use in debriefing conferences
- Conduct a debriefing conference, which is a time for participants and observers to engage in group discussion and learning-based on the actions taken by the participants. Rationales for clinical decisions can be discussed, suggestions for alternative actions made, feelings related to the situation shared, and mistakes identified. During the debriefing session, only selected portions of the videotape should be shown to make the desired point. Instructors should focus on the exact actions taken and evaluate the communication and interaction between participants.

Learning Objectives of the Simulation Process

The simulation procedure is commonly used to:
- Develop highly complex cognitive skills, such as decision-making, evaluating and synthesizing
- Impact positively on the learner's values, beliefs and attitudes
- Induce feelings of empathy in the minds of the students.
- Sharpen human relation skills and communication skills
- Unlearn negative attitudes or behavior.

Steps of Simulation Process [Designed by Goldstein and Pfeiffer (1983)]

The steps of the simulation process include:
- Experience
- Sharing
- Processing
- Generalization
- Application.

Experience

This stage involves experiencing or simulating the particular problem or situation. Four or five participants are selected and each one of them should identify their own purpose of the exercise and its ultimate goal.

Sharing

The second stage involves participants sharing their experiences after the exercise is concluded. Members are encouraged to share both their observations of what, when and how they felt about the activities or events. Often the feelings are important to reveal their comments about objective events.

Processing

This stage involves processing the information gathered during the sharing stage. Unlike sharing, which is done in small groups, this is generally accomplished with all the participants. The goal of this step is to identify commonly shared experiences or perceptions and to identify common themes among the group members.

Generalization

In this stage, the teacher guides the group into drawing broad implications from the experience and resulting discussion. This is the most important phase of the entire process, and if left out, the learning will appear incomplete.

Application

The final stage of the process is to help the participants to apply the new generalization to future situations. Overall application phase is designed to give the participants a chance to apply the new concepts, feelings and ideas in real-life situation.

Requisites for a good simulation process:

A successful simulation process should meet the following criteria:
- *Active involvement* of all the students.
- *Clarity*: The decisions made should be based on the clear consequences and causes of the simulation process and resulting discussion.
- *Feasibility*: It measures the cost in terms of materials, space, and time against outcomes.

- *Repeatability and reliability*: These qualities are important because it is essential that simulation be repeated with the same degree of reliability relative to its outcome. This will improve the accuracy of learning as well as the credibility of the simulation process.

Advantages of the Method

Simulation is a teaching device that motivates and involves students actively that stimulates them for the acquisition of purposeful activities. It has the following advantages:
- Simulation establishes a setting where theory and practice can be combined
- It develops the problem-solving skills of the student, helping him to resolve problem in a linear or nonlinear fashion
- The procedure makes it mandatory for application of knowledge by the student and improves their critical thinking skills
- It may be used in the classroom or in the laboratory as structural activity or as an independent study assignment, can provide immediate-feedback and/or corrective action
- It enhances decision-making skills, and content retention by the student
- It requires the teachers to be active participants in the process
- It promotes student-student, teacher-student, and student-teacher interactions
- It serves as a foundation for small or large group discussion. Students can experience "real" situation without client risk
- The feelings of self-confidence and competence of the students are increased
- There is no risk involved, as the decisions are made and carried out without physical or psychological harm to the students or the institution.

Advantages for Nursing Education

Simulation technology offers many advantages for nursing education. Fletcher (1995) listed several, including:
- The clinical setting can be realistically simulated
- There is no threat to patient safety
- Active learning can occur
- Specific and unique patient situations can be presented
- Errors can be corrected and discussed immediately
- Consistent and comparable experiences can occur for all students
- Enhanced cognitive, psychomotor, communication and discussion skills
- Improved learner organizational, observation and integrative skills
- Increased confidence, shift of attitude and smooth transition from the classroom or laboratory to the health care setting

- Benefits of immediate-feedback
- Increases the ability of the faculty to identify students' performance levels. In addition to these advantages, simulation was found to be fun, interesting and motivational to learning.

Disadvantages of the Method

- The whole process is time consuming to develop and of high cost
- Must be realistic enough for transfer of learning to real situation
- Teachers may feel that they have lost control of learning environment
- The technique must be structured so that all learners are become involved in the situation and problem-solving process
- There is a need for many simulators. But all the students may not be involved, who may not get the experience.

Computer-based Simulation Programs

Computer-based simulation involves the use of software developed to simulate a subject or situation. The software may be of low, moderate or high-fidelity, and can test many aspects of learning, such as skill, knowledge, and critical thinking. These systems are also convenient to use because students may have access to these programs outside of regular class hours, which gives them the ability to practice and learn independently. Tools have been developed that evaluate individuals for knowledge skill and critical thinking.

Advantages

- Controlled
- Cost
- Reproducible and predictable
- Programable
- Ease to use
- Simultaneous use by many students
- Entertaining
- May be less stressful for both students and faculty
- May not be location specific. Students may be able to use programs off site.

Full-scale Simulation

Full-scale simulation is probably the most recognized form of simulation in health care. Full-scale simulation attempts to recreate all of the elements of a situation that are perceptible to students.

This type of simulation can involve real people, real physiology, real interaction, real actions, and realistic responses and reactions. The environment is made to resemble the intended environment as closely as possible in order to immerse students in an experience that is the closest we can come to real-life. With full-scale simulation, students must act at a higher level and must call on myriad cognitive and technical skills during the scenario. The scenario can be a simulation of a crisis or of noncritical physiology, requiring students to respond in an appropriate way.

Actors, props, and other environmental elements must be considered and used when appropriate. Interpersonal interaction is also a key component of this form of simulation.

This method is usually manikin-based but can also include standardized patients and role play. The fidelity of manikin-based simulation must be high, both in appearance and response. The simulation unit is more costly. Full-scale simulation often involves debriefing after a scenario. In the debriefing process, students are allowed to self-assessment as well as receive peer assessment in the presence of a skilled facilitator. The debriefing uses a video recording of the scenario to initiate discussion, and the key learning objectives are culled from the session. Debriefing is very constructive but can also be psychologically traumatic for certain individuals or when used improperly. The debriefing process should be respected, and quality debriefing must always be a priority.

The advantage of full-scale simulation is that it facilitates three types of learning in approximately 1 hour.
1. Scenario participants learn by realistic experience
2. Individuals watching the live broadcast learn as observers (virtual "flies on the wall")
3. When scenario participants and observers gather as a group, they all learn by sharing their experiences in group discussion.

Microteaching

"A miniature teaching to practice teaching skills".

Definition

"Microteaching is a procedure which reduces the teaching situation to simpler and more controlled encounter achieved by limiting the practice teaching to a specific skill and reducing teaching time and class size". (Clift et al.)

Bush (1968) has defined microteaching as "a teacher education technique which allows teachers to apply well-defined teaching skills to a carefully prepared lesson in a planned series of 5–10 minutes encounters with a small group of real classroom students, often with an opportunity to observe the performance on videotape".

Characteristics of Microteaching

- Microteaching has the following characteristics
- Microelement: Microteaching reduces the complexities of the teaching situation in terms of:
  - Number of students to be taught
  - Duration of the lesson
  - Subject matter to be taught.

This enables the trainee or student-teacher to concentrate on a particular skill at a time.

Mastering of teaching skills and teaching strategies: Microteaching enables trainees to master the various instructional skills and perfect them in such a way as to master the teaching strategies.

Safe practice ground: A microteaching laboratory possesses all the inherent features of the real classroom. Teaching is performed under simulated conditions with a small group; the trainee is on a safe practice ground.

Availability of teaching models: The trainee gets many teaching models like demonstration given by the supervisor, or a tape or a film. This gives her the opportunities to identify the pattern of behavior desired by the students.

Feedback: Oral feedback by the supervisor, observation schedules filled in by the peer group participating in the microlesson, audio and videotape recording are certain reliable and authentic sources that provide necessary feedback to the trainee.

The Microteaching Process

- Microteaching is a scaled down sample of teaching. The complex art of teaching is broken down into simple components. Only one particular skill is attempted and developed during one microteaching session. The teaching act is scaled down in terms of the content of the lesson, the size of the class, and duration of the lesson. A student teacher teaches a short lesson of 5–8 minutes to a small group of students, usually less than 10.
- A single concept is taken in one lesson. At the end of the session, the student teacher discusses with the supervisor regarding the performance of the skill and gets feedback. She modifies her teaching accordingly, and reteaches her microlesson with a different group of students, under the same conditions in an attempt to improve her previous lesson. The process can be repeated till the desirable skill is developed.
- The success of microteaching depends on the teach–reteach cycle which can be completed in about 30 minutes.

The above description of microteaching aids to break it down into the following steps:
- Defining the skill to be attained or mastered at the end of the session
- Demonstrating the skill-videotape or film can be shown or a real demonstration of the particular skill can be done by the supervisor
- Planning the lesson
- Teaching the microlesson
- Discussion on the lesson delivered

- Identification of pitfalls and drawbacks by the student teacher
- Replanning and reteaching the lesson: In the light of the feedback and supervisor's comments, the student-teacher replans and reteaches the lesson, in order to acquire the skill more effectively
- Rediscussion and refeedback: The lesson is again observed or audio or videotaped. Feedback is again provided on the retaught lesson
- Repeating the cycle: The teach-reteach cycle is repeated till the desired level of skill is achieved
- The supervisor should be in a position to offer continuous consultation to enable the student-teacher to perfect her performance in the particular teaching skill.

Advantages of Microteaching

Microteaching possesses the following advantages:
- Microteaching helps the student-teachers to perfect their performance and improve it to a superior level
- Teaching skills are learnt in a real practice situation, not under simulated conditions
- Microteaching focuses on sharpening and developing of specific teaching skills (the practice of certain instructional skills, the practice of a particular method of teaching, etc.) and eliminating errors
- Microteaching provides increased control of the practice teaching session
- Microteaching is very effective in modifying teaching behavior
- Microteaching provides a safe practice ground for the student-teachers
- Microteaching provides a good prelude to a macro-lesson
- Microteaching provides for repeated practice without adverse consequences to the teacher or his students
- Microteaching provides accurate and powerful feedback on the performance of the student-teachers, by oral feedback by the supervisor, observation schedules filled in by the peer group, and audio and videotape recording
- Microteaching individualizes the training as it paces teaching according to the learning ability of the student teacher
- Microteaching lessens the complexities of the normal classroom teaching by "scaled down teaching"
- Beyond everything, microteaching increases the self-confidence of the student-teacher.

Disadvantages of Microteaching

The disadvantages of microteaching are:
- Microteaching is skill-oriented rather than content-oriented
- Much emphasis is laid on specific skills and broad-based patterns of behavior are not paid much attention
- Microteaching has a very narrow scope
- Microteaching is highly time-consuming
- Microteaching emphasizes only on acquiring independent and isolated teaching skills, but teaching involves a more complex and comprehensive process.

Computer Assisted Learning

Computers have become omnipresent and ubiquitous today and are found in every walk of life.

100 million words or 300,000 pages can be stored on a CD-ROM disk.

Computer as a Tool of Learning

Computer can be made to assist learning in many ways since it is capable of:
- Dense storage of data in an organized form, e.g. a large textbook could be stored in a classified manner on a 9 cm disk
- Quick access to the database in milliseconds: The 300,000 pages on a CD-ROM can be searched in seconds for word occurrences
- Multimedia capability: The new generation of multimedia computers add sound, animation, 3D and video to the text
- Logic function which can compare learner's responses and gives appropriate feedback and reinforcement
- Ability to keep track of the learner's performance, award marks and give instant feedback of evaluation.

> **Process of computer assisted learning:**
> - Choose a relevant topic.
> - Decide the cognitive level of the students, aimed by the module, viz. knowledge, understanding or problem-solving.
> - Decide the computer assisted learning (CAL) mode to be used.
> - Develop CAL sequence in the form of "frames".
>   - I—Frame or introductory frame gives directions to the learner
>   - L—Frame or learning frame presents the matter to be learnt
>   - T—Frame or test frame tests the learners and gives appropriate feedback.
> - Prevalidate the CAL by sharing them with peers and students and get feedback. "Too easy, rigid, difficult or boring" parts need to be revised.
> - Get the written CAL module converted to a computer program.
> - Do postvalidation of the CAL program and make corrections if needed.
> - Release CAL unit for learners to use and learn.

Modes of Computer Assisted Learning (CAL)

A variety of modes are possible giving a teacher much flexibility in using CAL effectively. They include:

Drill and practice mode: In this, the students learn facts and memorize them by drill method, e.g. using an MCQ bank for drill and practice. This method is useful for slow learners.

Tutorial mode: Here, a well-structured programed learning unit (or CAL module) provides interactive learning. This mode, if used well, could result in 90% retention of the content compared with 30% retention after the best lecture. In tutorial method, a module lesson consists of:
- Presentation of content in a structured way
- Task-prescription to elicit the learner's response
- Instant feedback and reinforcement to the learner.

Laboratory mode: Computer could be programed to simulate a variety of biological processes to supplement or do away with laboratory experiments. The learner explores various options and learns by inference.

Case-simulation mode: A variety of diagnostic and therapeutic problems and the patient management type could be effectively computerized. This has proved quite useful in learning problem-solving, the highest cognitive domain.

Consultant role: "Expert" programs have been devised, which could bring the expertise of a consultant within the easy reach of a primary care nurse.

Manager of educational process: Computer-based Management Information System (MIS) could keep track of student performances and offer suitable advice to make the educational process more effective.

Other than this, computers have become a store house of information. Several sources of reference like MEDLINE and POPLINE are available on the internet. This provides information on any subject that a teacher may desire. Internet also provides a platform for teachers to exchange notes, raise queries, and receive answers.

Limitations of CAL Method

Inherent limitations: CAL could be very effective on developing cognitive domain alone, especially problem-solving skills and has a very limited application to the other two domains.

Content: All topics and subjects are not suited for CAL (e.g. Literature. Only topics that are logical or that could be well-structured are suitable).

Program development: Developing a CAL module is tedious and time consuming process.
- Faculty involvement is limited.
- Evaluation of the use of CAL is not standardized.

Cost effectiveness: It involves high-cost to develop and utilize a program.

Developed educational programs may not be able to keep pace with the rapid advancement in technology.

Peer Tutoring

"Specialized, interpersonal relationship existing among tutor-tutee".

Peer tutoring in higher education is an effective strategy for promoting academic gains. Within nursing, peer tutoring has been used in the classroom and clinical setting. A peer tutoring program can be created to help to meet the needs of students. Peer tutoring is the process between two or more students in a group where one of the students acts as a tutor for the other group-mate(s). Peer tutoring can be applied among students of the same age or students belonging to different age groups. Peer tutoring is a flexible, peer-mediated strategy that involves students serving as academic tutors and tutees. Typically, a higher performing student is paired with a lower performing student to review critical academic or behavioral concepts. There are many tutoring patterns such as dyad, small group, skill based, assignment based, and question-based can be used successfully to help the students to learn the concepts and skills.

According to Keith Topping and Shirley Hill, peer tutoring can be defined as "people from similar social groupings, who are not professional teachers helping each other to learn and learning themselves by teaching".

A peer tutor is anyone who is of similar status as the person being tutored.

Types/Models of Peer Tutoring

In general, peer tutoring models are flexible and can be altered to meet individual student or class learning needs.

Incidental peer tutoring: Incidental peer tutoring often takes place, either at college or while working in the clinical areas or when students are socializing. Whenever students work or study together, one guides the others. This may be stated as a kind of incidental peer tutoring.

Structured peer tutoring: It refers to peer tutoring implemented with specific purposes and for specific subjects, following a well-structured plan prepared by the teacher.

One on one peer tutoring: In this, one exclusively acts as a tutor and the other one is a tutee.

Dyad peer tutoring: In dyad pattern, both of them support each other and both play a role of tutor and tutee.

Class-wide peer tutoring (CWPT): It involves dividing the entire class into groups of two to five students with differing ability levels. Students then act as tutors, tutees, or both tutors and tutees.

Cross-age peer tutoring: Older students are paired with younger students to teach and the positions of tutor and tutee do not change. The older student serves as the tutor and the younger student is the tutee.

Reciprocal peer tutoring (RPT): Two or more students alternate between acting as the tutor and tutee during each session, with equitable time in each role.

Same-age peer tutoring: Peers who are within 1 or 2 years of age are paired to review key concepts. Students may have similar ability levels or a more advanced student can be paired with a less advanced student.

Short-term peer tutoring: In which the tutor tutee relationship exists for a specific period of time.

Long-term peer tutoring: The tutor tutee relationship exists for a long period of time.

The reason for introducing peer tutoring:
- Students may find difficulties in studying a certain subject.
- Facilitate better understanding of professional roles to students.
- Acclimatize students to the demand of the profession and enhance their confidence and skills in dealing with role conflict.

Tutor is a person who extends support for the tutee and acts as a mentor. A peer tutor is anyone who is of a similar status as the person being tutored. Tutee is a person who seeks help from the tutor and willingly takes guidance for the professional growth. The relationship may be either one on one or dyad.

Importance of Peer Tutoring
- It is a widely-researched practice across ages, grade levels, and subject areas. The intervention allows students to receive one-to-one assistance
- Students have increased opportunities to respond in smaller groups
- It promotes academic and social development for both the tutor and tutee
- Student engagement and time on task increases
- Peer tutoring increases self-confidence and self-efficacy
- The strategy is supported by a strong research base.

Hints for Choosing Tutors
- Tutors should be motivated to be a tutor
- Tutors need an adult coach to observe in a tutorial situation
- Choose tutors, who want to help others and show compassion
- The tutor should be able to devote adequate time to meeting the "teacher/coach" to develop good teaching techniques
- Prospective tutors need to be able to show patience and the ability to give meaningful suggestions, praise and encouragement.

Benefits of Peer Tutoring

For the Tutor
- They will learn the subject matter that is being tutored
- They will learn how to tutor
- They will learn how to listen and communicate effectively
- They will learn about learning. Additionally, they will learn the need for developing a sense of responsibility
- Practice students' communication skills with junior students
- Give tutors great confidence to talk to the staff members while the line of communication is opened up for both of them.
- Give tutors an opportunity to develop their own leadership skills.

Helping another student will more often motivate the tutor to learn as well. It makes sense that a tutor would "feel important" and thus self-esteem would probably be enhanced through successful experiences.

For the Tutee

Help tutees feel more at ease, and concentrate better on the subject matter, with a peer tutor rather than a professional teacher or consultant.

According to Goodlad and Hirst (1989), there are four main benefits for tutees when they seek out peer help:
1. Tutorees receive individualized instruction
2. Tutorees receive more teaching
3. Tutorees (may) respond better to their peers than to their teachers
4. Tutorees can obtain companionship from the students.

For the Teachers
- Peer tutoring is also beneficial to teachers who may not have the time to spend with each of their students one-on-one
- Help the subject lecturer break the whole class into small groups so that students have the chance to learn in a more intimate environment, which allows them to take more initiative. For example, students ask more questions at the tutorials and that hardly happens in lectures.

Hindrances to Tutoring
- It takes "teacher/coach" time to implement and monitor
- Lack of readily available materials to "train tutors"

- The mindset that all teaching is best transmitted from adult to child
- Teacher resistance
- Parent resistance
- Administration resistance
- Possible implications of tutor selection process being criticized
- Apprehension of noise in the classroom
- Behavior problems tutors may possibly have to deal with.

Role of Peer Tutors and Tutees

Tutors
- Motivator
- Motivate students or tutees to learn
- Counselor
- Sharing personal experiences with tutees
- Advisor
- Provide comments on tutees' effort. The final answers lie with the subject lecturer
- Middle man
- A peer tutor is the bridge between tutees and subject lecturers.

Tutees
Tutees are expected to:
- Review relevant subject matters before tutorial sessions
- Raise questions before or during or after tutorial sessions
- Be cooperative and take active part in all tutorial activities
- Solve problems individually or as a team
- Be punctual and attend all tutorial sessions.

Humor

"Learn to laugh to learn easily".

Humor is also a way of saying something serious.
—TS Eliot

Humor is a complex phenomenon with a long and rich history. Humor is a communication that induces amusement. Thus, it must be shared. It makes the learning environment a shared and pleasurable experience. The use of humor in the classroom can be productive and promoting comfortable and safe interactions between faculty and students. In education, the most positive forms of humor are funny stories or comments, jokes and professional humor. The use of humor in nursing education improves outcome.

Humor is a teaching strategy that may enhance student learning. Learning is a process that involves both cognitive and affective functions. The best results are achieved when students learn in a nonthreatening, challenging, and relaxed atmosphere, with a rich sensory environment that engages all levels of the mind (Caine and Caine, 1989). Humor can help produce that environment by combining the cognitive and affective functions, while reducing anxiety.

Why do we Laugh?
Humor is much more than mere joke-telling or being funny. It is an attitude, a way of life. Humor is any act with an element of surprise embedded in it, which leaves everybody feeling good and relaxed. The key is the surprise element, which is crucial. Just as a joke fails if its punch line (which normally comes at the end of the joke) fails to deliver, similarly humor loses its teeth if the surprise element is taken out. This act of surprise, coming unexpected, leaves people with a smile, with a sense of relief from a tense situation.

Components of Humor
Humor is comprised of three components: wit, mirth, and laughter.
1. **Wit** is the cognitive process that elicits humor.
2. **Mirth** is the emotional experience or reaction to humor, joy and pleasure.
3. **Laughter** or smiling is a physical expression of humor.

Central Theories of Humor

Superiority Theories

Suggest that people laugh at others to whom they feel superior. The laugher always looks down on whatever he laughs at, and so judges it inferior by some standard. According to this view, all humor is derisive.

Relief Theories

People who have been undergoing a strain will sometimes burst into laughter if the strain is suddenly removed.

Incongruity Theories

The laughter or amusement occurs as an intellectual reaction to something unexpected, illogical or inappropriate in some way.

Brain Activity in Humor

The affective component of humor engages the limbic system, thereby enhancing short-term and long-term memory and increasing the willingness of the learner to apply knowledge and skills. The expression of feelings, such as empathy and anger, can be more constructive when approached in a witty manner. Both sides of the brain are actively engaged during laughter and the perception of humor. The right side of the brain involves reading and interpreting the visual, nonverbal information of humor while the left side of the brain interprets the language nuances of humor. Novelty, imagination, and visualization help move information into long-term memory through the engagement of multiple brain cells firing simultaneously.

Effects of Humor and Laughter on Health and Learning

Effects on Health

Humor reduces anxiety and tension, helps students focus their attention, makes learning fun, increases learning memory and strengthens social relationships. Humor reduces anxiety through release of tension by focusing or something other than the mere absorption and retention of facts. It also improves the relationship between students and their teacher. According to Watson and Emerson (1988), "this (humor) reduces the authoritarian position of the teacher, allowing the teacher to be a facilitator of the learning process" in partnership with students. Stimulating mental processes and controlling fear and anxiety through the use of humor help students retain the information they have learned. In addition, as anxiety is reduced, students are more likely to open their minds to learning and enjoy the experience. In short, humor is a legitimate teaching tool "that can be integrated into instruction to facilitate learning."

Physiological response produced by belly laughter is opposite to the effects of stress. Twenty seconds of guffawing gives the heart the same workout as 3 minutes of hard rowing. After humor, there is a slight rise in heart-rate and blood pressure followed by immediate recoil. Muscles relax and blood pressure comes down to prelaughter level, accompanied by the release of endorphins, the body's natural pain killer by the brain. More oxygen is pumped into the bloodstream and thus to the brain. All these help the body cope with stress.

Humor in teaching reduces stress; increases motivation; improves morale, enjoyment, comprehension, interest and rapport; and facilitates socialization into the profession. Humor should be appropriate to the topic and should be in context. Research showed that a charismatic and impressive teacher could be rated highly by students, despite the absence of content in the material presented.

It has been shown to increase teacher credibility. The effective use of humor promotes creativity, learning, retention and enculturation of professionals.

Humor can promote learning through the physical benefits of reduced stress, increased productivity, and enhanced creativity. It contributes to all necessary principles of learning—enjoyment; creativity; interest; motivation; a relaxed, open, warm environment; a positive student–teacher relationship; and decreased tension and anxiety. Humor used constructively builds a positive self-image. It serves as a vehicle for enhancing the learning environment through enlivening potentially dreary topics, keeping lectures engaging and enjoyable, and humanizing faculty in student's perceptions. The cultivation of abilities to laugh at oneself and others bridges many gaps between people and broadens the pathway from student to professional.

Effects on Learning

Humor can be used judiciously throughout a class session or course and in all types of classroom situations—lecture, laboratory, field work, and various course assignments. Positive and constructive humor can be used to put the learner and the teacher at ease with the subject matter. Faculty may need to collect jokes, cartoons, movie excerpts, and humorous exercises to insert in to their regular teaching activities to enhance the learner's receptivity to information and participation during content presentations.

Incorporating Humor in Everyday Activities

Surround oneself with humor. Find sources such as humorous video or audio recordings or cartoons, and analyze what one likes about particular types of humor. Nonmedical sources of humor include the newspaper, Reader's Digest, and popular comedians.

Laugh more often and tell jokes and funny stories, learn a new joke or story and practice it with a few friends. As one gains confidence, can add one or two jokes at a time until one has built up his repertoire.

Play with language; create puns and other verbal humor. Look for double meanings in words and incongruities in everyday situations.

Observe humor in everyday life. Improving one's sense of humor requires active participation. Develop a humorous perspective as one experiences daily events.

Tips for Using Humor in the Classroom

- Create a casual (and safe) atmosphere.
- Smile; adopt a laugh-ready attitude.
- Relax, use open, nonverbal posture; increase interpersonal contact through eye to eye and face to face contact.
- Remove social inhibitions; establish nonjudgmental forum for discussion.
- Begin class with a humorous example, cartoon, anecdote or thought for the day.
- Use personal stories, anecdotes, current events related to class content.
- Plan frequent breaks in content for application, humorous commercials or exaggerated examples; provide humorous materials.
- Encourage, give and take with students; laugh at oneself occasionally.

- Memorize the material. If one is concentrating on his notes, he may lose his audience's attention.
- Practice timing. Pauses allow the audience to picture the events and possible results of the joke or story.
- Involve the audience. Active participation increases student attention.
- Speak clearly and vary your voice. Students dread presentations by teachers who mumble or monotonously read their notes to the class. Volume and tone can emphasize humor.
- Use one's body to supplement the words. Facial expressions, gestures and walking around the room can emphasize the point and keep students attention. A movement of eye contact with a student as one begins a humorous event also will make the humor more personal. Move away from the podium and into the audience if this is permitted by the room arrangement.
- Use audio-visual aids. Overheard projector transparencies, slides, audiotapes, computer projections and other props are effective in presentations. Cartoons on overhead transparencies are a simple way to add humor.
- Learn to critique presentation style to analyze one's presentation to learn what was successful, what was not, and how one can improve it.

Humor Delivered Orally

Most forms of humor delivered orally contain three elements: Expected serious set-up with commonly understood situation or content, expected build-up of tension and unexpected twist—punchline. This is the humor trisect. All three elements are required for maximum winnings.

When students anticipate a joke is coming, clued by the teacher's set-up, body language or bullhorn announcement, have the benefit of building tension before delivering the punch. That build-up can affect the impact of the punchline. The delivery needs to be intentionally calculated with a pause just before the punchline. It needs to be practiced with anecdotes or any other longer joke forms.

Humor in Print

In contrast to the above, "script humor" has no build-up of tension. It is a bisect, just expected followed by unexpected twist. The reader does not have a clue when the punch is coming. He or she is reading seriously. The punchline is the point of collision between two conflicting trains of thought—serious sentence meets unexpected ending. The shock is our recognition of this incongruity. There is virtually no opportunity to warn the reader. The only exception is a multi-panel cartoon, where each panel builds tension—bubble after bubble—toward the final panel punch.

Strategies to Infuse Humor

There are basic strategies that can be used to infuse humor systematically into teaching. The strategies are categorized by level of risk: low, moderate, and high. The lowest level involves inserting punchlines into normal print material. The moderate and high-risk categories rely on oral delivery.

Humor Strategies

- Humorous material on syllabus
- Descriptors, cautions, and warnings on the cover of handouts
- Humorous problems/assignments: It includes humorous real or hypothetical situations in assignments and can be done in-class and out-of-class by individual and small group using problem-solving exercises, games, etc.

High-risk Humor Strategies

- Opening jokes: Forms of humorous material that can be delivered by the teacher or students: Stand-up jokes, quotations, proverbs, and questions ("thought for the day"), cartoons, multiple-choice items, anecdotes and one-shot handouts (e.g. medications, letters, articles, memos).
- Commercial interruptions: When the students' eyeballs begin glazing over, stop for a commercial: Stand-up joke, anecdote and humorous handout (e.g. picture, cartoon).

Rules to Remember

- Be oneself.
- Do not force humor. The students may not like forced humor in teachers and do not respect them because they appear fake.
- Use humor regularly. Add humor to class presentations routinely but not at consistent, preset intervals because students will only wake up for the jokes.
- Avoid offensive humor. Humor that is disparaging, stereotypical, sarcastic, or demanding can make the students less attentive to it and make the educational message less effective. When negative humor is used, students may tighten up, withdraw or become resentful, angry, tense or anxious. Negative humor also can cause students to turn off.
- Be sensitive to emotional students.
- Be spontaneous. Encourage students to engage in humor also.
- One can stimulate more interest and involvement through playful use of spontaneous students' humor
- Use relevant humor to emphasize an educational point. Students are focused on what they need to learn in class. If humorous material is not to course content, they can be used to return to the class topic.
- Add humorous material to syllabi, tests and handouts.

Laughter is likely to be greater in larger, more crowded classes, than in smaller classes in larger rooms. Laughter, like yawning, is contagious; so once a large group gets going it may take time to bring them back to focus. Humor is a part of communication and not dependent upon the natural comedic ability of an instructor. It is an attitude and permission for enjoyment of the educational process. It can be spontaneous or planned. Humor can be very useful in the enculturation of novices into one's profession, especially when dealing with elements of embarrassing intimacy and reality shocks that may occur in health care provision. Some ways to increase one's use of humor is by exposing oneself to humorous experiences, such as comics, joke books, and comedy clubs, collecting print and electronic humor samples, and even looking for the humor around oneself. This may include viewing the world through exaggeration or broad, silly perspectives. Let us incorporate humor in nursing education to maximize the benefits for nursing community.

MUDD Mapping

"My understanding through dialog and debate".

MUDD mapping is an innovative, interactive teaching-learning activity, wherein the main participant is the learner and the central activity is dialog. The overall goal of a MUDD mapping activity is to bring learners together so that they can engage in a purposeful dialog that will lead to an improved and sustained understanding of a subject matter. MUDD mapping is an acronym for My Understanding through Dialog and Debate.

MUDD mapping was designed by one of the authors in Newfoundland, Canada, as a teaching learning strategy aimed at improving the quality of learning in the classroom. The foundation of MUDD mapping is built on the conviction that dialog is the single, most important step in the development of partnerships in the teaching and learning arena of education. "Learning is facilitated opportunities to talk about and share experiences". Dialog in a MUDD mapping activity invites individuals to share their ideas, views, positions and propositions. Learners can affirm, validate, modify or add to their knowledge base through a dialog. Hence, MUDD mapping promotes dialog as a tool used by the learner to either affirm or refute existent knowledge or discover new knowledge.

MUDD mapping reflects the 5 principles of adult learning by knowledge. These principles of self-concept, experience, readiness to learn, orientation to learning, and motivation to learn provide a solid foundation for the teaching-learning strategy of MUDD mapping and are manifested at various levels in each individual's ability to participate in learning. Although MUDD mapping acknowledges and respects the self-esteem needs of the adult learner, it expects the adult learner to take risks, through dialog, in the quest to achieve the highest level of understanding on a given subject matter.

Invaluable Worth and Merit of Dialog in Teaching-learning

Dialog is a way of thinking out loud, hearing what others have to say. Dialog places value on learning as deliberate exchange of information, meaning, energy, feedback and reinforcement. It provides for the exchange and sharing of past experiences and previous learning. Dialog can create a learning situation wherein case studies, inviting description, analysis, application, and implementation of new learning can be applied.

In a MUDD mapping activity, it is the learner's responsibility to carry on the dialog.

Not all classroom dialog is meaningful. Therefore, it is important for learners to know how to talk effectively in educational settings. To help with this, MUDD outlines two effective modes of dialog experiential and hypothetical. In the experiential mode of talk, the learner shares past experiences that can relate back to the topic at hand. Experiential talk has the potential to foster a connection between past experiences enter into adult learning unless the learning experience or content is new to the learner. In the hypothetical mode of talk, the learner proposes (hypothesizes) what is. This mode of talk has the potential to foster a discovery for new learning. People are excited when new learning enables them to better understand their own themes and propositions. Irrespective of which of these two types of dialog the learner uses, it is important that the underpinnings of the dialog are appropriate and applicable to the topic.

The teacher is able to hear how the learner is processing his/her thinking, reaching his/her decisions. Every world in the acronym MUDD has been intentionally assigned. It embraces the learner and the learners needs.

The first letter in the word is M. It represents the pronoun "my", clearly indicating ownership.

"My" implies that the learner will be taking ownership for learning and will be doing so at the very outset of the activity.

"My" takes the attention away for the teacher.

"My" reflects the learner's acquisition of knowledge.

The letter U refers to "understanding", the second letter in the MUDD acronym. It denotes the teaching and learning. Simple memorization or rote learning to a more complex comprehension taxonomy.

The learner is encouraged to draw new conclusions from recognized knowledge sources (e.g. required readings, journals, etc.) as well as from their experiences. Understanding involves entering into a dialog that seeks to find answers to the question. Through dialog, the learner begins to exhibit many forms of hypothesizing (e.g. supposing, proposing, contemplating and entertaining).

The third word in the MUDD acronym, dialog, represents the concrete measurable expression of one's understanding (or even misunderstanding) about a concept or an idea.

The last word in the MUDD acronym, debate, is used to describe the magnification of dialog to its highest level that is putting one's position forward so as to enter into a debate with one who might hold a different position. At this point in a MUDD activity, the learner had already demonstrated a strong knowledge base, sufficient enough to engage in the rigor of the debate.

For MUDD mapping to be successful, the learner should understand the relationship between these principles and the expectations of MUDD mapping itself.

MUDD Mapping for Learnes

- Learners will acknowledge that they have:
  - Read the required readings
  - Completed any preassigned activities
- Learners will demonstrate willingness to dialog by presenting a word or phrase that connects to the central theme or concept
- Learners will be receptive to constructive and ongoing criticism of peers and the teacher
- Learners must come prepared to engage in dialog (experiential and hypothetical).

Therefore, before the session begins, learners are reminded that they must agree with these rules of engagement. Failure to do so means that the learner can be excluded from the session or asked to leave during the session. This is not a punitive action, but an affirmation to those who come prepared, that there will be purposeful and meaningful dialog, based on knowledge. You cannot have a MUDD session without a commitment to dialog.

MUDD Mapping for Teachers

- The teacher will explain the process of MUDD mapping (the principles of adult learning; experiential and hypothetical dialog)
- The teacher will secure the tools needed for MUDD mapping
- The teacher will begin the activity by identifying the central concept to be MUDD mapped
- The teacher will move outside learners seating circle, once the central concept is mapped, but will remain present to offer any needed redirection and/or clarification
- A teacher should not have a MUDD mapping session if he/she:
  - Does not support the principles of adult learning
  - Does not value learner dialog.

Clinical Teaching Methods

"Good teaching is more a giving of right questions than a giving of right answers".
—Josef Albers

The clinical learning environment, meant for practicum experiences, may be any place where students interact with patients and their families for purposes of acquiring clinical skills, critical thinking, clinical decision-making, and psychomotor as well as affective skills. This environment also provides the opportunities for students to apply theory into practice.

It is essential that the clinical environment be supportive and conducive to learning for the students to acquire the required clinical skills, qualities, and abilities to practice efficiently.

The methods of teaching employed in the classroom may not be appropriate in clinical set-up as the students have to deal with real patients in the latter situation. Therefore, clinical teaching methods that are more appropriate and effective in the clinical area should be used to teach the students.

Clinical teaching involves the careful design of an environment in which the students have opportunities to foster mutual respect and support for each other while they are achieving identified learning outcomes. Through appropriate clinical teaching methods a teacher can always help her students to acquire an appreciable level of nursing skills.

Let us now discuss some of the common clinical teaching methods that are used in nursing.

Nursing Case Study

"A study of breadth and depth of an individual patient".

A case study is one in which there is a comprehensive study of an individual patient to understand his needs and problems and plan and implement nursing care accordingly. It gives a total perspective of the patient and the care he requires and receives.

The nursing care study tries to give as much breadth and depth of an individual patient and places emphasis on the actual nursing care of the patient. The nursing care study provides the student opportunities to identify, gather and process the information required to solve the patient's problems.

Nursing care study can be defined as the blueprint of nursing care rendered by the student to a selected patient, for a particular period, by following the nursing process approach, with an intention to develop comprehensive nursing care abilities.

Development of the nursing care study is done in various phases:

- Selection of a suitable patient under the guidance of the teacher
- Collection of information and the facts about the patient, his disease condition and his social and personal history, etc. in a complete and comprehensive manner. This can be done only if the student establishes rapport with the patient
- With all the required data in hand, the student will now prepare a nursing care plan, identifying all his priority needs and problems
- Complete, supportive, and therapeutic nursing care will be given to the patient under the expert guidance of the clinical instructor
- All recordings and reporting has to be done and the nursing care plan has to be submitted in a written form for evaluation
- Throughout the care study, emphasis should be on the individual needs of the patient and how they are met
- The format and content for the care study varies from institution to institution, but an ideal care study invariably contains of descriptions regarding patient's demographic information, health profile, details about the disease condition, investigations, line of management, related literature, nursing care planned and implemented according to the nursing process approach, etc. The list is not an end on itself and the teacher can include other relevant aspects.

Advantages of Nursing Care Study

- The nursing care study is highly advantageous for the individual student to apply and practice nursing care activities, if properly selected, directed and supervised
- It provides an opportunity for the student to solve nursing problems, in an actual situation
- It helps the student to apply theory into practice
- It enables her to view the patient more comprehensively
- It stimulates the student to employ critical thinking skills, decision-making skills, and reflective thinking
- It helps the student to learn to see a patient as an individual person and not just as a case with so many symptoms or undergoing so many procedures
- It promotes group dynamics and enables the student to work as part of the health team
- It helps the student to integrate all her knowledge of the various subjects
- It contributes to the building up of a specific body of knowledge in nursing science. If the case studies are filed, they can be used for future references.
- The nursing care study serves as an excellent means for the student to demonstrate her nursing skill, her scientific knowledge, her sociologic and psychological insight into the problems of the patient and her skills in developing and maintaining interpersonal relationships.

Disadvantages of Nursing Care Study

- When adequate guidance is not obtained, the nursing care study may become a failure.
- The student may not have identified all the problems and needs present in the patient because of inexperience and negligence
- The case study may become distorted and unduly limited so that problems cannot be identified clearly
- It leaves no opportunity, once the study is completed, to branch out and incorporate new ideas
- It requires a great deal of time to write the case study in an acceptable form. Sometimes the student may not have good writing and presentation skills which may also distort the care study.

Bedside Clinic

"An informal discussion about a patient related problem".

The bedside clinic is one of the most effective methods of clinical instruction and it is mandatory that it is conducted in the presence of the patient. New knowledge is acquired through the observations made and study of an actual patient.

The bedside clinic is defined as "an informal discussion about a patient-related problem and free exchange of knowledge and experience about the same, identifying management strategies using problem-solving techniques". It can also be defined as "a course of action discussion, focusing on assessing the nursing problem, arriving at possible solutions, helping students to examine a patient's problems from his perspective".

Planning a Nursing-clinic

Clinics are necessarily preplanned to be most effective. Usually, the patient is not present for the entire discussion. Before he is brought into the ward or classroom, the group goes to the bedside, one of the students or staff nurses, who knows the patient, describes his personal characteristics, family background, his physical and mental condition, etc. The nursing care and the problems related to his treatment are also discussed. After this initial phase, the group interacts with the patient, asks him questions for clarification. When he is no longer needed, he is returned to bed. The discussion follows, questions are answered in the group. The material is summarized, important points emphasized and evaluation done as to the effectiveness of the clinic.

Planning of a bedside clinic consists of three phases that include: preparation, conduction and conslusion.

Preparation Phase

This phase involves:
- Determining the purpose of the clinic
- Selecting patients for the clinic and determining when they are going to be visited. Patient chosen for the clinic

should have typical rather than unusual conditions. The dramatic and typical condition may leave the student with erroneous impression
- Getting the consent from the patients
- Selecting the setting for conducting the clinic (patient's bedside or conference room)
- Instructing the students what they have to observe and the contexts in which they have to be well prepared
- Collecting all relevant and necessary patient related data well ahead.

Conduction Phase
The conduction phase consists of group discussion.

Introduction: During the introduction phase, the students have to be acquainted with the patient's background, other pertinent details about his management, purpose of the clinic, significant observations to be made and questions to be asked.

Patient-centered discussion: During this phase, the data collected should be analyzed, needs and problems of the patient have to be identified and a successful line of nursing management has to be outlined using the problem-solving approach. Patients have to be given opportunity to verbalize their concerns and how they meet a particular problem situation. If the patient is unresponsive or tired, the clinic should be better stopped.

Postclinical discussion: During the postclinic session, students have to discuss the various strategies in which the particular patient can be successfully dealt with, have to identify problem-solving techniques suitable for the patient, and design intervention strategies for him.

Conclusion Phase
The students and the supervisor conjointly come to a conclusion about the management of the patient and prepare a summary of the clinic. The group work together, and take solutions using the problem-solving approach and the responsibility to act on the problem is delegated to one or more of the students.

Advantages of a Bedside Clinic
The bedside clinic provides learning in real practical environment to the students.

It enhances the critical thinking and problem-solving skills of the students.

It mandates all the group members to participate in the conference.

It develops the skills in collecting relevant information from the patient and analyzing them.

It is advantageous to the patients, if properly conducted and guided.

Limitations of a Bedside Clinic
The bedside clinic, as the name indicates is conducted in front of the patient, all communications should be very carefully made. The patient should not receive any information that he should not. Nothing should be done or told which may hurt his feeling or embarrass him.

It may be time-consuming.

The group can accommodate only a small number of participants (not more than 8 to 10).

Nursing Rounds
"An extension of bedside clinic".

Nursing rounds is concerned with judging the adequacy of nursing care received by the patients and it is conducted under the leadership of senior nurses or nursing administrators with the active participation of nursing teachers, staff nurses and nursing students.

Nursing rounds is actually an extension of the bedside clinic. In the latter, only a single patient is concentrated and discussed about for a period of 30–40 minutes. Whereas in the former, the nursing management of almost all patients in the particular ward are discussed about, spending only a few minutes with each patient. The ideal duration of nursing rounds in a ward is 45 minutes and this time is sufficient to know about 20–25 patients.

The head nurse or the ward sister (whoever knows in detail about all the patients) may lead the nursing rounds and she briefs the treatment details and nursing care of the patients to all members of the group. The staff nurse or the nursing student who has been taking care of the patient are also allowed contributing some genuine points to the group. The group spends a period of 5–10 minutes with each patient and discusses the nursing care aspects in brief and may seek consultation from specialists if required. The senior nursing personnel in the group then conclude the discussion by giving some opinions, needed guidance and suggestions. She also assigns the responsibility of recording all the instructions and suggestions to a staff nurse or student. The group proceeds to all other patients of the ward in the same manner. All the group members are encouraged to contribute and participate in the discussion.

Nursing rounds motivates the students to:
- Learn nursing care in a real set-up, under the guidance of experienced and senior personnel
- Learn more about the nursing management by referring related literature and through discussion with experts
- Develop a positive attitude toward providing nursing care to patients
- Promote team spirit and professionalism among the members. The students develop an ability to categorize

patients into high-risk, moderate risk and low-risk groups, depending on the severity of the illness.

Conference

"An act of consulting together".

Conference is a two-way process, where teaching and learning goes on spontaneously. It is a method of teaching where a teacher meets a small group of students for the purpose of accomplishment of a clinical learning objective. The conference is held under the chairmanship of an expert, who is either a teacher or a senior member of professional group.

A conference is defined as the act of consulting together. Conferences are necessary to the practice of nursing to give and receive information. Nurses convene conferences for a variety of purposes including.

Direction giving conferences, in which the leader gives information and directions specific to the assignment. They are meetings called at the beginning of a work shift for the specific purpose of communicating job assignments, delineating areas of responsibility, and imparting information necessary for members to care for clients effectively.

Client-centered conferences, in which members identity problems and attempt to arrive at solutions and decide on course of action. They are meetings in which problem-oriented care is discussed and evaluated. It is designed to help overcome the decentralization of care. The focus of attention is usually on the analysis of one client or family situation for whom the nurse or group is caring. Client-centered conferences provide a means whereby all participants will benefit from the experiences of a few. Where possible, the client and other significant people are included in the sessions and the client is the focal point of discussion.

Content conferences, in which participants assemble to acquire knowledge about a specific subject. Constant input of knowledge enables client and caregivers to perform the tasks expected of them more effectively. One way of ensuring participants the opportunity to increase their learning is to provide them with time to meet for the sole purpose of exploring content.

Reporting conferences, in which participants give progress reports.

General problems conferences, in which individuals express their impressions about the work situation and try to resolve work or personnel problems.

Nursing care conferences, in which participants collaborate for problem-oriented nursing care.

Based on the number of participants, the conference may be of two types: individual and group.

Individual Conference

Individual conference is a clinical teaching method which focuses on the comprehensive development of the individual student with special emphasis to the development of clinical skills. It offers the teacher an excellent opportunity to discover the interests, the needs and the problems of the individual student and to help her to achieve a proper balance among them.

It is a dynamic interaction between the student and the teacher, with a purpose of educational guidance. The student is hoping to receive from the knowledge and experience of the teacher.

Individual conference is more similar to an interview process. But apart from obtaining facts or giving information, the former provides guidance to the individual student regarding her performance in the clinical area.

Principles of the Individual Conference

- Individual conference is a professional relationship between the teacher and the student with the purpose of educational guidance
- The teacher should display an attitude of willingness to listen with sympathy, interest and patience, understand and help the student
- She should have an attitude of concern for the self-development of the student and the solution of her problems
- She should have proper attitudes, and have a desire to help the student
- She should be skillful in observation, recognizing ambivalent feelings, and establishment of rapport
- She should present intellectual challenges to the student and stimulate her motivation
- She should be able to make constructive criticism while assisting the student in evaluating the learning experience
- Both the teacher and student should have recognized the value and importance of the method
- The conference should take place in a friendly and private atmosphere. The setting should be such that the learner feels comfortable, at ease and free from interruptions
- The teacher should guide the progress of the conference and keep it focused on the problem area
- Rapport must be established between the two; the student should develop confidence on the teacher
- The role of both the student and teacher are important in the conference method for making it a success.

Advantages of the Individual Conference

- The individual conference serves as a tremendous aid in helping the student to comprehend, associate or integrate the knowledge she has received

- It serves as a valuable tool in evaluating the progress of the learner and determining the future dealings with the student
- It serves as a valuable interaction between the student and the teacher, advantageous for both. (The teacher comes to know the student's abilities, potentialities, and shortcomings and the student gets the confidence and feeling of security by the individual attention and guidance she has received)
- It can be used to clarify class material, to supplement instructions, to explain answers to questions of individual students which do not concern the entire class.

Disadvantages of the Individual Conference
- The individual conference is time consuming
- Sometimes the student may be uncooperative, inattentive, or lacks skill or interest and she may not want to disclose facts to the teacher. In such instances, the conference becomes a failure
- The teacher may lack the skill to conduct the conference to a success.

Group Conference

Group conference can be defined as "a meeting of professional persons for the purpose of interchange of ideas and solve problems that are related to patients and their surroundings". All the members of the group are involved in accomplishing common, patient centered goals. It is a small group teaching method.

The main objective of the group conference is to assess the health needs of the patients and to attain these needs through comprehensive approaches by the contributions of all the members of the team.

Principles of Group Conference
- There must be a common objective or patient-centered goal to be accomplished
- The teacher in-charge or a senior student may serve as the leader of the group
- Topic selected for the discussion should have a clinical orientation and enrich the clinical skills of the students
- All the members of the group and the leader should be well prepared about the topic of discussion
- The time, place, duration, and purpose of the conference are to be announced well ahead to all concerned. All members should come well prepared with recent information especially
- All members should be encouraged to contribute and participate in the discussion
- The leader should see that the discussion goes in line with the clinical objectives to be accomplished and is not diverted
- At the end of the session, the points of discussion are to be summarized by a student or the leader and all interactions recorded promptly
- Date for the review conference has to be decided and announced.

Process Recording

"A written report of conversations".

Process recording is a written report of the conversations that occurred between the patient and the professional nurse, when they were working together toward a common objective. It can be defined as "a verbatim account of a visit for purposes of bringing out the interplay between the nurse and the patient in relation to the objectives of the visit" (Walker).

Purposes of Process Recording

The process recording may be used to assist the students in acquiring, understanding the importance and developing competence in maintaining interpersonal relationships.
- To learn about interpersonal relationships and to gain competence in related skills
- To improve the interviewing and conversational skill of the student
- To recognize the verbal and nonverbal cues to the patient's needs
- To evaluate nurse-patient interactions
- To increase observational skills of the student
- To identify thoughts and feelings related to self and others
- To improve the ability to identify problems and gain skills in solving them.

Phases of Process Recording

There are three important phases in process recording:
1. Preparing the student for process recording
2. Recording nurse-patient interactions
3. Evaluating the interactions by the instructor and the student.

Preparing the Student for Process Recording

The student must be helped to define clearly the appropriate objectives to be accomplished regarding the nurse-patient interactions. Then she should be motivated to use the process record to accomplish the desired goals. Later, the student should also be helped to write a process record.

Recording Nurse-Patient Interactions

It consists of four parts:
1. The exact verbatim of the nurse-patient conversation
2. The student's conscious feelings and her interpretation of the patient's feelings

3. Analysis for meanings and clues to patient's needs
4. The instructor's and the student's evaluations of the total process recording experience.

While making the recordings, the patient should be reassured that strict confidentiality will be maintained with the interview material. The student should be instructed to record all verbal interactions, and make notations on thoughts, feelings and actions that she experiences during the interaction. The nonverbal communications should also be noted.

Evaluating the Interactions by the Instructor and the Student

The interaction data so collected should be analyzed and the student should be given due guidance in doing the same. During the process of analyzing the recordings, the objectives of the learning experience should be clearly kept in focus.

Disadvantages of Process Recording

- The technique is highly time consuming
- It is highly complex and complicated for an average student
- The student is required to have very good communication skills
- The patient may not be cooperative for the technique.

Summary

- Education is a process, the chief goal of which is to bring about desirable changes in the behavior of the learner in the form of acquisition of knowledge, proficiency in skills and development of attitudes.
- The three main components of the educational process are development of educational objectives, organization of the teaching-learning activities and evaluation. This is called the educational spiral.
- There are four dimensions identified in the educative process. They were substantive dimension, procedural dimension, environmental dimension and human relations dimension.
- Learning is any relatively permanent change or modification of behavior that results as a result of practice or experience.
- Learning is the process of growth and development whereby the learner acquires a body of knowledge, develops ideas which she makes a part of herself and develops the ability to use her knowledge in the pursuit of her ideals. Learning is a part of education, learning brings modification of behavior.
- The pillars of learning are learning to know, learning to do, learning to live together and learning to be.
- Teaching is a system of directed and deliberate actions that are intended to induce learning through a series of directed activities designed to induce learning. Bevis (1989) defined teaching as an art and science in which the content is structured and the processes used enable student learning.
- Educational objectives are statements which tell us what the student should be able to do at the end of a learning period that he would not beforehand. Educational process aims at evaluation of the learner and not the teacher. It is advantageous to have objectives written in terms of learner behavior.
- A lesson plan reveals the knowledge and philosophy of the teacher, her understanding of students, objectives of education, the content to be taught and teaching ability to utilize appropriate method of teaching.
- Unit may be defined as a large subdivision of the subject matter. Planning the unit is known as unit planning.
- A course may be defined as a complete series of studies leading to graduation or a degree. It could also mean any of the separate units of instruction in a subject made of lectures and classes.
- Teaching methods are the stimulation, guidance, direction and encouragement for learning and also the means to achieve the desired educational objectives.
- A teaching-learning method will help the teacher to conduct teaching in an agreeable, student-friendly and successful manner by initiating and maintaining link between the subject matter and the student. Certain principles are to be followed in selection of methods of teaching.
- The various methods of teaching are classified into inspirational methods, expository methods, individualized methods, encounter methods, natural learning method, discovery methods, and group methods.

3. Instructional Media and Methods

"The foundation of all learning consists in representing clearly to the senses, sensible objects so that they can be appreciated easily".

—*Comenius*

Objectives
After reading this unit, you will be able to:
- Define audio-visual aids
- Classify audio-visual aids
- Apply the principles in using audio-visual aids
- Understand the advantages and disadvantages of audio-visual aids
- Explain the various types of audio-visual aids.

Introduction

Audio-visual aids are being increasingly used in modern day educational programs and has become inevitable to make the classroom teaching colorful and vivid. These are the devices by which the teacher helps the students to clarify, establish and correlate concepts and appreciate them through utilization of more than one sensory channel. They are means of communication that help to make learning more meaningful, more interesting and more effective. The term "Media" refers to the channel through which an idea or concept is communicated to the learners. In any instructional situation, media follows the method and both go hand-in-hand. Audio-visual media is highly exploited in the classroom situation for effective communication. Audio-visual aids supplement the teacher's explanation and are called "Teaching Aids" since teachers plan, prepare and use them in the classroom. It is to be remembered that in any situation, teaching aids can never be able to replace a teacher.

Definition

Audio-visual aids are any devices that can be used to make the learning experience more concrete, more realistic and more dynamic (Kinder).

Dent defines audio-visual aids as "all materials used in the classroom or in other teaching situations, to facilitate the understanding of the written or spoken words".

Mckown and Roberts define as "audio-visual aids are supplementary devices by which the teacher, through the utilization of more than one sensory channel is able to clarify, establish and correlate concepts, interpretations and appreciations.

Burton defines audio-visual aids as those sensory objects or images which initiate or stimulate and reinforce learning. An audio-visual aid is an instructional device in which the message can be heard as well as seen.

Audio-visual aids are defined as any device used to aid in the communication of an idea. This definition gives the idea that virtually anything can be used as an aid, providing it, successfully communicates the idea or information for which it is designed. Audio-visual aids are not a supplement to teaching and not a substitute for teacher or books.

Senses as Gateway of Learning

Researches in America have shown that we learn about:
- 1% through the sense of taste
- 1.5% through the sense of touch
- 3.5% through the sense of smell
- 11% through the sense of hearing
- 83% through the sense of sight.

Further, with regard to the retention of learning, elaborate researches have shown that we remember about:
- 10% of what we read
- 20% of what we hear
- 30% of what we see
- 50% of what we see and hear
- 80% of what we say, and
- 90% of what we say as we do a thing.

The traditional teacher depended too much on verbal exposition. The pupil hears and forgets. Further, unless the individual has pragmatic imagination, it will be difficult for the individual to visualize objects and events however vivid, the verbal description is. It is highly possible that concepts formed will depend upon the nature of background experience of the individual. It is highly essential particularly in science and technology that knowledge gained by an individual is accurate where considerable visualization of objects (Pupil see and remember) and processes (Pupil do and understand) are necessary and formation of accurate concepts essential.

Where to use Audio-visual Aids

- Where they add to the clarity of the subject
- Where the subject is too far to be actually seen, as in geography and astronomy
- Where the subject is too big to be handled or brought to the classroom
- Where the subject is too small to be seen by naked eyes, e.g. germs, atoms, etc.
- Where the concept of teaching is related to abstract and nonvisual subjects.

Classification of Audio-visual Aids

- Audio aids
- Visual aids
- Combined aids

Audio Aids

They are also known as auditory aids and can be only heard. They comprise of radio, tape recorder, microphones, amplifiers, earphones, etc. The tape recorders are extensively used as teaching aids (Flowchart 3.1).

Visual Aids

They can be broadly classified into projected aids and nonprojected aids. Those that are not requiring projection are nonprojected aids and are the most commonly used and important aids. This category includes graphic aids (including graphs, charts, diagrams, cartoons, flannel graphs, maps, flip charts, chalkboard, bulletin boards, etc.) and three-dimensional aids (including real objects, specimens, models, puppets, exhibits, etc.).

Combined Aids or Audio-visual Aids

They are a combination of audio and visual aids.

AV aids/media can be classified into three different perspectives as below:
1. Hardware/software — Projected and nonprojected
2. Dimension — Graphics and models
3. Technology advancement — Traditional and digital

Projected and Nonprojected Media

Projected media is one which requires hardware like OHP, slide projector, LCD projector, etc. for projecting the software to be presented. On the other hand, nonprojected media does not require any hardware and can be projected for presentation straight. Some examples of projected and nonprojected media are:

Projected	Nonprojected
• Slides/film strips	• Chalkboard
• OHP transparencies	• Charts
• Movie (35 mm/16 mm film)	• Magnetic cut-outs/displays
• Video projection	• Felt cut-out/displays
• Powerpoint slides	• Models
• Monitor	
• LCD	

Graphics and Models

The word Graphics emerged from the Greek word "Graphien" which means both writing and drawing. Pictorial representation was an earliest means of nonverbal communication. "One picture is worth a thousand words" is not a mere propaganda, but it is true. Graphics takes many forms such as program titles, diagrams, graphs, maps, etc. Graphics may also be used to catch the eye, to create atmosphere or to "humanize" a subject. Properly designed graphic images convey facts and ideas more economically and more elegantly than real images.

Traditional and Digital

A traditional media is one which is made by using common materials such as cardboard, hardboard, wood, plastics/perspex, transparencies, films, photographs, color cardboard, black cartridge paper, poster color papers, fluorescent papers, poster color paints, thermocole, and so on. It could be a chart, transparency, a set of slides or film strip or a model.

A digital media is one which is developed using digital devices and computers. Powerpoints, graphic animations

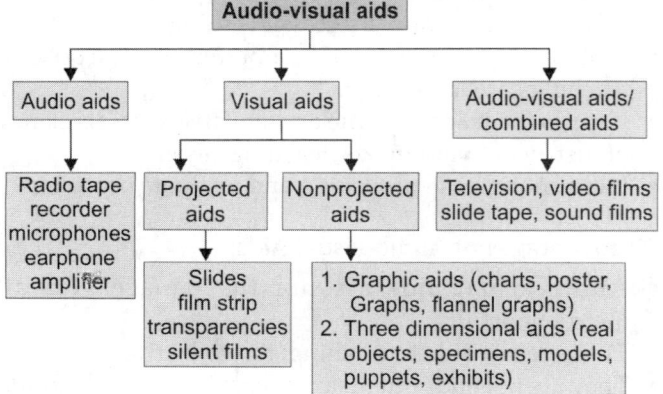

Flowchart 3.1: Classification of audio-visual aids.

(2D or 3D), Computer Based Teaching (CBT) materials, Computer Based Multimedia Learning Packages (CBMMLP) are some of the digital media.

Principles in the Use of Audio-visual Aids

The following principles are to be followed in the use of audio-visual aids:
- **Principle of selection:** The instructional aids selected should be suitable for the level of audience, the educational objectives, and the nature of content that is to be instructed
- **Principle of preparation:** This refers to cost-effectiveness in preparing the audio-visual aids. It will be better to make the aids by using locally available materials utilizing the creativity of the students
- **Principle of presentation:** Getting an instructional aid is of no value, when it is not presented in an attractive and acceptable manner
- **Principle of response:** The teachers should motivate the students to respond properly to the instructional aids
- **Principle of evaluation:** There should be a continuous evaluation of both the audio-visual aids and teaching techniques in the light of realization of the desired objectives
- **Principle of preservation:** All the aids that are used by the teachers or the students must be maintained properly and kept away from dampness, dusts, insects, moths, etc.

Requisites for an Effective Audio-visual Aid

An effective audio-visual aid should be:

Motivating
- Meaningful
- Purposeful
- Accurate
- Simple
- Attractive
- Facilitating group participation
- Up-to-date
- Easily portable

Self-explanatory
- Clear
- Creative and vicarious
- Realistic and provide variety

Reinforcing
- Meeting individual differences
- Following scientific principles
- Facilitates positive transfer of learning
- Makes the concept to be easily understood, easy to handle and manipulate

Uses of Audio-visual Aids in Teaching
- Best motivators
- Concrete
- First-hand experience
- Variety
- Greater retention
- Attractive
- Promotes learning
- Saves energy and time
- Realistic
- Vividness
- Meets the individual needs
- Aids in mass education
- Promotes scientific temper
- Develops higher faculties
- Reinforces learning.

Advantages of Audio-visual Aids
- They provide a concrete basis for conceptual thinking
- They stimulate interest among students and hold their attention. It sustains and focuses attention on to the content
- They make learning more permanent and realistic and it helps to retain learned content permanently
- They help to communicate ideas clearly and precisely
- They stimulate self-activity on the part of the students by offering a variety of experiences
- They promote group dynamics among the students
- They provide experience not easily obtained through other materials and contribute to the efficiency, depth, and variety of learning
- They economize time, effort, and materials
- They help in sharing experiences and motivate toward change of attitudes
- They are potent starters and motivators
- They provide variety of classroom techniques
- They give a true picture of the object/set-up/structure
- It relieves from boredom by breaking the monotony
- It supplies a concrete basis for conceptual thinking and hence reduces the need for verbal communication
- It contributes to growth of meaning and vocabulary development
- It provides experiences not easily secured by other materials and contribute to the efficiency, depth, and variety of learning
- It develops continuity of thoughts in teaching
- It is possible to show inaccessible things
- Motivates the teacher to do a better and purposeful teaching career
- It saves the teachers' time and enhances the efficiency of instruction and makes teaching easier
- It can motivate goal seeking and evaluate outcomes.

Disadvantages of Audio-visual Aids
- Audio-visual aids are not the panacea for all instructional ills
- They are not aids to teaching, but to learning
- They are not ends but means to facilitate good learning
- They should not be misused.

Criteria for Selection of Audio-visual Aids

The following criteria can be used in the selection of audio-visual aids:
- Type of objective to be achieved
- Entry behavior of the learners
- Size of the class
- Nature of the subject matter
- Availability of resources
- Availability of time
- Teacher's competency to use a specific method/media.

Problems in Utilizing Audio-visual Aids
- Apathy of the teachers
- Indifference of the students
- Ineffective aids
- Electrical problems
- Lack of knowledge in preparation and handling
- Language difficulty
- Financial problems.

Graphic Aids

"Visual way of presenting the information".

Graphic presentation is a visual art, based on the use of visual symbolic and visual abstract forms. Graphic aids make it easier to understand and read the written text. They present the text in an interesting, concise and visual way, information that would otherwise be given in long and complicated written text. These aids make the textbook more comprehensible by summarizing concisely the major points of the text, actually saving the time in reading.

Selection of Graphics/Images

Psychological, technical and esthetic factors are involved in selecting images. The typographical forms that will heighten the learner interest and focus on key information transmit clear and memorable information about structures, relationships, processes and other abstract ideas. Important subliminal statements and degrees of emphasis will be imparted through the choice of colors, dimension, scale, layout and type face. The designer must gauge the speed at which an idea can be grasped when it has been converted into a symbol or schematic image.

Graphics techniques can be used for greater impact, to hold attention and to distinguish finer points of emphasis and grasping. Some graphic devices become so institutionalized that they replace language altogether, e.g. the arrow or pointing hands as directional signs. Bold, original and surprising effects have strongest initial impact. Pictures can be used as part of this, to intrigue pupils and develop ideas or liven up the page. The concept of contrast in its various applications helps us to understand which graphic element will "stand-out" more strongly.

Leonardo do Vinci was one of the first writers in science and technology who recognized the importance of integrating pictorial representation with verbal description as a way to communicate factual information clearly and efficiently.

The planning of a graphic aid is primary part, to determine which type of graphic aid best meets the necessities for efficient transmission of information. The secondary part is to decide where to place the graphic aid. The graphic aids like tables, photographs of specialized subjects or situations, drawings and diagrams, graphs, posters and charts make a presentation more impressive than a written description.

Especially, graphic visual materials like graphs, pictures, tables, and diagrams contain visual material that is pertinent to the main ideas in the chapter which aids improve:
- **Concentration**: By visually attracting attention.
- **Comprehension**: By helping us to interpret the visual information into verbal language.
- **Retention**: By reinforcing our memory, as we learn information visually and verbally.

Graphic materials are designed to be clear and accurate so that they will help us learn unfamiliar concepts. To make the text easily understandable, these aids should consist of the following components:

Component	Description
Headings	Titles found above the graphic aid.
Legends	Symbols that explain a graphic aid.
Captions	An explanation accompanying a graphic aid.
Foot notes	An explanatory note found below a graphic aid.
Keys	Information used to interpret a graphic aid.

Graphic aids are the illustrative instructional material depicted on a two-dimensional surface combined with drawings, pictures, paintings, and words. They provide nonverbal or visual learning experiences resulting in the formation of mental associations between abstract and concrete ideas. The purpose of these pictures is to help us visualize, what is being described in the written text. They are included not only to illustrate a major point, but also to add interest to what we have already read.

Charts

"An illustrative visual media".

Charts may be defined as combination of graphic and pictorial material, designed for the orderly and logical visualizing of relationships between key facts and ideas. The main function of the chart is always to show relationships such as, comparisons, relative amounts, developments, processes, classification, and organization.

Charts can also be defined as a visual symbol summarizing, comparing, contrasting or performing other helpful services in explaining the subject matter. It is meant to depict pictorial and written information in a systematic way by effective arrangement of the key facts. They are visual displays arranged on thick sheets, poster paper, newsprint or cardboard.

Purposes of Charts

- It is used to motivate the students
- It serves as an illustrative visual media
- It depicts logical relationships between main idea and supporting facts
- It is useful in teaching situations where breakdown of a fact or a statement is to be listed
- It is useful in showing points of comparisons, distinctions and contrast between two or more things
- It is useful in learning situations for depicting organizational and hierarchical structures
- It is used for presenting abstract ideas in visual forms.

Classification of Charts

Generally, charts can be classified as:
- Tree chart
- Stream chart
- Narrative chart
- Tabulation chart
- Flowchart
- Genealogy chart
- Time chart.

Tree Chart

A chart depicted in the form of a tree with several branches is called as a tree chart. The main concept is represented as the trunk of the tree and various subdivisions/developments of the concept will be depicted as its branches. The possible consequences of a complex disease could be explained well with the help of a tree chart (Fig. 3.1).

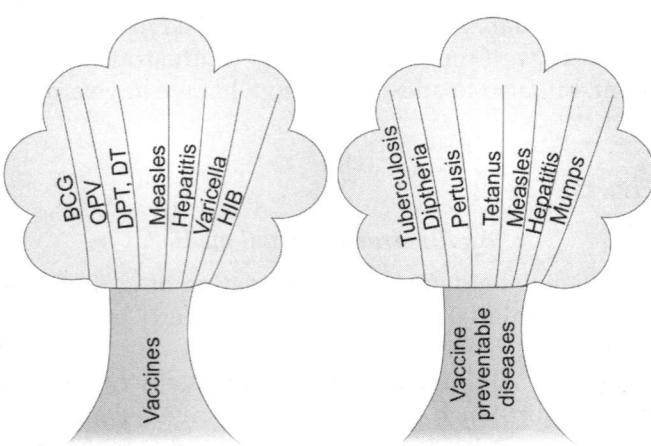

Fig. 3.1: Tree chart.

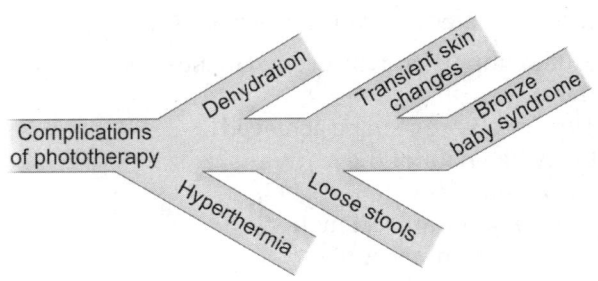

Fig. 3.2: Stream chart.

Stream Chart

In these types of charts, the main concept is explained in the form of a stream of river, and its subparts in the form of tributaries coming out of it. It is more similar to a tree chart (Fig. 3.2).

Narrative Chart

It is an extended left-to-right arrangement of facts and ideas used to express the concept(s). It is also used to explain the cause and effect.

Tabulation Chart

In these types of charts, the data is presented in a tabular form. They are commonly used for comparisons, or for listing advantages and disadvantages of a particular treatment or like. It presents information in ordinary sequence. They are very valuable aid in the teaching situation where breakdown of a fact or a statement is to be listed.

Advantages of essay	Disadvantages of essay
• Easy to construct	• More subjective
• Encourages creativity	• Time consuming to answer
• Helps in organizing ideas	• Offers less feedback
• Helps to assess writing skills	• Takes long time to score
• Allows for free expression	• Has limited range of application

Flowchart

These are helpful in learning situations that requires the study of organizational or hierarchical structures. In these, lines/rectangles/circles or other graphic representations are connected by lines showing the directional flow. While designing a flowchart, care must be taken to preserve a sense of order and sequence (Flowchart 3.2).

Genealogy Chart

This is used to represent the growth and development of an empire, dynasty or historical facts of this nature. Similar to a tree chart, these charts also take an analogy from the tree, the origin in a single line rectangle, circle or other

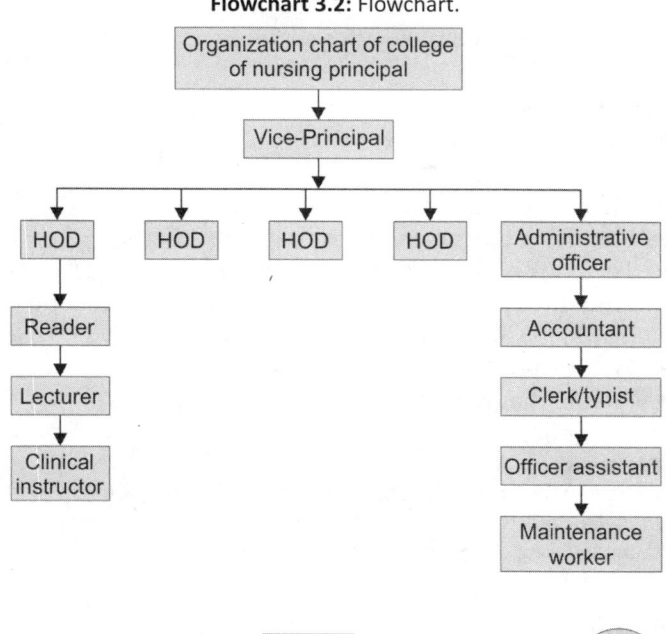

Flowchart 3.2: Flowchart.

Table 3.1: Time table for I year MSc (N) Program (for a week).	
8–10 AM	Nursing education
10–12 noon	Advanced nursing practice
12–1 PM	Nursing research
1–2 PM	Lunch
2–4 PM	Clinical specialty

- They are used to explain, clarify, and simplify the complicated subject matter
- They attract attention and reduce the amount of verbal explanation given by the teacher.

Principles of Preparing Charts

- Choose the appropriate material either thick or thin, depending on the purpose
- Decide on the information to be written or drawn
- Prepare a layout using the pencil. Draw margin in all four sides
- Decide on the size of the letter. Use of stencil will enhance the legibility of the work
- Draw picture neatly and artistically
- Use appropriate colors. Use dark color against a light color
- Decide on how to display.

Effective Uses of Charts

- Sufficiently large in size
- Explain only one concept
- Limited writing
- Neat appearance
- Provision for hanging the chart
- Use of pointer
- Proper storage, preservation and reuse.

Disadvantages of Charts

- Charts cannot be used for large groups
- They cannot be used for illiterate audience.

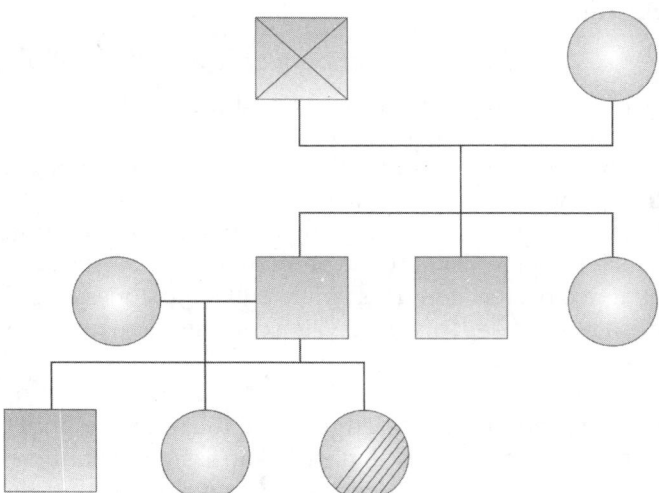

Fig. 3.3: Genealogy chart.

representation of the trunk and the various changes or developments are shown as the branches (Fig. 3.3).

Time Chart

They provide a chronological framework within which events and developments may be recorded. They develop time sense among the pupils, helping them to comprehend and visualize the pageant of time and its relationships (Table 3.1).

Advantages of Charts

- Charts are an effective tool for learning
- They arouse interest in the student
- They are prepared in a very low-cost
- They are portable and available for use and reuse
- They are easily prepared and maintained

Pictures

"Representations of beautiful dreams of reality."

Most learners are visual minded; so pictures are a great help in teaching. They remind the learner of the meaning and help her to communicate. They help the teacher save her voice. Also the same pictures may be used for several purposes and for review purposes (Fig. 3.4).

Pictures are the most interesting, easily available and understandable as well as interpretable graphic aids. They simplify the abstractions and help to create and maintain interest. They include photographs, paintings, illustrations clipped from periodicals (magazines, newspapers, newsletters, publicity materials or calendars).

120 Nursing Education: Principles and Concepts

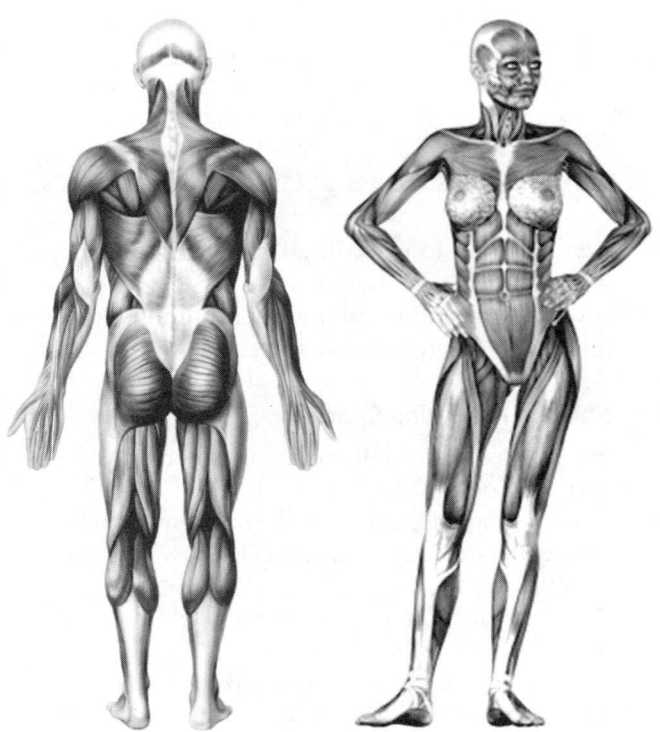

Fig. 3.4: Picture.

The selected pictures are to be relevant to the text in which it is presented and it should be more colorful, attractive, informative, clear, and accurate.

Too many pictures may distract the attention of the students, which is to be avoided. The displayed picture should be genuine and not misguiding. A picture is a cheap and inexpensive graphic aid that can serve as valuable instructional material if used properly.

The picture should be invariably captioned and labeled. It should arouse the curiosity, imagination, and thinking of the student. One should remember that:"A picture is worth more than ten thousand words".

Points to be kept in mind while selecting and showing pictures:
- The picture should be large enough for the entire class to see clearly
- The pictures should illustrate, at first glance, the point under the study
- The colored pictures are more effective than black and white ones and can be used for many purposes
- The pictures should fit into the cultural pattern of the learner
- The picture should tell the learner something familiar to connect it with real life
- The pictures should be labeled to ease classroom practice
- Pictures should not be confusing
- It should be relevant
- Sufficient time should be given to see the picture
- Too many pictures should not be shown at a time
- Adequate lighting should be provided
- It should be removed after showing.

Types of Pictures

Various types of pictures that can be used in teaching are:
- Picture post cards
- Pictures made on charts or pasted on charts
- Textbook and reference book pictures
- Pageant type aids (well-drawn and colored portraits)
- Picture assembly
- Picture diagram.

> **Dioramas**
> It is three-dimensional scene in depth incorporating a group of modeled objects and figures in a natural setting. It is very effective in the teaching of biological and social sciences.

Posters

"Visual representation of concepts".

A poster is an informational or educational tool with which many people in different locations can be reached easily. Posters incorporate visual combinations of images, lines, colors, and words. They are intended to catch and hold the viewer's attention long enough to communicate a brief image, usually a persuasive one. The most effective posters convey a single and simple message. A poster, when kept on display, is a continuing reminder of information being used.

Posters may be a method of communicating information and knowledge and educating the public and professional peers. A poster is an assignment nurses can relate to because posters are prevalent within the health domain.

Poster presentation requires students to know current information and understand a specific content area, as well as be able to reinterpret and organize information so it reaches the audience in a meaningful way. This requires complex skills, and this activity fosters and develops in a logical and applied way.

This approach fosters critical thinking, communication, creativity, analysis, and problem-solving skills, and it allows for different learning styles.

The activity engages students in a collaborative planning process that satisfies the need to know the how, what and why of learning.

Purposes of Posters

- To motivate the students to learn
- To convey information quickly and easily
- To create an esthetic effect
- To serve as an instructional aid both in the classroom and in the community.

Features of a Good Poster

A good poster should have the following features:
- Brevity : Message conveyed should be concise
- Simplicity : Message should be easily understandable
- Concept : Should be based on a single and relevant idea
- Layout : Should be simple and attractive
- Color : Poster should be attractive and eye-catching with suitable colors and color combinations

Preparation of Poster

Posters can be prepared using chart, drawing paper, poster board or thick chart. Posters are hand drawn using various colors or sketch pens. Posters vary in size and it depends upon the content and purpose. In general, overcrowding of letters is avoided and diagrams are used to convey the theme. Nowadays posters are designed and digitally printed using various materials.

Advantages of Posters

- Complex ideas and concepts can be conveyed more easily through posters
- Posters are very attractive and hence they convey the message more quickly
- Posters promote student's skill in creativity
- They can stand alone and are self-explanatory
- Assessment of the students' critical thinking abilities can be done through posters
- Posters provide students with feedback from peers and faculty
- Students get a sense of achievement from producing posters
- Evaluation of posters can be done immediately.

Disadvantages of Posters

- Posters involve faculty time to develop assignment and evaluation techniques
- Can be frustrating to students who are not visual learners
- Posters always may not give enough information
- When a poster is seen too often, it becomes a part of the environment and then no longer attracts attention.

Graphs

"Flat pictures which employ dots and lines".

Graphs are flat pictures which employ dots, lines or pictures to visualize numerical and statistical data, to compare and contrast different variables. Graphs make presentation of specific quantitative data for analysis, interpretation or comparison. A huge data and long list of figure is always boring but the same represented by a graph captures attention and makes students think. Just a single glance of a good graph can give a lot of valuable information. Graphs and diagrams are widely used in the presentation of statistical data either alone or in conjunction with other graphic aids. Graphs readily show a comparison between two or more variables or attributes.

Graphs are preferred to descriptive material as:
- They furnish a visual method of examining quantitative data
- They make a more lasting impression than detailed numbers
- They convey an idea forcefully
- They help us to have a real grasp of the overall picture rather than the details
- They capture attention and stimulate thinking
- They are easily understandable and interpretable.

In order that these graphs and diagrams present ideas truthfully and emphasize correct ideas, they must be drawn according to certain basic rules which are dependent partly on convention, partly on mathematical considerations, and partly on personal preferences.

Types of Graphs

There are four main types of graphs:
1. Line graphs
2. Bar graphs
3. Pie graphs
4. Pictorial graphs.

Line Graph

Line graphs are used when a considerable quantity of data is to be plotted or when the data are continuous. The concepts are represented with the help of simple lines vertically or horizontally drawn (Fig. 3.5). It is usually a free hand smooth line through various points indicating the instantaneous values of two variables at various moments. The line may be a straight line or

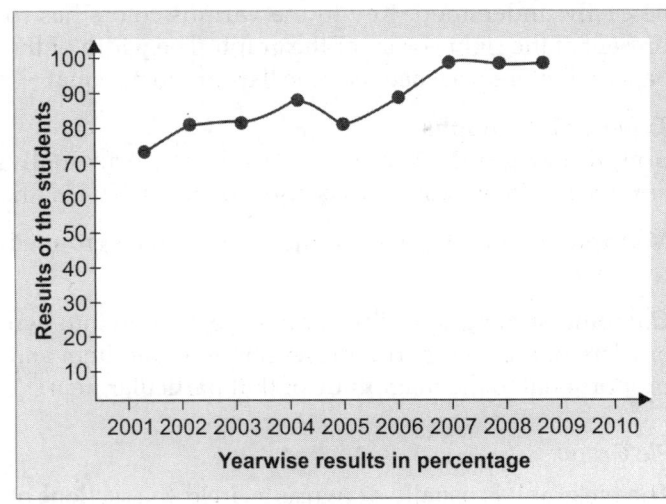

Fig. 3.5: Line graph.

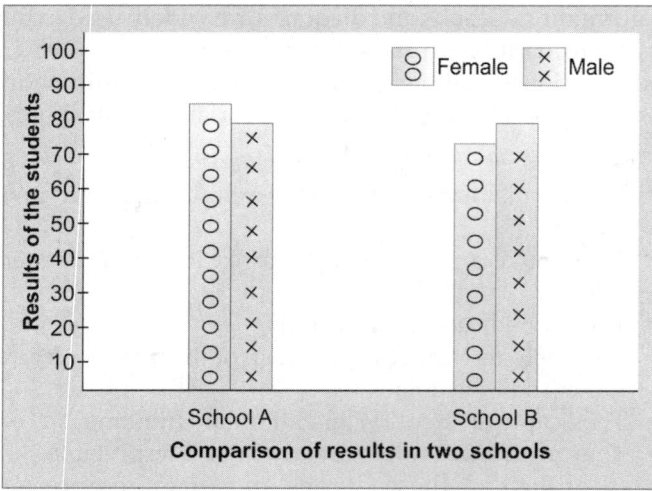

Fig. 3.6: Bar graph.

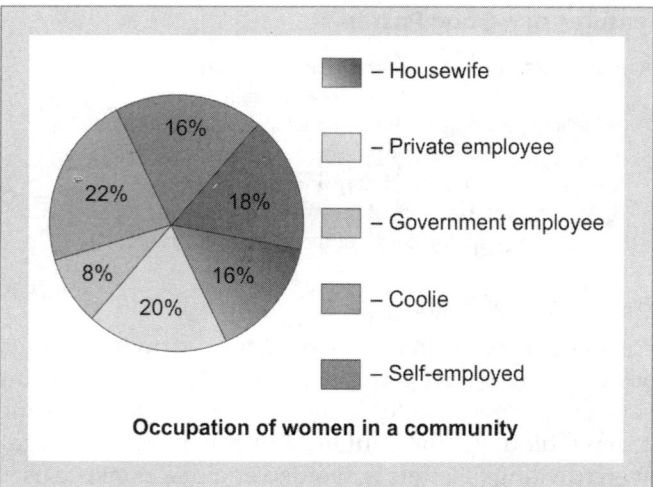

Fig. 3.7: Pie graph.

curved line indicating the relationship between two variables. Pictorial illustrations and cartoons can also be occasionally used on the line graphs to increase their interest and readability.

Bar Graph

A bar graph consists of bars arranged horizontally or vertically from a "zero" base. Two perpendicular lines from a point (called origin) work as the reference lines. The size, length, and color of the bars represent different values. Especially, the length of bars represents the magnitude of a given attribute, while the spaces between bars represent second variable which should be uniformly changing.

Bar graphs are especially useful in comparing and contrasting two variables or two groups of the same attributes (Fig. 3.6).

Bar graphs can be made more attractive by using different colors for different attributes, for them to be easily understood. Key to the various colors has to present at the right corner of the graph. The width of the bars and inter-space between the bars are to be equal.

Types of Bar Graphs

Simple bar graph: May be vertically or horizontally arranged. Suitable scale must be used to present bar length.

Multiple bar graphs: Two or more bars can be grouped together.

Component bar graph: The bar may be divided into two or more parts, each part representing a certain item and proportional to the magnitude of that particular item.

Pie Graph

The pie graph is usually drawn as a circle, the sections of which are used to represent component parts of a whole. The circle, that resembles a disk, is divided into sectors of different angles to represent the fractions or percentages of the divisions of a distributive attribute.

Method of construction of pie graphs:
- The surface area of circle is to cover 360°.
- The total frequencies or values are equated to 360° and then the angles equaling the component parts are calculated.
- After determining their angle, the required sectors in the circle are drawn.
- The numerical data may be converted into the angles of the circle (Fig. 3.7).

Pictorial Graph

Pictorial graph is an outstanding method of graphic representation. In this type, graphic pictures are used for the expression of ideas, thus more attractive and easily understandable. We can either use same type of pictures but of different sizes, proportional to the magnitudes of attributes represented or else, pictures of same size different in number to represent different magnitudes (Fig. 3.8).

Pictorial graphs are more attractive and effective in explaining the difficult concepts and are more appealing to the viewers, especially children.

Disadvantages of Graphs
- Too many representations are difficult to follow
- If percentages are very small fractions—it may be difficult to represent clearly
- If there are too many slices in the pie, the observer may become confused
- If percentages are too similar, an individual may have trouble in making distinctions
- Careful, concentrated, time consuming effort is needed to prepare the graphs.

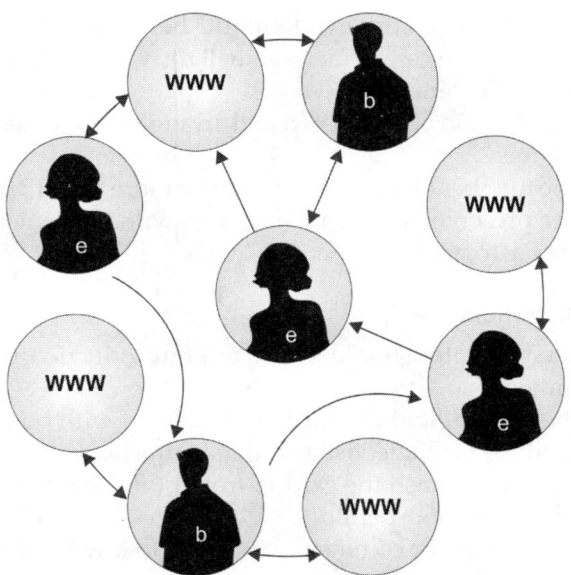

Fig. 3.8: Pictorial graphs (social graph).

Maps

"Graphic representations of the earth's surface".

Graphic representations of the earth's surface or portions of it are termed maps. They are common graphic aids for teaching social sciences. They are more valuable while teaching abstract ideas of distances, sizes, directions of different places, regions and lands, world and universe that are to be put into concrete reality. The basic problem, that of depicting the varied, boundless and nonflattened surface of the earth on a limited plane surface is a difficult one and has resulted in the development of many kinds of map projections and many types of maps (Hiedgerken).

A map is an accurate representation of plain surface in the form of a diagram, drawn to a scale, the details of boundaries of continents, countries, etc.

Various Aspects of Maps

The user should understand and interpret the key of index.
- The user should understand the lines—boundary lines, lines of communication, lines indicating the rivers, contours, meridians and parallels
- She also should understand the colors, tints, shadows, symbols in a map or a globe
- The top of every map is not north, but the direction of northern pole is north
- She should distinguish between various types of maps
- She should understand the position of earth in the universe.

Types of Maps

- Relief maps
- Historical maps (Boundary lines of various kingdom and symbol)
- Distribution maps (Population, language, race and economic maps)
- Geographical maps (Weather, archeological, rainfall maps).

Cartoons

"Humorous caricature which gives a subtle message".

A cartoon is a novel way of using pictures or symbols or bold exaggerations for presenting a message or a point of view concerning a personality, news, situations, or events. It is more attention drawing and, in a small space, gives a lot of imagination, particularly on the current happenings.

A cartoon is metaphorical representation of reality, and can be defined as a humorous caricature which gives a subtle message. In a cartoon, the features of objects and people are exaggerated along with generally recognized symbols. It makes strong appeal to the emotions thus enhancing learning.

The cartoon is an interpretative illustration which uses symbols to portray an opinion, a scene or a situation. It makes use of personalized humor, fantasy, incongruity, satire and exaggeration. In short, a cartoon is figurative and subtle graphic aid (Fig. 3.9).

Cartoons are meaningful in addition to be humorous. More clearly, they have a visual appeal along with a crisp message. Beneath a superficial exterior, they may portray a deep penetrating meaning.

The main sources of cartoons are periodicals. Newspapers carry cartoons daily which are either political or social in nature. Special periodicals and magazines may carry cartoons on science, management, economics, and education.

For a cartoon to attract attention:
- The quality of drawing should be high
- It should be suitable to the level of the learner
- It should be meaningful and intelligible
- It should be based on the educational objectives and background of students
- It should be simple and clear

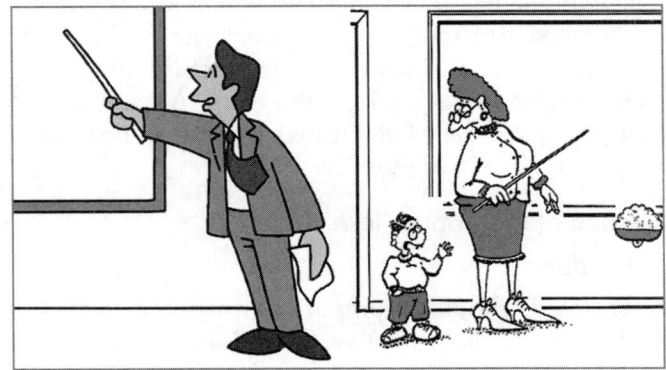

Fig. 3.9: Cartoon.

- It should explain the concept without too much explanation/too long a caption, or excessive dialogue
- The symbols used should be familiar
- The drawing should be intellectual though sarcastic and ridiculing.

Advantages of Cartoons

A cartoon can be effectively used:
- To initiate lessons
- To motivate students to start discussion
- For making teaching lively and interesting
- To reveal truth or reality about the people, events and incidents
- To modify the behavior and develop positive attitude in the learner.

Disadvantages of Cartoons

When the instructor decides to use cartoons as instructional aids, she has to choose them judiciously and discriminately, as certain cartoons can injure the personal feelings of students. The amount of sarcasm and ridicule has to be carefully watched so that it does not hurt anybody's feelings.

> The uniqueness and simplicity of the cartoons make them useful in appraising, interpreting, and emphasizing different concepts.

Flash Cards

"Flash of cards for communication".

Flash cards are a set of compact, pictured, paper cards of the same size, that are flashed one by one in a logical sequence. They can be self-made or commercially prepared and are made up of chart paper, drawing paper, and plain paper using colors or paintings.

The cards may be plain or laminated for long-term use. The size of the card for small group is 12 cm × 17 cm, 24 cm × 28 cm for the medium size group and 37 cm × 50 cm for large group. Either diagrams are drawn or cut out pictures are used to portray the theme for each card. Number the cards as per sequence. The letter should be legible in the flash card and use of minimum writing is encouraged. The message should be brief and up to the point in the card. A contrast color picture/diagram is used against a light background color. A margin in all four sides looks neat. For effective use, the group size can range from 5 to 15 in number.

Method of Presenting Flash Cards

Preparation
- The cards should be prepared in such a manner that they are simple, attractive, and colorful
- Bold lettering and illustration should be used on the cards
- The message conveyed should be brief and to the point. Unnecessary material will distract the attention of the viewers.
- They should be numbered and arranged in a sequential manner
- The number of cards should not be more than 15 or 20.
- The presenter should be thorough with the content of the flash cards.

Presentation
- The presenter should give a brief introduction to the audience
- She should hold the card at chest level with both the hands to facilitate visualization by the learners
- She should flash the card in front of the learners, just for a very short period
- Explanation or commentary should follow flashing of each card
- Language used should be simple and realistic
- Sequence should be followed while explaining the cards
- Important points should be stressed and distraction from the theme should be avoided.

Evaluation

Questioning and discussion may be encouraged at the end of the session.

Important points may be explained again and doubts cleared.

Advantages of Flash Cards
- They can be used easily for illiterate groups
- They attract attention and convey messages quickly
- They are easy to prepare, portable, and economic
- They are dynamic and flexible and maintain continuity
- They are helpful in overcoming the language barrier
- They are very effective to convey important messages in areas where people gather
- They can be used to introduce, present, and review a topic.

Disadvantages of Flash Cards
- Way of presentation influences the effectiveness of flash cards
- Maintenance of the flashcards for a longer time may be difficult
- They cannot be used for a bigger audience
- Viewers may lose interest when too many cards are used
- Literate and high class people may not be attracted by this method.

> The flash cards are called so because they are flashed or shown to the class just for a short time.

Pamphlets, Booklets and Leaflets

"Printed material in a crisp and concised manner".

Booklets, pamphlets, and leaflets are printed material containing relevant information in a crisp and concise manner. They may be used to supplement any classroom teaching method, especially lecture, or to disseminate information to the community in a short period. They provide opportunity for reading, learning, and referring a specific topic or subject.

A booklet is a small book with a cover page. It is particularly useful for topics which have a high degree of public interest like controlling obesity, care during pregnancy diabetic care, etc.

A leaflet is simple sheet carrying helpful information on useful themes.

A pamphlet is printed material consisting of only a few pages about a specific topic.

A pamphlet or leaflet should be:
- Colorful
- Attractive
- Illustrated with pictures
- Simple and precise
- Informative
- Self-explanatory
- Useful.

Advantages of Pamphlets, Booklets and Leaflets

- Information can be reached to a large group within a short time
- They are highly economic, flexible and portable
- Facilitates individualized learning
- Can be reproduced in any language
- Can be utilized for any group of people at any context
- Stimulates interest on the part of the learner.

Disadvantages of Pamphlets, Booklets and Leaflets

- Presentation is very important, if not found to be attractive, will be easily thrown out
- Receiving feedback from all those who got the pamphlet or leaflet is not possible
- It cannot be used for illiterates
- It cannot be preserved for a longer time
- Printed teaching material is sometimes described as a frozen language, which may not serve its objective.

Chalkboards

"Most familiar visual aid and a good friend of the teacher".

The chalkboard is the most familiar visual aid in the classroom. Chalkboards or display boards, the plain writing surfaces, are among the most common, cheapest and perhaps the most effective teaching resources. Despite other advanced visual aids, the chalkboard, usually called as the blackboard, remains the most commonly used visual aid in the classroom as well as in the laboratory.

The blackboard provides a sure, quick, and easily accessible means of visualizing important ideas—particularly those which arise during discussion and virtually demand visualization for complete understanding. The teaching atmosphere is created only in the presence of a blackboard. It provides a tremendous help to the teacher for explaining, illustrating, and describing the concepts.

Types of Chalkboards

The traditional blackboard was made with a large surface fabricated with wide planks and coated with dull black paint. It is held by an easel. This type of blackboard had only limited working area, but may be useful when classes are conducted in an open area. These are nowadays replaced by wallboards.

Wallboards: The wallboards consist of either the plank board fitted to wall surface or a rectangular portion coated with suitable paint. The modern chalkboard is made up of the following different types of writing surfaces.

Paint-coated pressed wood: Hard board or any plywood surface finished with dull paint.

Dull finished plastic surface: Any special or suitable colored plastic sheet, PVC or laminated plastic sheet may find special use. For general use, such boards are not suitable because of the high cost and furthermore the surface wears out easily.

Vitreous-coated steel surface: It is made up of steel and can be used as magnetic board also. On its surface, it is possible to use semi-permanent chalk or permanent chalk-ink. It serves as a very flexible and useful tool for teachers and students.

Ground glass board: It is the ideal board for the modern classroom, which is made in a variety of colors. The most important aspect to be considered is that there is no coating of any material on the writing surface to wear out. The writing surface is ground glass, whose thickness will depend upon the size of the board.

The roller board is like a mat, made of thick canvas wrapped on a roller.

White boards, which can be used for classroom teaching for a small group, can be wiped off easily when written with marker pens.

Tariff boards are used for price listing, reception, welcoming the delegates to a conference, etc.

Selection of color chalks for different chalkboard backgrounds.

Chalkboard background	Color chalks
Green	White, yellow, pink
Black	White, yellow, blue, green, pink
Red	Green, yellow
Orange	Blue or light green
Yellow	Blue
Rose	Purple, dark blue

Placement of Chalkboard

The height of the chalkboard is fixed with reference to the height of the human being using it. The lower edge of the board is placed at half the human height. The height of the board should generally be manageable by a human being by extending his/her hands above and below the mid-level of the board.

> **A teacher uses blackboard/chalkboard to:**
> - Illustrate the main points
> - List questions and problems
> - Explain abstract concepts
> - Stimulate students' interest
> - Draw diagrams, pictures and graphs
> - Review the whole topic taught

Guidelines for Use of Chalkboard

The chalkboard is similar to a store window display. Everyone knows that an overcrowded and dirty store window display has little value as compared to one that is clean and neat and displays a few well-chosen items that secure the attention of the public.

The following rules for using the chalkboard should definitely increase its effectiveness as a visual aid:

- Prelesson practice pays good dividends
- A clean chalkboard is a help
- Always hold the chalk between the thumb and the forefinger with nonworking end of the chalk pointing to the palm of the hand
- Hold the chalk at an acute (low) angle to the chalkboard in order to avoid uneven noise produced during writing.
- The fingers and thumb must act as a chuck for holding the chalk and should not contribute to forming the stroke shape
- The third and fourth finger nails may be used steadily on the chalkboard for special lines but over use of this practice will result in incomplete finger nails
- The strokes must be firm not feathery, whether they be light or heavy in intensity
- Develop the habit of slightly rotating the chalk as the stroke proceeds, and of changing to a new face of the chalk for a new stroke or work. This practice permits intensity without excessive thickness and helps in achieving an evenness of the chalkboard work.
- Always keep the chalk lengths in line with the stroke being drawn, so that chalk is pulled, unless one specifically requires a broad line. The technique sometimes necessitates the wrist being placed in an awkward position.
- Stand back so that the elbow is slightly bent, yet the reach to the board is easy
- Be comfortable and balanced
- Stand in front of the chalkboard such that the plane containing your body is approximately at an angle of 45°
- The stroke is made mainly through joint movement and to a lesser degree wrist, elbow and body movement.
- Use body sway to and fro to accommodate for differences of distance
- Use side sway of the body to obtain horizontal reach.
- Do not hesitate to bend the knees for low reach in vertical strokes
- Good balance is always essential
- Small circles are formed by wrist work and larger ones by a combination of elbow and shoulder movement
- The method which gives the best result is the right one to develop
- The qualities required in chalkboard writing are legibility and speed
- For chalkboard writing, use appropriate letter style, letter shape, letter size, spacing between letters, stroke thickness and levelness of lines
- Speed is essential for good coordination of chalkboard work and oral exposition but not at the price of legibility
- Printing is slower than writing, but it embodies a greater clarity and esthetic appeal and it is preferable to use it for headings and for emphasis
- The total work on the chalkboard should enable a teacher to consolidate his/her presentation in that session. This is known as the chalkboard summary.
- Do not overcrowd the chalkboard with too much matter. A few important points make a vivid impression.
- Make the material simple. Brief, precise statements are more effective than long sentences.
- Plan the work on the chalkboard in advance. Keep the layouts prepared for guidance.
- Gather everything needed for the chalkboard use before the group gathers (Colored chalks, ruler, eraser, etc.)
- Check the lighting conditions. Glare on the chalkboard should be avoided.
- Any writing on the board should be large enough to be visible at a distance and neat in order to be easily legible. Any diagram drawn should be large. Color chalks should be used only to emphasize or differentiate.

- Erase all unrelated material. Other work on the chalkboard distracts attention.
- Keep the chalkboard clean. A dirty chalkboard has the same effect as a dirty window.
- While writing or developing a picture, it is necessary/desirable, and essential that one should talk or narrate what is being done
- Never talk to the chalkboard; keep turning back and forth; speak to the students while writing on the board
- Stand on one side of the chalkboard while explaining to the students. Use a pointer to draw attention of the students.
- Chalk can be obtained in two forms, standard and dust-free. The dust-free chalk will not deposit dust on the teacher's clothing or other audio-visual media present in the classroom.
- Upper case letters are used as main headings and all other writing should employ lower case
- When writing on the board the teacher should stop talking, as the voice will not project to the audience. Some teachers feel this silence to be threatening, so they write as quickly as possible, with a resulting loss of legibility.
- The period spent writing on the board can be used as a minibreak for the learners, so that their arousal will increase when the teacher faces them again
- Emphasis can be achieved by upper case lettering, underlining, encasing or encircling and coloring the words
- The diagrams must be large enough to allow the audience to see the details.

Advantages of Chalkboard

A blackboard is the most commonly used teaching aid as it has its own advantages:
- It is the never failing friend of the teacher
- Very cheap, inexpensive teaching aid that could be used again and again
- Could be maintained very easily, at a lower-cost
- Could be used any time, without much prior preparation
- Could be used for a comparatively larger audience
- More convenient to use, does not require any technical knowledge to handle
- Very useful in drawing enlarged illustrations from textbooks.

Disadvantages of Chalkboard

- Most of the times, blackboard is fixed to a particular place, hence confined to that place. It cannot be carried over from place to place, limiting its use in a classroom lecture alone.
- Teacher-centered and teacher-based lessons are only possible with a blackboard

- Constant use leads on to wearing of the surface, making further use difficult
- It makes the lesson a dull routine
- Material once written cannot be presented for a long time (e.g. complex drawings)
- It is two dimensional only
- It cannot show motion
- It can be used for the limited audience
- Chalk dust is another disadvantage.

Effective Use of a Blackboard

B Be kind and gentle while using the blackboard
L Layout the plan in advance
A Arrangement check for:
- L-Lighting
- A-Angle
- G-Glare.

C Check for cleanliness
- C-Colored chalks
- E-Eraser/duster
- R-Ruler
- C-Cane (Pointer)
- Any other templates.

K Keep the board in a comfortable height
B Be judicious while using it
O Order SOS (Stand on side)
A Attract by CUPS
- C-Color chalks and capital letters when necessary
- U-Underline
- P-Pointer
- S-Style in writing

R Writing with a BRUSH
- B-Bright
- R-Readable
- U-Uniform
- S-Straight
- H-Horizontal.

D Drawings and pictures to be based on PEN
- P-Purposeful
- E-Easy
- N-Neat.

Checklist for Effective use of Chalkboard

Before the lesson:
- Devise the chalkboard plan
- Clean the board
- Clean the eraser
- Ensure that sufficient chalk is available in a variety of colors
- Check for glare spots by walking around room
- Check visibility using a sample heading and viewing from rear of room.

During the Lesson
- Adhere to chalkboard plan
- Use appropriate lettering
- Emphasize the important words
- Write legibly
- Stop talking when writing
- Erase only when more space required, or when material will cause interference with subsequent points
- Check with learners before erasing.

End of Lesson
- Use chalkboard material as a summary
- Erase completely for next class.

Flannel Board

"Displaying material on the flannel board".

The flannel board is a wooden or plywood board covered with a piece of flannel, terry cloth, or felt cloth, on which desired pictures or items can be displayed. The items displayed, e.g. pictures, drawings, etc. should have a flannel or sandpaper pasted on the reverse side. If items to be displayed are cut-out from flannel, blotting paper and sandpaper, no additional rough surfaced backing is required.

The flannel board can be used as a chalkboard, on which we place prepared items and remove them when needed. Students may be often asked to fix these to arouse their creative interest.

Purposes of Flannel Board
- It enables teacher to develop an idea step-by-step in a very dramatic and impressive manner
- It is an educative media for both literates and illiterates, more appealing to the children
- The flannel board helps to convey idea more expressively, avoiding boredom
- It can be effectively used for teaching arithmetic, grammar, hygiene, nature study, geography, languages, etc.

Guidelines for Effective use of the Flannel Board
- Display material on the flannel board in a sequence, as the lecture goes on
- Change pictures or cut-outs while talking to the learner. Students may also be asked to fix these to arouse their creative interest.
- Use appropriate pictures for teaching different subjects
- Make sure that the pictures to be displayed on the board are attractive and sufficiently large to be clearly seen by all who are listening
- Make sure the environment is well lighted for the pictures to be clearly seen
- Be thorough with the sequence of the pictures
- Avoid pictures that are not directly related to the concept being taught.

Advantages of Flannel Board
- Flannel boards are inexpensive, easily made from local materials
- They are flexible, dynamic, portable, convenient, and reusable
- Easily maintained and transported to remote areas.
- Prepared figures can be reused in various other presentations
- It is ideal for showing sequence of events and reviewing lessons
- Holds attention of students, and attractive, if properly used
- Can be adopted for group participation
- The display materials can be changed without use of drawing pins or paste.

Disadvantages of Flannel Board
- Requires considerable advance preparation
- Artistic ability is required in making homemade figures
- Can be used only for a small group
- May create confusion if sequence of pictures is changed
- Not useful for abstract learning.

Bulletin Board

Bulletin board is the display board which shows the visual learning material on a specific subject. They may range from expensive boards with protective glass doors and built-in lights to illuminate the material displayed, to those made of a wood panel covered with several layers of blotting paper, felt or other appropriate material to allow for the insertion of thumb tacks.

Purposes of Bulletin Boards
Bulletin boards have an important place in health education, as they often reach the audience very easily and effectively. The various purposes they serve in the college are:
- Attract the attention of the students
- Effective communication of the intended message
- Promotes the creativity of the students and the teachers
- Used as an effective educational media
- Can be used for a larger audience.

Classification of Bulletin Boards
The bulletin boards can be classified into two types:
1. Classification I
    - Classroom bulletin boards
    - All-purpose bulletin boards
    - Magnetic bulletin boards.

2. Classification II
   - An introductory bulletin board
   - Explanatory bulletin board
   - A summary bulletin board.

An introductory bulletin board is used to introduce the concept in a pictorial form. An explanatory bulletin board is made plain in a pictorial way a concept or principle that is hard to visualize from a verbal description alone. A summary bulletin board may be used to show applications of one or all of the generalizations studied. A magnetic bulletin board is made of light weight metal and the materials are held in place by means of small magnets. They are commonly used in homes to post grocery lists or remainders for family members, etc.

Principles to be followed to make the bulletin board display effective:

- *Location of the board*: Ideally the board should be placed, where:
  - The lighting is good
  - It can be easily seen
  - The potential audience passes by.
- *Height of the board*: The board should be placed at a comfortable height for the observer; boards intended for the children should be placed lower than those intended for adults.
- *Background* of the board should be neutral in color, so that when colored display materials are used, they will not clash.
- Classroom bulletin boards should be used only for teaching purposes; instructions for the employees, notices and similar items should be displayed elsewhere, so that they do not interfere with the teaching display.
- Careful planning has to be made regarding what to display on the bulletin board. The material displayed must:
  - Attract the observer's attention
  - Make clear what the display is all about
  - Project the message entirely on its own merits.
- *Content of the board*: The topic for the board must be appropriate for the potential audience and should include only one theme or idea at a time. Most of the people who may see the board are just passing by; the point is to catch their attention quickly and impress them with one idea.
- An effective display has a large, easily seen heading that states the subject of the display, and a central focus for the eye, such as an attractive colored picture and explanatory captions that are brief and to the point.
- The displayed materials are to be frequently checked and should be changed as appropriate to the situation.

Frequent assessments have to be done to check whether the boards are serving the purpose or not, attracts attention, people are interested enough to look at it closely, and whether the students are asking the teacher for more information about the topic being presented.

Advantages of Bulletin Boards

- A bulletin board display is one of the least expensive visual aids
- It makes available to students or public, those materials, of which there is only one copy
- It may be placed wherever required on a classroom wall, in the corridor of the college, or public building, or at an information center
- It stimulates interest
- It serves as a good supplement to normal classroom teaching
- It adds color and liveliness to the classroom as they have decorative value along with educational value
- Bulletin board displays can be effectively used as follow-up of chalkboard work
- Bulletin board displays can be used to introduce a topic as well as to review it.

Disadvantages of Bulletin Boards

- Bulletin boards cannot be used for all inclusive teaching
- It has to be used only as a supplementary aid
- At times the collection of relevant material for certain specific topics may be difficult
- Arranging the display material on the board may be a challenging task for the teacher, as it requires artistic and creative potentialities
- If not used properly, may fail in its purpose to convey the central theme.

Three-dimensional Models Objects, Specimens, and Models

Objects may be defined as real things which have been removed as units from their natural settings, for example: patient care equipment that are portable, coins and stamps, relics, etc.

"Substitute for real things, replica of the original" can be used effectively as objects in teaching various subjects.

A specimen may be defined as a typical object or part of an object, which has been removed from its natural setting and environment.

Models are concrete objects, may be replicas of the real objects (of the same size, or smaller, or bigger) mostly three-dimensional or sectional to explain clearly the structure or functions of the original.

Why real objects cannot be used?
- Too small to be observed, e.g. atomic structures, microorganisms, etc.
- Too large to be available, e.g. airplane
- Too concealed to be observable, e.g. interior of the organ
- Too fast to be perceived, e.g. flying objects

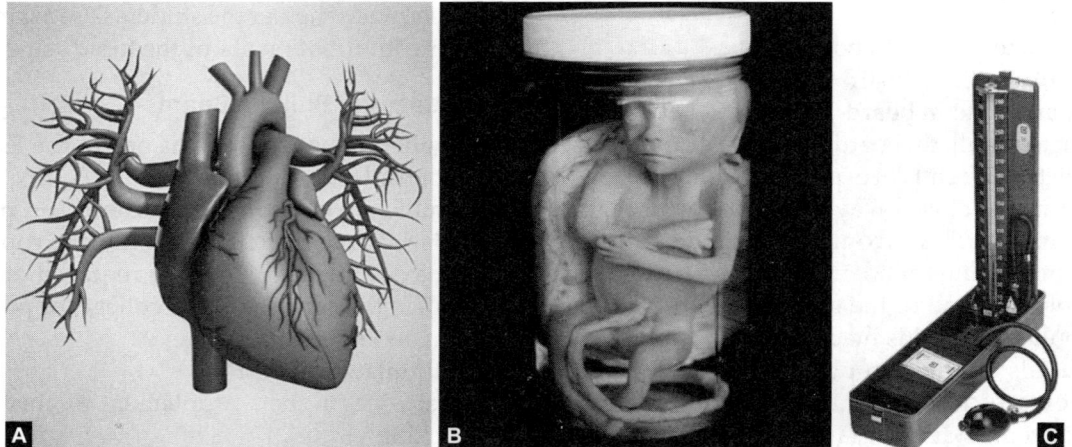

Figs. 3.10A to C: Objects, specimen and model: (A) Model of a heart; (B) Specimen of a fetus; (C) BP apparatus (object).

Objects and Specimens

Collections of real things for instructional use refer to objects. Specimen is any typical object representing a class or group of things. As both of them are real things, they impart direct learning experience to the students. Replica is full-sized copy of an object. It looks, feels, and acts like the object itself. A replica of a written or printed document or art is called Facsimile. The advantage of using a replica is getting an accurate picture of finer points and details and it also presents a multi-sensory approach in learning. The students get firsthand experience or information by looking at or handling the objects and specimens.

Models

The use of models for teaching/training purpose should definitely be highly effective. Models are concrete objects, some of them are larger than the real object and some of them are small replicas of objects which are too large to be seen as a whole, can be prepared. These may be mostly three-dimensional or sectional or assembly type to explain clearly the structure or function of the original (Figs. 3.10A to C).

In many cases it will be more practicable to use a model. Models can be classified as given in Table 3.2.

The construction of a model should be simple. It should not be made out of fragile materials as far as possible.

Models may be defined as three-dimensional representations of real things. They reduce large objects to a size convenient for observation and produce interior views of objects which are normally covered or invisible. Nonessentials are removed so that fundamentals can be more readily observed. Models can be handled, operated and seen from a number of angles and hence are generally more interesting and instructive than a picture or a chart which is two-dimensional. A model should have the essential qualities of accuracy, simplicity, utility, solidity, and ingenuity to be maximally useful.

Table 3.2: Classification of models.

Material	Size	Nature	Structure	
			Type	Shape
Wooden	Enlarged	Dynamic	Sectional	Three
Thermocole	Reduced	Working	X-ray	dimensional
Perspex	Normal	Static	Assembly	(or)
				Two
				dimensional

Models are advantageous than real objects because it helps to explain the details in a clear and leisurely manner which is not possible in case of real objects. It can be used to show the minute parts of a system or a process through a model which cannot be done when it is actually in operation. It is used to show the internal functioning of a system which is not visible from outside with the help of cross-sectional or dissectible models. We can also use with safety and convenience.

Materials used in preparation of models
- Cardboard
- Plastic
- Plaster of Paris
- Wax
- Wood
- Clay
- Thermocol

Classification of Models

Models may be classified as:

Scale models: In order to form a correct idea of an object, scale models are used. For example, models of organs of human body.

Simplified models: They are made of clay to give an idea of the external form of the object. Although they are not made to exact scale, they have educational value.

Working models: Such models are used to demonstrate in a simple way, an operation or process, for example, the working model of a human heart.

Cross-sectional model: Such models show the inside of an object. They are of immense use in the teaching of technical objects.

Models can be useful for generating student interest. They should be used in an interesting manner as possible. Students may be encouraged to examine the models, ask questions and make generalizations. They should be encouraged to produce models to illustrate objects, concepts, or ideas. These teaching aids are powerful interest arousing devices which possess the capacity of involving all the five senses—touch, sight, hearing, smell, and taste.

> **Mock-ups**
> A mock-up refers to a specialized model or working replica of the object being depicted. In a mock-up, a certain element of the original reality is emphasized or highlighted to make it more meaningful. A mock-up may or may not be similar in appearance. Mock-ups of airplane, ships, buses, etc. are used in technical institutions to explain their structure and actual working.

Merits and Demerits of Model

The advantages of a model are:
- Models help in simulating a real situation
- The size can be adjusted as needed
- Distance and time do not become a limitation
- It gives the learner visual, tactic, and oral stimuli which increases the learning experience
- It can explain concepts, structures, and working of parts
- They stimulate interest and capture attention
- It enables to have a correct concept of an object
- Working model will secure immediate attention and serve as motivation to learn.

The disadvantages of a model are:
- Models are quite costly
- Needs more storage space
- They are useful only for teaching small groups
- Requires skill and talent to prepare.

> - Objects are real things, visible, tangible aid, complete in itself.
> - Specimen is a part taken from the whole, so as to represent the whole.
> - Model is a recognizable imitation of a real object.

Slides and Films

"A small piece of film".

The use of slides and films is becoming increasingly popular in teaching contexts. They possess an attention focusing power which increases interest and motivation among the students.

Definition

A slide is still transparency of 70 mm, 35 mm, or 6 mm size which is optically enlarged and projected on a screen as a real image. It is actually a small piece of film or other transparent material on which a single pictorial image or scene or graphic image has been photographed or reproduced otherwise.

A film strip is a series of sequenced slides on a piece of film covering a large portion of a lesson. They are closely related to slides, but instead of being mounted as separate pictures, the film after processing remains uncut as a continuous strip.

Slides are small transparent visual aids which can be viewed with the help of a slide projector. They are effective promoters of discussions, making abstractions concrete and realistic.

Types of Slides

Normally, slides are of three types:
1. Photographic slides
2. Handmade slides
3. Computer made slides.

Handmade slides include the following types:
- Marker ink slides
- Cellophane slides
- Silhouette slides
- Etched glass slides.

Characteristics of a Good Slide

- *It is simple*:
  - Depicts one idea
  - Minimum description
  - Disseminate information in about 4 seconds.
- *It is legible*:
  - Area should not exceed 7.5 cm × 11 cm
  - Number of words is not more than 35
  - Number of lines is not more than six
  - Only two or three columns and rows are used for tables
  - Headings are depicted in bold letters.
- *It is accurate*:
  - There are no spelling mistakes
  - There are no factual errors.
- *It is appropriate*:
  - Content material relevant to subject
  - Depicts best visuals
  - Technically well executed
  - Properly exposed and developed
  - Properly mounted.

The slides and film strips are projected on the screen using an optical instrument called slide and film-strip projector. It works on the principle that when an illuminated object is placed between the focus and twice the focus of a convex lens, it produces an enlarged real image beyond twice of the focus on the other side of the lens.

Preparation and projection of slides and film strips:
- Depending upon the nature of instructional objectives, the content for slides and films may include written words, sketches, graphs, cartoons, pictures, etc. after deciding what the content is going to be, the slides/film strips are prepared in the following manner:
  - Only one concept should be depicted in one slide
  - Written descriptions, if any, should be legible, simple, and precise
  - Only key points are to be stressed
  - The size of the letters should not be less than 6 mm and a maximum of seven lines can only be included in one slide.
- The prepared slides have to be numbered according to the sequence and kept in order
- The slides should be positioned correctly before projection
- The slide/film projector should be placed on a rigid and stable table
- The screen should be placed on an appropriate place so that the whole class can see it
- Insert the slide carrier or filmstrip carrier in its place, and mount a slide of filmstrip in its carrier
- Darken the room in which projection is to be carried out
- Present the slides or frames sequentially accompanied by due explanations
- After completion of the projection, equipment should be replaced in its place and the class should be opened for discussion.

> **Materials needed for producing slides:**
> - Plain, colored or etched glass
> - Binding tape
> - Cellophane
> - Colored pencil
> - Colored inks.

Advantages of Slide and Film Projections

The common advantages of slide projectors include:
- They can be projected in a partially darkened room thus facilitating further class discussion and notes taking
- They may be enlarged to any amount of desired size
- They are convenient aids for making classroom teaching interesting
- The slides and filmstrips because of their repeated use are quite cheaper
- They provide a logical and sequential order of presentation and can be used according to convenience
- Slides and filmstrips are compact in size, and hence can be stored and transported easily. They can be preserved for a longer time.
- They produce an increased visual impact but cause less eye soaring
- A variety of printed, typed, or drawn material can be presented in different colors or combinations in the slides or filmstrips
- The image on the screen can be held for required amount of time
- They save the time of the teacher
- They capture interest and attention of the students
- It can be viewed by the entire class.

Disadvantages of Slide and Film Projections
- They are comparatively expensive
- They easily get dirty and smudged with finger prints.
- Projector bulbs do not stay long and are expensive to replace
- They require skill in operating
- The teacher may not have eye contact or direct interaction with the students as the classroom is partially dim. The size of the slide trays is not standardized, so a teacher's personal slide tray may not fit the projector used in a particular institution.

Slides can be obtained commercially, or made by the teacher. The former can be useful as many are produced specifically for nurses in a wide range of topics. Other outside sources that might be useful are the medical photography departments in the hospitals, who may be able to make slides for the use.

Checklist for Effective use of Slide Projector

Before the Lesson
- Position screen for maximum visibility
- Align projector so that required size of image is obtained
- Focus sharply using a slide
- Insert slides.

During the Lesson
- Switch off lights when showing slides
- Use a pointer on the screen.

After the Lesson
- Remove all slides, including the last one in the well
- Do not move projector until lamp is cool.

Puppets

"Education by entertainment".

Puppet show is a form of entertainment. In south India, especially in villages earlier, there were no fairs and festivals without puppet show. Traditional puppetry shows focused more on entertainment and teaching morals. It is one of the audio visuals used in educating not only the students but also the public. It is one of the recreational ways of education. Puppet is a doll which can be made to move. Puppetry involves creating puppets and making them to act.

Puppets are prepared from leather, fabric, carved wood, or bamboo. Nowadays, readymade puppets are available, prepared from waste papers. It needs skill and experience to prepare puppets.

Historical Background

It is believed that puppet theater began in India and China thousand years ago, and then spread to other parts of the world. Traditional Indian puppeteers make their puppets out of leather, fabric, carved wood, or bamboo. It needs years of training to make these puppets. If a puppet became old and could no longer be used, it was never just thrown away. It was taken to a river, and cast into the water with the chanting of sacred verses.

Types of Puppets

- Hand puppet
- Rod puppet
- Shadow puppet
- String puppet.

Hand Puppet

The puppeteer wears a hand puppet like a glove and moves it using his fingers. Tiny hand puppets, which are worn on the fingers, are called finger puppets. Usually the hand puppeteer sits at a lower level, behind a screen, and pushes the puppet up on the stage. So the audience sees only the puppet, while puppeteer remains hidden.

Rod Puppet

It is much bigger than hand puppet and is held by a central control rod which is attached to the head. It is also operated from below the stage.

Shadow Puppet

It is flat figure, usually made of leather. The figure is held close to a white screen which allows light to pass through. The puppet is then lit by a strong light from behind. The audience sits on the other side of the screen, and when the puppet is moved, they see its shadow moving. The different parts of the puppet are loosely joined together and moved using thin horizontal rods or wires held against the screen.

String Puppet

It has a main body with movable parts manipulated by strings. There is also a main string which the puppeteer holds, to stop the puppet from swinging about (Fig. 3.11).

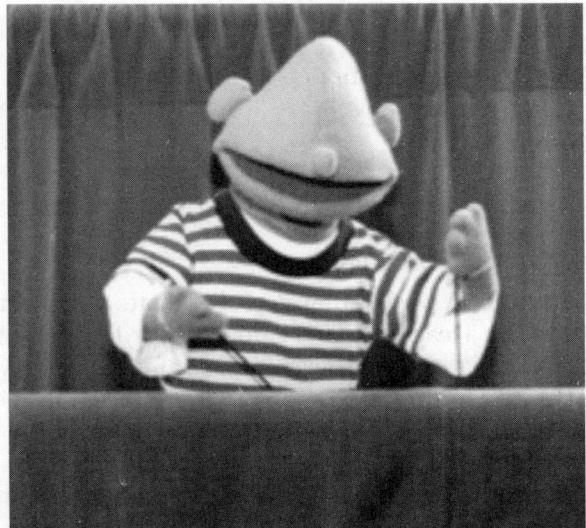

Fig. 3.11: Puppets.

Preparation of a Puppet

In olden days, they are prepared from leather, fabric, carved wood or bamboo. Nowadays readymade puppets are available. It is prepared form waste papers. The waste papers are immersed in the water. Then they are made into a solid paste after grinding. After adding some preservatives with this paste, puppets are made. After drying, these are painted. The other way to prepare a puppet is from plaster of Paris. With the help of many molds, puppets are made.

Advantages of Puppets

- They provide an entertaining way of education
- They are attractive and attention capturing
- They serve as audio-visual aids for all age groups, levels, and standards
- The message what they convey is easy to remember
- They improve the creative skills of the students
- They encourage observation, thinking, reasoning, and listening skills
- They are humorous
- Student teacher can express all inner qualities and capacities (singing, tone, mimicry, narrating a story, etc.)
- They are useful for health education in community, and in clinical set-up especially in children wards
- They are useful for advertisement.

Disadvantages of Puppets

- Puppetry is time consuming
- Requires skill in preparation and presentation
- It cannot be used as an audio-visual aid for all types of teachings
- It cannot be used for large group

- It requires coordination of voice of presenter and actions of puppet
- Need to use more puppets as more characters.

Handouts

"Learning in-hand".

Handouts or Reprographics

A handout is a well-planned duplicated document prepared by a teacher for her students in order to promote their participation in the teaching-learning process. Well-structured handouts can be very valuable in terms of interest, motivation and record of information.

One of the most common learning aids used in the classroom is the class handout. This consists of a sheet or sheets of paper given to each learner for permanent use.

Purpose

- To provide information
- As a lecture guide
- For further references and reading
- Assessment and questioning.

In the classroom, handouts enhance a lecture, serve as a platform for instruction, and ensure all students have access to the same information.

Handout provides organization and a reminder of what was said during the class session.

Adults prefer to come away with learning in-hand and with an opportunity to review material in a concise presentation, prefer receiving information in a printed form in handouts are given to stimulate critical thinking. Handouts may be styled for active and participatory learning.

Even in the internet age, handouts continue to be used, in either paper or electronic formats.

MacLean (1991) offered the following suggestions for using handouts:

- Use handouts as advance organizers
- Provide a technical terminology handout either at or prior to the start of the course
- Consider whether it is worthwhile to produce an introductory handout that provides basic information that the students should read before attending class
- Use the handout as a study guide
- Integrate the handout with the lecture flow, so students engage in a variety of learning activities during the course of the session
- Introduce a handout-reading break during class at a point when students' concentration on the spoken word begins to wane
- Use a handout in small group teaching to identify issues or questions to be addressed.

> Reprography is a branch of technology dealing with methods of duplication or reproduction. Duplication involves making a number of identical copies of the original. Reproduction enables preparation of one or more identical copies of the original, same size or different size in monochrome or color, e.g. duplicators.

In a discussion of peer evaluation to improve handout quality, McLeod and Tenenhouse (1988) listed the five most frequent evaluator comments, including:

1. Improve the clinical relevance handout data
2. Decrease unnecessary detail
3. Use more diagrams to illustrate points
4. Leave space to write notes
5. Break up text into paragraphs with headings, rather than using continuous prose.

When to Give Handouts?

- Much in advance of the presentation
- Just before the start of the session
- During the progress of the session
- Just after completion of the session
- Much after the presentation.

According Ellington (1985) and Heinich et al. (2002), there are various types of handouts, including:

- Complete notes on specific topics.
- Skeleton notes, containing blank spaces for learners to fill in.
- Shorter documents, often a single sheet, given out during a lesson to save student from copying complicated material, such as a diagram or map.

Characteristics of a Good Handout

When designing a handout, educators should consider variety (varying the style), balance (either formal with symmetrical elements, or informal with text and images placed asymmetrically on the page), and simplicity, it is clear and clean, with easy-to-find key point. In addition, development of quality handouts includes consideration of basic elements such as type and layout, purpose, focus topic, and visual appeal, and professional elements such as care in editing, inclusion of references, date of preparation, and copyright protection.

Focus Topic

Generally, a handout should have a single topic. Elements pertaining to the topic could be key points, definitions, story illustrations, pictorials, formulas, or statistical information. Interest can be added to the topic by including quotation from nursing scholars or leaders, quotations from popular literature, or poetry. The addition of appropriate light humor can make a handout delightful.

Visual Appeal

Adding, visual appeal to handout communicates an instructor's professional interest in the topic. With the aid of computer software, using clipart, borders, word art, interesting fonts, and color, makes it creative than ever before to be creative. Printing on color paper is visually appealing.

Educators must also consider spacing of material and design layout. Too many printed lines may be irritating to readers.

Using a font size of 12 to 14 and bold print can promote easier viewing. Handout length may vary according to their purpose, but it is worth noting that handouts can be a source of distraction when attendees have to move back and forth through multiple pages. Keeping handouts brief encourages the audience to follow the presentation points.

A handout which is prepared in a professional way will communicate the standard or quality of handouts to students and faculty members.

Care in Editing

It is imperative that faculty demonstrate care in editing, sound referencing practices, and consider other issues such as documenting the date of handout development and specifying if a handout is copyrighted.

Taking the time to carefully review handouts and make corrections communicates and models faculty's professional expectations and represents faculty's commitment to promote learning experience.

Spelling and grammar checking features may be useful for editing purposes. Asking a colleague to proofread the handout also helps to identify errors that may be missed because of the creator's familiarity with the document.

Inclusion of References

Accurate documentation communicates an expectation of academic honesty, and providing citations offers students an opportunity to build a bibliography as a learning resource.

Faculty may consider concluding handout content with a list of literature sources as a learning supplement. The listing clearly designates the usefulness of the reference to the learning experience.

Date of Preparation

Dating handouts serves as a quality checkpoint when the faculty reviews the course. Depending on content, a planned review schedule ensures the handout information in current.

Handouts are a common and practical instructional aid. The act of developing quality handouts involves applying education principles, while making the handouts purposeful to the learning experience.

Overhead Projector

The overhead projector is a versatile and popular device for projecting transparencies, with brilliant screen images suitable for use in a lighted room. It is a very vital teaching aid which has made projections so simple and easy.

Overhead projector permits daylight projection and face to face interaction with the students. It gives a bright evenly light image which attracts the student's attention. The operator has complete control over the presentation.

Parts of the Overhead Projector

Figure 3.12 shows the parts of an OHP:
- Projection head lens and mirror
- Focus wheel
- Projection handle
- Glass plate/transparency stage
- Fresnel lens
- Switch to intense or dimmer
- Switch for cooling fan
- Adjustment feet
- Overhead projector
- Metal box with a 1000 W/600 W halogen lamp.

Overhead Projector Transparencies

Overhead transparencies are easy to operate with the projector and are very simple to prepare. A standard size of acetate sheet measuring 18 cm × 22 cm is used to

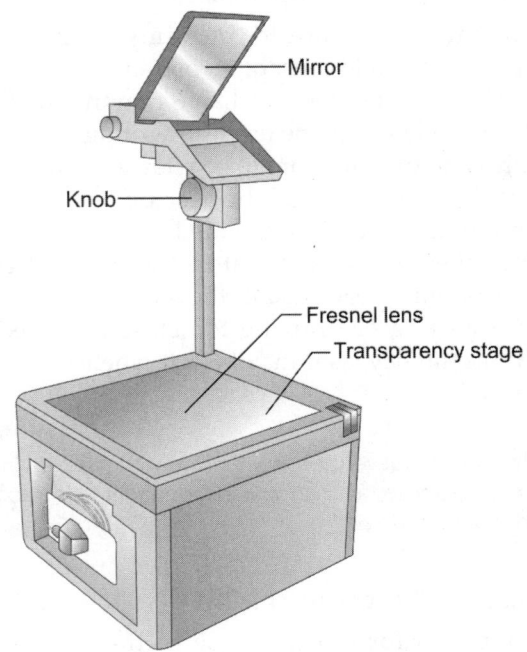

Fig. 3.12: Overhead projector.

print, write or draw materials relevant to subject matter. When it is placed on the platform of the projector, a large image is projected on a screen that is kept behind. Good transparencies can be preserved for the future use. Roll transparency: Besides single transparency, we can use roll of transparency on which writings and pictures can be made in a sequence and can be projected on OHP in a classroom. It can be moved backward forward as required.

Method of Preparing Transparency

Various methods are used to prepare a transparency. *They include*:

Hand-drawn transparency: As the name indicates, using marker pens the required material is either hand-drawn or written. The marker pens are available in water soluble forms or permanent form. Permanent ink can be erased by using spirit such as after shave, whereas soluble ink needs only a wipe with a damp cloth.

Photographic transparency: Employing reflex printing, negative or reflex printing paper can be made, where some complicated drawings are pictured. With these negatives, positives can be printed on sensitized positive acetate.

DIAZ process: It is a process used to make large number of copies of transparencies from chemical acetate.

Copying process: With the help of thermographic process, transparencies are prepared by the copying machines.

Preparation of OHP Transparencies

- Transparencies should be simple, preferably expressing a single concept on one sheet
- Letters should not be less than 6 mm in size. Simple lettering style should be used for writing.
- Figures and diagrams are to be relevant to the content
- Only key messages should be emphasized; overcrowding should be avoided
- Using different colors may attract student's attention
- Leave margin at each end of the acetate
- Avoid writing or drawing too close to the edge of the transparency, as it may be lost when the image is projected.

> When the OHP is kept very low, it will distort the image, i.e. image will get wider at the top and narrower at the bottom. This distortion is called "Key Stone Effect".

Principles for Effective use of OHP

The principles for effective use of the OHP can be discussed in following phases:

Preparation Phase

The screen should be so kept that all students can view it without difficulty; lower border of the screen should be in level with the heads of audience.

- Collect all required materials well ahead.
- Focus the projection lens until the image is sharp.
- Keep the transparencies in sequence.
- Use appropriate masking strategies; reveal the transparency only when it is required.
- Explain clearly and concisely.

Presentation Phase

Switch on the OHP only while showing the transparency to the audience. Overheating of the bulb may blow it off. *Switch off when*:

- Placing the transparency on table
- Removing the transparencies
- Explaining the concept or idea.

Use pointer to indicate, preferably on the transparency rather than on the screen.

Use mask to reveal points in a step-by-step fashion, whenever required.

Do not move the OHP when the bulb is switched on, as the filament of the bulb may break due to jerks during shifting.

When the content presented with the transparencies during presentation consume more than 3–4 minutes, switch off the OHP while giving the oral explanations or providing clarifications to the learners. Organize your presentation with transparencies in such a way that every 3–4 minutes the OHP should be switched off. Switch it on after a minute or two.

Aftercare of the Equipment

- Collect the transparencies and preserve them for further use.
- Never move the machine, while the lamp is still hot.
- Do not disconnect it from main supply while the fan is operating.
- Clean the lens with a moist pad and detergent cleaner.
- Cover the OHP and keep it safely.

Advantages of OHP

- The OHP produces a large projected image in a minimum of projection distance
- It helps the students in sequential learning, when the technique of progressive disclosure is used
- It can be used with other audio-visual aids more easily
- The teacher can have constant interactions with the class
- It can be used in a normally lighted room, hence the student can take down notes, and the teacher can observe the students' interactions
- The equipment is quite cheaper than other projected aids

- It saves a lot of class hours that could be used for other more important purposes, like providing more attention to weaker students, counseling students, etc.
- Operation of OHP is easy; it does not involve any complex technology
- It can be used for a large group of students.

Disadvantages of OHP

- Apparatus is quite costly; if the bulb blows of, a spare lamp is to sought for, which is costlier
- Electrical power consumption is high
- Requires extensive maintenance
- Teacher/students may become dependent on OHP.

Radio

"For ears by air".

Radio is a powerful mass medium used in action for disseminating information, imparting instruction, and giving entertainment: It serves with equal ease in both developed and developing countries. It spreads information to a greater group of population, thereby saving time, energy, money, and manpower in an effective way. Radio is a simple and cheap medium readily available as a small toy (Fig. 3.13).

Now, small and handy transistors are available with even poorest of people. A small transistor can carry the message to any place on the earth. It needs very little for maintenance and cheaper production can be taken up with more and more resources. Radio speaks to an individual so also to millions at a time. Hence, any listener can think the broadcast is meant for him whereas when listened in group all think the message directed toward them. Each student takes the broadcast as very intimate to him. Due to its portability and easy accessibility radio could find its place everywhere whether it was a field, a school, a kitchen or a study room. Radio is a blind man's medium and is meant for ears only. It plays with sound and silence, where the sound can be anything like voice or word, music and effect. When one hears radio, simultaneously one can imagine happenings in his/her mind. So it is called as theater of blind or a stage for the mind. Radio can be listened to simultaneously along with another work like reading also.

The radio has been and is being used to serve a variety of purposes from its very inception—to inform, to educate and to entertain people. Continued technological innovations have radio broadcasting increasingly available to a large number of people throughout the world.

The radio is the cheapest and the most easily accessible of the other three electronic media, i.e. audiocassette, television, and videocassette. It caters to people of different ages and levels of maturity ranging from a primary school child to grandfathers.

The radio lends itself to serve different purposes. For instance:

- It provides learners with new joys of learning
- It can develop their command over vocabulary
- Promote concentration and critical learning to supplement/enrich a concept
- Give additional views on a theme
- It improves fluency and confidence in speech and discussion
- It can be used for formal and informal education
- It supplements and enriches the formal school subjects.

Strengths of Radio/Medium

- Easy accessibility
- Wide coverage
- Low capital investment and operating cost
- Easy learner-reception
- Effective thought promotion
- Motivative, supportive facilities
- Easy production
- Effective creation/transmission of reality
- Feasible mode of learner enrichment
- Direct instruction.

Limitations of Radio/Audio Medium

- The radio is not a flexible medium
- There is no face-to-face interaction, dialogue or discussion between the listener and the speaker
- The doubts and queries arising in the mind of the learner cannot be attended immediately. There is no immediate feedback to the learner
- It may not be an effective medium for all types of course materials
- The more heterogeneous the audience, the more difficult it is to produce a radio program of common utility/appeal

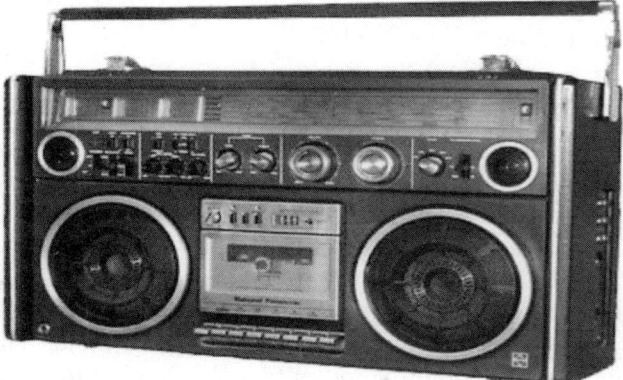

Fig. 3.13: Radio.

- The span of attention of the learner is short and the retention of factual information is generally low
- Radio programming demands experienced and creative personnel with a sound academic background.

Tape Recorder

Definition
A tape recorder is used to record sounds on magnetic tape which can be reproduced at will and as many times as required.

Audio Tape
It is a magnetic tape used for recording sounds.

Audio tapes can be adapted to any teaching/learning situation for any size of audience and also for self-learning. Audio tapes can be used to provide narrations for slide sequences, give commentary for silent films and filmstrips, demonstrate heart sounds and give instructions for use of equipment. Professionally prepared audio tapes are available which have recorded dialogues among subject experts on different topics. These audio tapes are good media for presenting discussion among experts on controversial topics.

Characteristics of Audio through Tape Recorder

Immediacy: Books can describe events that have happened, but recordings can describe events as they happen.

Emotional impact: The student's interest can be captured and her imagination stirred through the combined effect of voice, environmental sounds and music.

Authenticity: Through tape recorders, it is possible for experts to visit any classroom anytime.

Conquest of time and space: Through simulated programs, audio media can actually overcome the barriers of time and space.

One way communication: Tape is a one-way communication tool; this limits its usefulness for teaching since it provides no possibility of feedback to the students.

Audition: Tape programs can be auditioned to determine their educational value.

Needs and interest: Recording made by the teacher and the students can be used to meet their specific needs and thereby enhance the teaching-learning situation.

Advantages of Tape Recorder
- Tape recorder can be used to record educational broadcasts and for replay at suitable and convenient times
- It can be used for music and other sound effects for use during staging of dramas in the colleges and cultural performances
- It can be used to record the speeches of important visitors to the institution and this can be effectively used later
- Tape recorders are largely used in language laboratories for giving speech training and for correction of pronunciation defects
- Tape recorders can be used for appreciation or and for teaching music
- Instructions for doing experiments or any activity can be recorded on cassette and the individual can listen to it through the headphones and do the necessary operations without disturbance to others
- A tape recorder can be used very effectively during the microteaching sessions. It will provide the necessary feedback for discussions to improve the lesson.

Disadvantages of Tape Recorder
- There is no personal contact with the speaker
- It does not cater to individual differences
- Listening for a long time generally distract
- It encourages passive learning
- It is costly, and so all people cannot afford it
- It does not provide a laboratory experience, though instructions may be given.

The principle of audio tape recording is that plastic tape, covered in ferrous oxide or chromium dioxide, is pulled at a constant speed past two electromagnetic heads. The tape is capable of being magnetized and as it passes over the "erase" head any previous signal is wiped off. It then passes over the "record" head, where magnetic impulses from the sound source are recorded on it. When the tape is played back, the record head picks up these magnetic impulses and converts them back to the recorded sound via the loudspeaker. The erase head in nonoperational during play, to avoid wiping off the recording.

Audio tape recording can capture the feelings and experiences of patients, which makes it a good medium for adding interest to sessions on nursing care. Such recordings are relatively simple to make.

Tape recordings are outdated now which is replaced by recording by mobile phones.

Making Audio Tape Recordings
Audio tape recordings can be made by direct recording of sound sources such as radio or records, or by the use of microphones. The modern tape recorders have inbuilt microphones, though it is necessary to use external microphones in recording in a noisy environment. If the teacher is reading a script for a recording session, then he should be sitting comfortably at a table, with the microphone high enough to avoid having to speak down to it. The head should be held up and the script must not intervene between the face and the microphone.

Instructional Media and Methods

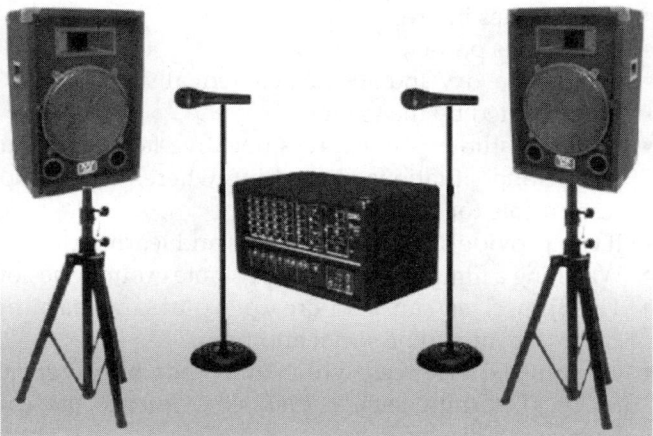

Fig. 3.14: Public address system.

Recording requires an assistant to switch the machine on and to monitor sound levels. It is important to position the tape recorder at some distance from the microphone so that amplifier hum is not picked up.

Public Address System

"A large group communication".

Public address system is required for communication in large groups (more than 30–50 students). This system aims at reproducing the original sound at a higher intensity. The quality of reproduction depends on the public address system and the acoustic qualities of the hall. The public address system consists of microphone, amplifier, and speakers (Fig. 3.14).

Microphone is a sound sensitive transducer that converts sound energy into electrical energy. The electrical energy is reconverted to sound energy by the speakers at a higher intensity. Microphone could either be mobile (collar microphone) or fixed to a table or a floor stand.

The speaker should maintain a distance of about 20 cm from the lips to avoid sound distortions.

Amplifier controls the volume and the tone of the sound. Tone control consists of low frequency (bass) and high frequency (treble) components and helps in giving the desirable quality of sound.

Television

"A mass education media".

Television constitutes an important medium widely used to disseminate information to its viewers. It has the advantage of serving as both audio and video aid, thereby having greater appeal than the radio and print media.

Television is being acknowledged as powerful medium of mass education. In India, television is being used for imparting information and distance education through the UGC programs and other educational programs. It

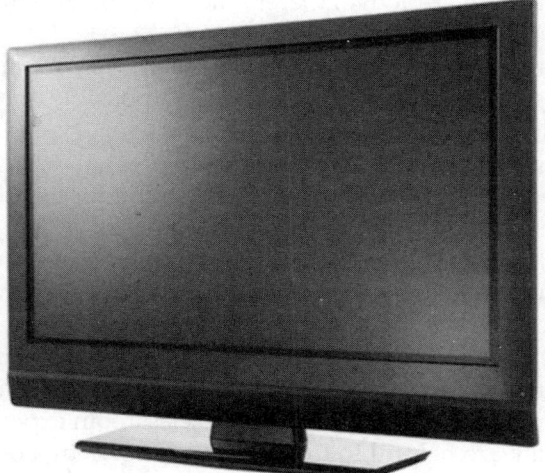

Fig. 3.15: Television.

has the ability to bring the events and happening to the viewer in action (Fig. 3.15).

Kinds of Television Broadcasts

Live Broadcast

Under this system, educational events are directly broadcasted. Immediate transmission of the programs to a large number of audiences is possible through the live telecast.

Recorded Broadcast

Under this system, prerecorded programs are telecasted as per the transmission schedule. The existing educational television services in the country depend mainly on the already produced programs. Such programs can be well planned and evaluated at each developmental stage. Recorded programs could be of a better quality than live broadcasts because all facilities in terms of time, manpower, equipment, etc. are exploited for producing these programs.

Closed Circuit Television Broadcast

Under this system, the prerecorded or live programs are transmitted on a closed circuit. It is the link between the studio and a series of classrooms, usually by means of cables installed in an institution to transmit educational programs. The system can link several classrooms or institutions, and allow transmission from any of the classroom studios.

Merits of Television as Educational Tool

- Television caters to the masses of people including people living in remote areas
- Television programs are well planned and presented, thus providing higher quality of instruction

- They are attractive, thereby holding the attention of the students
- Rapid and continuing change in curricula and instructional methods are made possible through educational television
- It reduces dependency on teacher
- Television provides in-service training for teachers to improve their teaching methods and skills
- It has proved its effectiveness/supremacy in teaching certain subjects such as agriculture, science, geography, etc.
- Television programs break the monotony of normal dullness of classroom instruction by the teacher. It provides novelty and variety to classroom experience
- They are helpful in updating the knowledge of both teachers and students as they include the latest information and findings
- It can impart experiences which are out of physical reach (other countries, people, events, etc.).

Limitations of Television as Educational Tool

- Television is a one-way communication device, and as such it does not provide for interaction
- Teaching through television is expensive
- Students differ in their learning speed and style. Hence, it cannot cater to the speed of every learner
- The learner remains as a passive spectator and not an active participant.

> Television induces effective learning as it appeals to the eye, ear and emotions of the learner and seeks total involvement from his part.

Films

"A variety entertainment".

Using feature films to teach nursing is a creative and under-utilized way to engage students in learning complex material. Films are widely used in other disciplines and films are taken seriously as a teaching strategy. Films have been used to teach a variety of college subjects including biology, communication, ethics history, philosophy, political science, psychology, and religion. Also films have been used extensively in teaching psychiatry and counseling.

Advantages of Films

- It increases the attention span
- It stimulates critical thinking
- It motivates the learner
- It helps in easy remembrance of the concepts
- It appeals to the visual learner
- It increases curiosity
- It increases observation skills
- It stimulates interest
- It increases participation
- It can make dry and abstract content alive
- It is accepted by the students
- It allows students to express negative feelings about people and situations in a setting where they are not responsible for care
- It can provide shared experiences and learning
- Watching a film in a group can promote group cohesion
- The film class can also create a pleasant learning environment and be social and fun
- Certain experiences which may not be given as practical learning such as disasters, violence, etc. can be given through films.

Disadvantages of Films

Teacher should have control over the students' learning. Otherwise, it will be a mere watching the movie. If not facilitated by the teacher, the student may not relate movie with the subject.

It is time consuming for the teacher. Selection, organization, displaying, and relating to learning is very difficult.

Not all the concepts can be taught by using the films.

Steps in Using Film

Planning

- Formulate the objectives
- Select the topic
- Check for feasibility and facilities available
- Plan for the content to be covered
- Choose the movie.

Preparation

- Access the movie
- Buy or download the movie and select the relevant portion for showing to the students
- Write the lesson plan
- Do the rehearsal.

Presentation

- Explain the purposes and what should be observed
- Inform objectives
- Project the film
- Discuss the issues
- Clarify the doubts and supplement.

Evaluation

- Evaluation of self
- Student learning
- Film as a teaching strategy.

Tips for Using Films Successfully
- Buy videos and DVDs selectively
- Familiarize with copyright matters
- Videos must be shown in an instructional room such as classroom or an auditorium
- Films can be shown only for educational and not for recreational purposes
- Videos, not illegal copies, must be used and the copyright notice has to be shown
- Have an alternate film, handouts and discussion questions prepared in case the video does not work
- Instruct the students to have pen and paper to note down questions or comments
- Instruct the students what to be observed for
- Explain what you are doing to other faculty. Do not let them hear rumors that you are cutting theory classes to watch movies.

Computer

"A master brain by master's brain".

It goes without saying that the importance of computers is felt in every field and has become the integral part of our society. Learning the high-end technology has thus become a necessity for people in various contexts. Computers have become ubiquitous today and are found in every walk of life. Eric Ashby, the historian, has called information technology, the fifth major revolution in education, after instruction by professional teachers, creation of the written word, printing and advances in educational science and technology.

Computer is an electronic data processing machine capable of performing millions of operations with tremendous speed. It has the capacity of storing large volume of data, which can be used in future. Computer only follows the instructions given by the user, without any strain, self-thinking or reasoning. With the above qualities, computer can be used in almost all fields. Nursing field is not an exception.

Computer is often compared with the human brain which can be called as the most powerful super computer. Computer can perform excellent job that is tedious and complicated without error, but it is the human brain that is behind the computer to make the machine work competently. The human can make sense out of disorganized nonsense, but computer can make sense out of sense only (Fig. 3.16).

Characteristics of a Computer

A computer possesses the following characteristics:
- **Speed**: Computers work at incredible speed. They can handle millions of instructions at one second.
- **Storage**: A large volume of information be can stored in memory.

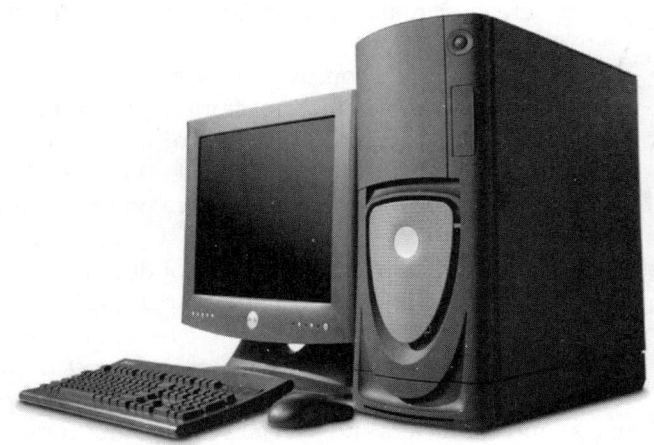

Fig. 3.16: Computer.

- **Accuracy**: A device that is nearly 100% accurate depends on the operator.
- **Ability to operate automatically**: Does not require prompt input from the operator at each stage of operation.
- **Diligence**: Computer does not get tired, bored or lazy.
- **Scientific approach**: The entire approach to problem solving in computers is scientific and logical.
- **Versatility**: The computer is a versatile tool for doing a variety of jobs.

Parts of the Computer

The computer basically consists of the following parts:
- Input devices
- Output devices
- A memory store
- A processing unit
- A control unit.

Input Devices

These devices help to feed the data to the computer. They include the following.
- **Keyboard**: They are the basic input devices through which data and programs are fed into the computer. They have numeric and alphabetic symbols, edit, control, and functional keys. A keyboard is very much like that of a standard computer.
- **Mouse**: It is used to position the cursor on the screen. Its manipulation on a flat surface moves the cursor in the same direction as the movement of the mouse. The box contains a ball underneath, which senses the movement and transmits it to the cursor over the screen.
- **Light pen**: This is a pen like device connected by cable to display. When pointed at the screen the computer revises the position of the point. It can be moved and repositioned as required. It helps to draw pictures

on the screen or make changes to an already drawn picture or figure.
- **Graphic table**: It is a computer-based terminal with additional features for creating, storing, and printing pictures. One can create an image of a picture by simply moving a stylus on the picture. As the stylus moves, the picture is created and drawn on the screen for checking.
- **Joy stick**: Moving a joy stick increases or decreases the voltage level in a resistor. It helps in playing games using a computer.
- **Optical character reader**: They are input devices used to read any printed text. They can interpret handmade marks and characters and special symbols and codes.
- **OCRs scan**: It reads the text optically, character by character and convert them into a machine readable code and store them into the system's memory. They can read at a rate of 2400 characters per second.
- **Voice input**: This is another means of communication via the computer. It incorporates the wave from which it is created, and analyzes it.

Output Devices

Output devices translate information back into understandable form. The data fed into the computer are processed as per the instructions given to the computer and returned in the form of output.
- **Printers**: It is the most commonly used output device. The paper copy obtained from the printer is often referred to as the print output.
- **Visual display unit**: When the program is keyed in, the screen displays the characters. The user can read the program line by line and make corrections before it is stored or printed. Screen sizes differ from system to system. The cursor on the screen is controlled by the cursor keys on the keyboard.
- **Computer output microfilm (COM)**: When large amounts of data are to be printed and stored for future reference, conventional paper output will not be economical. In such situations, computer output microfilm is used, which consists of photographed images produced in miniature by the computer.
- **Audio response unit**: Computer audio output or voice response units speak by arranging half-second records of voice sounds of prerecorded words.
- **Plotters**: They are used to produce output containing graphics or diagrams. With the availability of multicolor plotters, they are increasingly used for preparing financial documents, annual reports and engineering drawings.
- **Memory store**: It contains all the information, which has been fed into the computer through the input equipment.

- **Processing unit**: It operates and processes the information. It can add, subtract or multiply. It can also select particular information out of a large amount of stored information in terms of scientific criteria.
- **External storage devices**: The purpose of external storage device is to retain data and programs for future use. A number of files containing information can be stored in this manner.
- **Control unit**: This controls the actions of the processing units.
- **Floppy disks**: It is flexible plastic disk coated with magnetic material and works like a photograph record. Information can be recorded or read by inserting it into a disk drive connected to the computer.
- **Hard disks**: They are suitable for storing large volumes of information and are popularly known as the Winchester disks. A hard disk consists of two or more magnetic plates fixed to a spindle one below the other with a set of read or write leads. These are permanently sealed inside a casing to protect it from dust.

Computer as a Teacher

Computer can never replace a teacher. It merely complements a teacher's role. However, in some areas of instruction, it is even better than a human teacher. For example:
- It never gets bored or irritated
- It never makes mistakes on its own
- It permits individual attention (1:1 interaction)
- It permits a learner to decide his/her own pace of learning.

> Computer is an electronic device that is designed to accept, store and process the data according to the instructions to produce desired results.

Camera

Camera is a piece of equipment for taking photographs, moving pictures or television pictures (Fig. 3.17).

Photograph

According to Emmert, the still photograph represents a cross-section of a visual experience of that instant in time.

Purposes of Camera
- To impart knowledge
- To increase perceptual and conceptual learning
- To bring remote events closer
- To provide field type of learning
- To provide realism
- To convey the message easily

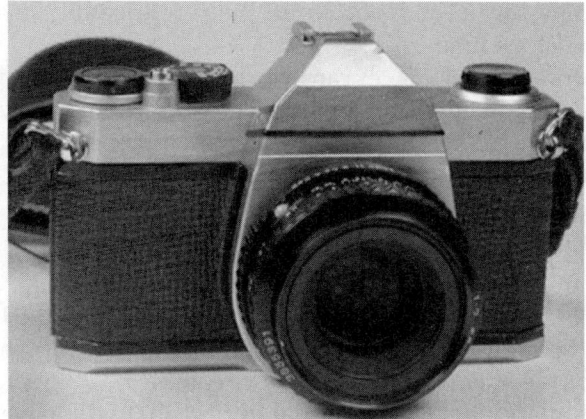

Fig. 3.17: Camera

- To attract group attention
- To start discussion or review.

Types
- Fixed focus simple box camera with single speed shutter
- Box camera with two speed shutter
- All metal reflex
  - Single lens
  - Double lens
- Miniature cameras with couple range finders
- Old model field cameras using plates
- Digital cameras.

Parts
- Lens
- Iris
- Shutter
- Rewinding mechanism
- Negative film
- Opaque box
- Press button.

Steps in Photography
- Loading the camera with suitable film
- Selection of shutter speed, lens aperture
- Required view
- Exposure
- Processing
- Printing
- Mounting.

Advantages
- Conveys message easily
- Helps in retention
- Holds attention and concentration
- Interesting, easy and fast

- Saves time
- Duplication is possible
- Entertainment
- Reality.

Disadvantages
- High maintenance
- High production cost
- Suitable for high audience only
- Considerable preparation and technical skills needed.

Liquid Crystal Display Projector

"Liquid Crystal Display".

LCD means liquid crystal display.

An LCD projector is a type of video projector for displaying video, images or computer data on a screen or other flat surface. It is a modern analog of the slide projector or overhead projector. The LCD projector was invented by New York inventor Gene Dolgoff (Fig. 3.18).

How Images are Displayed?

To display images, LCD (liquid crystal display) projectors typically send light from a metal halide lamp through a prism that separates light to three polysilicone panels—one each for the red, green, and blue components of the video signal. As polarized light passes through the panels (combination of polarizer, LCD panel and analyzer), individual pixels can be opened to allow light to pass or closed to block the light. The combination of open and closed pixels can produce a wide range of colors and shades in the projected image.

Metal halide lamps are used because they output an ideal color temperature and a broad spectrum of color. These lamps also have the ability to produce an extremely large amount of light within a small area.

Projection Surfaces

These small metal halide lamps have the ability to project an image on any flat surface. LCD projectors tend to be

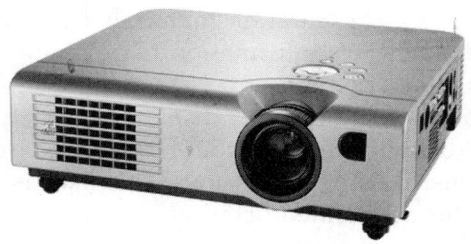

Fig. 3.18: LCD projector.

smaller and more portable than other types of projection systems. Even so, the best image quality is found using a blank white or gray surface, so dedicated projection screens are often used.

Perceived color in a projected image is a factor of both projection surface and projector quality. Since white is more of a neutral color, white surfaces are best suited for natural color tones; as such, white projection surfaces are more common in most business and school presentation environments.

However, darkest black in a projected image is dependent on how dark the screen is. Because of this, some presenters and presentation space planners prefer gray screens, which create higher perceived contrast. The trade-off is that darker backgrounds can throw off color tones. Color problems can sometimes be adjusted through the projector settings, but may not be as accurate as they would on a white background.

Educational Uses

- When watching educational videos in the classroom, images projected on a large screen allow students to catch every detail, even from the back rows.
- As images can also be projected in well-lit environments, students can refer to their texts or take notes at the same time, thus effectively allowing the class to gain a deeper understanding of the subject matter
- With computers now being introduced in more and more classes, computer screens can be output directly to projectors to supply students with pertinent information in real-time
- Projectors become powerful teaching tools, particularly when instructing a class in how to operate computers
- Projecting the example of teacher's computer screen onto a large screen allows class progress to be closely monitored so that support can be given where needed
- Moreover, by installing a fixed projector in a large capacity venue, such as a gymnasium or hall, the benefits of projecting images on the big screen can be magnified to reach even larger numbers during intramural events or other occasions.

Meetings and Small Conferences

- Displaying presentation materials by projector at meetings allows information to be shared equally among those present
- Problem points and issues displayed on a large screen can be easily verified and thus facilitate more effective, smoother flowing discussions. This likewise sets the stage for accelerated decision-making and speedier administrative processes.
- Easy set-up and portability help reduce the loss of precious time
- Moreover, as images can be projected for viewing even in well-lit environments, participants can also engage in note taking and refer to printed materials or other documents.

Mobile Presentations

When presentations are made out of the campus, the use of projectors enables us to present highly appealing and communicative deliveries, on a large screen, which holds the attention of the audience completely. Big screen presentations deliver a visual impact that will leave an impression on clients long after the presentation is over.

Large Conferences

Projectors are now indispensable for conferences and seminars at large venues. They enable presentations that demand the attention of those present and leave a vivid impression through the synergistic effect of the presenter's oral explanation combined with a dynamic rendering of presentation content on-screen through an ensemble of animation effects. Highly appealing presentations can put together at will to consist not only of PC generated materials but also elements of video and website content as well. Seminars and conferences can proceed smoothly, while paper and labor that would usually be expended in distributing detailed materials to attendees are also saved.

Exhibitions

Projector generated images coupled with explanatory panels allow the staging of more dynamic presentations to achieve a greater impact at events such as exhibitions. Moreover, projection enables a combination of presentation images to be employed for a wide range of applications. Projectors can thus be freely positioned to project from the ceiling, the floor or from the rear of projection surfaces and realize environments orchestrated to suit to every time, place and occasion.

Disadvantages

- Clarity and visibility of the projected images are reduced when used in well-lit environment
- Smooth, white, flat surface is required to project
- Projectors do not have self-playing capacity. It requires input from the computer
- Expensive and less affordability
- Technical knowledge and skill is essential to use the projector effectively
- Video output alone presented and requires audio supplementation by the presenter.

Powerpoint Presentation

Microsoft Powerpoint is a versatile tool for developing computer-based graphical presentations.

Criteria for Developing Powerpoint Presentations

- Powerpoint presentations are meant for use as a presentation aid with a speaker. It is not best for presentations without a speaker.
- Powerpoint slides comprising a presentation should support the message, not substitute for the presenter or for a more detailed handout
- A balanced and structured approach is needed for a presentation. Text to give context for the audience's understanding of what the presenter will be speaking about, and graphics and multimedia to touch the emotions of the audience.

Guidelines for Preparing Powerpoint Presentations

- Decide clearly the purpose of presentation.
- A structured presentation will be highly effective.
- Select colors that have high contrast so that the text and graphics can be easily seen. It is preferred to have dark backgrounds with light colored text or vice versa.
- Use fonts that provide clear visibility
  - Never use a font size below 24.
  - For titles and headings, use 36–44 font size.
  - Never use too many fonts.
- For title, either bold letters or underline can be used, never use both.
- Use bulleted points and short sentences, preferably phrases consisting of 5–6 words, to deliver the key ideas.
- Avoid using moving/flying text or graphics unless a purpose is there.
- The most preferred effect that is suitable in a presentation is the "appear" effect.
- Transition between slides should be smooth and appealing. Otherwise distraction may happen from the message being delivered.
- Use graphics, clip arts or photographs only if they add message to the slides.
- Avoid overly complex diagrams or charts.
- Do not use images that are not relevant to the topic of the slide.
- Charts, graphs and tables can be used to present information precisely and concisely.
- Never use annoying sounds.
- Never use poor quality of video or audio segments.

Tips for Effective Presentation

- Never read out the slides as it appears during the presentation. Simply reading the slides that are jammed with text is an insult to the audience.
- Elaborate the points, phrases, and key ideas present on the slides.
- Avoid abrupt jump of the content.
- Go back to previous slides, if required.
- Face the audience and not the projection screen.

Video Compact Disk

Video CD (abbreviated as VCD and also known as View CD, Compact disk digital video) is a standard digital format for storing video on a Compact disk. VCDs are playable in VCD players, most modern DVD video players, personal computers, and some video game consoles.

Advantages of Video Compact Disk

- Easy to store
- Large storing capacity
- Cheap and handy
- Copying is easier
- Self-playing capacity
- Durable
- Cannot be affected by fungus
- Combined audio and video output.

Disadvantages of Video Compact Disk

- Easily breakable
- Scratches affect the video quality.

Video Cassette Recorder

The video cassette recorder (or VCR, more commonly known in the UK and Ireland as the video recorder) is a type of video tape recorder that uses removable video tape cassettes containing magnetic tape to record audio and video from a television broadcast so it can be played back later. Most VCRs have their own tuner (for direct TV reception) and a programmable timer (for unattended recording of a certain channel at a particular time) (Fig. 3.19).

Advantages of Video Cassette Recorder

- Directly recordable
- Reproducible

Fig. 3.19: VCR.

- Copies can be taken
- Combined audio and video output.

Disadvantages of Video Cassette Recorder
- Affected by fungus
- Affected by magnetic force
- Not economical one
- Less durability
- Outdated
- Transferred to digital format.

Microscope

A microscope [Greek: *micron* = small + *skopein* = to look or see] is an instrument for viewing objects that are too small to be seen by the naked or unaided eye. The science of investigating small objects using such an instrument is called microscopy. The term microscopy means minute or very small, not visible with the eye unless aided by a microscope.

Parts of the Microscope

The parts of the microscope are shown in Figure 3.20.

Aperture Iris Diaphragm

This device is part of the substage condenser. It serves to control the angle of the cone of light emerging from the top of the condenser. When adjusted so that the back lens of the objective, as viewed through the eyepiece tube, is just filled with light.

Body Tube

This part supports the eyepiece and objectives. It is critical that the tube is constructed so that this optics shares a common axis. Mechanical tube length is the distance from the top of the eyepiece tube to bottom of the objective holder.

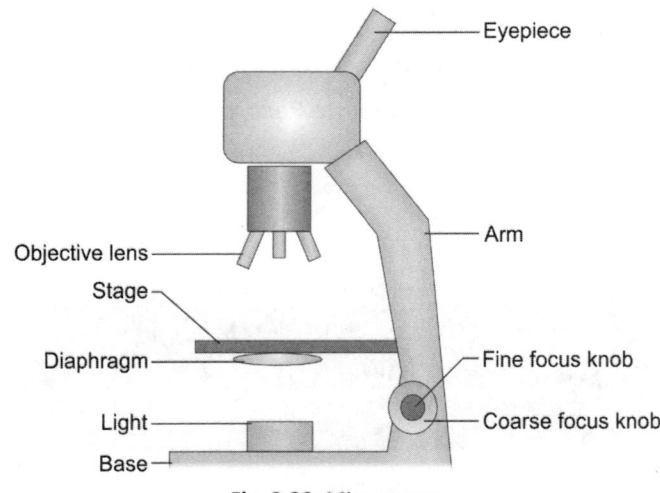

Fig. 3.20: Microscope.

Coarse Adjustment Knob

As the name suggests, this control (typically a pair, one on each side) moves either the body tube, or the stage/substage, up or down in a quick manner. This is accomplished by means of a rack and pinion assembly. The pinion is a toothed wheel (the knobs are attached to either end of the axial) that rides along a diagonally grooved bar or "rack", attached to the stage or body tube. A good coarse focus control will provide smooth, back lash free movement.

Condenser

It is a vital part of the illumination system, and is designed to collect, control and concentrate light from the lamp onto the specimen. As with objectives, the optical elements can introduce a variety of aberrations which are corrected to varying degrees, depending on the type of condenser one is using. Condensers (as well as filters and objectives) are available to provide specialized and contrast-enhancing illumination.

Condenser Focus Knob

This control is used to precisely adjust the vertical height of the condenser.

Eyepiece (Ocular)

Eyepieces are produced in a number of different designs. The top element is an achromatic doublet, and it provides a large, flat, and well corrected field of view.

Eyepiece Tube

A fixed tube, into which the eyepiece is inserted.

Fine Focus Knob

This control allows for precise focusing of the specimen. It is absolutely essential that this control works smoothly, with zero rebound effect, e.g. set the focus and leave for 5 minutes, the image should remain razor sharp.

Foot (Base)

It rests on the bench top and supports the stage and body of the microscope, and in many cases also houses the lamp. A well-designed base will ensure that the image does not dance about during focusing, or while manipulating the specimen. There are a vast number of different base designs.

Limb (Arm)

The arm is attached to the foot (in scopes without an inclined viewing head by means of an "inclination joint") and supports the body tube. The shape of the arm and the way in which the body is attached are often used to illustrate the history of the microscope's development. In modern stands the "body tube" has been replaced by two removal parts, a viewing head and an objective changer, with the top end of the arm forming the middle section. This type of arm is very strong and can better support additional equipment, such as video cameras.

Mirror (Or Internal Lamp)

The mirror serves to direct light into the condenser. Except for specialized mirrors, all are second surface mirrors, in other words the silver coating is applied to the back, rather than front glass surface.

Nosepiece (Objective Changer)

A rotating device to which objectives are attached. The quality of objective changer is often a good indication of a microscope's overall quality. It should move smoothly, and most important, should have a distinct click or feel when an objective is properly "seated".

Objective

This, together with the condenser, is the microscope. It is much better to start with two good quality objectives then four mediocre ones. In many cases the barrel of the objective is engraved with information on its optical characteristics. Objective lenses are very tiny and as a result great care is needed to form and assemble such lens systems. A revolving nosepiece permits rapid changeover between objectives. In practical terms it is essential that the focus of the image be preserved during the change of objectives.

Stage Clips

These are the basic stage slide holders. Supplied in pairs, they are adequate for general slide manipulation.

Stage

This is the platform or "stage" that supports the specimen (which are typically mounted on glass slides). To do this job properly it must be perfectly perpendicular to the optical axis, dead flat and of adequate size. A microscope with a dinged or out of line stage should be a void. As mentioned above mechanical stages are often supplied. They may be integrated into the stage itself (with the stage deck moving in one axis rather than the slide holder) or they can be attached see Figure 3.20 for the parts of microscope.

Types

"Microscopes" can largely be separated into three classes.
1. Optical microscopes
2. Electron microscopes
3. Scanning probe microscopes.

Optical microscopes are microscopes which function through the optical theory of lenses in order to magnify the image generated by the passage of a wave through the sample. The waves used are either electro-magnetic in optical microscopes or electron beams in electron microscopes.

Simple versus Compound Microscope

Simple Optical Microscope

A simple microscope, as opposed to a standard compound microscope with multiple lenses, is a microscope that uses only one lens for magnification. This use of a single convex lens to magnify objects for viewing is still found in the magnifying glass and the hand-lens.

Compound Optical Microscope

The compound microscope would have a single glass lens of short focal length for the objective, and another single glass lens for the eyepiece or ocular. Modern microscopes of this kind are usually more complex, with multiple lens components in both objective and eyepiece assemblies. These multicomponent lenses are designed to reduce aberrations, particularly chromatic aberration and spherical aberration. In modern microscopes the mirror is replaced by a lamp unit providing stable, controllable illumination.

Optical microscopes, through their use of visible wavelengths of light, are the simplest and hence most widely used type of microscope. A stereomicroscope is often used for lower-power magnification on large subjects. Various wavelengths of light are sometimes used for special purposes, e.g. in the study of biological tissue.

Electron Microscopes

Electron microscopes, which use beams of electrons instead of light, are designed for very high magnification usage. Electrons, which can be accelerated to produce a much smaller wavelength than visible light, allow a much higher resolution. The main limitation of the electron beam is that it must pass through a vacuum as air molecules would otherwise scatter the beam.

Transmission electron microscope: It passes electrons completely through the sample, analogous to basic optical microscopy. This requires careful sample preparation, since electrons are scattered so strongly by most materials. This is a scientific device that allows people to see objects that could normally not be seen by the naked or unaided eye.

Scanning Probe Microscope

In scanning probe microscopy (SPM), a physical probe is used either in close contact to the sample or nearly touching it. By moving the probe across the sample, and by measuring the interactions between the sharp tip of the probe and the sample, a micrograph is generated. The exact nature of the interactions between the probe and the sample determines exactly what kind of SPM is being used. Because this kind of microscopy relies on the interactions between the tip and the sample, it generally only measures information about the surface of the sample.

Direction to Use the Microscope

- To carry the microscope, grasp the microscopes arm with one hand. Place the other hand under the base.
- Place the microscope on a table with the arm toward you.
- Turn the coarse adjustment knob to raise the body tube.
- Revolve the nose piece until the low-power objective lens clicks into place.
- Adjust the diaphragm. While looking through the eyepiece, also adjust the mirror until one can see a bright white circle of light.
- Place a slide on the stage. Center the specimen over the opening on the stage. Use the stage to hold the slide in place.
- Look at the stage from the side. Carefully turn the coarse adjustment knob to lower the body tube until the low-power objective almost touches the slide.
- Looking through the eyepiece, adjust very slowly, the coarse adjustment knob until the specimen comes into focus.
- To switch to the high power objective lens, look at the microscope from the side. Carefully revolve the nosepiece until the high-power objective lens clicks into place. Make sure the lens does not hit the slide.
- Looking through the eyepiece, turn the fine adjustment knob until the specimen comes into focus.

Care and Handling

Transporting: When picking up the microscope and walk with it, grab the arm with one hand and place the other hand on the bottom of the base. Do not swing the microscope!

Handling and cleaning: Never touch the lenses with the fingers. Human being's body produces oil that smudges the glass. This oil can even etch the glass if left on too long. Use only lens paper to clean the glass. Toilet paper, kleenex, and paper towels have fibers that can scratch the lenses.

Storage: When finished with the "scope" assignment, rotate the nosepiece so that it is on the low-power objective, roll the nosepieces so that it is all the way down to the stage, then replace the dust cover. Do not forget to use proper transporting techniques.

Clean-up: Clean all slides, materials, and work area when it is done. Be careful with the slides and cover slips.

They are made of glass and if broken, one will get cut and will bleed.

Advantages

- Magnification
- Direct analysis
- Direct identification
- Some models work without power.

Disadvantages

- Cannot store the result
- No self-interpretation
- Not suitable for large groups
- Handling and preservation is not easy.

Summary

A wide variety of instructional media is used to impart education and make the learning process interesting and effective. They are namely charts, graphs, projects, models, overhead projectors, LCD projectors ,tape recorders, radio etc. Audio-visual aids are any devices that can be used to make the learning experience more concrete, more realistic and more dynamic (Kinder). Audio-visual aids can be classified as projected and nonprojected, traditional and digital, and graphics and models. It is also defined as audio aids, visual aids, and audio-visual aids.

Each audio-visual aid is unique in its purpose, principle followed and methods of preparation and handling/use. Although there has been a rise in variety of AV aids since the advent of technological advancements, the traditional methods of administering the content remains the basis of delivering the educational content effectively by almost all educators.

Audio-visual aids can supplement teaching, but are no substitute for teachers or books. Audio-visual aids should not be misused; they should be used properly to attain the educational and instructional objectives.

4. Measurement and Evaluation

"To observe without evaluating is the highest form of intelligence".
—J Krishnamurthi

Objectives
After completing this unit, you will be able to:
- Understand the difference between assessment, measurement and evaluation
- Explain the purpose and scope of evaluation
- Apply the principles of evaluation
- Explain the criteria for selecting evaluation techniques
- Differentiate between standardized and nonstandardized tests
- Discuss various types of evaluation tools and techniques.

Introduction

Testing, measurement and evaluation plays an important role in all educational institutions, including nursing educational institution. Students' achievement is profoundly influenced by the evaluation practices used by the teachers in the classroom. Student evaluation is a basic process of teaching. Evaluation is not an add-on feature of instruction but an integral part of it, since the information it provides allows teachers to make adjustments to outcomes and teaching methodologies. Instruction can seldom be effective without a comprehensive evaluation plan that is carefully and systematically implemented in the classroom. Evaluation consists of empirical observations. The evaluator follows a formalized procedure so that any other observer can confirm or replicate the evaluation. Evaluation involves the objective, gathering and analyzing of information to aid in decision-making. The nurse educator is responsible for evaluating students in order to improve their classroom and clinical performance. It also serves as a basis for guidance and counseling services. This unit describes the concepts of evaluation, methods and types.

Meaning and Definition

Evaluation, an integral part of an educational program, is the process of judging the effectiveness of educational experience through careful appraisal. Educational evaluation is made in relation to the objectives that have been determined previously by faculty, individual teachers and students.

Evaluation is the process of determining whether predetermined objectives have been achieved. This definition implies two things:
1. The existence of objectives, and
2. The use of an appropriate measuring instrument.

Evaluation is much more than testing; it is a continuous and comprehensive process, rather than a series of sporadic and independent events. Evaluation should guide student to learn daily rather than simply providing information for making decisions on promotion at the end of the year.

It is a process to judge the worth of all the educational outcomes brought almost as a result of the teaching-learning process.

According to Ralph Tyler (1950), evaluation is the process of determining to what extent the educational objectives are being realized.

According to NCERT (1963), evaluation is the process of determining the following:
- The extent to which an objective is being attained
- The effectiveness of the learning experiences provided in the classroom
- How well the goals of education have been accomplished.

Meaning of Measurement, Assessment, Evaluation and Testing

The term evaluation is frequently interchanged with the terms assessment, measurement and testing. These terms have distinct meanings.

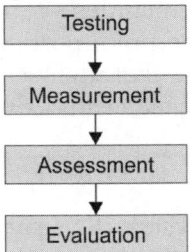

Terminologies	Definition
Measurement	A process of quantifying or assigning a number to performances
Assessment	A term used instead of measurement when a numerical value is not involved, e.g. checklists of behaviors
Evaluation	The process of judging the value or worth of an individual's characteristics or an outcome or a programme obtained by measurement or assessment
Test	An instrument or tool for obtaining measurements or assessments, e.g. an essay
Examination	A formal situation in which students undertake one or more tests under specific rules

Assessment

A teacher's day in the classroom is filled with situations in which she has to make decisions—some about individual students, some about the class as a whole, some about instructional matters and so on.

The process of collecting, synthesizing and interpreting information to aid in the process of this decision making is called *assessment*.

According to the American Federation of Teachers, assessment is defined as the process of collecting information to be used in making educational decisions about students, to give feedback to them, to make judgments regarding curriculum and instructional techniques and methods.

Assessment is a general term that not only includes the full range of information that a teacher gathers, but also ways in which she gathers this information.

Dimensions of Assessment

- Formal
- Quantitative
- Episodic
- Formative
- Teacher-centered
- Norm-referenced
- Informal
- Qualitative
- Continuous
- Summative
- Student-centered
- Criterion referenced

Measurement

Measurement is defined as a procedure for assigning numbers to a specified attribute in such a way that the numbers indicate the degree to which the person possesses this attribute (Nitko, 1996).

It is the process of quantifying or assigning a number to performance. It includes scoring that produces a numerical description of a particular performance. It is an act or a process that involves the assignment of a numerical index to whatever is being assessed.

Test

A test is a formal, systematic, usually paper and pencil procedure used to gather information about the students' behavior. Nitko (1996) defined test as an instrument or systematic procedure for gathering measurements. It is a device or procedure for confronting a subject with a standard set of questions or tasks to which the student is to respond independently and the results of which can be treated in such a way to provide a quantitative comparison of the performance of different students.

Evaluation

Finally, evaluation involves making judgments about the quality of the students' performance or a possible course of action.

Gronlund (1985) stated that evaluation puts a value upon assessment. Evaluation is a more comprehensive and inclusive term than assessment, measurement and testing. He also points out that evaluation may involve quantitative description (measurement) and qualitative description (non-measurement) of students, where the main emphasis is on the extent to which learning outcomes are achieved. Both types of evaluations and descriptions are necessary for comprehensive student evaluation.

Difference between Measurement and Evaluation are shown in table below:

Measurement	Evaluation
It is quantitative	It is qualitative
It is limited to quantitative testing	It goes beyond testing and measurement
It is more external	It is both external and internal
Every measurement is not evaluation	Without measurement evaluation does not carry much meaning
It measures only quantity	It takes into consideration both quantity and value judgment or quality
Evaluation is not a part of measurement	Measurement is a part of evaluation

Evaluation Process

The evaluation of the student does not take place in vacuum. It takes place in the context of teaching and learning, and many factors in this context have implications for student evaluation. Figure 4.1 shows

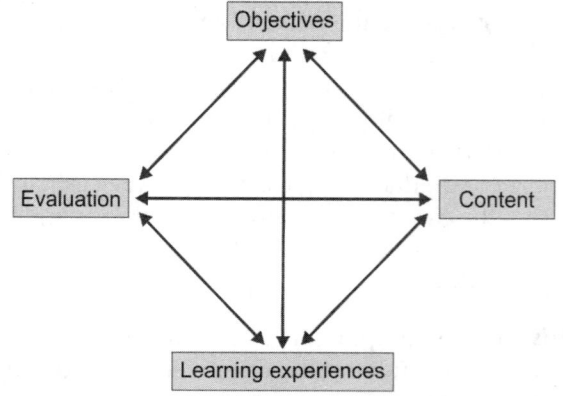

Fig. 4.1: Evaluation process.

the interrelationship between the objectives, content, learning experiences and evaluation.

Concepts of Evaluation

- Evaluation, in a general sense, is a process of assessment
- Evaluation is a continuous process
- It is a systematic process
- Evaluation differs from measurement
- It is an integral part of education.

Principles of Evaluation

- Evaluation takes its direction from a definition of education which, stated in its broadest sense, is to enable students to realize their potential as human beings.
- Evaluation is a means to an end, and never-an-end in itself.
- Evaluation, by definition, connotes value.
- Evaluation involves teacher judgment.
- Validity and reliability are of paramount concern in any evaluation activity.
- Evaluation is continuous in that it is taking place all the time and comprehensive in that it is concerned with the cognitive, psychomotor and affective domains of human development.
- Evaluation is an integral part of the teaching-learning process.
- Every evaluation should be made with reference to specified outcomes.
- Evaluation procedures should take into consideration individual differences among students.
- Evaluation of students involves more than a single appraisal at any one time.
- The process of evaluation begins with the outcomes of the educational program.
- The primary purpose of evaluation is to determine the extent to which students have achieved the intended outcomes of the educational program.
- Evaluation gives a picture of where students are, how they are progressing, and what their needs are.
- Evaluation is concerned with some attributes that are quantitative and some that are qualitative.
- Evaluation is a more inclusive concept than assessment. Assessment involves the collection of data needed for evaluation, but it is not evaluation per se.

Purpose of Evaluation

Evaluation occupies a very crucial and important place in the educational process. It occurs in each and every aspect of teaching-learning situation. The purposes of evaluation are varied that includes:

- To promote learning—alter behavior of the student as desired/as required to meet the specified objectives.
- To identify problems and shortcomings to diagnose learning deficits, ineffective teaching practices, defects in the curriculum and so on.
- To make decisions to assign grades, to determine merits by offering promotion or tenure.
- To improve products to revise a textbook, to add content to an independent study module.
- To judge effectiveness of the program to determine whether objectives, goals or standards are being met.
- To judge cost-effectiveness to determine that a program is self-supporting.
- To disclose facts to disclose students' needs, possibilities, strengths, weaknesses, and to suggest remedial measures for salvation of the problem. It also helps the student to realize where he exactly stands.
- To estimate the quality of teaching-learning techniques, instructional media, etc. whether the right methods and techniques are selected to attain the objectives of the program.
- To revise and modify the curriculum as and when required.
- To bring out the inherent capabilities of the student in addition to the conventional acquisition of knowledge, evaluation helps to bring out the attitudes, habits, appreciation and understanding, manipulative skills, etc.
- Evaluation, in addition to be instrumental in causing changes in the program and curriculum, it motivates the students toward better attainment and growth.

Educational	Administrative
Ensure quality of:	Develop accountability towards:
1. Learning – To monitor students' progress – To diagnose students' strengths and weaknesses – To determine the need for remedial work – To improve the quality of learning	1. Society – To meet the demands – To meet the needs and aspirations
2. Teaching – Assessing the effectiveness of teaching – Teaching strategy – Techniques, methods, and materials	2. Parents – To keep the parents informed of their children's education – To guide the parents
3. Curriculum – Improving courses – Improving texts – Materials used by teachers – Materials used by students	3. Educational system – To maintain quality and standards – To diagnose problems and take remedial steps

Scope of Evaluation

Evaluation and Teacher

Evaluation helps the teacher to adopt a student-centered approach in her teaching and to individualize instruction. It provides the teacher with adequate knowledge concerning the students' entry behavior, i.e. her ability for learning and what she currently knows. This knowledge helps the teacher in setting, refining and clarifying realistic objectives for each student.

Evaluation helps the teacher to organize appropriate learning activities for the students to realize the objectives and also to find out the extent to which objectives are realized. Evaluation assists the teacher to improve his classroom procedures and methods of teaching-learning in the light of feedback.

Evaluation and Students

Evaluation helps the students in many ways:
- It makes them aware of the objectives of the program.
- Evaluation increases motivation by informing about their performance, ultimately facilitating learning.
- Evaluation, being a continuous process, encourages students to adopt good study habits.
- Evaluation increases the abilities and skills of the students by giving them constant feedback about their strengths and weaknesses.

Evaluation and Administrators

Evaluation helps the administrators and others associated to take appropriate decisions in planning curricular and cocurricular program. It enables the educational personnel to determine the effectiveness of instruction and learning activities. Evaluation serves as a basis for summarizing and reporting the progress of students and institutions. For educational, personal and vocational guidance, systematic evaluation serves as an important basis.

Evaluation and Parents

A systematic and continuous program of students' evaluation keeps the parents well-versed with the performance of their children and helps them to take appropriate action for their further improvement.

Common Errors in Evaluation

- The **halo error** is the result of allowing one trait to influence the evaluation of other traits or of rating all traits on the basis of a general impression.
- A **logical error** is rating a nurse high on one characteristic because the nurse possesses another characteristic that is logically related.
- The **horns error** is the opposite of the halo effect. The evaluators are hypercritical. They rate lower than they should.
- The **contrast error** is produced by the tendency of supervisors to rate the nurse opposite from the way they perceive themselves.
- A small range of score may be a result of the **central tendency error**. They give average score for everything.
- When the rating on a preceding characteristic influences the rating on the following trait, a **proximity error** exists.

Functions of Evaluation

The basic functions of evaluation are:
- Diagnosis
- Modification
- Prediction
- Selection
- Motivation
- Guidance
- Testing
- Grading
- Feedback.

Types of Evaluation

Evaluation is classified into various types:
A. Based on the time during which the evaluation is done:
   - Formative evaluation
   - Summative evaluation.
B. Based on the purpose:
   - Criterion-referenced evaluation
   - Norm-referenced evaluation.
C. Based on the person who does evaluation:
   - Internal evaluation
   - External evaluation.

Formative Evaluation

Formative evaluation is concerned with judgments made during the design and/or development of a program which is directed toward modifying, forming or otherwise improving the program before it is completed (AJ Nitko, 1983).

Formative evaluation is used to:
- Monitor learning progress during instruction.
- Provide continuous feedback to both student and teacher.
- Detect learning difficulties.

Feedback to the student reinforces successful learning and identifies the learning errors that need correction. Feedback to the teacher provides information for modifying instruction and prescribing group and individual remedial work.

In order to be meaningful, tests which are part of formative evaluation should be frequent, cover small content areas; and give immediate feedback to students. Marks obtained in formative evaluation should not be counted for pass or fail in the final assessment.

It can be implied that:
- Formative evaluation is done during an instructional program. The instructional program should aim at the attainment of certain objectives during the implementation of the program.
- It is done to monitor learning and modifying the program if needed before its completion.
- Formative evaluation is for current students.

Characteristics of Formative Evaluation
- Its design is exploratory and flexible.
- It relatively focuses on molecular analysis.
- It is cause-seeking.
- It is interested in the broader experiences of the program users.
- It tends to ignore the local effects of a particular program.
- It seeks to identify influential variables.
- It requires analysis of instructional material for mapping the hierarchical structure of the learning tasks and actual teaching of the course for a certain period.

Summative Evaluation

Summative evaluation describes judgments about the merits of an already completed program, procedure or product (AJ Nitko, 1983).

Summative evaluation typically comes at the end of a course of instruction. It is designed to determine the extent to which the instructional objectives have been achieved and is used primarily for assigning course grades or certifying pupil mastery of the intended learning outcomes (NE Gronlund, 1985).

Summative evaluation is done at the end or completion of a particular instructional program whose duration may vary from a semester to whole year and to know whether the student is competent enough for certification. It provides feedback to the teacher for the success or failure of the program and of the student. Since the result is usually in the form of a single total score or a pass or fail, there is little scope of meaningful feedback either to the learner or to the teacher. The items in the test should cover a broad range of difficulty levels.

Characteristics of Summative Evaluation
- It tends to the use of well-defined evaluation designs
- It focuses on analysis
- It provides descriptive analysis
- It tends to stress on local effects
- It is unobtrusive and nonreactive as far as possible
- It is concerned with broad range of issues
- Its instruments are reliable and valid.

Criterion-referenced Test

The terms criterion-referenced and norm-referenced were originally coined by Robert Glaser.

A criterion-referenced test is one that provides for translating test scores into a statement about the behavior to be expected of a person with that score or their relationship to a specified subject matter. Most tests written by teachers are criterion-referenced tests. The objective is simply to see whether or not the student has learned the material. A common misunderstanding regarding the term is the meaning of criterion. Many, if not most, criterion-referenced tests involve a cutscore, where the examinee passes if their score exceeds the cutscore and fails if it does not (often called a mastery test). The criterion is not the cutscore; the criterion is the domain of subject matter that the test is designed to assess. For example, the criterion may be "Students should be able to correctly add two single-digit numbers", and the cutscore may be that students should correctly answer a minimum of 80% of the questions to pass.

The criterion-referenced interpretation of a test score identifies the relationship to the subject matter. In the case of a mastery test, this does mean identifying whether the examinee has "mastered" a specified level of the subject matter by comparing their score to the cutscore. However, not all criterion-referenced tests have a cutscore, and the score can simply refer to a person's standing on the subject domain.

Because of this common misunderstanding, criterion-referenced tests have also been called standards-based assessments by some education agencies, as students are assessed with regard to standards that define what they "should" know.

Norm-referenced Test

A norm-referenced test (NRT) is a type of test, assessment, or evaluation which yields an estimate of the position of the tested individual in a predefined population, with respect to the trait being measured. This estimate is derived from the analysis of test scores and possibly other relevant data from a sample drawn from the population. The term "normative assessment" refers to the process of comparing one test-taker to his or her peers.

By contrast, a test is criterion-referenced when provision is made for translating the test score into a statement about the behavior to be expected of a person

Table 4.1: Comparison of criterion-referenced and norm-referenced tests.

Criterion-referenced test	Norm-referenced test
• It would report the student's performance strictly according to whether or not the individual student correctly answered these questions	• It indicates whether the test-taker did better or worse than other people, who took the test. It would report primarily whether the student correctly answered more questions compared to other students in the group
• It measures the actual performance of the students	• It helps to relatively rank the students
• This test will use questions which were correctly answered by students who know the specific material	• This test will use questions which were correctly answered by the "best" students and not correctly answered by the "worst" students
• Tests that set goals for students based on a set standard (e.g. 80 words spelled correctly) are criterion-referenced tests	• Tests that set goals for students based on the average students' performance are norm-referenced tests
• Test-takers can fail in a criterion referenced test when they do not perform up to the criterion expected	• Test-takers cannot "fail" a norm-referenced test, as each test-taker receives a score that compares the individual to others that have taken the test, usually given by a percentile
• It can be used to certify a student that he has mastered in a particular subject	• It is used for selection and placement of a student
• It can be used to assess the progress of the students	• It cannot be used to assess the progress of the students
• It can enforce expectation from students that what all students should know or be able to do	• It does not seek to enforce any expectation of what all students should know or be able to do other than what actual students demonstrate
• Present levels of performance are taken into consideration to remove the defects in the system	• Present levels of performance and inequity are taken as facts, not as defects to be removed by a system

with that score. The same test can be used in both ways. Table 4.1 for comparison of criterion and norm-referenced tests.

Internal Evaluation

Evaluation by a teacher using various techniques such as teacher-made tests, standardized tests and observation is known as internal assessment. Assessment is done internally by the teachers teaching in the same institution. Internal assessment mitigates a major defect of the external examination. Instead of basing results of the assessment at any one time, internal assessment can be done as continuous as desired.

Internal evaluation enables us to diagnose pupils' difficulties in learning. It points out the potentialities of an individual and provides opportunities to find out the needs, goals and interests and aptitudes of an individual and shows him the way for his development. This has a motivating effect and this, in turn, induces him to utilize his resourcefulness which is otherwise cramped.

Advantages

- Teachers can evaluate better based on their continuous comprehensive observations and the performance of the student.
- Since internal evaluation is continuous, it builds regular study habits among students.
- It can test what is being taught.
- They may not have any fear or test anxiety.
- By assessing both the tangible and intangible attainments of students, internal evaluation supplements external assessment.
- It also helps in improving teaching-learning process.
- Internal evaluation provides a continuous feedback for undertaking diagnostic and remedial teaching and other measures.
- It can be flexible and can test various dimensions of the student's abilities and skills.

Limitations and Shortcomings of Internal Evaluation

- It can be misused by the teachers.
- It requires experienced, honest and sincere teachers.
- Its reliability and validity are questionable in view of several elements of subjectivity.
- It cannot replace external examinations. It can only supplement them.
- It requires lot of time to undertake several activities related to internal evaluation.

External Evalutation

External examination or assessment is organized and conducted by an external agency, other than the college. The questions mentioned below help to gain insight in conducting external examination.

- Do the examination questions address the aims and objectives of the course?
- Do the questions adequately cover the content and skills identified in the syllabus?
- Are the examination points or weighing allocated appropriately for the content and skills covered? A note should be made of any errors in question stems, distractors, or answer key.
- Are the questions clearly stated, and do they include sufficient background information to enable the student to answer the question fully?
- Do the syllabi, tests and grading fit together consistently.

Advantages
- It avoids subjectivity
- It is more objective
- The results are comparable from institution to institution
- Evaluation becomes more transparent and uniform
- A common certificate can be issued to everyone who takes up the examination.

Limitations/Disadvantages
- Teachers who evaluate may not know what their teachers taught.
- They do not know the background of the student or the performance of the student in general.
- It will focus only on that performance on the basis of which the external examiner may not be able to do complete justification.

Criteria for Selection of Evaluation

Initial Acceptance

Sources of evaluation data must be acceptable to teachers, student and parents. Unacceptable sources should be rejected and not used in evaluation activities. Acceptable sources move to the level of the framework where practicability becomes a concern. Acceptability, therefore, is a necessary, but not sufficient, attribute of any source of evaluation data.

Practicability/Feasibility

At the next level, practicability is of concern. If the gathering of data is enormous and time-consuming, conducting enough measurements to establish stability or reliability will be difficult and perhaps impossible.

Validity cannot exist in the absence of reliability and a method of measurement that has no potential for valid use is worthless. Hence, acceptability and practicability are both necessary, but not sufficient requirements of sources of evaluation data. Factors to be considered in deciding feasibility are time and resources required, availability of an equivalent form of the test for measuring reliability, and ease of administration, scoring and interpretation.

Reliability

Once acceptability and practicability have been established, sources of evaluation data should be able to produce measurements that are, within the limits of measurement error, stable. If the amount of an attribute does change, measurements of the attribute should not change. Measurements should be stable over time and across situations even where a source of evaluation data is being used in an invalid fashion. When the three attributes of acceptability, practicability, and reliability have been established, validity can be investigated.

Reliability refers to the stability or consistency of assessment information and is concerned with the question, "How consistent or typical of the pupil's behavior, is the assessment information, we have gathered?"

Reliability is a measure of reproducibility of the test. In other words, if the same or an equivalent test is given to the students, the scores obtained by individual students and the group as a whole would be similar. Reliability refers to the results of the test, not to the instrument itself. A reliable test does not indicate a valid one since the test can consistently measure something but not necessarily what is intended to be measured.

Measures to improve reliability:
- Increase length of test to optimum level
- Use appropriate levels of difficulty and discrimination to ensure widespread scores
- Maintain conditions of test constant
- Ensure objectivity of scoring
- Ensure validity of the instrument used.

Validity

Validity is the accuracy with which a test measures whatever it is intended to/supposed to measure. Validity is regarded as the absolutely indispensable property of any measuring instrument. Without validity, the instrument has no value. Validity is concerned with the general question: "To what extent will this assessment information help us make an appropriate decision?". It is a matter of degree, and it does not exist on an "all or nothing" basis. It should be considered in terms of categories—highly valid, moderately valid, and invalid.

Types of Validity
- *Content validity:* Does the test measure what was intended to be taught? Content validity is ensured by the following steps:
  - Prepare list of content matter or behavior changes to be tested
  - Assign weightage to above based on relative importance
  - Prepare a table of specifications.
  - Create test according to table of specifications.
- *Criterion validity:* Do students who are taught do better than those not taught? Criterion related validity is a measure of how well the test performance reflects either concurrent performance of the same behavior based on some other measuring instrument, or future performance obtained by another test given at some future time. Comparison of test scores with other scores obtained by other measuring instruments at the same time is called concurrent validity; and

comparison with subsequent scores obtained in future is called predictive validity.
- *Construct validity:* Does the score in the test correlate with presence of other qualities expected to be related to that which is being tested? Construct validity is really a comparison of the test scores with scores obtained by other measuring instruments which measure a related ability which is usually associated with that tested by the current measuring instrument. For example, a test which seeks to measure a student's skill at history taking may be expected to correlate with scores of a test which measures interviewing skill in general.

Factors Influencing Validity

Several factors affect validity. It is necessary for teachers to be aware of these to avoid the pitfalls which can decrease the validity of a test. These factors can be classified into those pertaining to the test itself and others pertaining to the students.

Test Factors
- Unclear directions
- Difficult and ambiguous phrasing of questions
- Poorly constructed items or questions
- Inappropriate level of difficulty
- Inappropriate item or question for the outcome being measured
- Improper arrangement of items (placing all difficult items at the beginning of a test)
- Identifiable pattern of answers, clues
- Too short a test
- Provision of insufficient time
- Adoption of unfair means by students
- Errors in scoring
- Adverse physical or psychological milieu.

Student Factors
- Emotional disturbance
- Lack of motivation.
- Correction of these factors would go a long way in increasing validity.

Objectivity

A test is objective, when the scorer's personal judgment does not affect the scoring. Several measures can be taken to increase objectivity of scoring of conventional examinations such as structuring of questions, preparation of model answers, agreeing on the marking scheme and having papers independently valued by two or more examiners.

Relevance

To what extent the test items conform to the objectives of the measuring instrument.

Specificity

The items in a test should be specific to the objectives.

Length

The number of items in the test should depend upon the objectives of the test.

Comprehensiveness

The total content and objectives have to be kept in mind while preparing items for the test.

Adequacy

A measuring instrument should be adequate by itself.

Precise and clear

Items contained in the test should be clear and precise.

Usefulness

Grading or ranking of the student should be possible with the items of the test.

Equity

Each of the educational objectives should be equally represented in the test. Easy to administer, score and interpret.

Economic

Conduction of the test should be cost efficient.

Steps of Evaluation

Several factors have to be considered in choosing the evaluation tool such as the purpose of evaluation, the domain to be tested, the number of students, feasibility as regards to resources, time and administrative issues, besides ensuring validity and objectivity. Steps of evaluation is shown in Flowchart 4.1.

Evaluation Methods for Different Domain

- **Cognitive domain**
  - *Written*: Essays, short answers, objective items such as supply and selection type, assignments.
  - *Oral*: Questions and higher order questions.
- **Psychomotor domain:** Practicals, OSCE/OSPE
- **Affective domain:** Rating scales, checklists, questionnaires, diary, logbook, group discussion.

Tools and Techniques of Evaluation

Various tools and techniques are used in evaluating the students' performance in clinical areas as well as in

Flowchart 4.1: Steps of evaluation.

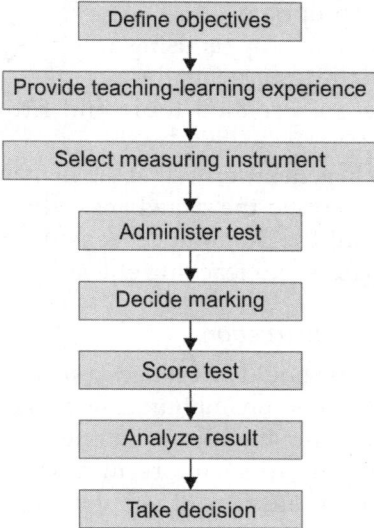

classroom. The choice of the type of examination depends upon the time available; setting in which the examination is conducted; the purpose of evaluation and the feasibility of evaluation.

Essay Examinations

Teacher-made tests are a source of evaluation data widely used in the classroom. Teachers need to have a clear understanding of types of test items, test assembly, test administration, testing practices, its validity and reliability. They are very useful in evaluating the students' progress to report parents and administrators.

Characteristics of Essay Type Evaluation

1. The essay type examination seeks to measure the integrated knowledge of the examinees and reveal certain traits such as originality, imagination, association of ideas, creativity, etc.
2. Essay questions are supply or constructed response type questions and can be the best way to measure the students' higher order thinking skills, such as applying, organizing, synthesizing, integrating, evaluating, or projecting while at the same time providing a measure of writing skills.
3. In this, the students write a response, which may be detailed and lengthy. The accuracy and quality of the response are judged by the teacher. Such questions let the student formulate her own answers and the teacher marks them according to the level it meets the criteria which have been laid down at the time of setting the paper. The degree of subjectivity that is inevitable with this type of questions can be minimized with careful preparation in advance of what is to be tested and by marking as objectively as possible.
4. As Dr Heidgerken remarks, "some of the mental processes which can be exercised and evaluated by means of the essay tests are functional knowledge, the ability to organize summarize, contrast, compare, evaluate and analyze critically".
5. Essay test has a distinct place in the assessment of cognitive skills. They are primarily used to assess higher level learning outcomes such as problem-solving ability or critical thinking which cannot be tested by other methods, or in other words it does not only assess the recall of knowledge and comprehension of information, but also the complex cognitive skills including analysis, synthesis, and evaluation.
6. Essay tests or questions should be aligned with objectives and instruction, like other types of assessments. If the teacher has not taught students what is meant by "compare" and "contrast" during the course of instruction, assessment in which they are called upon to do so in a new situation may be a test of their understanding and interpretation of the terms rather than their ability to demonstrate the higher level skills involved. In other words, instructors should prepare students for essay questions as in Flowchart 4.2.
7. Because of the time needed to answer and score essay questions and the limited amount of content that can be covered in them, essay questions should be used only when other types of questions cannot measure accomplishment of the objective(s).
8. They are particularly appropriate when there is some concern about test security and when the number of students being tested is small.
9. They can be useful when there is little time to prepare the assessment but more time in which to grade it.

Merits of Essay Type Examinations

The essay type examinations are advantageous as:
- They measure complex learning outcomes that cannot be measured by other means.
- They are easy to construct and conduct.

Flowchart 4.2: Types of written tests.

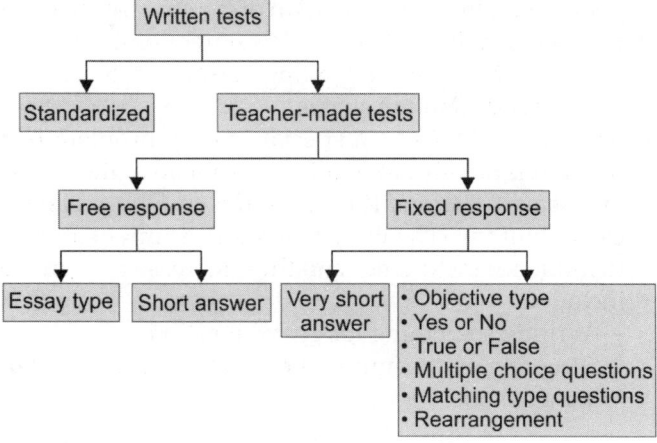

- They test a teacher's efficiency and a student's mental ability, including thinking and problem-solving skills, interpretation of facts, synthesis and analysis, etc.
- They help in organizing ideas and concepts.
- They promote application of knowledge in different spheres.
- They are useful to assess the knowledge of language and writing skills of the student.
- They provide the students sufficient independence in answering without hesitance or binding.
- They allow for free and effective expression.
- They give the students a good opportunity to express their individual ideas and talents, creativity and skills of presentation of a concept.
- It eliminates the possibility of the students' guessing the correct answer.

Demerits of Essay Type Examinations

The most common limitations of essay type examinations are:
- They stress only on intellectual attainment of the students, and do not measure their interests, aptitudes, etc.
- They examine the student in only one section of the curriculum. The composition of essay type examination may not be more appreciable, as factors like handwriting, language, presentation skills, etc. are influencing it and, therefore, lead to an error in interpretation.
- They do not aid in harmonious development of personality.
- A degree of subjectivity is inevitable in these examinations.
- They have limited range of application.
- It offers less feedback to the teacher.
- It takes a long time to score.
- It presents difficulties in obtaining consistent judgment of performance.

It leaves some scope for guess work by the students and the scoring pattern shows halo/an anti-halo effect (the first answer and its assessment influence the subsequent ones).
- Sometimes, the real evaluation of the students may not be possible with such type of examinations.
- There is a risk that the grading of essay responses can be subjective and unreliable.
- Sometimes, bluffing, a special scoring problem may occur. It is possible for students to obtain higher scores on essay questions than they deserve by means of clever bluffing. The ways that students might attempt to influence the teacher and thus, increase their marks include:
  – Writing something for every question.
  – Stressing on the importance of the topic covered by the question.
  – Agreeing with the teacher's views whenever it seems appropriate.
  – Being a name dropper using a famous personality's name in the test frequently.
  – Writing on a related topic and fitting it to the question.
  – Writing in general terms that can fit many situations.

Whatever may be the drawbacks, this method has been and is still the dominant means used to evaluate students' progress and teaching efficiency.

Guidelines for Construction
- The questions should be framed in such a way that the task is clearly and unambiguously defined and can be completed within the stipulated time.
- It is preferable to set more number of questions requiring short answers of about a page or two than a few questions requiring long answers of more than five pages.
- It is preferable not to give too many or too lengthy questions.
- Phrases like "Discuss briefly", "State everything that you know", etc. should be avoided.
- A range of difficulty and complexity should be maintained while setting the questions according to the level of students.
- It is preferable not to give overall choice on the questions (such as answer any 5 questions out of 8) but internal choice between two questions of the similar type can be given. In the previous one, construction of optional questions of equal difficulty is very difficult. The advantage of the second option is that the important questions are not skipped out by the students and comparisons of scores of two students become easy.
- Prepare a marking system acceptable to other examiners by prior discussion with a checklist of specific points against which marks are allotted.
- It is better to use point system of scoring based upon those elements that are expected to appear in the answer.

Sequential Steps in the Construction of Essay Type Test
- Check for the objectives of evaluation clearly.
- The objectives should be representative of entire areas of knowledge expected of students.
- Sampling of objectives must be done as it provides the basis for developing test items.
- Ensure the adequacy of sample.
- Give appropriate weightage to each behavioral domain, e.g.
  – Knowledge   50%
  – Skill   30%
  – Attitude   20%

- It is not possible to cover the entire content of the subject in the test. So sampling of the course content is done.
- Prepare a blueprint for the test.

Writing and Scoring Essay Questions

Essay questions designed to elicit lengthy responses are sometimes referred to as extended response items. Restricted response items, on the other hand, include in the directions, a limitation on the length of the answer (such as "in 75 words or less", "in one paragraph", or "in not more than two pages").

Constructing Essay Type Questions

When deciding whether or not to use essay questions in and when developing the questions, the following guidelines can be considered.
- Determine the level at which thinking is to be assessed (refer to the objectives and instructional methods).
- Keep in mind the reading and writing levels of the students.
- Use essay questions only for outcomes that cannot be measured by other types of questions.
- Two or more questions that are more specific and shorter are preferable to a single longer question.
- Define the task as specifically as possible without giving away the answer(s). From the directions students should be able to tell how the item will be scored (what is expected in the answersheet) and how much weight will be given to essay answers in determining the total test score.
- Provide more than one essay item and let the student select which one to answer if the items may not be of similar difficulty. Good students may select the difficult question but not do as well as they might have on the easier question. Some students may not know which question they can answer best.
- Suggest a (reasonable) time limit or page limit for each essay question.
- Decide in advance what is sought in the answer. Write a model response and/or develop a scoring system that includes the information to be rewarded in the answer.

Scoring of Essay Tests

The basis for scoring should be determined by the teacher prior to the administration of the assessment. Directions to the student should specify if penalties will be assessed for errors in spelling, punctuation, and grammar.

The following suggestions can help increase the validity and reliability of essay questions and the reliability of the scoring.
- The scoring of essay tests can be made more objective by preparing a model answer as a common basis with subdivision of scores for each element; checking the model answer against a sample and revising it, if necessary.
- The scoring for all answers to the same question should be done before proceeding to the next to avoid the carry over or halo effect.
- Review the text and class notes; list the main points to be covered in the essay response.
- Develop a model answer first to determine what is to be expected for.
- Score one essay item at a time for all students to increase consistency in scoring. (Score everyone's answer to essay question 1 before going on to essay question 2).
- Rearrange the order of papers randomly after scoring each item, and attempt to have students' identities hidden from the evaluator, when grading papers.
- If possible (and particularly if the score is important), have another person independently grade the answers to see, if their scores match each other.

Analytic Scoring

For analytic scoring, the score is based on the extent to which predetermined essential components are present. Because it is more structured than holistic scoring, scores are easier to justify because students can determine specifically where they made errors or wrote inadequate or incomplete responses.

In analytic scoring, essential parts of the answer are identified, and then parts are scored individually.

The main component(s) and subcomponents of the desired response are assigned a specific point value. If all are weighed equally, a checklist may suffice. If some components are worth more than others, a form may be needed to show the student the points earned for the various components.

After scoring the papers, there is still a question of how to convert the scores into meaningful information for the students. How many points does it take to earn an "A" or are the points converted to percentages (13 of 13 possible points = 100%).

Global or Holistic Scoring

The response is scored as a whole in comparison with characteristics of answers representative of the preestablished score levels. Holistic scoring tends to be more subjective than analytic scoring.

The first step in holistic scoring is to estimate the number of categories to which papers will be assigned. The characteristics of an answer in each category should be described. (This can be done through a rubric).

Next, the scorer reads a few (5) papers to sample the quality of the responses (and perhaps make adjustments in the scoring system).

All papers are then read and sorted into stacks representing the categories used in grading. (Excellent, good, fair, poor; A, B, C, D, E, etc.).

The papers in each stack are read, moving papers to other stacks if necessary.

Finally, the scores are assigned to the papers.

A Combined Approach

This involves scoring all responses holistically, then rescoring them analytically, focusing on the specific parts.

Improving the Objectivity in Evaluating Essay

Concealing the students' identity, averaging the scores of two examiners, avoiding distractions during scoring and ensuring adequate scoring time also contribute toward improving the objectivity of the essay tests. Objectivity can be further improved by framing short essay questions eliciting restricted response such as comparison of qualities of two similar items, listing of items more than two, or short explanations.

To sum up, it is apparent that essay type questions can be improved. Higher cognitive learning, i.e. ability to analyze, synthesize and solve problems of complex nature, have to be assessed by improving the essay test rather than abandoning the test totally in favor of objective type questions.

Mechanics of Question Paper Setting

Written examination is still the widely used tool of evaluation both in formative and summative evaluation. It cannot be replaced entirely by any other method. The instrument used in the written examination is the question paper.

The steps involved in question paper preparation are:
- Decision on the design of the question paper
- Preparation of a blueprint of the question paper
- Preparation of a model question paper
- Preparation of a marking scheme
- Refining the question paper
- Editing the question paper
- Review of the question paper.

i. **Decision on the design of the question paper:** In general, the design of the question paper will be done at the university level. The curriculum committee of curriculum department will decide on it, and it will follow a fixed format. In an educational institution, for conducting revision tests and other periodical tests, the principal along with other curriculum committee members can decide about the design. Many of the nursing institutions follow the university format in conducting model examinations.

  While deciding on the design of the question paper, the points to be remembered are:
   » Weightage to be given to different forms of questions, i.e. the number of essays, short answer type question, very short answer questions and multiple choice questions should be decided to make a balanced question paper. This also involves the number of question papers per subject, marks, duration and the number of section to be answered and method of answering, etc.
   » Weightage to be given to different learning objectives and to different topics or areas of the subject. If the educational objectives were already divided into must know, and desirable to know and nice to know categories, the same weightage can be adapted in the question paper. The question paper is also designed in such a way that it will find out or test whether the minimum knowledge required have been achieved by the student or not.
   » Guidelines regarding the use of options, nature of sections and difficulty level of the paper are also required to be decided.
   » Once the above decisions are made, it is advisable to write them in clear and simple terms. Such a document will help at a later stage to write the instructions to the question paper setters.

ii. **Preparation of a blueprint of the question paper:** Blueprint of a question paper, also known as table of specification, is a two-dimensional chart giving placement of different questions (in terms of marks and number of questions) in respect of objectives tested by the item(s), content area under which item is framed, and the form of question.

iii. **Preparation of a model question paper:** The model question paper can be written on an item card. It consists of:
   » Objective
   » Content area/Topic
   » Form of question
   » Marks
   » Estimate difficulty level
   » Estimated time
   » Model answer
   » Points of answer
   » Marks for the points

iv. **Preparation of a marking scheme:** Once a model question paper has been prepared, the next step is to evolve a marking scheme. The purpose of marking scheme is to assign proportions of marks to different parts of the answer. There are two types of marking schemes: Analytical (objective type and short answer type) and global (long answer type).

v. **Refining the question papers:** The following questions help the paper-setter to refine the questions:
   » Does the question test an important learning outcome?
   » Is it based on a predetermined objective?
   » Is the scope of the questions well-defined as regards to?
   » Clarity of directions.

- Language of the questions.
- Length of answer.
- Marking scheme.
- Appropriate difficulty level.

A question should be relevant to the set objectives of the course. The questions should not be related to trivial or insignificant, vague and diffuse topics. Questions on a rare phenomenon do not represent higher learning and do not necessarily judge the professional ability of the student.

The question paper should be set in such a way that even the average student should be able to answer, and there should be scope for all intelligent level students to answer the question. The mark allotted to the question should be directly proportionate to the length of the question and the difficulty level of the question.

It is ensured that there is a uniform coverage of the entire curriculum.

Special care should be taken to avoid making grammatical errors or spelling corrections which may cause confusion or even alter the meaning of the question.

The use of abbreviations should be avoided. "Open ended" questions will encourage rambling by a student. So a long answer question also is subdivided in order to make it more objective.

Even for the short answers, the question should be more specific than giving a topic as such, e.g. tuberculosis.

vi. **Editing the question paper:**
- While editing, the following points are to be checked
- Grouping of questions, e.g. all essays together, all short answers together
- Numbering questions
- Instructions for administration.

vii. **Review of the question paper:** The question paper can be reviewed with the following questions. They are:
- Has the paper covered the syllabus without giving undue weightage to a part of particular unit?
- Does the paper test the full range of abilities?
- Does the question paper adhere to the blueprint?
- Is there uniform coverage of the content?
- Whether it gives scope for the students of various abilities?
- Are the questions precise and unambiguous?
- Is there any excessive overlap between the questions?
- Is the time allotted adequate?
- Does the paper avoid the repetition of questions set in the previous years?
- Is there any spelling or grammatical error?
- Is it causing confusion anywhere?

Short Answer Questions

Short answer questions, as the name indicates, are short and direct questions and the students are expected to answer in a word or phrase or a numerical response to the question.

Principles of Constructing SAQs

- Word the item in such a way so that the required answer is both brief and specific.
- Do not take statements directly from the textbooks. Textbook statements are frequently too general and ambiguous to serve as short answer items.
- A direct question is generally more desirable than an incomplete statement.
- If the answer is to be expressed in numerical units, indicate the units in which the answer is to be expressed.
- When completion items are used, do not include too many blanks. Key words are to be omitted and the blank should come at the end of the sentence.
- Arrange spaces for recording answers on the right margin of the question paper.
- Give guidelines for answering each test item very clearly.
- The weightage for each question should be written with the question.

Types of Short Answer Questions

1. **Asking for a definition.**
   Example: How is nursing defined by ANA?
2. **Asking to draw a diagram.**
   Draw the structure of heart and mark the parts.
3. **Asking to complete an incomplete sentence.**
   The nurses' day is celebrated on……………..
4. **Asking for a unique answer to a direct question.**
   Who invented stethoscope?

Uses of SAQs

- Short answer questions are useful to test recall rather than recognition.
- They are used to test knowledge of factual information.
- In subjects where names of structures, substances and symbols have to be learnt, the short answer questions are valuable assessment tools.
- They are easy to evaluate, and reliability and validity are high.

Evaluation of test items should be carried out by a validation panel. The purpose of evaluation is to check the items for validity, reliability, clarity of language, absence of clues, and also to note the difficulty index and discrimination index of the test.

Objective Tests

The objective tests seek to measure more consistently and accurately the knowledge of terms, concepts, vocabulary facts and understanding and measure only what is intended to be measured. They are highly structured and require the student to supply a word or two or to select the correct answer from a number of alternatives. Objective tests are a set of standardized stimuli that elicit samples of behavior.

Types of Objective Type Test Item

Following the Objective type tests questions include the following:
A. Multiple choice items questions/select the best answer
B. True or false items
C. Matching type items
D. Sentence completion items.

Multiple Choice Questions/Select the Best Answer

It is an objective type of test, where student is provided with several alternatives or choices to a given question and asked to select the most appropriate one which is correct. It contains two parts:
1. The base or stem which presents the problem in the form of an incomplete statement or question.
2. The options list of possible/correct answer/ distractors/ alternatives.

The stem may be a statement, question, situation, graph or picture. The suggested answers other than one correct response or choice are called distractors. These incorrect alternatives receive their names from their intended function to distract those students, who are in doubt of the correct answer. The correct answer is the key.

Uses of MCQ

- It is one of the commonly used objective type tests
- It can measure a variety of learning outcomes from simple to complex
- It is adaptable to most types of subject matter content
- They are used for formative and summative assessment as well as for entrance examinations
- It is easier to score
- It makes comparison of the students more objective.

Principles for Preparation of Multiple Choice Questions

- The stem should be meaningful and it should present a definite problem.
- Use positive statements as far as possible. If negative statement is used in the stem, underline it.
- The stem should not be too long but the concept of the question should be completely expressed in it.
- Make the stem simple and brief.
- The item should be relevant.
- The alternatives should be grammatically consistent with the stem of the item.
- The distractors should be as short as possible.
- Make the distractors resemble the correct answer as far as possible.
- Try to avoid the phrases "all the above" or "none of the above", etc.
- The number of distractors should be uniform for all the questions.
- Arrange the distractors in such a way that there is no pattern evident about the correct answer.
- Represent only one concept in a single question.
- An item should contain only one correct answer.
- All distractors should be plausible.
- In a properly constructed MCQ, each distractor will be elected by some pupil. If distractor is not selected by anyone, it would be eliminated or revised.
- Provide a blank space against each item for writing the number of the correct answer.

Other points to remember are:
- The time to be allotted
- The weightage
- Difficulty index of questions.

Advantages of MCQ

- Can test large sample of knowledge in a short period of time
- Easy to score
- Objectivity and reliability in scoring is maintained.

Disadvantages of MCQ

- It does not test the students' ability to write logically and the capability of expression.
- It cannot test motor skills like communication and interpersonal skills.
- It does not give freedom to the students.

Type of MCQ

- One best response
- Multiple true and false
- Multiple completion type
- Relationship analysis type
- Matching

One Best Response

This is one of the most frequently used MCQs. A series of 4–5 choices is preferred to reduce the chances of random guessing. Instructions to the students should be given clearly to choose one right or appropriate response. "None of the above" and "All of the above" should be avoided. It usually tests the recall of facts. The greatest difficulty with this type is to find plausible alternatives. Reduction of five alternatives to four due to inability to find a fifth possible distractor greatly reduces the efficacy of the item since the possibility of getting the correct response by chance increases from 20% to 25%. Use of "All of the above" and "None of the above" does not always obviate the problem. Very often, a candidate, who knows that two of the options are both correct or both wrong automatically led to "All of the above" or "None of the above", respectively even though he knows nothing about the other distractors. Also, if he knows, that one of the alternatives is obviously wrong, he can eliminate that choices also "All of the above" and therefore the question is reduced to 1 in 3 choices.

Unintended grammatical clues play a very important role in this type of MCQ as also the excessive length of the correct response, as opposed to the distractors. Great care must be taken to avoid these errors.

Example
The World Health Day is celebrated every year on:
- 1st April
- 7th April
- 1st May
- 7th May

Multiple Completion Type

This is another common format used and is an improvement on the first type mentioned earlier and requires higher levels of cognition than mere recall of facts. The stem is followed by four completions, one or more of which are correct.

This type of item is useful to test higher levels of cognition. This format is also useful when an examiner can find only 4 plausible distractors instead of 5 for the one best response type of MCQ. Instead of reducing the one best response to one in four or adding a nonfunctional distractor, the same item can be rephrased to fit into the multiple completion type of format. The disadvantage of unequal lengths of alternatives, so important in the first type, is reduced in this format.

Example
Live virus is used in immunization against:
- Influenza
- The common cold
- Cholera
- Smallpox:
  - Responses 1, 2 and 3 are correct.
  - Responses 1 and 3 are correct.
  - Responses 2 and 4 are correct.
  - Response 4 is correct.
  - All four are correct.

Relationship Analysis Type

This type of item is useful to test higher levels of cognition as the candidate has to decide individually whether each statement is correct and then determine their cause-effect relationship. This is, however, becoming less popular due to problem in scoring. Items with correct response of A or B require the candidate to assess individual veracity of each statement and then to determine their relationship to one another, whereas in item with C, D, or E as correct response. He does not have to bother about a cause-effect relationship. A score of unity for all items with correct response of A, B, C, D or E would, therefore, be unfair as items with C, D, or E as the key require less intellectual effort on the part of the students. Besides, in situations where the student knows that either of the statements is false, he is automatically led to choices C, D, and E, the item thus gets reduced to one in three instead of one in five choices. Likewise, if the candidate knows that the first statement is true without knowing anything about the second statement, he is automatically led to choosing A, B or C and can ignore D and E, merely by exclusion.

Example
Cow's milk is preferable to breast milk for infant feeding. Because Cow's milk has a higher content of calcium.
- Both statements are true and causally related.
- Both statements are true but not causally related.
- First statement is true and the second is false.
- First statement is false and the second is true.
- Both statements are false.

Multiple True-false Completion Type

Each of these choices can be individually true or false and are not interdependent. Hence the item can have from nil to five true or false responses. The problems with the ordinary True–False item have been that of 50% probability of guessing which is not the case here.

The merits of this format are:
- The usual restriction of the ordinary multiple choice item in testing superlative situations such as "the best reason for", "the most accepted cause for", etc. which may sometimes call for an opinion, is desirably lifted.
- The restriction of having only one true or one false response is not operative.
- Since no coding is required, the candidates respond easily.
- Elimination of answers due to unlimited clues is less likely.

Some of the demerits of this format are:
- Unless care is exercised, the items formulated may only test recollection.
- The item tends to be a little too short and implicit rather than explicit.
- Each item in this format can score from 0 to 5 marks depending on the number of correct responses. The efficacy of the item in the ranking situation can be increased by giving a credit score to the item only if all five responses are correct. Greater use of this format

would, to some extent, reduce the difficulties inherent with other types of MCQs.

Example

The consequences of Total Parenteral Nutrition in children include:
- Oral aversion   T/F
- Electrolyte imbalance T/F
- Vitamin deficiency   T/F
- Weight loss   T/F
- Water retention   T/F

Matching Type

This type of item consists of a list of three to four parameters on the left hand side and a list of five suggested matches on the right hand side of which only four matches with one item each on the left. The number of choices on the right should be more than the items on the left so that the last item to be matched would still have three options to minimize guessing.

Example

Match the following vitamin deficiency diseases with its vitamin
- Scurvy   • Vitamin B
- Rickets   • Vitamin A
- Night blindness   • Vitamin D
- Beriberi   • Vitamin C
- Vitamin K

Rare types of MCQs such as the pictorial type are also used, but less often than the above five types.

Number of Items

For an MCQ examination to have validity as well as to ensure breadth of sampling, it is necessary to include sufficient number of items. Although there is no agreement on the exact number, probably 60–100 items are optimum for an examination of 60–90 minutes. There is a danger that with lesser numbers, the scores obtained may not indicate the depth of a candidate's knowledge. Using only 25–30 items as part of the written examination is, therefore, unreliable as a method of evaluation.

Time

One aspect that is frequently forgotten is that the time allotted should be sufficient for the candidate to attempt all the MCQ items in an examination as the primary purpose is to test knowledge and not speed of response, which though desirable, is less important. Provision of too much time is an incentive to guess and too little time makes it a test of speed of comprehension of language rather than response based on cognitive acquisition. Different formats require different time duration and this must be kept in mind in formulating the whole question paper. In general, appropriate time required for different items is as follows:
- One best response type   – 40 seconds
- Multiple true/false type   – 45 to 50 seconds
- Relationship analysis type – 50 seconds
- Multiple response type   – 50 seconds
- Case history type   – 60 to 90 seconds

Validating MCQ Question Paper

It is of two types:
1. Prevalidation
2. Postvalidation

Prevalidation: It is the process in which a constructed item is subjected to validation prior to appearing in an examination.

Postvalidation: It is the analysis of the item after it has appeared in a test.

Both steps are important in ensuring that the item is valid.

Prevalidation

First to decide on what educational outcome is sought to be tested by the item and whether an MCQ is the most appropriate tool for that purpose. Then to decide on the type of MCQ which is the most suitable for this purpose, e.g. if the outcome to be tested involves a cause and effect relationship, then the reason assertion type is the most suitable. A multiple response type may be more suitable for items with unequal length distractors. It is most important that having the item discussed in detail by 3 or 4 experts in the subject, who will look into the following aspects:
- Relevance with respect to the learning outcomes.
- Grammar of construction.
- Clarity, brevity and appropriateness of the stem.
- Plausibility of all distractors.
- A decision as to which of the alternative is correct and only one correct response is present.
- An estimate as to the level of cognition being tested by the item and the level of difficulty present.
- Lack of prevalidation because of an obsession with confidentiality leads to inclusion of defective items.

Postvalidation

The process of analysis of an item after it has appeared in an examination is called item analysis.

General Steps of Formulating an MCQ Paper

- Decide on the number of MCQs to be included.
- Select the appropriate number of various formats depending on the learning outcome to be tested.
- Group all similar formats together.

- Check for inclusion of different formats and with varying difficult levels in answering.
- Place some easy items at the beginning of the paper for the psychological support of the student.
- Make sure that all parts of an item are in the same page.
- Time should be adequate depending on the total number of different formats of MCQs. Instructions to the candidates as how to respond to individual items must be clear.

Checklists

The following questions in the checklist help the question paper-setter in improving the validity of the MCQ question.

Item as a whole:
- Is the direction clear?
- Is each item wholly independent of others?
- Are all unrelated details eliminated?
- Does the item test an important learning outcome/important content area?
- Is it specific?
- Is it brief?
- Is the level of difficulty appropriate?
- Is the time adequate?
- Are there clues which suggest the correct answer?
- Are negative statements used with care and appropriately emphasized?
- Is the type of item best for the particular problem?

Stem:
- Is it clear, concise and unambiguous?
- Does it ask for an opinion?
- Is it meaningful?
- Are all common elements placed in the stem?
- Are words like never, always, usually, sometime, etc. used with caution?
- Are double negatives avoided?

Options:
- Are they logical and plausible?
- Are they parallel and homogenous?
- Are options wherever appropriate arranged in numerical order?
- Do all options complete the stem grammatically?
- Are all distractors functional?
- Is care exercised in using all of the above/none of the above as distractors?
- In matching items, as number of responses sufficiently large so that the last of their premises can still have more than one option to choose from?

Key:
- Is it undeniably the only correct response?
- Are letters corresponding to the key equally distributed?
- Is key to an item provided as data in another item?
- Is care taken not to use words in key which are synonyms or very similar to words in the stem?

Item Analysis

Item analysis is the **process of analyzing the performance of a multiple choice item after it has appeared in a question paper**. The main purpose of this exercise is:
- To determine whether the item is of appropriate level of difficulty for the batch of students tested, and
- To determine whether the item is capable of discriminating between the knowledgeable and the poor students.
- To get the feedback on the "functionality" of alternatives to the correct response, since lack of functionality leads to a greater possibility of guessing.

Item analysis is a **measure of three important parameters** of a multiple choice item after it has been administered to a group of students. They are:
- Difficulty index
- Discrimination index
- Functionality

For calculation of these indices, it is necessary to have two groups for comparison such as the high achievers or the knowledgeable students and the low achievers or the ill-informed students. It is easy to divide the students' group into two halves, the top 50% and the bottom 50%. It may also result in problem since in the middle 10–20 percentile, there may be an overlap between their abilities. So it is more convenient to divide into three groups and use the top and the bottom third for comparison.

The essential steps of item analysis:
1. Score the whole test for all the students.
2. Rank the students in order of merit-based on their test scores.
3. Take the bottom third as the low achievers and the top third as the high achievers.
4. Prepare a table for each item as given below
5. Calculate the **difficulty index, discrimination index** and the **distractor effectiveness**.

Options	No. selecting the option against	
	High achievers (H)	Low achievers (L)
A	5	10
B	5	10
C	30	10
D	10	10
E	Nil	2
No response	Nil	8
Total (N)	50	50

In this item, correct response is "C". Based on the values given in the table, the difficulty index, discrimination index and the distractor effectiveness are calculated.

Difficulty Index

The difficulty index, item difficulty or facility value indicated by the symbol "P" is calculated by the

$$p = \frac{H + L}{N} \times 100$$

where
- H = No. of students answering the item correctly in the high achieving group.
- L-Similar number in the low achieving group or the poor student.
- N-Total no. of students in the two groups (including non-responders).

For the given example, the value of 'P' would be 40%. It is clear that the difficulty index value is merely the proportion of total students in the two groups, who have answered the item correctly.

Discrimination Index

It is calculated by the

$$d = \frac{H - L}{N} \times 2$$

where the symbols H, L, N represent the same values as before mentioned. It is a measure of the ability of the item to discriminate between good students and not so good students. For the given example, the value of 'd' would be 0.4.

The Distractor Effectiveness or Functionality

Any of the distractors in the item which has not attracted even 5% of the total response is said to be a nonfunctional distractor. In the item given as example, option number E is nonfunctional having attracted only 2% of students.

Interpretation

In general, items with a facility value (P) of 30–70% are acceptable (between 50% and 60% are ideal). Those with values over 70% are very easy and those with value below 30% are classified as difficult. Likewise items with a discrimination index of 0.25–0.35 are good, those with indices more than 0.35 are excellent and those with an index below 0.2 are poor. These criteria, however, hold true only for summative evaluation or for ranking students. However, discrimination index should never be negative as this indicates a defective item or a wrong key.

Item Difficulty and Item Discrimination

Analyzing Multiple Choice Question Responses

Understanding how to interpret and use information based on student test scores is as important as knowing how to construct a well-designed test. Using feedback from the test to guide and improve instruction is an essential part of the process.

Using statistical information to review the multiple choice test can provide useful information.

Three of these statistics are as follows.

1. **Item difficulty, P:** The percentage of students who correctly answered the item.
   - Also referred to as the P-value.
   - The range is from 0% to 100%, or more typically written as a proportion as 0.0 to 1.00.
   - The higher the value, the easier the item.
   - P-values above 0.90 are very easy items and should not be reused again for subsequent tests. If almost all of the students can get the item correct, it is a concept probably not worth testing.
   - P-values below 0.20 are very difficult items and should be reviewed for possible confusing language, removed from subsequent tests, and/or highlighted for an area for reinstruction. If almost all of the students get the item wrong, there is either a problem with the item or students did not get the concept.
   - Optimum difficulty level is 0.50 for maximum discrimination between high and low achievers.

   To maximize item discrimination, desirable difficulty levels are slightly higher than midway between chance (1.00 divided by the number of choices) and perfect scores (1.00) for the item. Ideal difficulty levels for multiple-choice items in terms of discrimination potential are:

   Ideal Difficulty Levels:
   - Five-response multiple-choice .60
   - Four-response multiple-choice .62
   - Three-response multiple-choice .66
   - True-false (two-response multiple-choice) .75

2. **Item discrimination, R(ID):** The point-biserial relationship between how well students did on the item and their total test score.
   - Also referred to as the point-biserial correlation (PBS)
   - The range is from 0.0 to 1.00.
   - The higher the value, the more discriminating is the item. A highly discriminating item indicates that the students who had high tests scores got the item correct, whereas students who had low test scores got the item incorrect.

   Items with discrimination values near or less than zero should be removed from the test. This indicates that students who overall did poorly on the test did better on that item than students who overall did well. The item may be confusing for better scoring students in some way.

   A guideline for classroom test discrimination values is shown below:
   0.40 or higher, very good items.
   0.30 to 0.39, good items.
   0.20 to 0.29, fairly good items.
   0.19 or less, poor items.

3. **Reliability coefficient (ALPHA):** A measure of the amount of measurement error associated with a test score.
   - The range is from 0.0 to 1.0.
   - The higher the value, the more reliable the overall test score is.
   - Typically, the internal consistency reliability is measured. This indicates how well the items are correlated with one another.
   - High reliability indicates that the items are all measuring the same thing or general construct.
   - Two ways to improve the reliability of the test are to:
     i. Increase the number of questions in the test
     ii. Use items that have high discrimination values in the test.

Reliability Interpretation

- 0.90 and above—Excellent reliability; at the level of the best standardized tests.
- 0.80 to 0.90—Very good for a classroom test.
- 0.70 to 0.80—Good for a classroom test. There are probably a few items which could be improved.
- 0.60 to 0.70—Somewhat low. This test needs to be supplemented by other measures (e.g. more tests) to determine grades. There are probably some items which could be improved.
- 0.50 to 0.60—Suggests need for revision of test, unless it is quite short (ten or fewer items). The test definitely needs to be supplemented by other measures (e.g. more tests) for grading.
- 0.50 or below—Questionable reliability. This test should not contribute heavily to the course grade, and it needs revision.

Distractor Evaluation

Another useful item review technique to use is distractor evaluation.

The distractor should be considered an important part of the item. Nearly 50 years of research shows that there is a relationship between the distractors students choose and total test score. The quality of the distractors influences student performance on a test item. Although the correct answer must be truly correct, it is just as important that the distractors be incorrect. Distractors should appeal to low scorers, who have not mastered the material whereas high scorers should infrequently select the distractors. Reviewing the options can reveal potential errors of judgment and inadequate performance of distractors. These poor distractors can be revised, replaced, or removed.

One way to study responses to distractors is with a frequency table. This table tells you the number and/or percent of students who selected a given distractor.

Distractors that are selected by a few or no students should be removed or replaced. These kinds of distractors are likely to be so implausible to students that hardly anyone selects them.

Points to Remember when Interpreting Item Analysis Results

- Item analysis data are not synonymous with item validity. An external criterion is required to accurately judge the validity of test items. By using the internal criterion of total test score, item analyses reflect internal consistency of items rather than validity.
- The discrimination index is not always a measure of item quality. There is a variety of reasons that an item may have low discriminating power:
  - Extremely difficult or easy items will have low ability to discriminate but such items are often needed to adequately sample course content and objectives.
  - An item may show low discrimination if the test measures many different content areas and cognitive skills. For example, if the majority of the test measures "knowledge of facts", then an item assessing "ability to apply principles" may have a low correlation with total test score, yet both types of items are needed to measure attainment of course objectives.
  - Item analysis data are tentative. Such data are influenced by the type and number of students being tested; instructional procedures employed; and chance errors. If repeated use of items is possible, statistics should be recorded for each administration of each item.

Uses of Item Analysis

Creation of Item banks

The primary use is to create an item bank of tested MCQs with known and consistent levels of difficulty and discriminating power, free of constructional errors and having functional distractors. One can prepare item cards for various subjects and keep it ready. So it can be used for testing students.

Use in Classroom Teaching and for the Teacher

For example, if a particular option is chosen by most of the students which is wrong indicates that the students have not learned the concept very clearly. This gives clue for the teacher to clarify the concept very clearly and correct any misunderstanding. It also gives the feedback to the teacher that all the students have learned the concept correctly if most of them have answered a question correctly.

In the ranking situation, usually items which have a good positive discrimination and moderate difficulty are chosen. In fact, teachers must aim at getting high facility values and low discrimination indices, as the aim of classroom teaching is not to distinguish between good and bad students but to ensure that all students have learnt the lesson correctly.

Although teachers use MCQs frequently to assess overall class performance, the total score of the candidate on the paper rarely gives the teacher a good feedback regarding individual learning difficulties. Item analysis can overcome this problem. This information can be used to improve teaching methods or resort to alternate methods, introduce audio-visual aids or use them more effectively or determine areas requiring emphasis and reinforcement. Item analysis also pinpoints the questions on which good students are confused and which students did not attempt. Teachers consequently can examine the amount of time allocated to those areas and/or clarity of teaching.

Frequent resort to administration of objective tests and performance of an item analysis as a routine procedure help tremendously to achieve better teaching, better learning and in the long-term better tests.

Though it requires a constant and consistent effort of the teachers, it helps them to learn a great deal more about their teaching and also to improve their MCQ items.

True or False Items

These are questions or statements followed by Yes/No or True/False responses. The student is asked to tick or mark the correct response. Here, the students are expected to accept or reject the statements by selecting these responses. These are easy to prepare, takes comparatively much less time than the other items.

They are used to test the misconceptions, beliefs and attitudes.

Principles of Preparation of True or False Items

- Only a single concept or idea should be represented in a statement.
- Write clear and direct statements. Avoid ambiguous statements.
- Avoid using clues like "usually", "sometimes", "none", and "nothing", "no", "should", "always", "may", etc.
- Avoid tricky and catchy items.
- Have equal number of true and false items.
- Determine the order of true and false by chance.
- Detectable pattern of answers should be avoided (T, F, T, F).
- If evaluation is to be addressed to the affective domain, the terms agree-disagree are used.
- The statement should not be taken directly from the textbook.
- The direction for answering the question must be clear.
- Avoid using negative statement. When it is used, underline the negative words.

Matching Items

The matching type items are prepared in two columns—one called as the stimulus column and the other one called as the response column. The student has to go through the stimulus column and match it with a correct response from the other side. These items are much easier to construct and evaluate.

Principles for Preparation of Matching Items

- The statements in the whole set of matching items should belong to the same kind or nature.
- The number of choices should be more than the required answers.
- Too many items may be confusing and distracting. Hence, the number of items should be limited to about 10.
- The stimuli and response columns should be on the same page.
- A single response should not be used for more than one stimulus.
- The terminology in one column should not give clues to the expected responses in the other column.
- Provide clear directions for matching.
- Arrange responses or both in alphabetical order, usually prevents clues to the responses. If the responses are in numerical quantities, arrange them in order from low to high.
- Use the longer phrases as stimulus and shorter as responses.
- Choose homogenous premises and responses for any matching cluster.

Merits of Objective Type Examinations

- Objective tests are reliable, valid, objective and practicable.
- They are "fool proof" and lead to a very detailed and minute diagnosis.
- The questions are precise, brief and clear.
- They cover a large area of study subjects.
- They help to test a large number of students.
- They are economical in terms of time and the effort to score the item.
- They are helpful for students, who have difficulties in written communication.
- They help in evoking each mental activity separately.

Demerits of Objective Type Examinations

- They take a lot of time and effort in preparing the test.
- They provide little or no opportunity for measurement of students' ability to organize and express thoughts.
- They do not measure the complex mental abilities of the students.

- Most of the time, the student do not use the reasoning skills to answer the questions, but resort to guessing.

Observation

Observation is the assessment method used most frequently in clinical performance evaluation. Performance appraisal of the students is done to compare the clinical competency expectations as designated in course objectives. Faculty analyzes the performance, provide feedback on the observation and determine whether further instruction is needed.

Observation can be defined as the direct visualization of performance of a talk or behavior. It involves watching students carry out some activity or listening to pupils' speech, reading, and discussing things.

The process of observing and recording an individual's behavior is called as "observational technique". It is useful for evaluation of clinical performance, skill competence, and development of attitudes and values. Observation allows for immediate feedback and opportunity for remediation.

On the basis of evidence drawn from observation of behavior, and listening to oral contribution, the teacher will draw inferences about a student's attitudes, personal qualities, abilities, motivation and commitment, learning speed and style, intelligence, attainments and progress. These inferences in turn will help the teachers to make certain judgments and decisions about students.

Observation may be planned or unplanned.

Principles of Observational Method

The following principles will make the observational method more objective:
- Observe the whole situation
- Select one student to observe at a time
- Students should be observed in the regular activities such as in the classroom, and in the clinical area
- As far as possible, observation from several teachers should be combined
- The observer must have an objective tool that can be used to collect information accurately and without bias, to obtain accurate results.

Types of Observational Method

Based on the fact, whether the observer makes his intention known to the persons observed or not, the observation method is classified into:
- Concealed observation
- Non-concealed observation.

Based upon the role of the observer, it is classified into:
- *Participant observation*: The observer is a part of the social setting, where the observation process takes place.
- *Nonparticipant observation*: The observer makes the observation from periphery of a social setting, he is not part of it.

Merits of Observational Technique

- It is more reliable and objective as it is being a record of actual behavior of the student.
- The information collected will be first-hand information that increases its reliability.
- It is the assessment of the individual in a natural situation and therefore, it is useful than the restricted study in a test situation.
- It can be employed to all categories of students, in all contexts.
- The technique does not require any special training or equipment for its conduction. Hence all teachers can use it in all situations.
- It allows for immediate feedback and opportunity for remediation.
- It is adaptable to both individuals and groups.
- Frequent observation of a student's behavior can provide a continuous check on his progress.
- Observational data provide teachers with valuable supplementary information.

Demerits of Observational Technique

- The observational process is more complex and numerous factors are influencing in interpretation of evaluating the data.
  - Lack of specificity of the particular behavior to be observed.
  - An inadequate sampling of behavior from which to draw conclusions about a student's performance.
- There is a great scope for personal prejudices and bias of the observer.
- Observer may not record with 100% accuracy.
- It is very difficult to observe everything that a student does or says.
- It reveals overt behavior only, behavior that is expressed and not that is within.
- Direct observation, is an inherently subjective technique, and only to the extent of subjectivity of direct observation is reduced, can the reliability and validity of evaluation be increased.
- The student, knowing he or she is being observed, will often inadvertently distort accuracy of data collected because of anxiety.
- In addition, distortion of one problem observed can affect results of future observed outcomes.
- If there are no objective criteria for observation, observations become biased, opinions that may skew results.

If the student is aware of objective criteria before evaluation, he or she has a clear understanding of expected behavior. Prior preparation will decrease anxiety among students, enabling a fair assessment. Faculty may provide a list of skills to be observed and the criteria for competence to the student. The student has a responsibility to prepare for the observation according to the criteria specified. This will give the student a sense of control over his or her educational experience and evaluation, hence decreasing anxiety.

Common methods of documenting the observed behaviors during clinical practice include:
- Unstructured, e.g. logs and field notes, and anecdotal records.
- Structured, e.g. checklists and rating scales.

Unstructured Techniques

Logs are record of events and conversations and usually are maintained on a daily basis by field worker.

Field notes may include daily log but tend to be much broader, more analytic and include more interpretation than mere listing of occurrences.

Sociometry

Definition and Meaning

The word sociometry comes from the Latin "socius," meaning social and the Latin "metrum," meaning measure. As these roots imply, sociometry is a way of measuring the degree of relatedness among people. Measurement of relatedness can be useful not only in the assessment of behavior within groups, but also for interventions to bring about positive change and for determining the extent of change. For a work group, sociometry can be a powerful tool for reducing conflict and improving communication because it allows the group to see itself objectively and to analyze its own dynamics. It is also a powerful tool for assessing dynamics and development in groups devoted to therapy or training.

> Jacob Levy Moreno coined the term sociometry and conducted the first long-range sociometric study from 1932 to 1938 at the New York State Training School for Girls in Hudson, New York.

Sociometry is defined as a methodology for tracking the energy vectors of interpersonal relationships in a group. It shows the patterns of how individuals associate with each other when acting as a group toward a specified end or goal. Moreno himself defined sociometry as "the mathematical study of psychological properties of populations, the experimental technique, of and the results obtained by application of quantitative methods".

Sociometry is based on the fact that people make choices in interpersonal relationships. Whenever, people gather, they make choices—where to sit or stand; choices about who is perceived as friendly and who not; who is central to the group; who is rejected; who is isolated. Moreno says, "Choices are fundamental facts in all ongoing human relations, choices of people and choices of things".

Sociometric Criteria

Choices are always made on some basis or criterion. The criterion may be subjective, such as an intuitive feeling of liking or disliking a person on first impression. The criterion may be more objective and conscious, such as knowing that a person does or does not have certain skills needed for the group task.

When members of a group are asked to choose others in the group based on specific criteria, everyone in the group can make choices and describe why the choices were made. From these choices, a description emerges of the networks inside the group. A drawing, like a map, of those networks is called a sociogram. The data for the sociogram may also be displayed as a table or matrix of each person's choices. Such a table is called a sociomatrix. A simple example of applied sociometry is to have group members make a selection on the basis of a simple, nonthreatening criterion. Ask everyone in the group to stand up and then say: "Whom in this group would you choose to take orders to buy snacks from everyone in this room; go to the bakery; and come back with the right snacks and the right change? Show your choice by placing your right hand on the shoulder of the person you choose.

Move about the room as you need to in order to make your choice. There are only two requirements:
1. You may choose only one person.
2. You must choose someone.

Typically the group members will make their choices after only a little hesitation.

This exercise may be repeated several times in the period of just a few minutes using different criteria each time. The exercise graphically illustrates not only the social reality of choice-making, but also the fact that different criteria evoke different patterns of choices.

Regardless of the criterion, the person who receives the most hands on his or her shoulder is what is known as the sociometric star for that specific criterion. Other sociometric relationships which may be observed are mutuals, where two people choose each other; chains, where person A chooses person B who chooses person C who chooses person D and so on; and gaps or cleavages when clusters of people have chosen each other but no one in any cluster has chosen anyone in any other cluster.

Here are some other sample criteria that could be used for this exercise. Whom in this room would you choose…
- To generate creative ideas?
- For support in taking risks?
- To relay messages accurately?
- To run a business for profit?
- To keep a confidence?

This "hands-on" exercise can be very helpful for teaching a group about sociometry and about the reality of the informal organization.

A More Complex Example

Suppose we want to know how much interpersonal trust exists within a small group of six members. Let's call the group members Ann, Kala, Clara, Deena, Edna, and Sheeba. For the purposes of this example, we will use the following criterion: "I trust this person to keep oral agreements and commitments, and not to undercut me or go behind my back." We will use the symbols "+" to indicate "High Trust", "O" to indicate "Moderate Trust" and "–" to indicate "Distrust/Conflict".

Next we interview each group member individually. When we have established rapport, and have explained that all responses will be kept confidential, we ask the person we are interviewing to rate every other person in the group, based on the criterion.

Say, we are interviewing Ann. Ann rates the others as follows:

- Kala   +
- Clara   –
- Deena   O
- Edna   +
- Sheeba   O

This means that Ann has high trust on Kala and Edna; distrusts or is in conflict with Clara; has moderate trust on Deena, Sheeba and so on.

In the course of the interviews, we can elicit details about all of these relationships. We can ask Ann, for example, why she distrusts Clara, and Ann's ideas about what Clara could do to improve the situation. After conducting all the interviews and obtaining ratings from everyone, the next step is to chart all the responses in the sociomatrix.

Here is the sociomatrix for our sample group:

	Ann	Kala	Clara	Deena	Edna	Sheeba
Ann		+	–	O	+	O
Kala	O		–	+	+	O
Clara	–	O		+	+	+
Deena	O	+	–		O	O
Edna	+	+	O	+		O
Sheeba	+	+	O	O	+	

We can see that Ann's choices have been charted in Ann's row: Ann's High Trust (+) rating of Kala is in the cell where Ann's row intersects Kala's column, her Distrust/Conflict (–) rating of Clara is in the cell where Ann's row intersects Clara's column, etc.

This matrix already tells us a great deal about the group dynamics. With a little analysis, the matrix becomes something like an X-ray or CAT scan of the group's interpersonal relationships. Columns showing a large percentage of +'s can identify the informal leader(s) of the group. Columns showing -'s can identify those people the group may be close to rejecting. Rows showing all O's or all +'s may highlight people who fear self-disclosure or people, who are undifferentiated in social relationships.

Another important pattern to look for is what is called mutuals. A mutual occurs when I rate you at the same level you rate me. A positive mutual is when we both rate each other +; a negative mutual is when we both rate each other. Positive mutuals show bonding in a group. Negative mutuals show areas of conflict. The identification of negative mutuals gives the consultant or therapist insight as to where to start to repair a dysfunctional group.

Here are the column totals, and mutuals for our sample group:

	Ann	Kala	Clara	Deena	Edna	Sheeba
Total +	2	4	0	3	4	1
Total O	2	1	2	2	1	4
Total –	1	0	3	0	0	0
Total choices received	5	5	5	5	5	5
Not chosen by	0	0	0	0	0	0
Mutuals +	1	2	0	1	2	0
Mutuals O	1	0	0	2	0	1
Mutuals –	1	0	1	0	0	0

We can see that the informal leaders are Kala and Edna because they both received the most +'s and received less 'O's. A closer look at the sociomatrix shows that Ann and Clara have mutual Distrust/Conflict.

If these were a work group and we were asked to improve the functioning of this group, we could start by improving the relationship between Ann and Clara before bringing the group together for team building.

Constructing a sociomatrix for a small group like this one is a simple task, but when the number of people in the group is more than about five or six, the clerical work and calculations become quite tedious and open to error. With a large matrix, the identification of mutuals begins to resemble a migraine headache. Fortunately there are computers. Software exists to automate all the tedious calculations involved in creating a sociomatrix of up to 60 people. The software produces not only the sociomatrix itself but also several useful group and individual reports.

Criterion Selection

The selection of the appropriate criterion makes or breaks the sociometric intervention. As in all data-collection in the social sciences, the answers we get depend on the questions we ask. Any question will elicit information but unless the right question is asked, the information may be confusing or distracting or irrelevant to the intervention's objective.

A good criterion should present a meaningful choice to the person in as simple a format as possible.

The criterion must be like a surgeon's knife: most effective when it clearly isolates the material of interest. In responding to the question, each person will choose based on an individual interpretation of the criterion. These interpretations, or subcriteria, for this particular question could include: do I want a person who works hard, who is amiable, who is helping, etc. A clear statement of the criterion will tend to reduce the number of interpretations and will, therefore, increase the reliability of the data.

Some Principles of Criterion Selection

- The criterion should be as simple as stated and as straightforward as possible.
- The respondents should have some actual experience in reference to the criterion; whether ex post facto or present otherwise the questions will not arouse any significant response.
- The criterion should be specific rather than general or vague. Vaguely defined criteria evoke vague responses. (Note for example that "friendship" is actually a cluster of criteria).
- When possible, the criterion should be actual rather than hypothetical.
- A criterion is more powerful, if it is one that has a potential for being acted upon. For example, for incoming college freshmen the question "Whom would you choose as a roommate for the year?" has more potential of being acted upon than the question "Whom do you trust?"
- Moreno points out that the ideal criterion is one that helps further the life-goal of the subject. "If the test procedure is identical with a life-goal of the subject he can never feel himself to have been victimized or abused. Yet the same series of acts performed of the subject's own volition may be a "test" in the mind of the tester (Moreno). Helping a college freshman select an appropriate roommate is an example of a sociometric test that is in accord with the life-goal of the subject.

As a general rule, questions should be future oriented; imply how the results are to be used; and specify the boundaries of the group (Hale, 1985). And last, but not least, the criteria should be designed to keep the level of risk for the group appropriate to the group's cohesion and stage of development.

Examples of Criteria for Use in a Work Setting

A. I trust this person to:
- Keep oral agreements and commitments
- Work for win-win solutions
- Not to undercut me or go behind my back.
+ = High Trust
O = Moderate Trust
− = Distrust/Conflict

B. Based on ability to work effectively as a team member, whom would you choose to work with you on an important team project?
+ = I definitely would want to have this person in my team.
O = I would not mind having this person in my team.
− = I definitely would not want to have this person in my team.

C. Consider each of your coworkers listed below and rate them as to how much or little you trust each of them.
+ = High Trust
O = Moderate Trust
− = Distrust/Conflict
Note: Example C is an example of what Moreno called "near-sociometric" because the criterion is somewhat vague. You "trust" your coworkers to do or not do what? Keep secrets? Perform procedure on me? Example A is more, specific.

D. Consider each of your coworkers listed below. What is your level of trust to share your feelings with each of them about issues at the workplace?
+ = High Trust
O = Moderate Trust
− = Distrust/Conflict

Examples of Criteria used in other Settings

If you had left to go home what person (or persons) would you want to invite to your home and what person (or persons) would you not want to invite to your home?

Steps in Sociometric Intervention

The typical process for a sociometric intervention in an organization follows these basic steps:
- Identify the group to be studied
- Develop the criterion
- Establish rapport/warm-up
- Gather sociometric data
- Analyze and interpret data
- Feedback data, either:
  - To individuals, prior to group meeting
  - In a group setting
- Develop and implement action plans
- Post-test (optional).

Application of Sociogram among Students

A sociogram is a device that is used to provide additional information regarding a student and how he/she interacts with peers. It is a valuable tool for determining how a student is viewed by his/her classmates. Students respond to a teacher-provided direction such as "List the two classmates with whom you would most like to sit"; "Write the name of the person with whom you would enjoy working on a project"; "If you were going on a vacation, which of your classmates would be nice to have along, and why?"

We might also assess interaction and social perceptions using negatively worded statements or questions such as "Who would you not want to play with during recess?"

The results are then tabulated to determine how many times each student was chosen and by whom. This information is graphically plotted to identify social isolates, popular students, disliked youngsters, and changes in interaction patterns over time. The sociogram can be useful in a number of ways. Allowing a student to work with a chosen peer may be a motivational tool. Social isolates (those not selected by others) could be placed in interaction situations with accepting peers or could be made the center of attention in positions such as leader or team captain. Those, who are negatively perceived by others, could be provided training in social skills. Additionally, interaction and friendship changes, and a student's progress in becoming more acceptable to others can be monitored via frequent administration of the sociogram technique. Caution and professionalism are vital when using this technique because of the possibility of harming the youngster's self-esteem.

How to Use Sociograms

- Devise a question. State it in simple, easy-to-understand language. Words of the question to be consistent with the information you desire to obtain (e.g. who to assign as field trip partners; who is unpopular and in need of social skills instruction).
- Have students write their answers to the question or statement. Allow and encourage the students to make their choices privately. Clearly explain any limitations on choices (e.g. number of choices, classmates only).
- On a listing of the names of the students, write next to each student's name the number of times he/she was selected by another (tally the responses).
- Make a large diagram of concentric rings so that it looks like an archery target. Have one more ring than the greatest number of times any student was chosen. Start outside the last ring and number the spaces from the outside toward the inside starting with "zero".
- Write each student's name inside the ring space corresponding to the number of times he/she was chosen.
- Draw arrows from each student to the student selected by them.
- Survey the diagram to assess popularity and interaction preferences. This information should remain confidential.

Anecdotal Records

Anecdotal or progress notes are objective written descriptions of observed student performance or behavior. They are the factual description of the meaningful incidents and events that the teacher has observed while dealing with the students. It is also used for describing a nurse's experience with a person or group especially in the clinical setting. Each incident should be written down shortly after it happens.

Anecdotal records can be defined as a brief description of an observed behavior that appears significant for evaluation purposes. It is a factual record of an observation of a single specific, significant incident of the behavior of a student.

Anecdotal records are objective descriptions of behavior recorded on plain paper or a form. The notation should include who was observed, by whom, when and where. The notation comprises a description of the setting or background and the incident and interpretation and recommendations may be included. Value-laden words such as good and bad should be avoided.

The format for these can vary from loosely structured "plus/minus" observation notes to structured lists of observations in relation to specified clinical objectives. They may be recorded on separate cards or as running accounts, one for each student, on separate pages of a notebook.

A good anecdotal record keeps the objective description of an incident separate from any interpretation of the behavior's meaning. These written notes initially serve as part of formative evaluation. As student performance records are documented over time, a pattern is established.

Characteristics of Anecdotal Records

- It is a factual recording only of the actual event, incident or observation, uncolored by the feelings, interpretations or biases of the observer.
- It is a record of only one incident.
- It is a record of an incident which is considered important and significant in the growth and development of the student.
- It should include:
  - a description of a particular occasion
  - a delineation of the behavior noted, indicating who, what, why, when, where and how
  - the evaluator's opinion or estimate of the incident or behavior.

Advantages of Anecdotal Records

- Anecdotal records can be maintained in those areas of behavior that cannot be evaluated by other, more rigorous systematic methods.
- It is useful in supplementing and validating observations made by other means.

- It can be used by students for self-appraisal and peer assessment.
- It is easy to develop and highly economical. It does not require any mechanical resources or equipment.
- It can be used for providing formative feedback.
- It provides insight into the behavior of the students.
- Frequent and brief observations make it possible to discover trends of behavior over a period of time.

Disadvantages of Anecdotal Records

- It is a highly subjective measure to assess the behavior of the students.
- There is a total lack of standardization.
- It is quite difficult to score the recordings.
- It is time consuming and has very limited applications.
- Interpretation of the recordings is very difficult and differs from one person to another person, thereby making evaluation difficult.

Effective use of anecdotal records could be made by:
- Determine in advance the behavior to be assessed and limit observations to those categories or qualities.
- Record enough of the situations to decrease subjectivity. Record the incident as soon as possible after its occurrence.
- Minimum time gap to record is necessary to avoid too much dependence on memory. This will increase its objectivity, validity and reliability.
- Limit each anecdote to a brief description of a single specific incident.
- Record both positive and negative incidents and consider both while making inferences.
- Relate anecdotal records directly to the clinical objectives.

For maximum clarity, an anecdotal notation should include:
- A description of the particular occasion.
- A delineation of the behavior noted, indicating who, what, why, when, where, and how.
- The evaluator's opinion or estimate of the incident or behavior.

Basic Elements of Anecdotal Records

- Students name, class and section
- Date of observation
- Name of observer
- Setting or background of the information
- Incident
- Signature of the observer
- Interpretation of behavior and recommendations concerning behavior.

Critical Incident Records

The critical incident technique is a method for collecting purely factual information. A critical incident is any important observable bit of human behavior sufficiently complete in itself to permit inferences to be made about the person performing the act. It differs from the anecdotal record in that no evaluative or judgmental statements are made. The evaluator records specific critical incidents of effective and ineffective behaviors. There are two sides or aspects of a performance record when this method is used—one for recording effective performance and the other for ineffective performance. The incidents present only the facts of the performance.

> Psychologists John Flanagan first introduced use of critical incident during World War II while attempting to evaluate men in the armed forces.

Effective behaviors include positive behaviors which especially contribute to patient care service, i.e. completion of an assignment or achievement of an objective and maintenance of quality in nursing care of patients.

Ineffective behaviors are negative behaviors which interfere with good nursing care or lead to poor nursing care.

Criteria for Using Critical Incidents

- The actual behavior must be reported rather than general traits.
- The behavior must be actually observed by the reporter.
- All relevant factors in the incident must be given.
- The observer must make a definite judgment about the behavior that is considered to be critical.

A collection of critical incidents is made on the basis of day-to-day observation of nurses in providing nursing care, as soon as possible after they occur. The following procedure may help in keeping records of critical incidents that are relevant and useful:
- Determine whether the incident observed was critical.
- Decide if the behavior was effective or ineffective.
- Relate the behavior noted to a specific standard and objective for the performance of the activity surveyed.
- Record the incident indicating the date, time and a brief description of the incident. Use as few words as possible.

Recording of Critical Incident

- The student's performance can have two parts.
- Number of incidents, effective and ineffective can be summarized.
- The period of observation can be mentioned in the form.
- Signature of the evaluator, signature of the person who is being observed and evaluated, and comments should be included.

Structured Techniques

Checklists

Checklists are lists of items or performance indicators requiring dichotomous responses such as satisfactory or unsatisfactory, pass or fail, yes or no, present or absent, etc.

Gronlund (2005) describes a checklist as an inventory of measurable performance dimension of products with a place to record a simple yes or no judgment.

A checklist is a grouping of items by which something may be confirmed or verified. It can be called as a behavioral inventory. It is basically a method of recording whether a particular attribute is present or absent or whether an action had or had not taken place. It consists of a listing of steps, activities or behavior which the observer records when an incident occurs. The educational and instructional objectives should be kept in mind when preparing and using a checklist.

Construction of Checklists

While constructing or preparing checklists following points to be kept in mind:
- Express each item in clear, simple language
- Avoid lifting statements verbatim from the text
- Avoid negative statements wherever possible
- Review the items independently.

Utilization of Checklists

- Use checklist only when one is interested in ascertaining whether a particular trait or characteristics is present or absent.
- Use only carefully prepared checklist for more complex kind of trait.
- Observe only one student at a time and confine one's observation to the points specified in the checklists.
- Have separate checklists for each student.
- The observer must be trained, how to observe, what to observe and how to record the observed behavior. To make a valid judgment he should omit recording those behaviors for which he has insufficient information.
- Checklists require the observer to judge whether certain behavior of a student and clinical practice has taken place. They can be used most effectively when components of clinical performance can be specified. It is possible for the observer to simply note whether the prescribed behavior has taken place or not. The actual physical, psychomotor skills involved can be jointly, precisely stated.

Merits of Checklists

- Short and easy to assess and record.
- Useful for evaluation of specific, well-defined behaviors and are commonly used in the clinical simulated laboratory setting.
- They can be used for both process and procedure evaluation.
- They are adaptable to most subject matter areas.
- They allow inter individual comparisons to be made on a common set of traits or characteristics.

The checking process implies that standards and criteria are available for gauging items. The inspection procedure requires scrutiny of behavior under investigation. Checklists are most useful for determining the status of tangible items, such as inventory and maintenance of equipment and supplies. They have the advantage that items to be observed can be determined in advance and will be the same criteria used in each situation. But there is no guarantee however, that the observed behavior is a persistent one and that the procedure will provide a representative picture of the individual being evaluated.

It is recommended that only significant behaviors essential for a successful performance be included on the checklist.

Limitations

It does not indicate the quality of performance. Only a limited component can be assessed.

Rating Scale

Rating means the judgment of one person by another. A rating scale is a method by which we systematize the expression of opinion concerning a trait. Rating scale is a common evaluation tool used in describing observed skills and performance. More than noting the presence or absence of a behavior, the rating scales locate the behavior to a point on a continuum and also involve judgments regarding quantitative and qualitative abilities. In simple words, it consists of a set of characteristics or qualities to be judged and a scale for indicating the degree up to which the particular attribute is present.

A rating scale can be defined as "a standardized method of recording interpretation of behavior, which is totally based on observation, strictly in line with the educational objectives".

A rating scale is a device used to evaluate situations or characteristics that can occur or be present in varying degrees, rather than merely be present or absent as in the instrument so designed as to facilitate appraisal of a number of traits or characteristics by reference to a common quantitative scale of values.

Rating scales resemble checklists but are used when finer discriminations are required. Instead of merely indicating the presence or absence of a trait or characteristic, it enables us to indicate the degree to which a trait is present. Rating scale provides systematic procedure for obtaining, recording and reporting the observer's judgment that may be filled out while the observation is made, immediately after the observation is made or as often in the case, long after the observation.

Rating scales consist of a set of characteristics or qualities to be judged and some type of scale for indicating the degree to which an attribute is present.

Types of Rating Scales

Various types of rating scales that are commonly used are:
- Descriptive rating scales
- Graphic rating scales
- Numerical rating scales
- Behaviorally anchored rating scales.

Descriptive Rating Scales

These types of rating scales use descriptive phrases to identify the points on a graphic scale. The descriptions are brief details that convey in behavioral terms for each trait (how pupils behave at different steps along the scale). The rater selects the one most applicable to the person. A space for comment is also frequently provided to enable the rater to clarify the rating or to record behavioral incidents pertinent to the rating. For example,

Observation of working hours		
usually late	sometimes late	usually on time
Completion of work assignments		
usually late	sometimes late	usually on time

The descriptions may take the form of:
- Abstract labels—such as A, B, C, D, and E
- Frequency labels—such as always, usually, frequently, sometimes, never.
- Qualitative labels—superior, above average, average, below average.

Graphic Rating Scales

The rater indicates the performer's standing in respect to each trait by placing a check mark at an appropriate point along the line. In this, each line is followed by a horizontal line. The rating is made by placing a tick on the line. A set of categories identify specific positions along the line, but the rater can also click between these points. Here the degree of each character is arranged so that the rater can make as fine distinctions as he wishes to make. Graphic rating scale in Figure 4.2.

Numerical Rating Scales

In this, the extent or degree to which a particular attribute is present in an individual is indicated by numbers. The observer puts a tick or circle on the number to which the student possess that attribute. Each number is given a verbal description that remains constant for a particular character. It includes numbers against which a list of behaviors is evaluated. This is not a very reliable tool because of the inconsistent value attributed to the number. It can be partially overcome by adding a few quantitative terms. For example,

Ability to get along with others	1	2	3	4	5
Punctuality	1	2	3	4	5
Clinical performance	1	2	3	4	5
Communication skill	1	2	3	4	5

1 = Never, 2 = Sometimes, 3 = About half the time, 4 = Usually, 5 = Always, Or

5 = Outstanding
4 = Above average
3 = Average
2 = Below average
1 = Dissatisfactory

The numerical rating scale is useful when the characteristics or qualities to be rated can be classified in to a limited number of categories and when there is a general agreement concerning the category represented by each number.

Behaviorally Anchored Rating Scales

BARS is an acronym for Behaviorally Anchored Rating Scales, sometimes known as BES, Behavioral

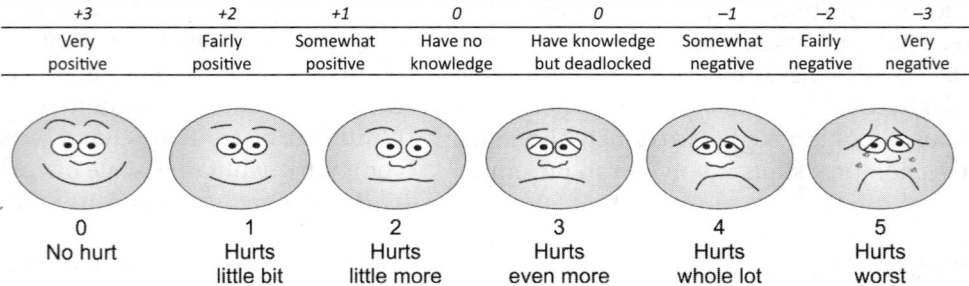

Fig. 4.2: Graphic rating scale.

Expectation Scales. BARS evaluates behavior relevant to specific demands of the job and provides examples of specific job behaviors corresponding to good, average, and poor performances. This reduces the amount of personal judgment needed by the rater. Separate BARS are needed for each job. BOS is an acronym for Behavioral Observation Scales. This system capitalizes on some of the strengths of BARS while avoiding some of the disadvantages. The evaluator lists a number of critical incidents for each performance dimension and rates the extent to which the behavior has been observed on a five point scale ranging from almost never to almost always.

| Punctual | Almost never | 1 | 2 | 3 | 4 | 5 | Almost always |
| Gets along | Almost never | 1 | 2 | 3 | 4 | 5 | Almost always well with others |

Principles in Preparing Rating Scales

- Rating scales should directly relate to learning objectives.
- They need to be confined to performance areas that can be observed.
- Three to seven rating positions may need to be provided.
- The scale may be made more objective, valid and reliable by getting a pooled rating from more than one observer.
- All raters should be oriented to the specific scale as well as the process of rating in general.
- As errors are common due to subjective judgment made by the observer, rater should be conscious enough to avoid them.
- A rating scale provides the instructor with a convenient form on which to record judgments indicating the degree of students' performance. This differs from a checklist; in that it allows for more discrimination in judging behaviors as compared with dichotomous 'Yes' or 'No' options.

Advantages of Rating Scales

- Rating scales are easy to administer and score.
- They can be used for large number of students.
- They have a wide range of application.
- They give a clear feedback to the students.
- They are used to evaluate skills, product outcomes, activities, interests, attitudes and personal characteristics.
- It is used to observe and record qualitative and quantitative judgments about observed performance.
- They tend to be adaptable and flexible.
- They are efficient and economical in the use of time.
- They can help to reduce the subjectivity and unreliability that are usually associated with the observation method.
- It will direct observation toward specific aspects of behavior.
- It will provide a common frame of reference for comparing all pupils on the same set of characteristics.
- It will provide a convenient method for recording the observer's judgments.

Disadvantages of Rating Scales

However, be careful, a degree of subjectivity is inevitable while using the rating scales.

Practical Examinations

The practical examinations are meant to assess the professional competence gained by the students over a period of time and whether it meets the requirements and expectations specified by the statutory boards. Completing the program successfully does not mean the students' mastery of the subject matter alone but also competency in actual practice and developing clinical efficiency.

Purposes of Practical Examinations

The central purpose of the practical examination is to assess the clinical competence of the students and to confirm whether it is in par with the stipulated criteria. The student has to get a pass mark in the practical examinations along with the written examinations for the completion of the program. The practical examinations are useful in assessing.

- Expertise and skill of the student in performing procedures and techniques.
- Skills in proper recording and reporting.
- The ability to employ the learnt skills in real, practical situation rather than in paper.
- Critical thinking, decision-making and problem-solving skills.
- Attitude of the students toward patients.
- Ability to work in a group.
- Ability to correlate theory with practice.

Procedure of Practical Examination

- The practical examination should be planned well in advance and executed according to the plan.
- Examiners should be clearly intimated regarding the date and venue of the examination.
- The examination should be conducted in a real set-up as far as possible. If not, a simulated setting can be used.

- Students should be intimated clearly which batch they belong to and the time they have to report at.
- Examiners should give proper and clear instructions to the students regarding what they expect from them.
- Both the examiners should evaluate all the students separately to increase the objectivity of the procedure.
- The examiners must try to create an atmosphere of nonstress situation.
- They should assess the students' knowledge and skills in a comprehensive manner. Assessment should be done in a manner, keeping in mind all the factors that influence the conduct of examination in the real situation.
- The students should be informed about the outcome of the examination and the corrective measures they have to take.
- Safety of the patients is to be considered while the students care for them.

Advantages of Practical Examination
- They provide the opportunity to test all the senses in a realistic situation.
- They are helpful to grade or promote the students to the next level.
- They provide opportunity to observe and test attitudes and responsiveness to a complex situation.
- They provide opportunity to test the ability to communicate under pressure.
- They are helpful in assessing the critical thinking, problem-solving and decision-making skills of the students.

Characteristics of Practical Examination
- They are held toward the end of the course or module.
- They are held on a fixed date in advance.
- They are frequently of long duration and require 5–6 hours.
- They comprise one or a small number of compulsory tasks, each of which may have several parts.
- Can test several areas of syllabus together and assess the students' ability to bring together a number of different skills learned in various units.
- It requires the examiner to observe carefully to evaluate the students' performance.

Procedure for Organization of Practical Examination
- It requires advance planning.
- Define the objectives of practical examination in relation to the course objectives.
- Decide in advance the students' level of learning and the levels of skills to be tested such as basic nursing skills and advanced nursing skills.
- Decide percentage of weightage and criteria for evaluation.
- Decide the wards or the clinical area where the examination is being conducted.
- Inform the ward in-charge and patient regarding the practical examination in order to get cooperation.
- Schedule the examination, i.e. the number of days and the number of students per day to be examined. The number of students per day is limited to 10–15 students.
- Prepare various documents including instruction to the students, answer sheets, evaluation formats, and marks statement.

On the Day of Examination

The person who is organizing practical examination should be present in the ward at least 1 hour prior to the scheduled time for examination. The organizer should check for:
- Availability of all desired equipment and supplies.
- Place for the examiners to hold viva and students to wait for their turn.
- Cleanliness of the ward.
- Arranging for some refreshments for the examiners, helpers and students.
- Transport if necessary.

After the Examination
- Students' performance should be discussed amongst the examiners; weak areas must be pointed out; and suggestions to be made are discussed.
- The mark scored by each student is written in words as well as in figures in a sheet of paper and examiners prepare a brief report on the performance of students.
- All the documents are signed by both examiners; sealed; and dispatched to the concerned authority.

Drawbacks
- It is subjective, as the student's score depends on the whims, fancies and mood of the examiner.
- It is time consuming and there is a lack of standardized conditions in bedside, which affects students' scores.

Proposed external basic criteria for appointment of external examiners:
- Proposed external examiner should not have been a member of staff or a student in the institution in the last 5 years.
- Expertise and experience in teaching the subject to be examined.
- Competence in assessing student knowledge.

- Equivalence between the level of the subject to be examined and the qualification of the potential external examiner.
- Experience as an external examiner (preferred).

Viva Voce/Oral Examination

Knowledge is tested in theory examination and skills are evaluated in clinical/practical examination and oral examination is meant to evaluate the following qualities: depth of knowledge, ability to discuss and defend one's decisions, attitudes, alertness, ability to perform under stress and professional competence.

Oral examination should primarily aim at testing, problem-solving, alertness, ability to develop and answer, and ability to come to a decision quickly, besides giving an opportunity to clarify wrong answers in the theory examination, so that the candidate can defend or change his views. Viva voce examination or oral examination is a face-to-face question-answer activity between the examiner and the student. One or more than one examiner ask questions to the student, which he attempts to answer. Generally this may be conducted simultaneously or after finishing the clinical examination.

Definition

A viva voce may be defined as an examination consisting of a dialog of the examiner with the examinee, where the examiner questions to which the candidate must reply.

The purpose of this examination is to assess the communication skills and professional attitude to certain extent.

Advantages

- It allows a direct contact between the examiner and the examinee; it provides an opportunity for studying personal characteristics and permits flexibility in questioning.
- There is less scope for cheating or unfair practice by the examinee.
- It can be a good learning experience as there is scope for an immediate feedback.

Disadvantages

- Oral examinations involve two persons, the examiner and the examinee in a face-to-face situation, and hence there is bound to be a degree of subjectivity.
- The appearance, the language, the accent and the institute to which a candidate belongs sometimes influence the judgment.
- Orals are time consuming and costly in terms of professional time.
- Most of the time, the examiners do not have a prior discussion as to what constitutes an adequate answer.
- It lacks validity, reliability and objectivity.
- Lack of clarity in questioning and questions of variable levels of difficulty are common.
- Uniformity in questioning students will not be maintained.
- Sometimes the examiners expect a predetermined correct answer and are unwilling to consider the candidate's answer as a possible alternative.

Characteristics of Viva Voce Examination

- It takes place on a fixed occasion.
- Examiners should prepare questions on varying degrees of difficulty, prior to the examination.
- Adequate and equal duration of time should be given to each student.
- Examiners should score the students independently according to the predetermined scheme.
- The questions asked should be in par with the level of the students, with the educational objectives and relevant to the subject being examined.
- The examiner should maximum try to reduce the level of subjectivity while examining the students.

Improving Oral Examination

- Prepare a list of tasks and abilities to be tested. These tasks can be in the cognitive, effective or communication areas.
- List the usual questions asked from memory.
- Revise whether they test the abilities intended to be tested.
- Check for clarity of the questions.
- Give adequate time for the students to think and answer and always remember the individual difference.
- Be courteous and do not contradict and show impatience.
- Do not distract the candidate.
- Otherwise make an attempt to know what the student knows.
- Do not hurry up.
- Consistency in scoring can be achieved by subdividing tasks into series of subtask and allotting marks for the answers.

Objective Structured Practical Examination (OSPE)/Objective Structured Clinical Examination (OSCE)

The traditional system of practical examination in nursing consists of either assigning a procedure to a student or a patient for identifying the needs and problems. This depends upon students' ability and availability of the patient for a particular procedure.

Realizing the problems related to the conventional practical examinations, the department of Physiology (Nayar et al., 1986) at All India Institute of Medical Sciences, introduced a new pattern of practical examination called OSPE, which has greater objectivity, reliability, and validity. The nursing curriculum requires students to be able to integrate theory with practice.

The OSPE is a tool which is used to assess laboratory skills of students in the preclinical stage of a health science curriculum. It is a concept in practical assessment of basic medical sciences which is well applied in nursing curriculum. It is a hands-on and real-world approach to learning that keeps examinees engaged, allows them to understand the key factors that drive the decision-making process, and challenges the professional to be innovative and reveals their errors in case-handling and provides an open space for improved decision-making, based on evidence-based practice for real-world responsibilities.

Objective Structured Practical Examination (OSPE) is a new pattern of practical examination, in which each component of clinical competence is tested uniformly and objectively for all the students who are taking up a practical examination at a given place. Through OSPE, one gets a reasonable idea of the extent of achievement of each student in every practical skill related to a particular discipline. It can be used for formative and summative evaluation.

History of OSPE

OSPE is an extended form of OSCE which was described in 1975 and in greater detail in 1979 by Harden and his group from Dundee. OSPE was first introduced as a teaching and evaluation tool in 1986 by Nayar and colleagues at All India Institute of Medical Sciences (AIIMS) to assess the practical skills of students in a physiology course.

OSPE/OSCE revolves around the following:
- The patient/activity
- The Examinee
- The Examiner

Difference between OSCE and OSPE

OSPE is supposed to test the higher level of knowledge and psychomotor skills whereas OSCE should test psychomotor skills of the students. OSPE is done in the laboratories and OSCE is done in the clinical settings. Real patients are required in OSCE whereas standardized patients can be used in OSPE. Examiners are required for each station in OSCE whereas an examiner for each station is not mandatory in OSPE. Though there are differences, in practical, both OSCE and OSPE are used synonymously.

Characteristics of OSPE

- OSPE is a new concept in assessing the practical skills of students.
- It is a modified form of OSCE.
- Multiple stations are designed and each station has a specific objective which needs to be tested.
- OSPE is more objective, reliable, and a valid tool to assess practical aspects of learning.
- Organization of OSPE requires team work and logistics, but at the same time a large number of students can be tested with standard setting in a short period of time.
- It is motivating, inspiring, and interesting.
- The objectives tested in an OSPE assess higher cognitive and psychomotor skills.
- Besides testing high cognitive and psychomotor skills, OSPE helps to assess the capacity for observation, analysis, and interpretation.

Types of Stations and Patients

Procedure Station

It requires a student to perform a task, e.g. administering intramuscular injection. When a student performs the task, simultaneously she is observed and marked against the checklist being prepared in advance, by a silent but vigilant examiner. Eventually, the student gets a score according to the skill demonstrated by her.

Example: Mrs Mala, a 25-year-old primi delivered a male boy with full term normal vaginal delivery with left mediolateral episiotomy. You are instructed to follow the aseptic precautions and to identify the apex correctly and suture the episiotomy in layers on the given mannequin.

Question Station

The student answers the question being asked on the answersheet provided and leaves it in the place specified.

Example: Carefully observe various pictures of newborn given and write the reflexes elicited by the newborn.

Linked Stations

Two stations can be linked and are possible with process. For example, physical examination is tested at one station and in the next station, the examinee answers questions or prepares a report on what was found at the previous station. A linked station is otherwise known as "couplet" station.

A second type of linked station is where an examinee is asked to undertake part of a procedure at the first station and complete it at the second station. For example, the examinee can insert a Ryle's tube in one station and feed the patient in the next station.

Another type of linked station is to provide information about the patient in first station to be ready for performing task by prioritizing the problem. In the second station, the examinee is expected to perform tasks based on the information given in the previous station. For example, in the previous station, student is given information about the patient such as vital signs and subjective and objective data. In the next station, the student has to perform the task such as cold compress/sponging if patient suffers from fever or positioning and oxygen administration if patient has breathing difficulty.

The fourth type of linked stations is one where the examinee undertakes some activity or observes an activity, for example, a recorded interview with a psychiatric patient at the first station, and discusses this with the examiner at the second station. The list is not the end in itself. One can use creativity in designing stations.

The following can be used in stations:
- Real patient
- Simulated patients
- Simulators
- Video recordings
- Patient Medical Records and Investigation
- Text description of a patient

While Using Real Patients
- Obtain consent from the patient
- Select the patient who can spend/spare his time in the stations
- Give clear instruction to the patient about his role
- Arrange for refreshments
- Orient the patient to the environment
- Standardize the history of the patient
- Arrange for transportation of the patients

Simulated Patient

Simulated patient is a person who is carefully trained to re-create the history, physical findings, and psychological and emotional responses of the actual patient in a realistic manner. Faculty and students can act as stimulated patients and they require less training to enact. The simulated patient is expected to replicate his/her portrayal consistently for each candidate both verbally and nonverbally with gestures, facial expressions and eye contact. If stimulation requires more than one person, especially in pediatric patients, the person accompanying the patient also needs training.

Video recordings of patients can be used to assess the students' decision-making abilities with regard to patient care.

The patient's records and their investigations may also be used in an OSCE, where examinees are asked to discuss and interpret the results of an investigation, such as an ECG or abnormal blood results.

Timing of Stations

It can vary from 5 minutes to 15 minutes per station depending upon the nature of the task. The coordinator must ensure that the tasks in all stations are set in such a way that all require equal timing for completion of the task.

Conduction of OSPE
- Preparation for OSPE should start well ahead before the date of examination.
- There should be a coordinated activity of staff at all levels.
- Constitute the examination coordinating committee and the coordinator and members.
- Prepare a list of skills, behavior and attitudes to be assessed in all subjects.
- The questions for stations should be written in accordance with the blueprint.
- Objectives tested with MCQs and SAQs should not be repeated in OSCE/OSPE.
- The answer key should be prepared before examination. The OSPE questions (stations) should be reviewed by a multidisciplinary committee before they are administered.
- Check for the availability of patients/stimulated/standardized patients and equipment.
- Develop checklists and criteria for scoring.
- Decide on the number of examinees and examiners.
- Inform the examinees about the objectives of the examination.
- Train the examiner for the roles they have to play in the stations.
- Decide the examination site and arrange the stations.
- Check for adequate space for all stations and the space for movement for examinee/examiners.
- Decide on number and type of stations.
- Decide on the time allocation for each station.
- Ensure realism as far as possible.
- Decide on instruction to be given to the examinees.
- Prepare directions arrows and stations identification cards.
- Prepare a smaller set of cards with station numbers.
- Prepare a list of candidates.
- Appoint a timekeeper or automatic time signal.
- Decide on giving feedback to the students.

- Organize resources.
- Conduct OSPE as planned.

Instructions to Students

Before the start of OSPE, instructions are given to students on the following:

- Stationery items they should bring to the stations
- Electronic devices which are prohibited in the stations
- Writing of identification details
- How to proceed to stations
- Starting and ending time in each station
- Direction of rotations and number of stations
- Clear instructions on do's and don'ts at each station.

Role of the Examiner

- Checking resources at the station including the patient or stimulated patient
- Greeting the examinee and checking his/her number
- Observing the examinee and completing the checklist and/or rating scale
- Scoring the response
- Providing comments as feedback on the scoring sheet
- Ensuring the timing/time keeping of all concerned
- Keeping a record of any problems that arise in the examination
- Deciding the outcome for each examinee
- Providing feedback to examinees individually or in a group
- Evaluating the stations and the examination process.

Test Security

When more than one group of candidates is assessed on the same examination over a period of time, there is a threat to the examination. The prompting by candidates will lead to lack of test security and this can be managed by quarantining/corralling of students.

Variables in designing OSPE/OSCE

In conduction of OSPE, one can vary with the following:

- Number of stations
- Length of time for stations
- Number of circuits
- Types of stations—procedure vs skill stations and the use of double and linked stations
- Organizations of the station in the circuit
- Provision of feedback to the examinee.

Merits of OSPE/OSCE

- It is objective, reliable, valid, and discriminatory
- All students are exposed to same standardized questions/tasks
- It covers a wide spectrum of learning domains
- It tests a wide range of skills in a short period of time
- Learning objectives can be achieved
- The content and complexity of the examination can be controlled by the examiners
- It gives a reasonable idea of the achievement of the student in every objective of practical exercises
- Helps to test the analytical abilities of the students
- Large number of students can be examined in a short time
- It ensures interaction of teaching and learning.

Limitations of OSPE

- OSPE is used only in simulated situations due to nonavailability of patients for the same procedure.
- The simulated situation may not reflect the real life situation.
- Empathy toward the patients cannot be evaluated.
- The skill of the student in providing holistic nursing care cannot be assessed.
- It may be time consuming to construct an OSPE.
- It needs more resources in terms of manpower, time and money.
- There is no interaction between the examiner and the student.
- There is a risk of fatigue.
- Breaking clinical skills into individual competencies may be artificial and not meaningful.
- Careful organization is required since all stations require equal time.

Problems in Conducting OSCE

- Nonavailability of many faculty members
- Lack of enthusiasm of the teachers to try out new methods
- Students' apprehension for having to learn even the smallest detail of the subject
- Lack of physical facilities and cooperation in the clinical settings
- Controversies over the evaluation criteria.

Strategies to Overcome

- Training the faculty members in using OSPE.
- Preparation of the students from the beginning of the course for this type of examination.
- Proper communication with the administrators of the clinical areas regarding OSCE.
- Ensuring the reliability and validity of the evaluation criteria.
- Adequate planning and organization of the whole exercise.

Attitude Scale

An attitude scale measures how the participant feels about a subject at the moment when he or she answers the question. Several popular types of attitude scales are used in evaluation of nursing education.

Types of Attitude Scales

There are various types of attitude scales used in evaluation of students, they are:
- Point scale
- Differential scale (LL Thurstone scale)
- Summated (Likert) scale
- Semantic differential attitude scales.

Likert Scale

The Likert scale is an ordered, one-dimensional scale from which respondents choose one option that best aligns with their view.

Likert scale is designed to determine the opinion or attitude of a subject and contains a number of declarative statements with a scale after each statement. The original version of the scale included five response categories. Each response category was assigned a value, with a value of 1 given to the most negative response and a value of 5 to the most positive response.

Likert scaling is a bipolar scaling method, measuring either positive or negative response to a statement. Sometimes a 4-point scale is used; this is a forced choice method since the middle option of "Neither agree nor disagree" is not available.

> **Why this scale is known as Likert scale?**
> The scale is named after its inventor, psychologist Rensis Likert.

A Likert item is simply a statement which the respondent is asked to evaluate according to any kind of subjective or objective criteria; generally the level of agreement or disagreement is measured. Often five-ordered response levels are used, although many psychometricians advocate using seven or nine levels. The format of a typical five-level Likert item is:
1. Strongly disagree
2. Disagree
3. Neither agree nor disagree
4. Agree
5. Strongly agree

Response choices in a Likert scale most commonly address agreements, evaluation or frequency.
- **Agreement options** may include statements such as strongly agree, uncertain, disagree and strongly disagree.
- **Evaluation responses** ask the respondent for an evaluative rating along a good/bad dimension, such as positive or negative or excellent to terrible.
- **Frequency responses** may include statements such as rarely, seldom, sometimes, occasionally and usually. The terms used are versatile and need to be selected for their appropriateness to the stem.

Use of uncertain or neutral category is controversial because it allows the subject to avoid making a clear choice of positive or negative statements. Thus, sometimes only four or six options are offered, with the uncertain category omitted. This type of scale is referred to as a forced choice version. The difference between a Likert scale and a Likert item is as follows:

Likert scale	Likert item
The Likert scale is the sum of responses on several Likert items. It is the summated scale	A Likert item is simply a statement which the respondent is asked to evaluate according to any kind of subjective or objective criteria; generally the level of agreement or disagreement is measured. It is otherwise known as an individual item

The Likert scale is the sum of responses on several Likert items. Because Likert items are often accompanied by a visual analog scale (e.g. a horizontal line, on which a subject indicates his or her response by circling or checking tick marks), the items are sometimes called scales themselves. This is the source of much confusion; it is better, therefore, to reserve the term Likert scale to apply to the summated scale, and Likert item to refer to an individual item.

The phrasing of item stems depends on the type of judgment that the respondent is being asked to make. Agreement items are declarative statements such as "I feel good about my work on the job." Frequency items can be behaviors, events or circumstances which the respondent can indicate how often they occur. A frequency stem may be, "I read research articles in journals", "I do exercises and yoga". An evaluation stem could be, "The effectiveness of computer as an aid in promotion of students' learning". Likert scale usually consists of 10–20 items each addressing an element of the concept being measured. Half the statements should be expressed positively and half negatively to avoid inserting bias into the responses. Scale value of negatively expressed items must be reversed before analysis. Usually the values obtained from each item in the instrument are summed to obtain a single score for each subject. Although the values for each item are technically ordinal level data, the summed score is often treated as interval level data, thus allowing more sophisticated statistical analyses.

Likert scales may be subject to distortion from several causes. Respondents may avoid using extreme response categories (central tendency bias); agree with statements as presented (acquiescence bias); or try to portray themselves or their organization in a more favorable light (social desirability bias). Designing a scale with balanced keying (an equal number of positive and negative statements) can obviate the problem of acquiescence bias, since acquiescence on positively keyed items will balance acquiescence on negatively keyed items; but central tendency and social desirability are somewhat more problematic.

Advantages
- Questions used are usually easy to understand and so lead to consistent answers.
- Easy to use.

Disadvantages
- Only a few options are offered, with which respondents may not fully agree.
- People may become influenced by the way they have answered previous questions. For example, if they have agreed several times in a row, they may continue to agree.
- They may also deliberately break the pattern, disagreeing with a statement with which they might otherwise have agreed.

Semantic Differentials

The semantic differential was developed by Osgood and colleagues (1957) which measures attitudes or beliefs. It consists of two adjectives with a 7-point scale between them. The subject is to select one point on the scale that best describes his or her view of the concept being examined. In a semantic differential, values from 1 to 7 are assigned to each of these spaces, with 1 being the most negative response and 7 the most positive response. Placement of negative responses to the left or right of the scale should be randomly varied to avoid global responses (in which the subject places checks in the same column of each scale). Each line is considered one scale. The values for the scales are summed to obtain one score for each subject.

The Semantic Differential (SD) measures people's reactions to stimulus words and concepts in terms of ratings or bipolar scales defined with contrasting adjectives at each end. An example of an SD scale is:

Good	_	_	_	_	_	_	_	Bad
	3	2	1	0	1	2	3	
				or				
Good	_	_	_	_	_	_	_	Bad
	7	6	5	4	3	2	1	

Usually, the position marked 0 is labeled "neutral"; the 1 positions are labeled "slightly"; the 2 positions "quite"; and the 3 positions "extremely". A scale, like this one, measures directionality of a reaction (e.g. good versus bad) and also intensity (slight through extreme).

A number of basic considerations are involved in SD methodology:
- Bipolar adjective scales are a simple and economical means for obtaining data on people's reactions. With adaptations, such scales can be used with adults or children, persons from all walks of life, and persons from any culture.
- Ratings on bipolar adjective scales tend to be correlated; and three basic dimensions of response have been labeled as Evaluation, Potency and Activity (EPA).
- Some adjective scales are almost pure measures of the EPA dimensions, e.g. good-bad for evaluation, powerful-powerless for Potency, and fast-slow for Activity. Using a few pure scales of this sort, one can obtain, with considerable economy, reliable measures of a person's overall response to something. Typically, a concept is rated on several pure scales associated with a single dimension, and the results are averaged to provide a single factor score for each dimension. Measurements of a concept on the EPA dimensions are referred to as the concept's profile.
- EPA measurements are appropriate when one is interested in effective responses. The EPA system is notable for being a multivariate approach to affect measurement. It is also a generalized approach, applicable to any concept or stimulus, and thus it permits comparisons of affective reactions on widely disparate things.
- The SD has been used as a measure of attitude in a wide variety of projects. Osgood et al. (1957) report exploratory studies in which the SD was used to assess attitude change as a result of mass media programs.

Differential scale dimensions		
Evaluation dimensions	Potency dimensions	Activity dimensions
• Nice-awful	• Big-little	• Fast-slow
• Good-bad	• Powerful-	• Alive-dead
• Sweet-sour	powerless	• Noisy-quiet
• Helpful-unhelpful	• Strong-weak	• Young-old
• Hot-cold	• Deep-shallow.	• Passive-active
• Pleasant-unpleasant		
• Beautiful-ugly		

Thurstone Scale

In psychology, the Thurstone scale was the first formal technique for measuring an attitude. It was developed by Louis Leon Thurstone in 1928, as a means of measuring attitudes toward religion. It is made up of statements about a particular issue, and each statement has a numerical value indicating how favorably or unfavorably it is to be judged. People check each of the statements to which they agree, and a mean score is computed, indicating their attitude.

Thurstone was one of the first and most productive scaling theorists. He actually invented three different methods for developing a unidimensional scale—the method of equal appearing intervals; the method of successive intervals; and the method of paired comparisons. The three methods differed in how the scale values for items were constructed, but in all three cases, the resulting scale was rated the same way by respondents.

Construction of Thurstone Scale (Method of Equal Appearing Intervals)

Developing the focus: First decide on the concept or theme to which the respondent has to rate. Define the focus for the scale and the purpose for which it has to be created. The description of this concept should be as clear as possible so that the person(s) who are going to create the statements have a clear idea of what will be measured.

Generating potential scale items: The next step is to create a large set of candidate statements (e.g. 80–100) because the final scale items are selected from this pool. All of the statements are worded similarly—that they do not differ in grammar or structure.

Rating the scale items: The next step is to have the participants (i.e. judges, i.e. approximately 50 or more) rate each statement on a 1-to-11 scale in terms of how much each statement indicates a *favorable* attitude toward a particular concept. It is not that the judges rating their attitudes toward a concept, or whether they would agree or disagree with the statements toward a concept. It is to rate their "favorableness" of each statement in terms of an attitude toward a concept, e.g. AIDS, where 1 = "extremely unfavorable attitude toward people with AIDS" and 11 = "extremely favorable attitude toward people with AIDS".

Computing scale score values for each item: The next step is to analyze the rating data. For each statement, from 50 judges' values, the median and the interquartile range is computed. The median is the value above and below which 50% of the ratings fall. The first quartile (Q1) is the value below which 25% of the cases fall and above which 75% of the cases fall—in other words, the 25th percentile. The median is the 50th percentile. The third quartile, Q3, is the 75th percentile. The interquartile range is the difference between third and first quartile, or Q3–Q1. These values can be computed easily with any introductory statistics program or with the most spreadsheet programs. To facilitate the final selection of items for the scale, sort the table of medians and interquartile range.

Select the final scale items: The statements that are selected should be at equal intervals across the range of medians. Within each value, the statement with the smallest interquartile range is selected. This is the statement with the least amount of variability across judges. And also, look over the candidate statements at each level and select the statement that makes the most sense. If the best statistical choice is a confusing statement, the next best choice is selected.

Administering the scale: The final selected items make a single Thurstone scale to measure the attitude toward a concept. This is given to the samples to measure the attitude. The participants have to either agree or disagree with each statement. To get that person's total scale score, get the average value for the scores of all the items that person agreed with.

Question Bank

A large number of questions can be created and pooled from which the faculty can select appropriate questions based on the test blueprint. Test banks also are created easily by using a word processing program that is used to store test items and make item revision easier. All the questions would be vetted by course team members for quality and then they would be indexed and banked. These questions, when pooled in a bank, are called a question bank.

The advantage of question bank is that questions which work out well in practice can be reused on a number of later situations. Thus, new questions do not have to be generated at the same rate from year to year and the quality of questions gradually improves. The question bank is, thus, a planned library of test items pooled through the cooperative efforts under the aegis of an institution for the use of evaluators, academics, and students in partial fulfillment of the requirements of the teaching-learning process.

In the absence of stock of readymade questions, the quality of question papers is liable to suffer. That is why preparation of quality questions in different subjects has to be entrusted to experienced teachers who are well conversant with the content and techniques of framing questions. Under these conditions, it is necessary that a readymade stock of questions is built up and made available to teachers and testers. Such a pool of test materials can be of immense use if developed according to predetermined objectives.

It is always good to revise tests with some frequency to avoid giving the similar test year after year. Preparing a new set of question paper is a very tedious and time consuming job. At the same time, if questions are often repeated in the question papers, then students prefer to study the questions which are asked very frequently. The paper setter when composing questions for the test must determine their difficulty level, determine course coverage, etc. so as to ensure that the test will neither be too hard nor too easy. By using computers for question banking the steps for the above processes are bypassed. Question banks are large database of suitable questions that are coded by subject area, instructional level, instructional objectives measured, and various other pertinent question characteristics (e.g. difficulty level and discriminating powers). Questions in the question banks are often called "items".

However, question banks are not sufficient for all measurement problems. Persistence and good judgment must remain vital aspects in any test construction and test usage effort. Every effort should be taken to include only quality questions in the question bank. The same care and effort must go into item writing. Questions submitted by item-writers must be evaluated carefully for matching with the course/curriculum as well as for technical quality. Question banks equate various tests and items. Practically it becomes little difficult to equate tests that cover entirely different subject matter. In order to avoid this, item review process must also include a careful evaluation of the skills assessed by each question and tests must be carefully formulated. Any institution undertaking an item banking project should have full understanding of the practical as well as mathematical theoretical aspects of question banking. In order to develop a question bank, many tests are to be calibrated, equated and organized. This requires a great deal of work in terms of preparation and planning and in terms of computer time and expertise. Once the item bank is established, test development time, effort, and loss are reduced substantially.

Advantages
- It is storage of large number of questions.
- It saves time and energy over conventional test development.
- It provides platform for discussing curriculum goals and objectives.

Disadvantages
- It requires great deal of time in preparation and development of the question bank.
- All the items should be analyzed before including in the question bank.
- Item analysis involves the use of various mathematical and statistical procedures.

Planning a Question Bank
Planning for a question bank involves the following activities:
- Defining processes for preparation of individuals who develop question bank.
- Preparatory work for the question bank.
- Identifying what has to be established with the question bank.

The two major objectives of planning a question bank can be:
1. To increase the value of measurement
2. To increase the pedagogical value of evaluation.

Development of Question Bank
The type of questions in the question bank may range from written examination questions to oral examination questions, practical examination questions or the questions of all three types.

Blueprinting for Developing Question Bank
The blueprint can be prepared for:
- The behavior/objective aspect
- The content/subject area aspect.

The objective aspect refers to the expected learning outcomes in terms of abilities like recall, recognition, translation, extrapolation, application, analysis, synthesis, evaluation and other abilities. The content aspect includes the unit and the subunit. A good question pool will be one that contains questions on all the topics in a subject testing all abilities. A mere collection of a large number of questions will not constitute a question pool of quality, unless all such items fit into a predetermined structure. Questions may be collected from old question papers set in various examinations, from standardized tests, experienced teachers, examiners and paper-setters. It can also be collected from the practicing teachers.

Preparations of question banks require a lot of cooperative efforts. Expertise has to be tapped from all the available sources (from within and outside the university) and pooled together. Writers and reviewers of questions for the bank should have, besides their expertise in the subject content and teaching experience, sufficient grounding in evaluation methodology. Even persons selected to act as paper-setters, moderators or evaluators should have not only prescribed experience of teaching the subject, but also adequate background of modern evaluation methods. Having identified such personnel, subject/course wise question bank task groups may be formulated.

Every task group will be guided by one faculty and consists of 4–6 persons selected from among course-writers, teacher counselors, and experienced item-writers available from other institutions.

Screening of Questions
After the questions are written, it can be passed onto other members of the group for their comments. Then, these comments are passed on to the question paper setter or the

author of the questions for corrections. Then, it can be passed on to a committee or a team to review and finalize it.

Item Review

Review, editing, and revalidation of items submitted by the item-writers should be done in presence of item-writers under the guidance of content and evaluation specialists. Generally the target of number of items per course at the optimum level is taken as 10 times the total number of items to be taken in the question paper. There is no upper limit to question bank size. Each question or item to be deposited in QB for a particular course must be well-characterized in terms of the following aspects:
- The section/chapter and unit number of the book
- Type of item and subtype
- Estimated level of difficulty from the point of view of average learner
- Maximum marks
- Time (in minutes) required to answer the question paper
- The marking scheme for supply type questions and "key" answers for selection type questions
- The level of educational objectives which is intended to possibly test (in the taxonomy hierarchy).

Items available for different courses should essentially pass through the revalidation process particularly content and evaluation-edition at the time of their usage for paper-setting. Postvalidation of question used in evaluation involves determining the descriptive statistics such as mean, standard deviation, marks distribution, standard error of measurement of marks secured by the students (population sample) in the examination of each course and item analysis. Item analysis is the statistical study of the performance in each question by the student group as against the performance in question paper as a whole. This is a necessary feedback for the future improvement of the question bank. This can be achieved with the help of a computer and using standard method of analysis.

Descriptive statistics from the test analysis is extremely useful in making decisions such as pass/fail, grace marks for borderline cases, grading, and so on. The results of item analysis are essentially important for improvement of question banks for deciding on the reuse of "good" questions for future examination and improvement or rejection of poorly functioning questions.

Process of Item Analysis

Item analysis indicates which items may be too easy or too difficult and which may fail to discriminate between the better and poor examinees. Item analysis suggests why an item has not functioned effectively and how it might be improved. A test is more reliable if item analysis has been developed. Item analysis consists of the following steps. They are:

Step 1: Conduct a test on the items prepared.

Step 2: Evaluate the answersheets objectively.

Step 3: Arrange answersheet based the score obtained in descending order.

Step 4: Identify an upper group and a lower group. Upper group is highest-scoring 25% and lower group is lowest-scoring 25%.

Step 5: For each item, count the number of examinees in the upper group, who have chosen each response alternative. Do similarly for the lower group.

Step 6: Calculate the items difficulty (called the p-value).

Step 7: Calculate the index of discrimination (D-value).

Discrimination index can be used in the selection of the best items (i.e. most highly discriminating) for inclusion in an improved version of the test. Analysis of a wide variety of classroom test suggests that the indices of item discrimination for most of them can be evaluated in the following manner. If index is greater than or equal to 0.40 then the items are very good items. If index is between 0.30 and 0.39, the items are good but possibly need improvement.

If index is between 0.20 and 0.29, items are marginal and need improvement. Below 0.19, the items are poor and liable for rejection. Hence it becomes clear that a test with higher average index of item discrimination will always be more reliable and better.

The sum of the indices of discrimination for the items of a test and the variance of the scores on the test is expressed in the formula by Ebel:

$$S_x^2 = (\Sigma D)^2/6$$

where 'D' is the discrimination index and 'S_x' is the standard deviation of scores. Hence, one can say that score variance is directly proportional to the square of the sum of discrimination indices, $(\Sigma D)^2$. The larger the score variance for a given number of items, the higher is the reliability of the scores. The formula also indicates that the greater the average value of the discrimination indices, the higher the test reliability is likely to be.

The possibility of preparing valid, reliable and useful questions is greatly enhanced if a few basic steps are followed. They are:
- Determining the purpose of testing
- Developing the test specifications
- Selecting appropriate questions
- Preparing relevant questions
- Assembling the test
- Using the results.

Preparing the Question Cards

It is the easiest method where an institution can prepare for its own. The finalized questions may be written on the card using various colors for essay, short answer and objective type questions and also for various units for easy identification. Then these cards can be properly arranged with the details of topic, estimated difficulty level, subject specification, estimated time limit, etc.

Filing and Storage of Questions

It can be stored in file cabinet kept under lock. It is good to have a duplicate of it. Duplicate can be issued to the teachers or testers whereas the original can be kept intact for official use and reference.

Review and Removal of Unwanted Questions

A question bank may become a store of outdated material after some years, if not evaluated at regular intervals. Enrichment of questions by updating, replacing, discarding, modifying, adding new questions, regrouping and classification is to be an ongoing process to give the question bank a dynamic look.

Computer expertise is an essential requirement of question banking. One should be capable of modifying computer programs, establishing a database system, and capable of running packaged programs. For planning a question bank, evaluation pattern of the program has to be specified.

Computerized Question Banks

One essential activity for the "On demand" examination system is the preparation of question banks. The difficulty of a test is determined by difficulty of the items that comprise it. Item analysis is thus a good exercise to do. As long as differences in student learning exist, and as long as the purpose for testing is to identify such differences, the distribution of test scores should exhibit high variability. The larger the standard deviation of the score, the more successful the test construct or has been in capturing the individual differences in achievement. The reliability of the scores of a group is an important measure of the quality of the scores. All these characteristics are important to consider in evaluating the quality of a test and the evaluation of each can provide clues regarding the ways in which the test items might be revised and improved, for further use.

Computerized question banks are very useful in test development. Items are classified according to relative difficulty. Once items are inserted in the question banks, new set of question papers can be made with known or desired characteristics. The effect of including or excluding particular items can also be predicted. A question bank can store as many questions as possible so that generation of randomized tests is done without any difficulty.

Question banking thus provides substantial savings of time and energy over conventional test development. In a conventional setup, questions can be described relative to the other items within the test and between the students who took it, whereas question banks are not specific, questions are described by their relative difficulty across grade levels and drawing them from the question bank allows one to make fairly accurate predictions concerning composite test characteristics. A question bank also helps in providing a platform for discussing curriculum goals and objectives. The items put in the question banks can be made to inherit properties like common mistakes made by the students, their capabilities and incapabilities, etc. This provides a way to discuss possible learning hierarchies and ways to better structure curriculum.

Test

Purposes

Before instruction:
- To determine readiness
- To place the candidate or categorize
- To assess existing knowledge.

During instruction:
- To assess learning
- To use as diagnostic tool.

After instruction:
- To assess the learning outcome
- To assess the level of mastery
- To grade.

General purpose:
- To direct, stimulate, and motivate
- To assess teaching effectiveness.

Types of Tests

Criterion-referenced Tests

Criterion-referenced tests are those that are constructed and interpreted according to a specific set of learning outcomes. This is useful to measure mastery of subject matter.

Norm-referenced Test

Norm-referenced tests are those constructed and interpreted to provide a relative ranking of students. This type of test is useful for measuring differential performance among students.

Table of Specifications

It includes map, test grid, and test blueprint. The purpose of developing table of specifications is to ensure that the test serves its intended purpose.

Step I. Define the specific learning outcome to be measured. It can be derived from course and unit objectives. It is written as a statement that specifies the behavior that students should be able to perform on completion of instruction. Bloom's taxonomy is used as a guide for developing and leveling general instructional and specific learning outcomes.

Step II. Determining the instructional content to be evaluated and the weightage to be assigned to each area. This is done by developing a content outline and using the amount of time spent teaching the material as an indicator for weighing. This is calculated by using the below mentioned formula.

No. of items/section = Percentage of teaching time × Total no. of items.

Percentage of teaching time for each content is calculated from course plan. The total number of items is planned by the teacher.

For example:

Sl. No.	Content	Teaching time (%)	No. of items/section
1.	Gastrointestinal disorder	20	10
2.	Genitourinary disorder	20	10
3.	Neurological disorder	25	12–13 (12)
4.	Cardiovascular disorder	20	10
5.	Integumentary disorder	15	7–8 (8)
		100	50

Total number of items = 50

Step III. Developing a two-way grid.

Outcomes (content)	Knowledge	Comprehension	Application	Total
Gastrointestinal disorder (20%)	2	4	4	10
Genitourinary disorder (20%)	2	4	4	10
Neurological disorder (25%)	2	5	5	12
Cardiovascular disorder (20%)	2	4	4	10
Integumentary disorder (15%)	2	3	3	8
	10	20	20	50

Two-way grid is developed with content areas being listed down on the left side and learning outcomes listed across the top of the grid. Each cell is assigned a number of questions based on the weighing of content and cognitive level of learning outcomes.

Selecting Item Types

Items may be selection type which provides a set of response from which to choose or supply type, which requires the student to provide an answer. Common selection type items include true-false, matching, and multiple choice. Supply type items include short answer and essay. The choice of type of item depends on what we want to measure from the student. Generally lower level outcomes (knowledge, comprehension, and application) can be easily evaluated by selection type items whereas higher level outcomes (analysis, synthesis, and evaluation) require the use of supply type items.

Characteristics of Selection and Supply Type

Sl. No.	Characteristics	Selection type	Supply type
1.	Easy to create	No	Yes
2.	Easy to score	Yes	No
3.	Objective	Yes	No
4.	Measuring higher level skills	No	Yes
5.	Broad sampling	Yes	No
6.	Eliminates noncontent skills	Yes	No

A general guide for planning is to allow 1 minute for each moderately difficult multiple choice item.

Editing and Validating Test Items

It is very essential to edit the items and make any needed corrections. At this stage, peer review of questions is helpful for refining the question, ensuring accuracy, testing for reliability and eliminating grammatical errors.

Assembling and Administering a Test

Once the items are written and edited, they must be assembled into a test. This step includes arranging the items, writing test directions, and responding and administering the test.

Arranging Items

The following points to be considered in arranging the items:
- Grouping similar item types together.
- Place items within each group in ascending order of difficulty.
- Begin the test with an easy question. Follow simple to complex, and known to unknown.

Writing Test Directions

The written test directions should be self-explanatory. It should include the following information:
- Time allotted to complete the test.
- Instruction for responding (choose the most appropriate answer).
- Instruction for recording the answer in answersheet.
- Marks assigned to each questions.

Reproducing the Test

The test should be easy to read and follow. The following guidelines are suggested:

- Type test neatly
- Space items evenly
- Number items consecutively
- Keep item stem and options on the same page
- Place introductory material (e.g. graph or chart) before item
- Keep matching lists on the same page
- Proofread after compiling and before duplicating.

Administering the Test/Role of the Faculty

- Provide conducive physical environment.
- Conducive physical environment includes adequate lighting, comfortable room temperature, and sufficient space for each candidate, minimal interruptions, away from loud noise, comfortable furniture, and ventilation. Faculty should maintain non-threatening attitude and avoid unnecessary conversation before and during examination.
- Faculty should avoid giving unintentional clue to the students.
- Maintain confidentiality.
- Maintain the test security (locking up the question paper).
- Do not give the same question paper each year.
- Inform earlier the consequence of cheating.
- Ensure close supervision throughout the examination.
- Ensure careful seating arrangements and spacing of students.

Sample Test Item Analysis for a 30-item Scale

P (item difficulty)/ D (item discrimination)	>.50 .40-.49 .30-.39 .20-.29 Negative total
Very difficult P = 50% or less	
Difficult P = 51%–69%	
Average P = 70%–80%	
Easy P = 81%–100%	

Grades

In the evaluation system, grading is a recent phenomenon; earlier and even now in many courses of study the scoring system is still used. Grading when compared to traditional system of scoring has some pertinent advantages.

Drawbacks of Traditional Scoring System

- Marking involves subjectivity and bias.
- Results are declared as either pass or fail.
- All scores have to be summated at the end for assigning a particular division.

The traditional grading system was to assign a single letter grade for each subject. For example—A, B, C, D, E.

- They are a combination of achievement, effort, work habits, and good behavior.
- The proportion of students assigned each letter grade varies from teacher to teacher.
- They do not indicate a student's specific strengths and weaknesses in learning.

While assigning grades the following queries have to be clarified:

- What should we include in letter grade?
- How do we convert a client data into grades?
- How do we create a frame for grading?

Basically, letter grades are meaningful if they represent achievement, but if it is mixed up with the other external factors like effort, works, etc. it gets contaminated as they do not consider quality aspects. However, teachers feel even these factors should be considered while giving grades. It is very difficult to assess exactly a student's efforts/potential; also it is hard to distinguish between aptitude and achievement. Some students are good at certain aspects and others are good in some other aspects. This means if grading is considered differently for different students it may send wrong messages that may be unfair at times.

While converting scores into grades different components have to be given different weightages and the composite score should be generated for which grade should be decided. For instance, 60% weightage to the final examination, 20% to the presentation, and 20% to the assignment can be given. Likewise the weightage can be decided and together the composite score should be generated for 100. But in the above example, the weightage given to different components being different, the strengths of the students in each area may vary and affect their aggregate score. The other way may be to take less number of aspects, e.g. two aspects or assign equal weightage to different components; thus the scoring and grading becomes more objective. In fact a more refined weightage could be using standard deviation as a measure of variability. If teachers are equipped with computing skills then measurement becomes very simple and more objective.

According to Jacobs and Chase (1992), the characteristics of a good grading system include:

- Informing students of the specific grading criteria at the beginning of the course (stated clearly in the prospectus/syllabus).
- Grades should be assigned only based on the learning outcomes and not taking into consideration of the factors such as attendance and effort.
- Collecting sufficient data before assigning a grade.
- Recording data collected for grading purposes quantitatively (e.g. 90% not A).
- Following uniform grading systems for all students.
- Using statistically sound principles for assigning grades.

Assigning Grades

Grading the students not only gives feedback and it also motivates the students. Each institution might have grading policy or scale.

The two basic methods for assignment are the **absolute and the relative or comparative scales**.

Absolute Scale

This grading is very convenient when the course objectives have been clearly specified and standards and mastery level approximately set; the letter grades in an absolute system may be defined as the degree to which objectives have been attained. This rates performance relative to a standard. The students' earned marks in percentage are compared with the standard and grades are assigned.

They can be discussed in the following ways:
- Preestablished percentage score
- Criterion-referenced grading
- Numerical rating.

Pre-established Percentage Scores

The different range of percentage marks for assigning grade letter is used. The test and the assessment designed to yield scores in terms of percentage of correct answers; the absolute grading can be decided as given below:
- A = 95% to 100% correct
- B = 85% to 94% correct
- C = 75% to 84% correct
- D = 65% to 74% correct
- E = below 65% correct.

For example

Range	Assigned grade
90–100	A
80–89	B
70–79	C
60–69	D
<60	E

Criterion-referenced Grading

The criterion standard has been fixed either by the teacher or the authorities beforehand in view of the difficulty of the test, and standard or quality of learning performance needed from learners, i.e. decision with regard to the students' performance in terms of behavioral changes, on the basis of which letter grades are gained. This can be represented as:

Grade	Performance	Level of performance
A	Outstanding	Student has mastered **all** the courses, major and minor instructional goals.
B	Very good	Has mastered **all** the courses, major instructional goals and **most** of the minor ones.

Contd...

Contd...

Grade	Performance	Level of performance
C	Satisfactory	Student has mastered **all** the courses, major instructional goals but **just a few** minor ones.
D	Very weak	Student has mastered **just a few** of the courses, major senior instructional goals, and basically has essentials needed for the next highest level of instruction. Remedial work would be desirable.
E	Unsatisfactory	Student has not mastered any of the lower major instructional goals. Does not need next higher-level instruction. Remedial work is needed.

The Grading System

A+, A, A–
Full mastery of the subject; in the case of the grade of A+, the student must be of extraordinary distinction.

B+, B, B–
Good comprehension of the course material; a good command of the skills needed to work with the course material; and the student's full engagement with the course requirements and activities.

C+, C, C–
Adequate and satisfactory comprehension of the course material; the skills needed to work with the course material; the student has met the basic requirements for completing assigned work and participating in class activities.

D+, D, D–
Unsatisfactory, but some minimal command of the course materials; some minimal participation in class activities that is worthy of course credit toward the degree.

E
Unsatisfactory and unworthy of course credit toward the degree.

Range of marks	Letter grade
85–100	A+
75–84	A
70–74	A–
65–69	B+
60–64	B
55–59	B–
50–54	C+
45–49	C
40–44	C–
35–39	D+
30–34	D
25–29	D–
00–24	E

Numerical Grading

Here, each objective or benchmark is represented with a numerical rating. This can be seen as follows:

Acquired Proficiency

4 = Skill developed, good proficiency
3 = Skill developed satisfactorily, proficiency could be improved
2 = Basic skill developed low proficiency, needs additional work
1 = Basic skill not acquired.

Advantages

- The objective-based grades are determined based on students' performance.
- Performance-based grade is assigned.
- If all students demonstrate the same level of mastery, all of them will receive high grades respectively.
- A comprehensive report generally includes a checklist of objectives to inform both parents and students.
- Report provides detailed information to indicate which skill is acquired and which has not been acquired.
- All standard procedures are followed.

Limitations

- Teachers have no flexibility to prepare as per the local needs.
- Objective-based performance may not be seen all the times.

Relative Scale

A relative scale rates students according to their ranking within the group. The faculty has to record the scores of all students in a descending order. Grades may then be assigned using a variety of techniques. One method is to assign the grades using natural "breaks" in the distribution. This method has disadvantage of being subjective. The other method is to find out the measures of central tendency (mean or mode). In a bell-shaped curve (normal distribution), mean and mode will be the same and in skewed distribution, median can be used as a measure of central tendency (Fig. 4.3). Then determine the standard deviation. The C grade will be set as the mean plus or minus one-half the SD (encompassing 40% of the scores).

Grade	Calculation
A	>Upper B
B	Upper C + 1SD
C	Mean ± .5SD
D	Lower −1SD
E	<Lower

Or

Grade	Percentage of class assigned with grades
O	Top 7% of a class group
A	Top middle 24 % of a class group
B	Middle 38% of a class group
C	Bottom middle 24% of a class group
D	Bottom 7% of a class group

Depending on any of the performances in terms of the numerals the marks may be arranged in descending order and the letter grades should be assigned as shown above, i.e. top 7% with "O" grade, top middle with 24% with "A", middle 38% with "B", bottom middle 24% with "C", and bottom 7% with "D".

Advantages

- It is based on normal curve distribution, which gives clear direction to teachers while taking decisions on assigning grades.
- The faculty can set general guidelines for grading.
- They can evolve separate distribution for the introductory and advanced level groups.
- Distribution can be flexible from course to course and from time to time.
- The pass and fail is based not on the relative performance; it can set certain absolute standards.

Limitations

- Real potential abilities are not tapped exactly.
- They are not comparable elsewhere or equated with other groups.
- A lot of flexibility may have a stake for quality and standard.
- Teachers may find it difficult to make decisions without any set standard rules.
- Classroom designed test and instruments may not yield normally distributed scores.
- It needs more sensible decision-making as grades.
- It is more subjective and depends on the teacher's standard. Various techniques and tools are generally used to evaluate a student in a learning situation. The most commonly employed are the achievement tests.

Achievement tests are important tools in evaluation and as the name indicates, they encompass the achievements, attainments, and accomplishments of any student in the line of instructional and educational objectives. It places an important role in grading and promotion of the student, and measuring instructional progress.

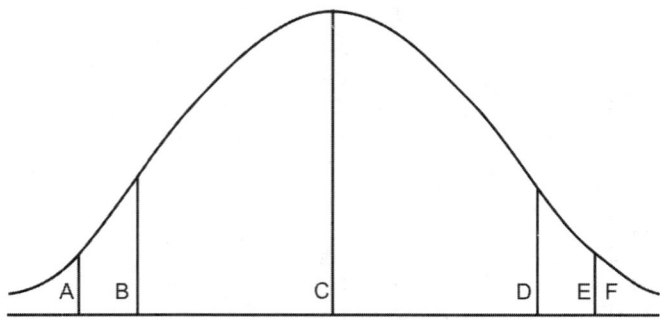

Fig. 4.3: Normal distribution.

According to Gronlund, an achievement test is a "systematic procedure for determining the amount a student has learned through the instruction".

Commonly, the ability to do something is called as achievement, and this can be learned only by watching the student at work. The main purpose of the achievement record is to estimate students' progress and to give them the help they need.

Standardized Tools or Tests

Meaning

A standardized test is a test administered and scored in a consistent manner. The tests are designed in such a way that the questions, conditions for administering, scoring procedures, and interpretations are consistent and are administered and scored in a predetermined, standard manner.

The standardized test is designed for general use. The items and the total scores have been carefully analyzed, and validity and reliability have been established by statistical controls. Norms have been established based upon the performance of many subjects of various age groups living in many different types of communities and geographical areas. Not only the content of the test has been standardized, but the administration and scoring have also been set in one pattern so that those subsequently taking the tests will take them under like conditions. As far as possible the interpretation has also been standardized.

The commonly used tests are **psychological tests**. A psychological test is an instrument designed to describe and measure a sample of certain aspects of human behavior. Tests may be used to compare the behavior of two or more persons at a particular time or one or more persons at different times. Psychological tests yield objective and standardized descriptions of the behavior, quantified by numerical scores (Table 4.2).

Objectivity

It is an important aspects of a psychological test. The purpose of standardizing a test is to give it objectivity, which is to devise an instrument that as far as possible will be free from subjective judgment regarding the ability, skill, knowledge, trait or potentiality to be measured and evaluated.

The following things make a test objective:
- There will be uniform and specified set of instructions to be followed by everybody who administer the test.
- Uniform scoring is done.
- Norms of the test are based on scientific sampling scientifically devised.
- Content of the test under construction is subjected to analysis by means of established techniques of test standardization.
- Objectivity is maintained in administering and scoring the test.
- Every test is designed for use with a specified population or group.

Classification of Psychological Tests

- Performance tests vs paper and pencil tests
- Power versus timed or speed tests
- Standardized versus nonstandardized tests.

Performance Tests versus Paper and Pencil Tests

Performance tests, usually administered individually, require that the subjects manipulate objects or mechanical apparatus while their actions are observed and recorded by the examiner. Paper and pencil test, usually administered in groups, require the subjects to mark their response on a prepared sheet.

Power versus Timed or Speed Tests

Power tests have no time limit, and the subjects attempt progressively more difficult tasks until they are unable to continue successfully. Timed or speed tests usually involve the element of power, but in addition, they limit the time, the subjects have to complete certain tasks.

Standardized versus Nonstandardized Tests

The test that the classroom teacher constructs is likely to be less expertly designed than that of the professional,

Table 4.2: Difference between the teacher-made tests and standardized tests.

	Teacher-made tests	Standardized tests
Learning outcomes and content measurement	They are used to evaluate the outcomes and the content of the local curriculum	They are used to evaluate the outcomes and content common to a number of colleges
Quality of test items	Quality is lower than that of the standardized tests	Quality is high
Reliability	Usually unknown	It is high
Administration and scoring	Uniform procedure is possible but it is usually flexible	Administration and scoring procedure is standardized
Interpretation of scores	Scores can be compared and interpreted only in the context of the local situation	Compared to norm groups

although it is based upon the logic and skill that the teacher can command and is usually "tailor made" for a particular group of pupils.

Classification of psychological tests in terms of their purpose is as follows:
- Achievement tests
- Personality inventories
- Aptitude tests
- Intelligence tests
- Interest inventories.

Design and Scoring of Standardized Tests

In practice, standardized tests can be composed of multiple-choice and true-false questions. Such items can be tested inexpensively and quickly by scoring special answersheets by computer or manually. Some tests also have short-answer or essay writing components that are assigned a score by independent evaluators who use rubrics (rules or guidelines) and anchor papers (examples of papers for each possible score) to determine the grade to be given to a response. Most assessments, however, are not scored by people; people are used to score items that are not able to be scored easily by computer (i.e. essays).

Scoring Issues

There can be issues with human scoring, which is a reason for the preference given to computer scoring. Agreement between scorers can vary between 60% and 85% depending on the test and the scoring session. Sometimes two or more scorers read each paper to improve reliability, though this does not eliminate test responses getting different scores.

Score

There are two types of standardized test score interpretations, a norm-referenced score interpretation or a criterion-referenced score interpretation.

Norm-referenced score interpretations compare test-takers to a sample of peers. Criterion-referenced score interpretations compare test-takers to a criterion (a formal definition of content), regardless of the scores of other examinees. Norm-referenced test score interpretations are associated with traditional education, which measures success by rank ordering students using a variety of metrics, including grades and test scores, while standards-based assessments are based on the belief that all students can succeed if they are assessed against high standards which are required of all students regardless of ability or economic background.

Standards

The considerations of validity and reliability typically are viewed as essential elements for determining the quality of any standardized test. However, professional and practitioner associations frequently have placed these concerns within broader contexts when developing standards and making overall judgments about the quality of any standardized test as a whole within a given context.

Advantages

One of the main advantages of standardized testing is that the results can be empirically documented; therefore, the test scores can be shown to have a relative degree of validity and reliability, as well as results which are generalizable and replicable. Another advantage is aggregation. A well-designed standardized test provides an assessment of an individual's mastery of a domain of knowledge or skill which at some level of aggregation will provide useful information. That is, while individual assessments may not be accurate enough for practical purposes, the mean scores of classes, schools, branches of a company, or other groups may well provide useful information because of the reduction of error accomplished by increasing the sample size.

Disadvantages and Criticism

"Standardized tests cannot measure initiative, creativity, imagination, conceptual thinking, curiosity, effort, irony, judgment, commitment, nuance, goodwill, ethical reflection, or a host of other valuable dispositions and attributes. What they can measure and count is isolated skills, specific facts and function, the least interesting and least significant aspects of learning."—Bill Ayers.

Though many educators recognize that standardized tests have a place in the arsenal of tools used to assess student achievement, critics feel that overuse and misuse of these tests is having serious negative consequences on teaching and learning. They also feel that this disfavors higher order learning.

Steps in Constructing Scales

Scale construction is a complex procedure that should not be undertaken lightly. It requires careful work. The steps in constructing the scales are as follows:

Defining the Concept

A scale cannot be constructed to measure a concept until the nature of the concept has been delineated. The more clearly the concept is defined, the easier it is to write items to measure it (Spector, 1992). Concept analysis helps in defining the concept clearly.

Design the Scale

Items should be constructed to reflect the concept as fully as possible. The process of construction will differ somewhat depending on whether the scale is a rating scale, Likert scale or semantic differential scale. A blueprint can be prepared to ensure coverage of all elements of the concept. Items should be constructed keeping in mind the potential respondents. It should be clearly stated, and express only one idea. The number of items constructed needs to be considerably larger than planned for the completed instrument because items will be discarded during the item analysis step of scale construction. Nunnally (1978) suggests developing an item pool at least twice the size of that desired for the final scale.

Seek Item Review

As items are constructed, it is advisable to ask qualified individuals to review them. Feedback can be obtained in relation to accuracy, appropriateness or relevance to test specifications, technical flaws in item construction, grammar, appearance of bias, and level of readability. Based on the critique and suggestion of the expert, items can be revised.

Conduct Preliminary Item Tryouts

Items can be tested on a limited number of subjects (15–30) who are the representatives of the target population. Observe the reactions of respondents during testing to note behavior such as long pauses, answer changing, or other indications of confusion about specific items. After testing, a debriefing session needs to be held during which respondents are invited to comment on items and offer suggestions for improvement. Statistical analyses are performed on data from these tryouts while noting means, response distributions, items left blank, and outliers. Revise these items on the basis of this analysis and comments from respondents.

Perform a Field Test

Administer all the items in their final draft form to a large sample of subjects representative of the target population. Spector (1992) recommends a sample size of 100–200 subjects. However, the sample size needed for the statistical analysis to follow is somewhat dependent on the number of items. Some recommend including 10 subjects for each item being tested. If the final instrument is expected to have 20 items and 20 items were constructed for the field test, as many as 400 subjects could be required.

Conduct Item Analyses

The purpose of item analysis is to identify whether the items are internally consistent, and eliminate items that do not meet this criterion. Internal consistency implies that all the items measure the same concept. Negatively worded items need to be reverse scored. Some statistical computer program such as SPSS performs item analysis. This package performs item-item correlations and item-total correlation. In some cases, the value of the item being examined is subtracted from the total score and an item remainder coefficient is calculated. The latter coefficient is the most useful in evaluating items for retention in the scale.

Select Items to Retain

Depending on the number of items desired in the final scale, items with the highest coefficients are retained. Alternatively, a criterion value for the coefficient can be set and all items greater than this value is retained. The greater the number of items retained, the smaller the item remainder coefficients can be and still have an internally consistent scale. After this selection process, coefficient alpha can be calculated for the scale. This value is a direct function of the number of items and the magnitude of intercorrelation, thus one can increase the value of coefficient alpha by increasing the number of items or raise the intercorrelations through inclusion of more highly intercorrelated items. The value of coefficient alpha varies from 0 to 1. The alpha value should be at least .70 to indicate sufficient internal consistency. An iterative process of removing or replacing items, or both, recalculating item remainder coefficients and recalculating the alpha coefficient is repeated until a satisfactory alpha coefficient is obtained. Deleting poorly correlated items will raise the alpha coefficient, but decreasing the number of items will lower it.

The initial attempt at scale development may not achieve a sufficiently high coefficient alpha. In this case, additional items will need to be written, more data collected, and the item analysis redone. This scenario is most likely to occur when too few items were developed initially or when many of the initial items were poorly written. It may also be a consequence of attempts to operationalize an inadequately defined concept.

Conduct Validity Studies

When scale development is judged to be satisfactory, studies must be performed to evaluate the validity of the scale. These studies require the collection of additional data from large samples. As part of this process, scale scores need to be correlated with scores on other variables proposed to be related to the concept being put into operation. Hypothesis need to be generated regarding variations in mean values of the scale in different groups. Exploratory and then confirmatory factor analysis is usually performed as part of establishing validity of the instrument.

Evaluate the Reliability of the Scale

Various statistical procedures need to be performed to determine the reliability of the scale.

Compile Norms on the Scale

Determination of norms requires administration of the scale to a large sample representative of the groups to which the scale is likely to be given. Norms should be acquired for as many diverse groups as possible. Data acquired during validity and reliability studies can be included for this analysis. To obtain large samples needed for this purpose, many researchers give permission to others to use their scale with the condition that data from these studies should be provided for compiling norms.

Publish the Results of Development of the Scale

Scales are often not published for a number of years after the initial development because of the length of time required to validate the instrument. Some researchers never publish the results of this work. Studies using this scale are published, but the instrument development process may not be available except by writing to the author. This information needs to be added to the body of the knowledge, and instrument developers need to be encouraged by their colleagues to complete the work and submit it.

Various Tests

Interest Inventories

An interest is a subjective attitude motivating a person to perform certain task. It affords pleasure and satisfaction. It results in curiosity toward the object of interest, enthusiasm to be attached to the object, strength of will to face difficulties while engaged in the task of one's interest, a definite change in behavior in the presence of the object characterized by attention and concentration.

Jones states, "Interest is a feeling of likening associated with a reaction, either actual or imagined to a specific thing or situation".

Bingham defines "interest is a tendency to become absorbed in an experience and to continue it, while an aversion is a tendency to turn away from it to something else".

According to Jones, interest is of two types. They are:
1. **Intrinsic interest**
2. **Extrinsic interest**.

The extrinsic interests are pleasurable emotions connected with a purpose or goal of an activity. It may involve fame, name, money, victory or such external motives of conduct. But the latter are connected with the activity itself, being basic and real attraction without any external motive. This intrinsic interest is continuous and permanent, even if the immediate goal is reached. The extrinsic interest dies as soon as the goal is reached.

The other classification of interest is as follows:
- Expressed interest
- Manifests interest
- Measured interest.

Expressed Interest

In the expressed interest the person expresses his personal likings through such sentences as "I love sports". Though it is the first source of knowing a person's interest, it may not be reliable and the interest may vary from time to time depending upon the maturity of the person.

Manifests Interest

Manifest interest is the interest that is not expressed but observed by others while the person is engaged and absorbed in an activity. Newton forgot his meals while engaged in scientific experiments.

Measured Interest

The measured interest is the estimate and account of a person's interest as revealed by some psychological test or interest inventories.

Measurement of Interest

Interest inventories attempt to yield a measure of the types of activities that an individual has a tendency to like and to choose. One kind of instrument has compared the subject's pattern of interest to the interest patterns of successful practitioners in a number of vocational fields. A distinctive pattern has been discovered to be the characteristic of each field. The assumption is that an individual will be happy and most successful in working in a field which he likes the most. It may be his or her own measured profile of interest.

Another inventory is based on the correlation between a number of activities from the areas of school, recreation and work. These related activities have been identified by careful analysis with mechanical, computational, scientific, persuasive, artistic, literary, musical, social service, and clerical areas of interest. By sorting the subject's stated likes and dislikes into various interest areas, a percentile score for each area is obtained. It is then assumed that the subject will find his or her areas of greatest interest where the percentile scores are relatively high. Interest blanks or inventories are examples of self-report instruments in which individuals note their own likes and dislikes. These self-report instruments are really standardized interviews in which the subjects, through introspection, indicate feelings that may be interpreted in terms of what is known about interest patterns.

Inventories of Standardized Interest

Some of the standardized interest inventories are:
- Strong vocational interest blank
- Kuder preference record
- Thurstone's vocational interest schedule.

Strong Vocational Interest Blank

Prof Strong of Stanford University, California designed and standardized this checklist. It contains 400 separate items. It is presented to the individual and he is simply asked to indicate whether he likes, dislikes or is indifferent on a 3-point scale. The test reveals the interest of the individual, his masculinity and of feminity, and his occupational level. It is useful for both educational and vocational guidance.

Kuder Preference Record

This has been prepared by G Frederic Kuder. This test covers a wider field, comprising of nine separate scales of occupations such as mechanical, computational, scientific, persuasive, artistic, literary, musical, social, and clerical. A detailed scoring system is employed for analysis and interpretation. A percentile of 75 or above is considered significantly high. If a person goes beyond 75 in any one of the areas, all the occupations in that area are attractive for him.

Thurstone's Vocational Interest Schedule

The test has been devised by Thurstone. He administered a comprehensive test to 3,400 college students who expressed their Likeness (L), Indifference (I) and Dislike (D) to each of the items in the test. He analyzed the test scores and through the techniques of factor analysis, arrived at eight factors of interest such as Commercial Interest, Legal, Athletic, Academic, Descriptive, Biological, Physical Science, and Arts.

Limitation of Interest Inventories

- Some of the tests reveal ability rather than interest. But interest is not the same thing as ability.
- The tests can reveal the subject's interest present at the time of test and not afterwards. The interest revealed may not remain permanent. The interests are cultivable also.
- The interest inventories reveal facts on the basis of the report given by the subject. The accuracy of the report is still a problem. Some people do not reveal the facts.

Achievement Tests

Achievement tests attempt to measure what an individual has learned from his or her present level of performance. Most tests used in schools and colleges are achievement tests. They are particularly helpful in determining individual or group status in academic learning. Achievement tests scores are used in placing, advancing or retaining students at particular grade levels. They are used in diagnosing strengths and weaknesses and as a basis for awarding prizes, scholarships or degrees.

An achievement test is essentially a tool or device of measurement that helps in ascertaining quantity and quality of learning attained in a subject of study or group of subjects after a period of instructions by measuring the present ability of the individual concerned. Achievement test is a systematic procedure for determining the amount a student has learned through instruction. Achievement test is a measure of knowledge and skills in a content area.

There are individual and group achievement tests. Some of the achievement tests are—Tests of Achievement and Proficiency, National Teacher Examination, and Metropolitan Achievement Test. Frequently, achievement tests scores are used in evaluating the influences of courses of study, teachers, teaching methods, and other factors considered to be significant in educational practice.

Functions of Achievement Testing

- To identify the individuals with specific achievement deficits and learning disabilities.
- To help parents to provide individual remedial efforts at home.
- To plan for specific instructional activities.
- To appraise the success of educational program.
- To group students with similar achievement for specific purposes.
- To assign grades.

Aptitude Tests

Aptitude is a condition or set of characteristics regarded as symptomatic of an individual's ability to acquire with training some knowledge, skill or set or responses such as ability to speak a language, to produce music, etc. Aptitude is something more than the ability. It is ability plus suitability of performance. Aptitude tests attempt to predict the degree of achievement that may be expected from individuals in a particular activity. To the extent that they measure past learning, they are similar to achievement tests. To the extent that they measure nondeliberate or unplanned learning, they are different. Aptitude tests attempt to predict an individual's capacity to acquire improved performance with additional training. According to Bingham, "Aptitude refers to those qualities characterizing a person's way of behavior which serve to indicate how well he can learn to meet and solve certain specified kinds of problems".

According to Freeman, "An aptitude is a combination of characteristics indicative of an individual's capacity to acquire (with training) some ability to speak language, to become a musician, to do mechanical work".

Nature of Aptitude Test

We generally observe among people that some are very good in art, some at music and some in dance with or without training, i.e. inborn talent. We also hear of extremely talented people who are good at mathematical abilities and some other specific technical skills. Another simple example to understand the importance of aptitude is that a mango seed will give a mango tree not the other tree, i.e. the seed has the basic potential of the plant hidden in it. Similarly human beings have some hidden talents and potentials in them, which can be nurtured to excel in that area without much difficulty.

While choosing a profession or assigning a task to an individual or choosing a course of study or an occupation it is quite important to understand the potential of that individual in that area to make them successful individuals in excelling in that area without much difficulty. It may be heredity, which will make them excel but at times we observe environment also creates work interest in that area and develops proficiency in that area. Thus, both environment and heredity are responsible for the aptitude. So, in order to know the aptitude of an individual our day-to-day achievement tests may not be adequate to measure. They not even require intelligence tests. But they need to have specific tests while taking up a profession or occupation for which many tests were designed and evaluated to establish their validity and reliability.

Difference between Ability and Achievement

Aptitude and present ability do not mean the same thing. A person may not have the present ability to drive a car but he may have a high aptitude for driving, which means that his chances of being a successful driver are good provided he receives the proper training. In this way, the aptitude has future reference and tries to predict the degree of attainment of an individual after an adequate training. Achievement is past oriented. It looks into the past and indicates what an individual has learned or acquired in a particular field.

Difference between Intelligence and Aptitudes

Intelligence tests usually test the general mental ability of an individual whereas aptitude tests concerned with specific abilities. The knowledge of intelligence of a person predicts his success in a number of situations involving mental function or activity whereas the knowledge of aptitude of a person predicts his special abilities or capacity to succeed in a specific field or activity.

Difference between Aptitude and Interest

Interest and aptitude go hand-in-hand. Though both are essential for the prediction of the success of an individual in a given activity, they are not one. A person may have aptitude to drive a car but he may not be interested. A person may also have interest in doing a particular activity but he may not have aptitude for it.

In a nutshell, achievement looks to the past, indicating what has been done.

Ability concerns the present, indicating the powers now.

Aptitude looks to the future, predicting what he may become.

Aptitude tests have been designed to predict improved performance with further training in many areas. These inferred measurements have been applied to mechanical and manipulative skills, musical and artistic pursuits and many professional areas involving many types of predicted ability.

Types of Aptitude Tests

Broadly, aptitude tests can be divided into:
- Specialized aptitude tests
- General aptitude tests.

Aptitude tests may be used to divide students into relatively homogenous groups for instructional purposes, identify students for scholarship grants, screen individuals for particular educational programs, or help guide individuals into areas where they are most likely to succeed.

Specialized aptitude tests are generally classified as follows:
- Mechanical aptitude tests
- Musical aptitude tests
- Art judgment tests
- Scholastic aptitude tests
- Professional aptitude tests
  - Teaching
  - Clerical
  - Medical
  - Engineering.

General aptitude tests are:
- Differential aptitude tests
- General aptitude test battery
- Armed services vocational aptitude battery

- Postgraduate selection tests
  - Graduate record examination (GRE)
  - Medical college admission test (MCAT)
  - Law school admission test (LSAT)
  - American college test (ACT).

Some important aptitude tests are:
- Minnesota mechanical aptitude test
- Minnesota clerical aptitude test
- Multiple aptitude test
- Seashore musical aptitude test
- Horne art aptitude inventory
- Stanford scientific aptitude test
- Preengineering ability test
- Minnesota engineering analogical test
- Teaching aptitude test.

Aptitude tests are the backbone of the guidance services. It helps the youth in the selection of special courses of instruction, fields of activities, and vocations. They can be safely used for the purpose of educational and vocational selection. They help us in making scientific selection of the candidates for various educational and professional courses as well as for specialized jobs. This, when combined with the other information received through interest inventory, personality tests, intelligence test and cumulative record, etc., can help to a greater extent in avoiding the huge wastage of human as well as material resources by placing the individuals in their proper places and lines of work.

Uses of Aptitude Tests in Evaluation

These tests have wide area of application. They are:
- Guidance
- Selection for jobs
- Admission
- They are the backbone of guidance services.
- The results of the aptitude tests are useful in predicting the success of the individual in the area concerned.
- It helps in selecting suitable courses of instructions.
- It helps in identifying suitable candidates for admission into various professional courses and specialized jobs.

Personality Tests

The term personality is derived from the Latin word "persona", which means a mask that actors used to wear for portraying different characteristics. Personality is the sum total of all the biological innate dispositions, impulses, tendencies, appetites and instincts of the individual and the disposition and tendencies acquired by experience (Morton Prince, 1929). Personality is the sum of activities that can be discovered by actual observations over a period of time to give reliable information.

Nature of Personality Testing

Personality is a complex characteristic that is difficult to measure for the following reasons:
- Personality is not a thing, it is an idea and abstraction and attempt to measure it.
- It is not static.
- It may not be exactly the same from time to time.

Personality inventories are designed to assess the relatively stable and enduring characteristics of a person that may affect job performance and workplace behavior. Personality scales are usually self-report instruments. The individual checks responses to certain questions or statements. These instruments yield scores which are assumed or have been shown to measure certain personality traits or tendencies. The five basic personality factors include:
- Extroversion
- Conscientiousness
- Agreeableness
- Openness to experience
- Neuroticism.

Typical characteristics of personality inventories are:
- They are quite long.
- They are paper and pencil test but offered in computer-based format.
- No right or wrong answers.
- Contains questions in a forced choice format rather than free response.
- Questions are often quite vague.

Minnesota Multiphasic Personality Inventory

It is a practical test of personality measurement. It consists of 550 verbal items, to which the person has to respond in "true", "false" and "cannot say". This scale is useful in measuring anxiety, hostility, hallucinations, phobias, and suicidal impulses. It also differentiates various types of neurotic and psychotic behavior. The 10 personality scales normally scored on the MMPI are as follows: Hypochondriasis, Depression, Hysteria, Psychopathic deviation, Masculinity-Femininity, Paranoia, Psychasthenia, Schizophrenia, Hypomania, and Social introversion.

The criticisms against MMPI are:
- Subjects make responses, which are acceptable to others, which may not be actually true. This reduces the validity of the scores obtained.
- Since the test items may not provide uniform meaning to all persons, it may produce different results from time to time.

Intelligence Tests

According to Woodsworth and Marquis, "Intelligence means intellect put to use. It is the use of intellectual abilities for handling a situation or accomplishing any task". According to Wagon, "Intelligence is the capacity to learn and adjust to relatively new and changing conditions". In general, intelligence is the ability to:
- Learn
- Deal with abstraction
- Make adjustment or to adapt to new situations
- Make appropriate responses to certain stimuli in a given situation.

According to David Wechsler, "Intelligence is the aggregate or global capacity of an individual to act purposefully, to think rationally, and to deal effectively with his environment".

Classification

Intelligence tests may be classified as:
- Individual tests vs group tests
- Verbal tests vs nonverbal tests.

Stanford-Binet scale is an example for individual verbal test for intelligence and the Alexander's Battery of performance test is an example of individual performance test for intelligence.

Army Alpha test is an example of group verbal intelligence tests, and the Army Beta test and the Chicago nonverbal test are examples of group nonverbal intelligence tests.

Wechsler Adult Intelligence Scale (WAIS)

It is a general test of Intelligence Quotient (IQ). Wechsler adopted from the Army tests. The WAIS-IV was standardized on a sample of 2,200 people in the United States ranging in age from 16 to 90 years. An extension of the standardization has been conducted with 688 Canadians in the same age range. The WAIS-IV measure is appropriate throughout adulthood and for use with those individuals aged 16 to 90. For persons under 16, the Wechsler Intelligence Scale for Children (WISC, 6–16 years) and the Wechsler Preschool and Primary Scale of Intelligence (WPPSI, 2 1/2–7 years 3 months) are used.

Uses of Intelligence Tests

- For measuring general learning readiness.
- To find out the differences in IQ among the children of same chronological age.
- To define more accurately the degree of intelligence quotient.
- To identify gifted children.
- For educational and vocational guidance.
- For study of mental growth.
- For homogeneous grouping.

Socioeconomic Status Scale

It is a tool to assess the socioeconomic status of a person or family. This scale is used in many community-based studies. This scale in general takes into consideration of the educational status, occupation and the family income. Based on the above data, we can classify a person's socioeconomic status as lower, middle and upper class. For example, Kuppuswamy's socioeconomic status scale classifies the socioeconomic status of person as lower, upper-lower, lower-middle, upper-middle, and upper class. He has assigned a separate score for various educational status and variations in occupation and monthly income. This scale is used in many correlational studies and also classifies the people based on their socioeconomic status.

Summary

- Evaluation, an integral part of an educational program, is the process of judging the effectiveness of educational experience through careful appraisal. Educational evaluation is made in relation to the objectives that have been determined previously by faculty, individual teachers and students.
- Evaluation is classified into various types. Based on the time during which the evaluation is done, it is classified into formative evaluation and summative evaluation. Based on the purpose, it is classified into criterion-referenced evaluation and norm-referenced evaluation. Based on the person who does evaluation, it is classified into internal evaluation and external evaluation.
- The terms criterion-referenced and norm-referenced were originally coined by Robert Glaser. A criterion-referenced test is one that provides for translating test scores into a statement about the behavior to be expected of a person with that score or their relationship to a specified subject matter. Most tests written by teachers are criterion-referenced tests.
- A norm-referenced test (NRT) is a type of test, assessment, or evaluation which yields an estimate of the position of the tested individual in a predefined population, with respect to the trait being measured. This estimate is derived from the analysis of test scores and possibly other relevant data from a sample drawn from the population.

- Some of the criteria for constructing tests are objectivity, validity, reliability, usability, practicality, feasibility, etc.
- The different types of evaluation tools used are essay, short-answer questions, multiple choice questions, rating scale, checklists, OSCE/OSPE, sociometry, anecdotal record, attitude scale, critical incident technique, etc.
- Item analysis is the process of analyzing the performance of a multiple choice item after it has appeared in a question paper.
- A standardized test is a test administered and scored in a consistent manner. The tests are designed in such a way that the questions, conditions for administering, scoring procedures, and interpretations are consistent and are administered and scored in a predetermined, standard manner.
- Some of the standardized tests are aptitude test, interest inventory, personality test, achievement test, socio-economic status scale, and tests for special mental and physical abilities and disabilities.

5. Nursing Educational Programs

"A teacher is one who makes himself progressively unnecessary".
—Thomas Carruthers

Objectives
After completing this unit, you will be able to:
- Appreciate the perspectives of nursing education at global and national level
- Understand the patterns of nursing education and training programs in India.

Introduction

Health for all implies both a revolution and decentralization, demanding changes in the role of all health professional at every level of the healthcare system. It also requires a preparation of healthcare worker, especially the nurses at various levels. In abroad and in India, nursing as a profession has undergone so many changes. Change is inevitable in any profession. Likewise in nursing, there were so many changes in the areas of education, practice, and research from the period of the nightingale to till today. The syllabus of all nursing courses has undergone many revisions according to the changes in the health plans and policies of the government and changing trends and advancements in education, nursing, health sciences, and medical technology.

Nursing Education at Global Level

There are various levels of nursing education in United States. They are:

Licensed Practical Nurse/Licensed Vocational Nurse Programs

This program prepares for LPN/LVN license. It is usually offered in high schools, hospitals, vocational, and technical schools and of 9–12 months duration. The aim is to teach basic technical bedside care. Each state board of nursing sets responsibilities and scope of practice. They usually work under the supervision of registered nurse or other licensed person and the scope of practice focuses on technical nursing procedures and treatments. They usually get employed in hospitals, nursing homes, and other structured settings. The LPN should pass the National Council Licensure Examination for Practical Nurse (NCLEX-PN).

Hospital-based Diploma Programs

It was one of the oldest and most traditional of nursing education programs. They began as training programs taught by physicians. Initially it was only a few weeks in length and then gradually extended to several months to one year and later two years to three years. It prepares for RN license. It is mostly offered in hospitals and some in conjunction with college. The diploma programs have declined since most colleges and universities do not recognize the diploma in nursing as an academic credential and also the growth of associate degree in nursing and Bachelor of Science in Nursing does not attract the candidate to the hospital-based diploma programs. The other factors are inability of the hospitals to continue finance nursing education, accreditation standards, and increased complexity of health care, which has required nurse to have greater academic preparation leads to decline in hospital-based diploma programs.

Associate Degree in Nursing

It is a two-year program in nursing. A LPN can take up the course of Associate Degree in Nursing and become a registered nurse. This also prepares for RN license. It is offered in community and junior college. They get employed primarily in institutions and provide basic technical care.

Bachelor of Science in Nursing

It is a four-year program and BSN is the basic qualification to enter into Master's Program in Nursing. It offers education for both basic students who are preparing for licensure examination and for registered nurses returning to school to obtain BSN (2 years duration).

Basic programs [like Basic BSc(N) in India] are offered in senior colleges or universities. After graduation, they have to undergo National Council for Licensing Examination for Registered Nurse. Then, they assume beginning practice and ultimately leadership positions in any healthcare settings including hospitals, community agencies, schools, clinics, and homes.

Master of Science in Nursing

The aim of master's program is to prepare advanced nurse practitioner and clinical nurse specialists. They are otherwise known as nurse practitioner. It is offered in universities and of 1–2 years duration. The scope of master's degree is advanced clinical practice, management, education, and leadership positions. Nurse practitioner writes prescriptions, receives reimbursement for care and does independent nurse practices, and operates health centers. The new option in master's education is the RN/MSN track, which allows registered nurse prepared at the associate degree or diploma level and who meet graduate admission requirement to enter a master's program leading to master's degree rather than a baccalaureate degree.

Combined degrees or a program such as MSN/MBA are available for nurse administrators.

Doctoral Programs

Doctoral programs are offered at universities and its purpose is to prepare for advanced nursing for research, clinical practice, and leadership positions. There are various kinds of programs or titles available at this level.

Doctor of Philosophy (PhD) is offered for those interested in research. It is an academic degree and prepares scholars for research and the development of theory.

Doctor of Nursing Science (DNS or DNSc) is offered for those who are interested in advanced clinical nursing practice. It is a professional practice degree and conceived as an advanced practice degree with an emphasis on clinical research. The DNS is extended to bridge the gap between the practice and research.

Doctor of Nursing (DN) is offered for those with higher degrees in nonnursing fields, who want to pursue a career in leadership.

Doctorate in Clinical Nursing practice prepares graduates for advanced clinical practice and clinical leadership.

Doctor of Nursing Education (DNEd) is offered for those who pursue research degree in nursing education.

Some of the other degrees offered are DEd (Doctor of Education) and DPH (Doctor of Public Health).

Certification Programs

It is a credential that has professional but not legal status. Specialized programs were developed to recognize nurses for advanced practice often lead to certification. These programs provide concentrated study in specific areas and last from several weeks to several months or even years. A comprehensive examination is required. Certified nurses have greater earning potential, wider employment opportunities, status, and prestige and in some states, they are eligible for insurance reimbursement, just as physicians are. Requirements for admission to certification programs vary, with some requiring only registered nurse licensure and others requiring either a baccalaureate or a master's degree.

Certification means that a certificate is awarded by a professional group as validation of specific qualifications demonstrated by a registered nurse in a defined area of practice. It includes Nurse Practitioner preparation programs such as Pediatrics, Gerontology, Family Health, Woman's Health care, Nurse Midwifery, and Nurse Anesthesia. The American Nurse Credentialing Center (ANCC), a subunit of the ANA, provides a number of certification programs for registered nurses. Some of the areas of certification offered by the American Nurse Credentialing Center are:
- Community health nurse
- Home health nurse
- Medical surgical nurse
- Pediatric nurse practitioner
- School nurse practitioner
- Family nurse practitioner.

Issues in Nursing Education

The LVN-to-BSN program is designed to merge with the RN-to-BSN program. Academically, LVN students differ from their generic counterparts. They frequently come from backgrounds where few parents or family members have university education. Many LVNs receive all of their prerequisite course work at community colleges, where academic standards may be less rigorous than those at 4-year university course.

LVNs experience academic challenges on admission to BSN programs. English is a second language, which compounds the challenge. Cultural diversity is also often an issue and students may struggle with a majority of professional value system incongruent to theirs, especially in the areas of time management, priority setting, interpersonal relationships, and personal presentation.

One additional challenge LVN students face is discrimination from multiple sources. Their employers may treat them as expendable, replaceable conveniences and offer less educational opportunity or support than is offered to their RN peers.

The LVN-to-BSN track builds from a focus on the care of acutely ill individuals in structured setting to a culminating focus on community-based care in less structured, less predictable settings. The program focuses initially on the role of professional nurses in providing care, then moves through the management of available resources, and finally establishes the role of the nurse as a member of the profession, leader, and change agent.

Specifically, the first semester in the LVN-to-BSN track includes a professional bridge course with an acute care clinical component, as well as deliberately tailored skills, laboratory course designed to cover RN-specific skills, and generally verify the student's skills competency.

For LVN students, the challenge is not in learning what nursing is, it is in stepping out of the follower, task oriented role in which they are successful and know well. They must assume a more autonomous, complex, strategic, and critical thinking leadership role. The challenge for the faculty is in developing the educational strategies that facilitate this professional metamorphosis.

Professional Socialization

LVNs approach the BSN program with a belief that they are really already functioning as RNs and have little new to learn beyond RN-specific tasks and that they are essentially just getting the credential to support their current practice. This creates two challenges. The first is a need to develop educational strategies specifically designed to facilitate their true role transition. The second is dealing with the frustration.

The LVN-to-BSN students need significantly less skills, laboratory and general acute care clinical time than do generic students. Instead, LVN students need clinical experiences that move them out of their comfort zone of familiar practice. Practice is structured to force LVNs into strategically focused, critical thinking leadership roles. Clinicals provide for some degree of autonomy, pushing the LVN students to go beyond a task-oriented behavior to be successful. Small group work and community learning projects allow students some choice in the specific area or topic on which they will focus and success depends on the student's ability to negotiate with clinical leaders to define both the vision and scope of the project and its implementation.

LVN students benefit from development as adult learners because their academic backgrounds are generally traditional and basic. General adult learning principles have been applied in the classroom, including a clear explanation with easy theory module, of the importance of understanding the material, opportunities through theory application assignments and projects for LVN students to use their own knowledge and experiences, and reflective learning assignments and projects embedded in real-life situations.

Course activities are also designed to strengthen areas in which LVNs are traditionally weak, such as reading comprehension, verbal and written articulation and presentation, and critical thinking. Case studies are used in all courses to refine and reinforce critical thinking and professional nurses roles as managers and providers of care.

There are associate and diploma programs that graduate nurses in 2–3 years, the traditional 4 years Bachelor of Science in Nursing (BSN) programs, and accelerated BSN programs that take 12–18 months.

Entry into-practice-master's degree prepares nurses to provide direct patient care in a variety of settings. It should be noted that this master's degree is a prelicensure program and is not an advanced practice degree. These programs are gaining popularity among adult learners.

To be admitted to the MN program, students complete 8 prerequisite courses—Anatomy and Physiology, Microbiology, Chemistry, Statistics, Psychology, Sociology, Lifespan Development, and Nutrition. A cumulative grade point average (GPA) of 3.0/4.0 in their undergraduate degree and prerequisite coursework and a successful interview with the program director are required.

The program spans 15 months or 4 consecutive semesters (6 graduate credits) beginning in one summer semester and ending in the following summer. The curriculum is unique in that it includes all theoretical content covered in a prelicensure program, provides a variety of clinical experiences in which the student can develop clinical reasoning and practice skills, and immerses the student in areas such as professional issues, research, nursing theory, leadership and management, and healthcare policy, consistent with graduate nursing education, by providing coursework and professional experiences in their areas.

In the first semester, students learn all of the nursing skills, including physical assessment and medication administration skills, with the exception of critical care skills and IV insertion. Theoretical content related to the skills is also presented.

Another key course in this first semester deals with professional roles and issues. Here, students learn about the profession, legal/ethical issues, and regulatory information. Students debate various issues facing the profession, including level of entry into practice, nursing shortage strategies, and consequences of impaired nurses, unionization and others.

The second semester has a heavy focus on medical-surgical and mental health nursing. In addition, students have a course on community nursing and research and theory. The clinical and theoretical courses have a heavy emphasis on evidence-based practice, which is threaded throughout the curriculum.

In the third semester, all students have a pediatric and obstetric theory course, a leadership course, and another research/theory course. The final summer semester focuses on critical care and role transition. In addition, a healthcare policy course is taken. The final 6 weeks is a preceptorship, where the students assume the role of a professional nurse, working for 192 hours (or sixteen 12-hour shifts) one-on-one with an experienced nurse on a unit of their choice.

Academic expectations are high because of the graduate status and accelerated nature of the degree. Students entering second degree option programs come as mature adult learners, who have excellent study habits and a hunger for learning. They bring their prior degree knowledge, work experience, and academic skills to this new educational endeavor. After taking the graduate coursework, the MN graduate has a broader vision and understanding of what nursing is and how he/she can contribute to the profession than a BSN graduate. Thus, the degree awarded reflects that the graduates abilities are beyond the BSN level.

The MN degree offers several advantages for the student. After graduates gain patient care experience, they are in a better position to take on leadership roles in their institutions. Second, students with a baccalaureate degree would prefer to obtain a master's degree, they see this as a vertical advancement of their education rather than a horizontal move. A third advantage is that more financial aid opportunities are available for students pursuing a master's degree. A final advantage is related to transferability of coursework. Given that the MN program is accredited as a "graduate" program, some of the coursework may be transferred, if the student goes on to pursue an advanced practice master's degree.

Five themes in the responses emerged most frequently are developing leadership/management skills, having a broader vision of the profession beyond patient care, understanding evidence-based practice, being more professional, and having a better understanding of research. The graduates noticed a difference between themselves and other new graduate nurses. The trends in these responses suggested that the program is accomplishing its goal of graduating an entry-level nurse who thinks about the profession more broadly than a BSN graduate does.

Nursing Education in United Kingdom (UK)

Many undergraduate, postgraduate, PG diploma, and doctoral programs are offered at United Kingdom for various durations to prepare nurses to work in the field of nursing.

Undergraduate Program in UK

The undergraduate program is of 3 years duration and is offered in various specialties as follows:
BSc (Hons) Nursing—Adult
BSc (Hons) Nursing—Child
BSc (Hons) Nursing—Mental Health
BSc (Hons) Nursing—Community Public Health Nursing
BSc (Hons) Nursing—Learning Disability Nursing
BSc (Hons) Nursing—Orthopedic Nursing
BSc (Hons) Nursing—Critical Care Nursing

For those who have a bachelor degree already and would like to choose nursing as a career, MSc Graduate Entry Nursing course is offered for 2 years duration. The examples of courses are Graduate Entry Nursing—Adult, Graduate Entry Nursing—Child, and Graduate Entry Nursing—Mental Health.

Postgraduate (PG) Diploma in Nursing

This course has been offered for graduates from any degree subject background who would like to become a nurse. The examples of course are as follows:
PG Dip Nursing Mental Health
PG Dip Nursing Adult
PG Dip Nursing Child
PG Dip Nursing Learning Disability

Postgraduate Nursing Program in UK

Postgraduate in Nursing is offered either full time or part time, the full time being 2 years duration and the part time is up to 5 years duration. The examples of courses offered are as follows:
MSc Clinical Nursing
MSc Advanced Nursing Practice
MSc Primary Care Nursing

Doctoral Program in Nursing in UK

Doctoral programs in Nursing are offered either full time for 3–4 years duration and part time for 5–7 years duration. There are online courses available. PhD in Nursing, Doctorate of Nursing Practice, and Interdisciplinary doctoral degrees are offered.

Nursing Education in China

China has a multitier nursing education system. Several programs lead to the title of registered nurse including:
- Diploma and Advanced Diploma
- Associate Programs
- Baccalaureate Programs
- Master's Programs

Diploma and Advanced Diploma

Diploma is offered by Schools of Health for students from junior high schools which is a 3-year nursing program designed to teach technical skills. Advanced Diploma is offered by colleges and universities with students from high schools and schools of health.

Associate Programs

A three-year Associate Nursing program is offered for general training alongside nursing theory and skills.

Baccalaureate Nursing Programs

This is offered by universities for students drawn from high schools and Diploma programs. Students enroll in a 5-year Bachelor of Nursing program providing a broad nursing foundation and this equips students to work at an advanced level of nursing in higher ranking hospitals or in management positions.

Master's Programs

The Masters of Nursing programs facilitate the development of expertise in either clinical practice or in research. Graduate nursing programs at the master's level are 3 years duration. There is a criticism that the Masters of Nursing course does not focus exclusively on professional nursing. Masters of Nursing course draws heavily on the medical-focused curriculum and includes other areas of study such as Political Theory, English Language, and Statistics.

Doctoral Programs

The Doctoral Nursing programs in China are a relatively recent phenomenon and the first Doctoral program was instituted in 2003. The Doctoral Nursing programs aim to train nurses in education, research, and management. Currently, there are two types of Doctoral Nursing programs in China—PhD by Research and Clinical Doctorate.

Students enrolled in doctoral programs are able to focus their research on Nursing management, Nursing education, Clinical practice, and specialized clinical field, such as Community Nursing or Mental Health Nursing. Enrolment in Doctoral programs is challenging for nurses for two reasons, such as shortage of current nursing-oriented learning resources and shortage of qualified nursing professionals to supervise postgraduate students.

Patterns of Nursing Education in India

The Indian Nursing Council is a statutory body that regulates nursing education in the country through prescription, inspection, examination, certification, maintaining standard, and uniform syllabus. They have also ensured easier measures for equivalence, exchange, and practice for nurses in any part of the country. There are various patterns of nursing education in India today. They are:

Nonuniversity Programs

- Auxiliary Nurse and Midwife
- General Nursing and Midwifery.

University Programs

- BSc(N)
- Post Basic BSc(N)
- MSc(N) in various specialties
- MPhil in Nursing
- PhD in Nursing.

Auxiliary Nurse and Midwife

The INC is committed to the position that the health worker training program must fit into the higher secondary education system. Auxiliary Nurse Midwives (ANMs) are regarded as the first contact person between people and organization, between needs and services, and between consumer and provider.

It is through their activities that people perceive health policies and strategies. It is through them that planners at the upper level gain insights into health problems and needs of the rural people. Considering their status as grass-root level workers in the health organizational hierarchy, a heavy responsibility rests on them.

The role of ANMs has been changing with the times. In the "50s" and "60s", training courses for ANMs focused on Midwifery and Maternal and Child Health (MCH) as 9 months out of 24 months were earmarked for these subjects. India's Second Five-Year Plan described the role of auxiliary health workers as those activities that supplemented the contributions made by doctors and other highly trained personnel for promoting preventive and curative health activities (GOI, 1986).

The Mukherjee Committee (1966) recommended a system of targets and incentives and identified ANMs and other village level workers as agents for the popularization of the program. In 1973, the Government of India (GOI) integrated the various functions of the health services, thereby changing the role of ANMs (Kartar Singh Committee, 1973).

In 1975, Srivastava Committee called for an expansion of the training to prepare them for multipurpose health work. ANMs were now required to provide child health services and primary curative care to villagers. In turn, the Indian Nursing Council (INC) approved an expanded syllabus in 1977. With this came the decision to reduce the training period from 24 months to 18 months.

The National Education Policy (1986) included the ANM program under the stream of Vocational Education. The INC again reviewed the curriculum for the +2 level and submitted its recommendations to the Ministry of Health and Family Welfare. However, only a few states have adopted this course at the higher secondary level as a vocational course.

Objectives of the Program

General: At the end of the training program, Auxiliary Nurse Midwife should demonstrate ability to plan and carry out job responsibilities assigned to her.

Specific: The ANM should demonstrate ability to:
- Explain the principles of healthful living related to all age groups in the community.
- Perform basic healthcare activities in community and institutional settings.
- Plan and carry out nutrition and health education activities in the home, clinic, and community.
- Provide basic maternal and child healthcare including immunization service, family healthcare, and family planning services.
- Perform basic midwifery procedures and basic nursing techniques with special emphasis on domiciliary and home nursing procedures.
- Participate in prevention and control of communicable diseases, assist in execution of national health programs, promote village and environmental sanitation, and perform basic nursing techniques.
- Provide first aid and emergency nursing care, elementary medical care includes treatment of minor ailments.
- Participate as a responsible member of health team.
- Identify community resources, which would be utilized for health promotion, health maintenance, and prevention of disease.
- Assist in the training community/village level health worker.
- Promote community development activities.

Admission Requirements
- The minimum age for admission should be 17 years.
- The maximum age for admission shall be 35 years.
- The minimum educational requirements for admission shall be successful completion of 12th class from a recognized board. Pass certificate will be required to support application.

Clinical Requirements for ANM Course
A school for training of the ANMs should be located in a community Health Center (PHC annexure) or a Rural Hospital (RH) having minimum bed strength of 30 and maximum 50 and serving an area with community health programs. The school should also be affiliated to a district hospital or a secondary care hospital in order to provide experiences of secondary level health care and an extensive obstetrics and gynecology care.

An organization having a hospital with 150 beds with minimum 30–50 obstetrics and gynecology beds and 100 delivery cases monthly can also open ANM school. They should also have an affiliation of PHC/CHC for the community health nursing field experience.

Existing ANM schools attached to District Hospitals should have PHC annexure (accommodation facility for 20–30 students) for community health field experience.

School has to be affiliated to district hospital or a secondary care hospital with minimum 150 beds.

Bed occupancy on the average should be between 60% and 70%.

Subjects Taught
The subjects taught are Nursing Foundations, Community Health Nursing, Maternal and Child Health Nursing and Basic Medicine, etc.

Duration of the Course
The total duration of the course is 2 years.

Diploma in General Nursing and Midwifery
The General Nursing and Midwifery course is conducted in many places in the country. The syllabus has undergone many revisions according to the change in the health plans and policies of the government and changing trends and advancements in general education, nursing, health sciences, and medical technology. The latest revision of syllabus by INC in 2015 has reduced the duration of the course from three and half years to three years. The basic entrance has become intermediate or class 12 instead of earlier class 10. Both science and arts students are eligible. The focus of general nursing education is the care of sick in the hospital. Schools of nursing are generally attached to teaching hospitals. Three board examinations are conducted, one at the end of each year. On passing, the candidates are registered as registered nurse and midwife by the respective state nursing councils.

Aims of DGNM Program
The basic Diploma course in General Nursing and Midwifery is geared to the health needs of the individuals, family, community, and the country at large. The aims of the Diploma in General Nursing and Midwifery program are:
1. To prepare nurses with a sound educational program in nursing to enable them to function as efficient members of the health team, beginning with the competencies for first level positions in all kinds of healthcare settings.
2. To help nurses develop an ability to cooperate and coordinate with members of the health team in the prevention of disease, promotion of health, and rehabilitation of the sick.
3. To help nurses in their personal and professional development, so that they are able to make maximum contribution to the society as useful and productive individuals, citizens as well as efficient nurses.
4. To serve as a base for further professional education and specialization in nursing.
5. To prepare nurses to keep pace with latest professional and technological developments and use these for providing nursing care service.

Student's Admission
- Age for the entrance shall be 17–35 years, provided they meet the minimum educational requirement, i.e. 12 years of schooling.
- Minimum education—all students should pass 12 classes or its equivalent, preferably with science subjects.
- Admission of students shall be once a year.
- Students should be medically fit.

The selection committee should comprise tutors, nurse administrators, and educationalist/psychologist. The principal of the school shall be the chairperson.

Training Program
It is of 3 years duration with 40 hours per week for 46 weeks. The first year course includes Biosciences, Behavioral Sciences, Nursing Foundations, Community Health Nursing, English, and Computer Education. The second year course includes Medical Surgical Nursing I and II, Mental Health Nursing, and Child Health Nursing. The third year course includes Midwifery and Gynecological Nursing and Community Health Nursing. Also, internship is placed in third year during which besides clinical posting in all specialty areas, theoretical hours for Nursing Education, Administration, Research, and Professional Trends and Adjustments are given. The INC has issued notification regarding phasing out of DGNM in the year 2021. Last admission year for GNM training program shall be 2020–21 academic year and no admission shall be made to GNM program thereafter.

Bachelor of Nursing Course
Graduate nursing education was started in India in the year 1946 in CMC, Vellore and in the RAK College of Nursing at Delhi University. At present, several universities in India offer the course.

Aims of BSc(N) Program
The aim of the undergraduate nursing program is to:
- Prepare graduates to assume responsibilities as professional, competent nurses, and midwives in providing promotive, preventive, curative, and rehabilitative services.
- Prepare nurses who can make independent decisions in nursing situations, protect the rights of and facilitate individuals and groups in pursuit of health, function in the hospital, community nursing services, and conduct research studies in the areas of nursing practice. They are also expected to assume the role of teacher, supervisor, and manager in a clinical/public health setting.

Eligibility for Admission
A candidate seeking admission should have:
- Passed the 2-year of preuniversity examination or equivalent as recognized by concerned university with science subjects, i.e. physics, biology, and chemistry.
- Obtained at least 45% of total marks in science subjects in the qualifying examination, if belongs to a scheduled caste or tribe, should have obtained not less than 40% of total marks in science subjects (percentage of total marks is subject to change as per INC norms).
- Completed 17 years of age at the time of admission or will complete this age on or before 31st December of the year of admission.
- Be medically fit.

Course of Study
The course of study leading to bachelor degree comprises four academic years. Table 5.1 lists the course details of the program.

Bachelor of Nursing Course (Postcertificate) for Qualified Nurses
The goal of postcertificate degree program leading to Bachelor of Science in Nursing is the preparation of the trained nurse as a generalist who accepts responsibility for enhancing the effectiveness of nursing care.

Eligibility for Admission
The candidate seeking admission must:
- Hold a certificate in general nursing.
- Be a registered nurse.
- Have passed preuniversity examination in the Arts/Science/Commerce or its equivalent which is recognized by the university.
- Be medically fit.
- Have a good personal and professional record.
- Have working knowledge of English.

Program of Study
Duration: The program of the study is two academic years from the date of commencement of program. Terms and vacations shall be as notified by the university from time to time.

Objectives: The goal of the postcertificate program leading to the Bachelor of Nursing is the preparation of the trained nurses as a generalist who accepts responsibility for enhancing the effectiveness of nursing care.
- Administer high-quality nursing care to all people of all ages in homes, hospitals, and other community agencies in urban and rural areas.
- Apply knowledge from the physical, social, and behavioral sciences in assessing the health status of individuals and make critical judgment in assessing the health status of the individuals and make critical judgment in planning, directing, and evaluating primary, acute, and long-term care given by themselves and others working with them.
- Investigate healthcare problems systematically.
- Work collaboratively with members of other health disciplines.

Nursing Educational Programs

Table 5.1: BSc(N) Program (4 years duration including internship).

Objectives of the program	Admission criteria	Subjects taught	Examination
To prepare graduates to assume responsibilities as professional competent nurses and midwives in providing promotive, preventive, curative, and rehabilitative services in the hospital, community, and other settings and also to prepare to assume the role of teacher, supervisor, manager, and researcher in various settings	Age shall be 17 years on or before 31st December of the year of admission. A pass in +2 (HSCE) or Senior School Certificate Examination (10+2), predegree examination (10+2), or an equivalent with 12 years schooling from a recognized board or university with Science, Physics, Chemistry, Biology, and English with minimum of 45% aggregate marks	**I year** Anatomy, Physiology, Nutrition, Biochemistry, Nursing Foundation, Psychology, Microbiology, Introduction to Computer, and English **II year** Sociology, Pharmacology, Pathology, Genetics, Medical Surgical Nursing I, Community Health Nursing I, and Communication and Educational Technology **III year** Medical Surgical Nursing II, Child Health Nursing, Mental Health Nursing, and Nursing Research **IV year** Midwifery and Obstetrical Nursing, Community Health Nursing II, and Management of Nursing Services and Education **Internship (Integrated Practice)** Midwifery and Obstetrical Nursing, Community Health Nursing II, Medical Surgical Nursing, and Child Health, Mental Health	**I year** **Theory** Anatomy and Physiology, Nutrition and Biochemistry, Nursing Foundation, Psychology, Microbiology, Introduction to Computer, and English **Practical and Viva Voce** Nursing Foundations **II year** **Theory** Sociology, Pharmacology, Pathology and Genetics, Medical Surgical Nursing I, Community Health Nursing I, and Communication and Educational Technology **Practical and Viva Voce** Medical Surgical Nursing I **III year** **Theory** Medical Surgical Nursing II, Child Health Nursing, Mental Health Nursing, and Nursing Research **Practical and Viva Voce** Medical Surgical Nursing II Child Health Nursing, Mental Health Nursing **IV year** **Theory** Midwifery and Obstetrical Nursing, Community Health Nursing II, and Management of Nursing Services and Education **Practical and Viva Voce** Midwifery and Obstetrical Nursing Community Health Nursing Theory examination will be conducted in all subjects. There will be an internal and external assessment

- Teach and counsel individuals, families, and other groups about health and illness.
- Understand human behavior and establish effective interpersonal relationships.
- Teach in clinical nursing situations.
- Identify underlying principles from the social and natural sciences and utilize them in adapting to, or initiating changes in relation to those factors.
- Acquire professional knowledge and attitude in adapting for leadership roles.

Course of Study for PBSc(N)
I year
- Nursing Foundation
- Nutrition and Dietetics
- Biochemistry and Biophysics
- Psychology
- Maternal Nursing
- Child Health Nursing
- Microbiology
- Medical and Surgical Nursing
- English.

II year
- Sociology
- Community Health Nursing
- Mental Health Nursing
- Introduction to Nursing Education
- Introduction to Nursing Administration
- Introduction to Nursing Research and Statistics.

Degree of Master of Nursing

Objectives
Graduates of Masters of Nursing program demonstrate:
- Increased cognitive, affective, and psychomotor competencies and the ability to utilize the potentials for effective nursing performance.
- Expertise in the utilization of concepts and theories for the assessment, planning, and intervention in meeting the self-care needs of an individual for the attainment of fullest potentials in the field of specialty.
- Ability to practice independently as a nurse specialist.
- Ability to function effectively as nurse educators and administrators.
- Ability to interpret the health-related research.
- Ability to plan and initiate change in the healthcare system.
- Leadership qualities for the advancement of practice of professional nursing.
- Interest in lifelong learning for personal and professional learning advancement.

Eligibility
The candidate seeking admission must:
- Have passed BSc Nursing/Postcertificate BSc, or Nursing degree of any university.
- Have a minimum of one year of experience after obtaining BSc in hospitals or nursing educational institutions or community health setting.
- For BSc, nursing postcertificate, a one-year experience is needed prior or after graduation. The candidate shall be a registered nurse and registered midwife.
- The candidate shall be selected on merit judged on the basis of academic performances in BSc Nursing, Postcertificate BSc, or Nursing and selection tests.

Specialties
Candidate will be examined in any of the following branches:
- Branch 1: Medical Surgical Nursing (now there are so many subspecialties in the II year such as Neuro-Sciences Nursing, Cardiovascular Nursing, Orthopedic Nursing, etc.)
- Branch 2: Pediatric Nursing
- Branch 3: Obstetric and Gynecological Nursing
- Branch 4: Community Health Nursing
- Branch 5: Psychiatric Nursing
- See Table 5.2 for course details.

Master of Philosophy Program in Nursing

In 1980, RAK College of Nursing started MPhil program as a regular and part time course. Since then several universities started taking students for the MPhil course in nursing. Prominent among these are: the TN Dr MGR Medical University, Rajiv Gandhi University of Health Sciences, SNDT Women's University and Delhi University, and Manipal Academy of Higher Education.

Objectives
The objectives of MPhil degree course in nursing are:
- To strengthen the research foundation of nurses for encouraging research attitudes and problem-solving capacities.
- To provide basic training required for research in undertaking doctoral work.

Duration
Duration of the full time MPhil course will be one year and part time MPhil course will be two years.

Course of Study
At the time of admission, each candidate will be required to indicate her priorities in regard to the optional courses. A candidate may be offered one course from MPhil program from the Department of Anthropology, Education, Sociology, and Psychology or any suitable department. The MPhil studies will be divided into two distinct parts, part 1 and part 2.
- Part 1: It consists of 3 courses, i.e. Research Methods in Nursing, Major Aspects of Nursing, and Allied Disciplines.
- Part 2: After passing the part 1 examination, a student shall be required to write a dissertation. The topic and the nature of the dissertation of each candidate will be determined by the advisory committee consisting of three members. The dissertation may include results of original research, a fresh interpretation of existing facts, and data or a review article of critical nature.

Doctor of Philosophy in Nursing

A candidate for admission to the course for the degree of Doctor of Philosophy in the faculties of medical science must have obtained MPhil degree of a university or have a good academic record with first or second class Master's degree of an Indian or a foreign university in the concerned subject.

The candidate shall apply to the university for the admission stating his qualifications and the subject he proposes to investigate enclosing a statement on any work he has done in the subject. Every application for the admission of the course must be analyzed by the Board of Research Studies.

Eligibility Criteria
The candidate should be Postgraduate in Nursing with more than 55% of aggregates of marks.
- Should have research background
- May or may not have published articles in journals

Table 5.2: MSc(N) (2 years duration).

Objectives of the program	Admission criteria	Subjects taught	Examination
To prepare graduates to assume responsibilities as nurse specialists, consultants, educators, administrators, and researchers in various settings. To prepare nurses with advanced nursing knowledge and clinical practice skills in a specialized area of practice	BSc(N) or Post Basic BSc(N) with minimum of one year experience in College, School of Nursing, Hospital, or Community. She should be a registered Nurse and Midwife.	**First Year** Nursing Education Advanced Nursing Practice Clinical Specialty I Nursing Research and Statistics **Second Year** Nursing Management Dissertation Clinical Specialty II	**First Year** **Theory** Nursing Education Advanced Nursing Practice Clinical Specialty I Nursing Research and Statistics **Practical and Viva Voce** Nursing Education Clinical Specialty I **Second Year** **Theory** Nursing Administration Clinical Specialty II **Practical and Viva Voce** Clinical Specialty II Dissertation and Viva

- The course duration for regular PhD is three years and for the part time is four years.

Post Basic Diploma Programs

Purpose

The course is given to train nurses to render quality care to patients and also manage and supervise patient care in clinical and community settings. They also expected to teach nurses, allied health professionals, patients, and communities in areas related to their specialty and conduct research.

Admission Criteria

RN and RM with one year of clinical experience.

Duration: One Year.

Courses offered

The post basic diploma courses offered are:
- Cardiothoracic Nursing
- Critical Care Nursing
- Emergency and Trauma Nursing
- Neonatal Nursing
- Neurological and Neurosurgical Nursing
- Oncology Nursing
- Operating Room Technique and Management
- Psychiatric Nursing
- Renal Nursing.

Summary

- In abroad and in India, nursing as a profession has emerged after so many changes. Change is inevitable in any profession. Likewise in nursing, there were so many changes in the areas of education, practice, and research from the period of nightingale to till today.
- There are various programs such as Licensed Practical Nurse/Licensed Vocational Nurse Programs, Hospital-based Diploma Programs, Associate Degree in Nursing, Bachelor of Science in Nursing, Master of Science in Nursing, Doctoral Programs, and Certification Programs, which are provided at global level.
- In India, Nonuniversity Programs such as Auxiliary Nurse Midwife and Diploma in Nursing and University Programs such as BSc(N), Post Basic BSc(N), MSc(N) in various specialties, MPhil in Nursing, and PhD in Nursing are provided.

6 Continuing Education in Nursing

"There is an inborn desire or motivation in all of us that cries to be nourished and satisfied above and beyond merely to survive".

—Tough (1979)

Objectives
After completing this unit, you will be able to:
- Understand the importance and steps in organizing continuing nursing education program
- Appreciate the need for research in continuing nursing education
- Analyze the various modes of distance education in nursing.

Introduction

Continuing education provides information and skills of current issues, prepares for discussions, and helps to develop problem-solving skills. The word "problem" is derived from the Greek word "problema" and "proballein" meaning something, which is thrown in front of you that obstructs your path. Continuing education in the broadest sense is all additional education or learning gained by the individual to increase knowledge and skills. The concept of continuing education is growing up very fast in nursing services. Literature says that nursing was the forerunner in offering continuing education for staff development in foreign countries. This resulted in high standard of nursing service and nursing education. Today, the expanded role of nurses calls for intelligent assessment of the nursing, which needs planning for intervention and implementation of these interventions to meet the assessed needs and evaluation of these interventions. Maintenance of accurate records and reports in imparting health education to the patients are also the nurse's responsibilities. The impetus for continuing education within the discipline of nursing has resulted from nursing's desire for continuous growth and development. Every developing profession demands constant educational and information renewal.

Meaning and Definition

According to the ANA, continuing nursing education is defined as "planned educational activities intended to build upon the educational and experiential bases of the professional nurse for the enhancement of practice, education, administration, and research or theory development to the end of improving the health of the public".

Continuing education in nursing is defined as "planned learning experiences beyond a basic nursing educational program". The learning experiences are designed to promote the development of knowledge, skills, and attitudes for the enhancement of nursing practice, thus improving healthcare to the public (ANA, 1974).

According to the American Society for Healthcare Education and Training (ASHET), continuing education that is broad in scope and designed to build upon previously learned knowledge and skills.

Concept of Continuing Education

The term "continuing education" implies that education is a lifelong process. It is not something that takes place at a certain age alone. It is a continuous lifelong process. It is from womb to tomb. Technological changes and researches in every field of life demand education in order to keep up and not to become back numbers. The integrated process of keeping abreast of new realms of knowledge from prekindergarten to the postretirement age can be given the title of continuing education.

Another important aspect of this term continuing education is that it does not take place in a classroom or in an institutional or formal way alone. It can occur in all places and at all hours. The expression of continuing education has a comprehensive connotation. It may include formal education as well as nonformal education. Continuing education can be syllabus oriented or need-oriented affair.

Continuing education (CE) for health professionals can be defined as processes aimed at improving healthcare outcomes through learning, either by individual efforts or as part of activities, products, and services developed by the employers, professional bodies, or CE provider units.

Continuing education is "any extension of opportunities for reading, study, and training to any person and adults following their completion of or withdrawal from full-time school and college programs", i.e. continuing education means all education that takes place beyond basic nursing school or college. It is, therefore, education for adults provided by specific schools, centers, colleges, or institutions that emphasizes flexible rather than traditional academic programs. It is often on part-time basis, voluntarily, and purposeful efforts toward the self-development of the individual by public or private agencies. Continuing education is a planned activity directed toward meeting the learning needs of the nurse following basic nursing education, exclusive of formal postbasic education. Continuing education is a part of lifelong education and made mandatory under staff development programs.

Need for Continuing Education

"In sandy soil, when deep you delve, you reach the springs below; the more you learn, the freer streams of wisdom flow".
—Thiruvalluvar

Nothing is permanent in the universe. Everything would undergo a change either for worse or for better. If we do not grow in knowledge and perception, our ideas shrink so that we were reduced to mere frogs in the well. It is only education that enables and empowers one to meet the emerging challenges as well as to develop the vision and meaning in life.

Dr Rabindranath Tagore, while describing a true teacher, observed "if the teacher does not possess learning, how can he/she impart it to others?" The idea of lifelong education was triggered off in our country by the Kothari Commission (1964–1966) and was strengthened by a report of the International Commission on the Development of Education (1971–1972).

Traditionally, human life is segmented into three stages. They are—the first segment is devoted to learning, the second to earning, and the third to enjoying. The ability to comprehend and manage life skillfully in the fast changing complexity has become imperative and inevitable. In today's environment, the current healthcare picture consists of rapid changes, cost-containment measures, staffing shortage, and an increased emphasis on quality of nursing care.

Farewell (1988) suggests that the half-life of nursing knowledge ranges from 2 years to 5 years. Therefore, continued professional development is vital to the delivery of quality care. Continuing professional education in nursing has benefits for nurses, clients, and the service. Therefore, it is necessary for nurses to:
- Keep pace with new development.
- Enhance professional knowledge base through sharing or practical experiences.
- Increase their opportunities to participate in problem-solving and decision-making.
- Learn ways to collaborate and participate in decisions affecting our profession and population we serve.
- Enhance their practical reasoning skills through action-research process.
- Thereby, nurses maintain professional competence throughout their career.

The need for continuing education comes from the phenomena of change. Professional roles are altered as society changes and as new knowledge and technology emerge. The individual, who wishes to avoid obsolescence, cannot leave to chance his acquisition of new knowledge or his ability to adapt to changing demands. If nursing profession is to respond effectively to the challenge of developing wise leadership and competent practitioners, current social changes must be accepted and future ones are foreseen. There are forces within the nursing profession as well as in the larger society, which highlight the need for planned programs of continuing education. The delivery of health care depends to varying degrees on three major sources of input: the patient, the healthcare system or care setting, and the healthcare professional. Competence and performance of healthcare professional and of the patient, in conjunction with the condition and performance of the care system, collectively determine the outcome of the intervention (health care).

Purposes of Continuing Nursing Education

Continuing Nursing Education
- Leads to improved professional practice.
- Aids in updating knowledge and skills at all levels of the organization.
- Keeps abreast of the latest trends and developments in techniques.
- Equips with knowledge of current research and developments.
- Helps in learning new knowledge and maintain old competencies.
- Develops interest and job satisfaction among the staff.
- Develops sense of responsibilities for being competent and knowledgeable.
- Creates supportive environment with opportunities for growth and communication.
- Helps in adjusting to change.
- Aids in developing leadership skills, motivation, and better attitudes.
- Encourages in achieving self-development and self-confidence.

Forms of Continuing Education Programs

Continuing education programs can be formal and informal and in service or outside the organization. In the United States, it is mandatory for all registered nurses to undergo CEs in specific areas for getting relicensure. But in India, it is not made mandatory to undergo CEs for registration in all States. In the State of Tamil Nadu, it is mandatory for the nurses to undergo CE programs to earn credit hours for the renewal of their license. Journal clubs, ward libraries, discussion forums, online certification programs, and case report studies are kinds of continuing education programs and informal learning includes self-learning, subscribing to journals, etc. Formal continuing learning includes undergoing organizational staff development programs, short-term courses related to the professional areas, etc. Recognized forms of postsecondary learning activities within the domain include degree credit courses by nontraditional students, nondegree career training, workforce training, formal personal enrichment courses (both on campus and online), self-directed learning (such as through internet interest groups, clubs, or personal research activities), and experiential learning as applied to problem solving.

Continuing education is an encompassing term within a broad spectrum of postsecondary learning activities and programs. Within the domain of continuing education, professional continuing education is a specific learning activity generally characterized by the issuance of a certificate by the Continuing Education Units (CEUs) for the purpose of documenting attendance at a designated seminar or course of instruction. Licensing bodies in a number of fields impose continuing education requirements on members, who hold licenses to practice within a particular profession. These requirements are intended to encourage professionals to expand their knowledge base and stay up-to-date on new developments. Depending on the field, these requirements may be satisfied through college or university coursework, extension courses, or conferences and seminar attendance. In general, CEs are implemented under in service education and staff development programs, which include orientation, skill training, leadership, and management development and continuing education.

Philosophy of Continuing Education

It is believed that the system of higher education, which provides the basic preparation for the members of a profession, must also provide opportunities for practitioners to keep abreast of advances in their field. Adult learners must be encouraged to update regularly the obsolete and the desire for constant renewal, which can be facilitated and reassured that there are many interesting ways to accomplish this goal.

Planning Continuing Education Programs

The learning needs of the adults are far different from the needs of the children. Adults have already completed the basics and established a large reservoir of experiential learning that makes them independent and responsible for their own learning needs. A systematic approach is necessary to provide quality continuing education activities and services. Planning for continuing education programs follow the familiar medical model for patient care, which includes diagnosis, treatment planning, treatment implementation, and follow-up. Planning for continuing education begins with an identification of needs, followed by setting objectives, setting educational activities, and evaluation. A congruence must be established among needs, objectives, activities, implementation, and evaluation.

Characteristics of Continuing Education

Program Content

The content of continuing education programs consists of concepts, principles, research findings, or theories related to nursing that build on the nurses' previously acquired knowledge, attitudes, and skills. In addition to content that ultimately improves patient care, the content of continuing program may also afford nurses the more general benefit of improved professional development as well as career advancement. Clinical topics might include areas such as working more effectively with families, creative approaches to discharge planning, modifying dressings for unique patient needs, working collaboratively with other hospital departments, simplified method of dosage calculations, and reducing the potential for legal liabilities. Topics related to leadership development also need to be widely applicable. Leadership topics appropriate for continuing education might include problem-solving, decision-making, delegation, critical thinking, organizing workloads, or establishing priorities of nursing care.

Preparation of Content

The most challenging aspect of continuing education is the need to foster innovative and creative approaches to nursing care of patients. Its purpose is to achieve more effective behavior in nursing practice to improve the patient care. At the other side, it brings out the potentials of the staff and helps in deciding which persons are able to assume more responsibility in their respective jobs according to the levels at which they function. The content may be developed on the basis of:
- Contents on the clinical areas like neonatal nursing, pediatric nursing, mental health nursing, cardiopulmonary nursing, surgical nursing, etc.
- Level of group of nurses like graduates, undergraduates, postgraduates, etc.
- Designations like staff nurses, ward supervisors, nursing tutors, etc.
- Experience like a new graduate or a nurse with three years experience in a specific clinical area and so on.

Program Duration

They are shorter in duration than orientation programs and longer than in-service offerings. The duration of continuing education offering is usually related to the scope of content covered and the format used to present the learning experience.

Program Format

It refers to the method we adopt to deliver the educational program. It may include brief sessions (lasting less than one hour) or more lengthy formats such as a workshop, seminar, conference, course, symposium, or self-study.

A workshop is a brief (often only a single day) but in-depth educational program for a relatively small group of participants. Teaching strategies such as small group exercises, group discussion, case studies, role plays, and various forms of audio-visual media may be used.

A seminar consists of a small group of learners, who come to the learning experience prepared to exchange information about a specific topic. The subject for the seminar is determined in advance and participants are expected to come prepared to discuss the topic following their own reading and study.

A conference involves participant discussion related to a single problem, situation, or an issue. A conference leader or coordinator may facilitate exchanges among and between groups and subgroups in attendance.

A course usually consists of an ordered series of classes or other learning experiences related to the same topic area. In contrast to academic courses that last for a number of months, short-term continuing education courses may last only a few days.

An institute consists of an intensive program of instruction related to a particular field in which expert consultants present information to the participants.

A symposium usually involves two or more experts presenting content related to an identified theme, followed by a summary of their comments by a symposium moderator and then a question and answer period. A symposium can accommodate a fairly large audience but often aims for 10–20 audience members.

Self-study includes programmed instruction, self-learning packages, reading books or journals, or using audio visuals or computer-assisted instructional programs.

Methods of Delivery

The methods of delivery of continuing education can include traditional types of classroom lectures and laboratories.

However, much continuing education makes heavy use of distance learning, which not only includes independent study, but which can include videotaped/CD-ROM material, broadcast programming, and online/internet delivery. In addition to independent study, the use of conference-type group study, which can include study networks (which can, in many instances, meet together online) as well as different types of seminars/workshops, can be used to facilitate learning. A combination of traditional, distance, and conference-type study, or two of these three types, may be used for a particular continuing education course or program.

Evaluating CE Activities

Continuing education programs are evaluated by the providing units. The issues related to continuing education evaluation are:

- Is there some logical relationship between the planned educational project and the identified needs of participant in relation to their practice responsibilities?
- What is the evidence that the program actually attended to the learning needs of participants?
- Are the project's goals and objectives stated appropriately?
- What evidence is there that the goals and objectives of the project have been achieved?
- Are the selection, orientation, and motivation of the faculty effective?
- Did the faculty demonstrate appropriate instructional and interpersonal skills in conducting the activities?
- Did the practice nurse who attended the project have the background and experiences that were anticipated when the project was planned?
- Are the planned activities based on the logic and on the principles and generalizations of management and educational psychology?
- Are the planned physical facilities appropriate?
- Do the instructional materials meet accepted criteria?
- Were the instructional materials used as planned?
- What was the impact of the evaluation?
- Is the program cost-effective?

Providers of Continuing Education Program

The five major providers for the continuing education are the following:
1. Universities and professional educational institutions
2. Professional organizations
3. Employers
4. Independent providers
5. Healthcare institutions such as hospitals, etc.

Elements Essential for Successful Implementation of Continuing Education

- A recognized need for continuing nursing education.
- The availability of nursing faculty with diverse areas of expertise.

- A working relationship between an accredited provider of continuing nursing education program and nursing faculty.

Relationship between Practice and Need for Continuing Education

As advances and changes in healthcare system such as shorter hospital stays, more outpatient department, and community services take place, patients are experiencing interactions with several nursing professionals from variety of organizations.

Patient's stories are a way to enhance continuing education. For example, patients may view cancer treatment from prediagnosis to completion of treatment as a continuum during which time they interact with nursing professional in several stages and locations. When these patient stories and their experience in the healthcare system are contrasted with research results, several issues emerge. Thus, it increases knowledge, changes attitudes, and patient behavior related to cancer treatment.

School and college of nursing education program in conjunction with continuing nursing education program is coprovided. It helps in improving the interaction between the nurses in clinical setting and the faculty. It also helps to change the views of the faculty members thereby it benefits the faculty members, their clients, etc. The faculty members can also assist the staff nurses to keep themselves current about changes in health care.

Implications of Continuing Education

Continuing education sessions are ideal place for representatives from each agency to speak about their experience with patients with a specific health problem.
- It helps to explore formal and informal communication methods, e.g. nursing process application, planned nursing rounds, etc.
- It helps in understanding the institutional structures that manage health service to determine the changes that are required.
- It expands the notions of health care and health services.
- It develops the issue of consumer rights of patients.
- It examines the positions of nurses and their rights as employees.
- It upgrades the ethical issues of nursing profession as well as the health profession in general.
- It identifies the critical issues facing the health sector and the role of nurses in facilitating changes.

Areas to be Addressed by Continuing Education

Traditionally, continuing education is a formalized presentation on a topic relevant to the nurses employed by a particular organization or who share a particular practice. It has been focusing only on clinical performance and improving learner's competence in their current positions. Today, the changes in the system of healthcare delivery, cost containment, and questions about the role of nursing are also the areas to be addressed by continuing education.

Currently, professional practice issues related to new skills, expanding responsibilities, and increasing autonomy are addressed. Theoretical concepts used in nursing staff development are drawn from a variety of discipline as adult learning, human resource development, adult education, nursing theory, systems and organizational development, etc. There is also the focus toward human development, which includes skills in information management, decision and planning research and investigation, communication, human and interpersonal relationship, critical thinking, management and administration, valuing, time management, public relationship, new teaching techniques, stress management, preretirement counseling, and personal development and learning. Rather than focusing only on clinical, administrative, and academic performance, broader issues facing the nursing profession have become increasingly vital, especially in the context of globalization, liberalization, and the unprecedented thrust and manipulation of market economy, which has become the major determining factor for both health and health care. Some of them are:
- Global, national, and local economies
- Policies of multilateral agencies such as World Bank, the national and state policies affecting health care
- Managed care practices
- Health industry and healthcare competition
- Political economy of health
- Human rights and consumer rights specifically
- Changes in demographics
- Current community efforts to ameliorate social, political, and economic problems
- Team building
- Conflict management
- Critical thinking courses.

Recommendations

Practice should be incorporated as an integral component of the faculty to help them keep in touch with the realities of the clinical world. Budden (1994) states that nurse educators are perceived as "living in ivory towers" because they spend most of their time in classroom.

All schools and colleges of nursing should be encouraged to integrate continuing education program by combining services offered by the institution.

The educational services and health services should be integrated administratively that in effect with the healthcare institutions or at least the nursing services should be under the administrative control of the schools or College of Nursing.

There should be a well-structured continuing nursing education department with specific objectives and faculty with diverse expertise in order to respond to the learning needs identified.

The scope of continuing education should extend beyond the conventional nursing topics to broad and specific subjects that have implications on health and health services.

Principles of Adult Learning

Adult Learning (Andragogy)

Malcolm Knowles (1978, 1990) is the theorist, who brought the concept of adult learning. He has argued that adulthood has arrived, when people behave in adult ways and believe themselves to be adults, then they should be treated as adults. He taught that adult learning was special in a number of ways. For example:

- Adult learners bring a great deal of experience to the learning environment. Educators can use this as a resource.
- Adults expect to have a high degree of influence on what they are to be educated for and how they are to be educated.
- The active participation of learners should be encouraged in designing and implementing educational programs.
- Adults need to be able to see applications for new learning.
- Adult learners expect to have a high degree of influence on how learning will be evaluated.
- Adults expect their responses to be acted upon when asked for feedback on the progress of the program.

Burns (1995) said that by adulthood, people are self-directing. This is the concept that lies at the heart of andragogy. Andragogy is, therefore, student-centered, experience-based, problem-oriented, and collaborative very much in the spirit of the humanist approach to learning and education. The whole educational activity turns on the adult learner since.

- Adult learner are autonomous and self-directed.
- Adult learner have accumulated a foundation of life experiences and knowledge.
- Adult learner are goal-oriented.
- Adult learner are relevancy-oriented.
- Adult learner are practical.
- Adult learner need to be shown respect.

According to **Stephen Lieb** (1991), one aspect of adult learning is motivation. At least six factors serve as sources of motivation for adult learning:

1. **Social relationships:** To make new friends, to meet a need for associations and friendships.
2. **External expectations:** To comply with instructions from someone else; to fulfill the expectations or recommendations of someone with formal authority.
3. **Social welfare:** To improve ability to serve mankind, prepare for service to the community, and improve ability to participate in community work.
4. **Personal advancement:** To achieve higher status in a job, secure professional advancement, and stay abreast of competitors.
5. **Escape/stimulation:** To relieve boredom, provide a break in the routine of home or work, and provide a contrast to other exacting details of life.
6. **Cognitive interest:** To learn for the sake of learning, seek knowledge for its own sake, and to satisfy an inquiring mind.

Elements of Learning

There are four critical elements of learning that must be addressed to ensure that participants learn. These elements are:

- Motivation
- Reinforcement
- Retention
- Transference.

Motivation

The instructor must establish rapport with participants and prepare them for learning, this provides motivation. Instructors can motivate students via several means:

- Set a feeling or tone for the lesson
- Set an appropriate level of concern
- Set an appropriate level of difficulty
- Feedback must be specific, not general
- Participants must also see a reward for learning.

Reinforcement

Reinforcement is a very necessary part of the teaching/learning process; through it, instructors encourage correct modes of behavior and performance.

Positive reinforcement is normally used by instructors, who are teaching participants new skills. As the name implies, positive reinforcement is "good" and reinforces "good" (or positive) behavior.

Negative reinforcement is the constant removal of a noxious stimulus that tends to increase the behavior. The constant presentation of a noxious stimulus that tends to decrease a behavior is called punishment.

Retention

Students must retain information from classes in order to benefit from the learning. The instructors' jobs are not finished until they have assisted the learner in retaining the information. In order for participants to retain the information taught, they must see a meaning or purpose for that information. They must also understand and be able to interpret and apply the information. This understanding includes their ability to assign the correct degree of importance to the material.

The amount of retention will be directly affected by the degree of original learning. Simply stated, if the participants did not learn the material well initially, they will not retain it well either.

Retention by the participants is directly affected by their amount of practice during the learning. Instructors should emphasize retention and application. After the students demonstrate correct (desired) performance, they should be urged to practice to maintain the desired performance. Distributed practice is similar in effect to intermittent reinforcement.

Transference

Transfer of learning is the result of training, it is the ability to use the information taught in the course but in a new setting. As with reinforcement, there are two types of transfer—positive and negative.

Positive transference, like positive reinforcement, occurs when the participants use the behavior taught in the course.

Negative transference, again like negative reinforcement, occurs when the participants do not do, what they are told not to do. This results in a positive (desired) outcome.

Transference is most likely to occur in the following situations:
- **Association**: Participants can associate the new information with something that they already know.
- **Similarity**: The information is similar to material that participants already know; that is, it revisits a logical framework or pattern.
- **Degree of original learning**: When participant's degree of original learning was high, transference is most likely.
- **Critical attribute element**: The information learned contains elements that are extremely beneficial (critical) on the job.

Andragogy has 5 components such as self-concept, experience, orientation, readiness, and motivation. These can be applied to videoconferencing in many ways.

A mature self-concept is something that nurses must possess. They must be very self-directed and self-aware. There is a wide range of experiences that nurses must have including a background in Sciences, Maths, and English. As soon as a course begins, they are rapidly oriented in various nursing concepts to which they must be prepared. Readiness to learn is apparent in them because they are usually not forced to attend class. They are present of their own will, and attentive, and ask questions. They are motivated and driven to succeed in programs where attrition is very high.

Steps in CE Program Development

In order to increase the probability that CE programs have an impact on professional competence performance, the following steps are helpful:
- Identify problems that focus on health care.
- Analyze needs or problems to determine if there is a potential educational solution.
- Identify potential facilitators of and barriers to the learning process.
- Select educational needs based on a priority system.
- State educational goals and objectives for the selected needs.
- Select or design a learning experience to meet the goals and objectives.
- Implement the learning experience.
- Evaluate the extent to which learners achieved objectives.
- Determine the extent to which the original problems have been reduced.
- Identify any additional tasks necessary to meet the need based on evaluation data.

Steps in Conducting Continuing Education in Nursing

- Conduct needs assessment
- Establish overall goals
- Conduct task analysis
- Specify objectives
- Develop assessment strategies
- Select methods and media
- Produce materials
- Conduct formative evaluation—revise as required
- Conduct summative evaluation.

Conduct Needs Assessment

Needs assessment is a critical part of a systematic approach to developing educational projects within the organization. The approach to needs assessment in continuing education for the health professionals is systematic process based on a carefully developed plan.

The plan calls for describing the purpose of the needs assessment activity, the uses of the findings, the issues that will be examined, and specification of the resources are required. The purpose of needs assessment is to determine better the nature, extent, and priority of educational needs to develop continuing educational programs that address the needs of the learners within the limited resources. No matter the size or setting of continuing education program, an educational design process must be based on learning theory and the principles of adult learning.

Learning Needs Assessment

Ongoing education for the nursing workforce is necessary to ensure current knowledge in order to enable evidence-based client care. The cost of education is high to the organization and the individual and must therefore be cost-effective, relevant, and appropriate. According to research, education for nurses is not always systematically planned and developed and often relies on the interest area and assessment of the nurse educators.

Learning needs assessment, which is a crucial stage in the educational process that leads to changes in practice and has become part of government policy for continuing professional development. It might be to help curriculum planning, diagnose individual problems, assess student learning, demonstrate accountability, improve practice and safety, or offer individual feedback and educational intervention. Published classifications include felt needs (what people say they need), expressed needs (expressed in action), normative needs (defined by experts), and comparative needs (group comparison). Other distinctions include individual versus organizational or group needs, clinical versus administrative needs, and subjective versus objectively measured needs. The defined purpose of the needs assessment should determine the method used and the use made of findings.

Questionnaires and structured interviews seem to be the most commonly reported methods of needs assessment.

Types of Needs Assessment

Methods of needs assessment can be classified into seven main types, each of which can take many different forms in practice.

Gap or Discrepancy Analysis

This formal method involves comparing performance with stated intended competencies by self-assessment, peer assessment, or objective testing and planning education accordingly.

Reflection on Action and Reflection in Action

Reflection on action is an aspect of experiential learning and involves thinking back to some performance, with or without triggers (such as videotape or audiotape) and identifying what was done well and what could have been done better. The latter category indicates learning needs.

Reflection in action involves thinking about actual performance at the time that it occurs and requires some means of recording identified strengths and weaknesses at the time.

Self-assessment by Diaries, Journals, Log Books, and Weekly Reviews

This is an extension of reflection that involves keeping a diary or other account of experiences. However, practice might show that such documents tend to be written nearer the time of their review than the time of the activity being recorded.

Peer Review

This is rapidly becoming a favorite method. It involves nurses assessing each other's practice and giving feedback and perhaps advice about possible education, training, or organizational strategies to improve performance. The last of these is the most formal, involving rating forms completed by nominated colleagues and shows encouraging levels of validity, reliability, and acceptability.

Observation

In more formal settings, nurses can be observed performing specific tasks that can be rated by an observer, either according to known criteria or more informally. The results are discussed and learning needs are identified. The observer can be a peer, a senior, or a disinterested person, if the ratings are sufficiently objective or overlap with the observer's area of expertise (such as communication skills or management).

Critical Incident Review and Significant Event Auditing

Although this technique is usually used to identify the competencies of a profession or for quality assurance, it can also be used on an individual basis to identify learning needs. The method involves individuals identifying and recording, say, one incident each week in which they feel they should have performed better, analyzing the incident by its setting, exactly what occurred, and the outcome and why it was ineffective.

Practice Review

A routine review of notes, charts, prescribing letters, requests, etc. can identify learning needs, especially if the format of looking at what is satisfactory and what leaves room for improvement is followed.

Needs assessment is not the same as assessment in the sense of examination of learning. Assessment systems that lead to academic or professional awards should show certain minimum characteristics, including measurement of performance against external criteria and standards, a decision on adequacy by an assessor, and standardized data gathering. Needs assessment might sometimes have these characteristics, but it also might be based on practice, reflection, professional judgment, discussion, and informal data. Needs assessment methods that are limited by the standards of assessment will fall into the trap of assessing only a narrow range of needs.

Establish Overall Goals

After assessing the needs, the organizer such as a hospital personnel department must formulate the overall goals for organizing continuing nursing education program. The goals must be based on the needs assessment of their employees and it should be practical, agreeable, and attainable.

Conduct Task Analysis

Organizing continuing nursing education is a challenging task, which requires a careful analysis. This involves various small activities, which should be carefully analyzed. This involves the program content, preparation, delivery, audio-visual materials and methods, budget for the program, the output to be achieved, etc. Each one of these requires careful planning and implementation. So, a task analysis helps the organizer to be prepared for the program.

Specify Objectives

The specific objectives can be formulated, which should be measurable, observable, and verifiable. The specific objectives formed should be directly related to the needs assessment of the learner. This directs the organizer to prepare for the content and to choose the methods of teaching and materials used for teaching. It also helps them in developing the evaluation strategies.

It helps the learner to recognize and realize what to be learned out of participating such continuing nursing education program.

Develop Assessment Strategies

The next step is selection and formulating assessment strategies to evaluate at the end of the program. The evaluation strategies are decided based on the topic, content, the level of the learner, the domain to be evaluated, the time factors, etc. A well-planned and prepared evaluation tool helps in assessing the learner, which gives the organizer the effectiveness of such program in fulfilling the objectives and goals.

Select Methods and Media

The methods for continuing nursing education might be a seminar, workshop, demonstration, panel discussion, etc. Any methods of teaching can be used, but it should help the learner to achieve the specific objectives. It also should be based on the number of participants, the content, and the duration of the program. The media includes audio media, video media, and the print media. Any one or the combination of these can be used.

Produce Materials

It is the phase where the actual education program is conducted using the predetermined methods and media. It involves the actual participation of the learners.

Conduct Formative Evaluation—Revise as Required

Formative evaluation is an ongoing evaluation, which is done while the program is in progress. It gives the immediate feedback to the organizer. Based on the evaluation, revisions can be done when it is required.

Conduct Summative Evaluation

It is the final evaluation done at the end of the program. It helps the organizer to review the whole program and to analyze the success of the program. It also helps them to identify the areas of improvement, modification, budgetary controls, and others.

The learning needs of the adults are far different from the needs of the children. Adults have already completed the basics and established a large reservoir of experiential learning that makes them independent and responsible for their own learning needs. A systematic approach is necessary to provide quality continuing education activities and services. Planning for continuing education programs follow the familiar medical model for patient care, which includes diagnosis, treatment planning, treatment implementation, and follow-up. Planning for continuing education begins with an identification of needs, followed by setting objectives, setting educational activities, and evaluation. Congruence must be established among needs, objectives, activities, implementation, and evaluation.

The following points must be considered when planning CEs:
- Most individuals are motivated to continue their learning beyond their professional education.
- Participation in continuing education is strongly influenced by individual's past experiences.
- Continuing education should support health professionals' natural desire to learn. Health professionals should be encouraged to accept the personal responsibility for learning.
- CEs must be planned according to adult learning principles.

Research in Continuing Nursing Education

Research is searching for the facts or truth. Research in continuing nursing education (CNE) is broader in scope, which gives us many insights. Research in this area is often ignored and does not seek much importance. The emergence of new knowledge and changes in all the fields demand one to update him or her in order to be an effective nurse. It is one of the nurses' responsibilities to update with the latest information and technology to meet the demands of the society. Nurse administrators and educators should play a crucial role in conducting research in the area of continuing nursing education.

Aims of Research in Continuing Nursing Education

- To assess the need for organizing continuing nursing education program.
- To objectively assess the needs of the learner.
- To identify the areas of learning required.
- To assess the impact of conducting such continuing nursing education program.
- To evaluate the effectiveness of the program.
- To correlate the effectiveness of continuing nursing education program with the output expected.

Areas of Research

Research can be conducted in the following areas. They are:
- Need assessment of the learner
- Content for CNE
- Teaching methods and materials
- Evaluation
- Variables influencing the effectiveness of CNE
- Immediate and long-term benefits or outcomes of attending such CNE
- Cost-effectiveness in organizing and conducting CNE.

Need for Research into Needs Assessment in Nursing Education

The below mentioned questions will answer the need for research into needs assessment:
- What are the effects of and responses to needs assessment alone for students, trainees, and senior nurses at different stages of nursing education?
- What is the relative validity, reliability, or utility of different formal and informal methods of learning needs assessment in nursing education at any level?
- To what extent, do needs assessment methods identify all important learning needs?
- What are the relative effects and efficacy of identifying group and individual learning needs?
- What methods of planning effective learning experiences are most effective on the basis of needs identified?
- What human characteristics or behaviors influencing in the effectiveness of CNE?
- What are the environmental variables influences in the effectiveness of CNE?
- What is the perception of nurses toward the need for participating in CNE?
- What are the employer's difficulties in organizing CNE?

Distance Education in Nursing

Distance education is defined as any learning experience that takes place a distance away from the parent institutions, home campus, or central headquarters (Keating SB, 2006).

Distance education is defined as students receiving instruction in a location other than that of faculty (Clark CE, 1998). This separation of teacher and student could be as close as within the same community or campus or as far as across states or continents.

Types of Distance Education Programs

Satellite campuses are defined as those programs that offer the curriculum in whole or in part in off-campus sites from the parent institution. The majority of the teaching and learning takes place in classrooms and involves in person interaction between the faculty and students. Faculty members who teach in the parent institution serve as on-site faculty or act as consultants to off-site faculty who teach the same curriculum. In the instances of off-site satellite campuses, the course content and materials for both theory and clinical are identical to that of the home campus. Activities are planned to link the off site and home campuses to foster the socialization process for students and faculty, so that there is a feeling of belongingness to the same institution. They use web-based instruction and videoconferencing.

This technology requires an "uplink" from the origination site to communicate with the orbiting satellite and a "downlink" at each of the sites selected to receive the transmission from a distance source. The visual component is only from the origination site. A satellite origination classroom is usually simulated in the production studio located at the uplink site. Technical staff is necessary to support the studio classroom. Use of satellite requires that students cluster at each downlink location for classes.

Videoconferencing and Broadcasting through Teleconferencing

Videoconferencing and teleconferencing require an infrastructure for cable TV or closed-circuit TV, dedicated classrooms that both broadcast and to receive communications, and technological support staff who manage the broadcasting and hardware and software for instructional support purposes.

Videoconferencing: It combines a television picture with audio or computer transmission. The video image can be real-time or freeze frame, with the cost of transmission directly proportionate to the sophistication of equipment. The visual image is often carried on telephone, microwave, or fiber optic lines and enhances the audio-conference or computer correspondence. Videoconferencing configurations are either one-way video and two-way audio or two-way video and two-way audio. Equipment is required at both the origination and the receiver sites to enable the videoconferencing facility.

Audioconferencing: Instruction transmitted over phone line is referred to as audioconferencing. A teacher located at the origination site, not necessarily a classroom, interacts with students in one or more receiving sites. Courses to be offered through this medium must be selected carefully to ensure that they can pedagogically be delivered without live video. It is good if students are encouraged to identify themselves and their location when they speak during the audio class sessions. Student should be oriented to the use of microphone or speaker phone. Because the teacher is unable to identify nonverbal cues, teaching strategies should include more questioning to determine class understanding of content being addressed. The minimum number of students per site is 8–10 and the maximum should not exceed 35–45 students.

Computer Conferencing

It uses the computer to establish a network on a mainframe or file server in which an unlimited number of individuals can communicate with each other using personal computers linked by a local or wide area network or modems. It may be used as an adjunct to on-campus courses or as the communication support for the courses offered totally on the World Wide Web. It is a medium that supports many-to-many student interactions without requiring participants to be gathered in a central place at a specified time. Personally-directed email messages also can be sent only to selected individuals.

Web-based course development: Web-based teaching and learning require a learning management system, computer access to the web by faculty and students, technological support through the use of instructional support staff, and training sessions for faculty and students who are not familiar with the system. Multiple learning activities are available through the internet, such as real-time chat rooms when students and faculty meet at a prearranged time and discuss topics or review questions about course assignments. Asynchronous entries (occurring at various times) about selected topics provide the students and faculty with opportunities to discuss topics and present their ideas and views on them. Flowchart 6.1 explains the process of web-assisted classroom instruction. Another form of asynchronous communication is "threaded discussions". It allows students and faculty to interact on one topic within the course and to track the interactions related to that topic or thread. Flowchart 6.2 explains the individual learning in web-assisted instruction.

Faculty can post a lecture through PowerPoint presentation that includes notes, illustrations, references

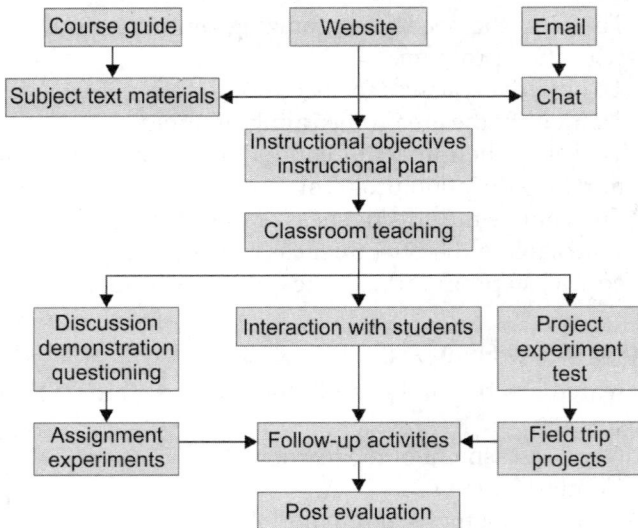

Flowchart 6.1: Web-assisted classroom instruction.

Source: University News, November 19–25, 2001.

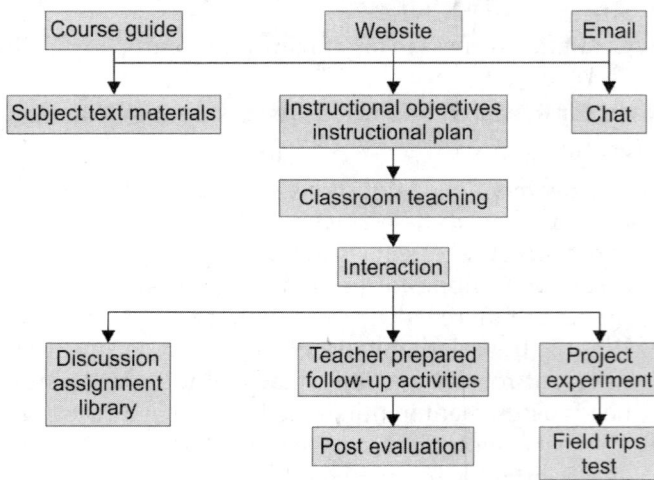

Flowchart 6.2: Individual learning.

Source: University News, November 19–25, 2001.

to URLs, videotapes, movies and other audio-visual media, and postthought questions for discussions related to the lecture. Group work assignments are possible through the use of chat rooms, threaded discussions, and email communications.

Clinical Courses and Distance Education

Faculty develops the clinical courses including skills laboratory courses. Students are assigned to clinical laboratories for the acquisition of assessment and clinical skills as well as to healthcare agencies for supervised clinical practice. They are under the supervision of faculty members who either directly supervises a group of students in the clinical setting or coordinate student preceptorships, where students are assigned to qualified staff nurse preceptors.

With careful planning, it is possible to provide clinical experiences for students enrolled in courses through videoconferencing or teleconferencing and web-based instruction. Assignments, examinations, and pre- and postconferences can also take place through technology and can be synchronous and asynchronous. The faculty can be hired or the institution faculty can travel to support and supervise the students.

When hired, setting standards for the qualification of the preceptors, orienting the preceptors to the curriculum, the course and the role of preceptors, and providing guidance to them are very important. Supervising preceptors, developing a communication network, participating with preceptors and students in the assignments of grades, and evaluating and revising the program are mandatory.

Correspondence Instruction

It can provide college level instruction that is efficient, economical, and sensitive to the changing needs of traditional and adult learners. They are sent a syllabus that contains specific guidance for meeting the academic objectives. Course materials are sent and the students are intimated about the examination. The examination papers are evaluated by the university appointed faculty members and the results are published. It is a successful learning option for independent and highly motivated students.

Needs Assessment for Distance Education

The needs assessment for distance education is done in respect to the external and internal factors influencing the effectiveness of distance education. They are:

External Factors

Feasibility, demand for the course, location and receptivity to the course, technology, infrastructure facilities, political climate, competitive issues, healthcare system, and health needs are some of the external factors determining the need for distance education.

Internal Factors

Mission, philosophy, purpose, goals of parent institution, economic factors, self-sufficiency, off-site offices, laboratories, classrooms, clinical experience facilities, technological support systems for videoconferencing, teleconferencing and web-based instruction, administrative faculty and staff expenses, library, academic and student services, and congruence with curriculum model are some of the internal factors determining the need for distance education.

Development of Distance Education Programs

The faculty members have to play the following functions in organizing and implementing the distance education programs:
- Planning
- Preparation
- Implementation
- Evaluation (delivery model selection).

Issues and Challenges in Distance Education

Funding, faculty development, legal and ethical issues such as intellectual property and privacy issues, quality, increased student access to education through technology, and competition are some of the issues and challenges in distance education.

The multimedia approach adopted for distance education makes use of innovative methods, some of which are listed below:
- Human contact: Face-to-face sessions.
- Audio-visual cassettes: Recording and demonstrating the material in a lively manner.
- Educational telecast, covering the major ideas relating to the subject in an interesting manner.
- Newsletters: In these, articles written by experts on different areas of study are published.
- Computers.

Webcast

Webcasting is a new instructional technology used to deliver audio and video presentations via the internet, enabling learners to participate in a live class via a personal computer.

Webcasting allows synchronous discussion and questions and answers between students and instructor, an interactive learning environment is facilitated.

A webcast delivers synchronous broadcasting to students in their homes, places of employment, or local libraries using web-based streaming video and synchronized multimedia presentation.

To produce a webcast, the following are needed: a room with a camera, microphone, presenter's computer, a Mediasite live capture workstation, and internet access and dedicated video and web.

Audio from the microphone is sent into the capture workstation via the inputs on the sound card and video from the rear wall-mounted camera is sent into the video capture card. Presentation images from the presenter's computer are also sent to the capture workstation by way of a Video Graphics Array (VGA) capture card. The capture workstation application sends the video and audio to the video server and the presentation images are sent to the Web/File Transfer Protocol (FTP) server.

The Mediasite live software combines these components into the Mediasite live navigator, which is what the viewers (students) see in their browser on their personal computers.

The Mediasite live navigator has two unique ways to communicate in real time with viewers of the presentation: poll questions and the Q and A forum. Poll questions are created by the presenter and entered into the presentation configuration prior to giving the presentation. Poll questions are then activated by the presenter at the appropriate time during the presentation and are posted to all viewers. Viewers can choose from multiple answers for the question and instantly see the results of the "voting." The presenter can also monitor the poll results from the Mediasite live tools page where the poll questions were entered. They can give their e-mail address, if they would like their question answered privately.

The moderator (instructor) is responsible for monitoring the Q and A forum so all questions are answered to ensure a positive, interactive, and virtual classroom experience. The instructor is also responsible for activating the poll questions when needed. The technological infrastructure, faculty development, student support, and curricular effects must be addressed during the implementation phase.

Technological Infrastructure

Support from information technology specialists is the backbone to achieve positive faculty and student outcomes. A considerable amount of time and energy must first be spent developing the necessary technological infrastructure to produce a webcast.

To produce a webcast, the following are needed:
- A room with a camera
- Microphone
- Presenter's computer
- A Mediasite live capture workstation and the internet access
- Video and web services.

Benefits

Students can ask for immediate clarification of any concept. The instructor can solicit student feedback and participation.

Webcast classes can be linked through the web platform. During the live webcast, students can complete group work in a bulletin board and then the instructor can comment on their work live, thus providing immediate feedback.

The webcasting system automatically archives classes. If the students cannot attend the live class, they can watch it at their convenience for as long as it is stored on the server.

Videoconferencing

Videoconferencing is a way of transmitting information to a distant site. Videoconferencing is a way to teach via distance education (DE) that includes totally online courses, hybrid or blended courses, voice technology, and video technology. Distance education has emerged in colleges of nursing around the country, making education available, accessible, and convenient for those seeking basic to advanced degrees.

Videoteleconferencing allows students to obtain instruction from a distance and has been successfully employed in multiple disciplines including nursing education. Videoteleconferencing can enable optimization of resources and will likely continue to expand its role in educational programs.

Lecture Presentation

When presenting lecture, the faculty should refrain from addressing class issues until all on-site students are present and connectivity is confirmed. If on-site students present questions to camera, those questions should be made available to all students. Faculty should address distance-site students specifically to facilitate an overall impression of class cohesiveness and inclusion. Faculty is also responsible for preparing material and addressing any technical issues that may arise. Room scheduling must allow time for setup as well as instructional class time.

One must verify connection to the distance site and confirm adequate audio and visual reception. It is also important to adjust placement and volume of microphones for optimal reception. A preliminary test of any display devices or software should be conducted before committing the presentation to one of these options. Finally, the speaker should test the presentation on the computer he/she will be using for the class.

Even with the best audio equipment, it is important that the speaker or students in the class speak clearly and loud enough for adequate reception.

What to Consider before using Videoconferencing?

Before undertaking videoconferencing, it is important to complete a needs assessment and find where to transmit the lectures.

What rooms are capable of videoconferencing and can they be used exclusively for this purpose? It is important to identify a group of flexible faculty members open to a different method of teaching. What extra personnel will be needed to train, monitor equipment, and troubleshoot problems? Budgetary issues are given considerations. Videoconferencing will bring in more students and this can help offset the costs of the necessary equipment.

Instructors, who are technologically savvy, should be the ones to help train and support faculty. Training should start with an informational class on videoconferencing and how it works. A second class should include how to use the equipment. All equipment needs to be user friendly to ensure that anyone with basic computer skills can use it. It would be helpful if the faculty goes to a distant site and observes the class. This will increase understanding and comfort tremendously.

The home site needs to have an instructional technology person to setup and turn on the equipment about 15 minutes before the class begins. Once faculty is comfortable with the equipment, they may want to do this. The distant site needs a moderator to sit in the class. This person takes attendance and monitors the students. Moderators need to know how to work with the equipment and have basic computer skills.

The following must be done by the organizers of videoconferencing:
- Complete a needs assessment to include possible transmission sites, hospitals/colleges.
- Get faculty input and ideas. Hopefully support.
- Contact IT department to find out what equipment is needed.
- Check firewalls if transmission is to hospital/college sites.
- Get prices of equipment (codec, monitors).
- Is there a dedicated room for videoconferencing?
- Get bids on installation of equipment.
- Each distant site needs a moderator and a fax machine.
- Write a timeline for the year with dates for meetings, evaluations.
- Introduction class for faculty. What is videoconferencing (1 hour) and how to prepare for transmission?
- Have faculty visit another site that is using videoconferencing.
- Start faculty training one week before class begins.
- Make photo guide with simple directions for equipment use.
- Create handout for students of videoconferencing etiquette.
- Have list of phone numbers for moderators/sites/IT personnel.
- Meet weekly with instructors and monthly with students for evaluation/problem/ideas.

How to Adapt Teaching Strategies?

When transmitting lectures by videoconference, a PowerPoint presentation is advisable. Slides should have a light background with dark font 24–32 in size and in Times New Roman or Arial with only 5 lines of text. Photos that are scanned into PowerPoint do not transmit well because of pixilation problems. The photo should be an original of good quality.

Interactive learning takes much preparation. To ensure that the courses run smoothly, the following items and support are necessary. Course material should be posted on the internet at least 24 hours before class on a program such as blackboard. Faculty should be ready and capable of offering virtual online office hours using e-mail or instant messaging. Students must be able to contact instructors and have college resources readily available to them. Instructors must be accessible to their students.

Examinations can be administered on the computer via the internet with platforms such as blackboard. They should be administered in a computer laboratory with a proctor at each distant site. If a paper examination is desired, it can be faxed to the moderator to administer and returned via fax or courier.

There is usually a 3–5 seconds delay in transmission of sound or voice. Although there may be increased participation at the home site, good communication between the instructor and distant students will create equality and a good experience for both groups of students.

Room Setup/Equipment

Because of the availability of the internet, there are three ways to videoconference—ISDN line, IP lines, or T one (T1) lines. In the use of three, ISDN lines produce near television quality audio and video interference, dropped calls or packet loss, and a decreased quality of transmission of PowerPoint are problems with an ISDN line. An IP line uses a broadband connection and the speed is much faster and more precise. The IP connection can be dedicated to one or more sites. Another possibility for transmission is a digital signal 1 (DS-1) line.

Other equipment includes cameras, TVs speakers, and microphones, which are setup around the room. It is helpful if a camera is voice activated and follows the lecturer around the room. A control panel in the form of a touch pad would be in front of the room for instructor use. Touch screens are easier to use than "remote controls" for the codec system operation.

The class starts when the remote sites are dialed. A computer is connected to a projector that transmits the camera input on a screen in front of the room. This picture is then transmitted to the distant site. A screen or television in the back of the room allows the instructor to see the students.

Common Problems and Possible Solutions

It is most important to choose a square room to use for distance education because a square room has better sound and transmission. Also, if two rooms are designed, it is best to equip them with the same supplies. Another suggestion to prevent problems is to hire an installer to setup the room. The installer is a specialist and if the room is equipped correctly from the start, problems will be limited.

Equipment breakdown and technical problems will occur. Reverberation and echo may need to be occasionally adjusted. This may require the installer to return and make the repairs. Any return visit from the installer will be expensive.

It is best to videocast lecture classes because skill demonstrations do not transmit well. Arrange skill courses at each remote site. One instructor does case studies and writes the answers on a whiteboard where the camera is directed to transmit. DVDs and VCRs transmit well and small items can be videocast with the use of a document camera (ELMO visual presenter).

A data port for an internet connection should be available for the laptop.

A committee can meet monthly from all sites to discuss progress. The most challenging aspect is becoming familiar with the new method of teaching in front of a camera. A recent dilemma is how to get students to feel connected and being part of the same cohort. The majority of students may not consider students at other sites to be members of their sites to be members of their learning community.

Team-building exercises and, if possible, meeting together at the beginning and the end of each semester are some suggestions. Instructors should keep dialog open and facilitate communications at each site.

Usage of Technology in Distance Learning— the Benefits of e-SIM

While the distance education system claims to be adopting the multiple media approach for instructional delivery which includes printed Self-instructional Material (SIM), audio-video cassettes and CDs, counseling, teleconferencing, and radio interactive counseling, the printed material still reigns the instructional package. The digitization of SIM and its delivery through electronic means cannot only resolve the problem of voluminous material printing, storage, handling, and dispatch, it will also drastically reduce on cost incurred on these accounts. Therefore, electronic Self-instructional Material (e-SIM) will play a substantial role in reaching the different segments of the distance learners while making the process of money transaction through web-based payment gateway easy at the same time.

Benefits of e-SIM

The e-SIM is going to be the cost-effective resource. It will have an advantageous edge over the printed SIM in the following ways:
- The e-SIM will be easy to download once payment is made online. It will be instant and available round the clock.
- The learners will be able to assimilate the knowledge and show their understanding in answering the questions as against reproduction of the same text crammed from the printed SIM. The learning objects and knowledge modules will enhance the grasping power of the learners.
- Institutional cost on the e-SIM will be considerably less when compared to the printed SIM on costs in relation to paper, printing, storage, handling, packaging, forwarding, transportation, etc. The benefit of lower cost can very well be passed onto the learners.
- It will be user-friendly. Being digital in nature, it is easy to search the e-SIM through the pages and skip undesired pages and straight away to go to the desired text location.
- It will have the facility for hyperlink glossary, PowerPoint presentations, audio-video special effects, graphics, diagrams, etc. It can provide links to other digital and e-resources including e-libraries.
- There is a facility for font resizing, which will make it easy to read.
- A normal memory card will be able to store lot of e-SIM material, which is also portable.
- The learners may form their portable digital library by storing the e-SIM in their Personal Digital Assistance (PDAs) or mobiles.
- Instant content updation will be very easy with e-SIM.
- Universalization and socialization of higher education will be very easy with the help of development of e-SIM modules and learning objects.
- The interest of learners in technological gadgets, i.e. mobiles, laptops, and computers will help them take full advantage of their curiosity by reading e-SIM at their own convenient pace, place, and time.

Format of the e-SIM

The e-SIM may be embedded with the following components:
- Text matter hyperlinked with glossary and definitions
- Empirical activities
- Animations and presentations
- Simulations
- Audio-visual clips with light and sound effects
- Virtual reality
- Online/instant continuous evaluation.

The delivery of e-SIM could even be through internet or other electronic mode on enrollment of the student and/or payment of the fee. The e-SIM can be accessed from any computer having access to internet. Alternatively, the PDAs and mobile phones can also be used to access the SIM from the main server and stored in mobile in simple but user-friendly format. The process of downloading of e-SIM will be a one-time measure. Therefore, special e-SIM reading devices would also be appropriate to use as an independent standalone appliance without having 24-hour internet connectivity. It can also be downloaded through internet to a computer and then saved in PDA/mobile phone/e-SIM reader. In order to read the e-SIM, one need not stay online, but stay offline and also can take a printout from a normal printer at one's own convenience. It will help the concept of e-SIM penetrate in rural and remote areas where 24 hours internet connection may not be available or possible due to electricity problems.

Challenges for the Institutions in Providing e-SIM

The major challenges before the institutions will be:
- To create multimedia facilities for creation of e-SIM.
- To transform the existing SIM to e-SIM.
- To provide expertise for development of learning objects for e-SIM.
- To create teams of content developers and learning object developers who could work in close coordination with each other.

Tutor Competencies for Online Teaching

The experiences revealed that the online teaching cannot be organized in the same manner as classroom-based teaching. The tutor should possess variety of skills and experiences to make online teaching a success. The role of a tutor in online education is a very crucial and that before participating in an online teaching program, a tutor should be equipped with following competencies:

Technical Skills

The technical skills include:
- Ability to use search engines like Google, Yahoo, etc. to access additional learning materials on the internet.
- Ability to upgrade the content consistently and be able to assist the students to different websites for more information.
- Ability to use online communication tools such as whiteboard, online chat, broadcast videoconferencing, and teleconferencing to be able to demonstrate ideas to the student.
- Ability to undertake resolution of the technical/operational challenges faced due to failure in the communication system on a real-time basis.
- Ability to use word processor and basic typing skills.
- Ability to develop multimedia presentations with embedded audio and/or video to demonstrate his or her ideas to the students.

Management Skills

Management skills include ability to:
- Establish the rules of communication with the learners.
- Develop a harmonious professional relationship with the learners.
- Guide the learner by helping his/her to set challenging but achievable goals.
- Provide encouragement to learners to sustain their interest on a continuous basis.
- Develop and monitoring the learner's plan to complete the learning material for the course.
- Enforce controls to keep the learners on track.

Subject Content Specialization Skills

Subject content specialization skills include:
- A deep understanding of the subject, so that he/she is able to generate content to supplement classroom materials, to fill in any gaps, and to clarify any misunderstandings.
- Ability to supplement and act as a backup to content that is presented elsewhere.

Teaching Skills

Teaching skills include ability to:
- Develop capacity in learners to solve problems, generate creative thinking, and help in conducting research to avoid from becoming completely dependent on the online instructor.
- Ask the right questions that stimulate learners to think for themselves, lead those to more powerful insights than could ever be obtained from regular teaching methods.
- Help the learners achieve their learning goals by challenging, encouraging, and providing constructive feedback.
- Respond to questions received in email, chat sessions, or the practical assignments based on multiple choice questions.

Communication Skills

Communication skills include ability to:
- Handle learners from different culture, accent, ethnic, and religious backgrounds.
- Be sensitive to the linguistic background of learners undergo accent neutralization process.
- Initiate discussion topics and questions to get things going.
- Control discussions, so that students do not deviate from the objectives of the course.
- Encourage all members to participate in the discussion.
- Be articulate in responding to the question posed by students and deliver in the format acceptable by them.
- Be a good listener and respond to the question asked by the students.

Assessment Skills

Assessment skills include ability to:
- Assess the learning outcomes and ensure that the learners are able to master up to 90% of the learning objectives of the course.

- Provide the learner with objective and constructive feedback based on specifics and not based on his/her personal opinion or values.

Summary

- According to the ANA, continuing nursing education is defined as planned educational activities intended to build upon the educational and experiential bases of the professional nurse for the enhancement of practice, education, administration, and research or theory development to the end of improving the health of the public.
- The idea of lifelong education was triggered off in our country by the Kothari Commission (1964–1966) and was strengthened by a report of the International Commission on the Development of Education (1971–1972).
- While preparing for continuing nursing education program, one should apply and follow the principles of adult learning. There are four critical elements of learning that must be addressed to ensure that participants learn. These elements are motivation, reinforcement, retention, and transference. Research into the areas of continuing nursing education is must and it is important.
- Distance education is defined as any learning experience that takes place a distance away from the parent institutions, home campus, or central headquarters (Keating SB, 2006). Videoconferencing, audioconferencing, and teleconferencing are some of the latest technologies used in the distance education.
- Nurses, who are well-informed on issues, are facilitated to manage obstacles and approach problems creatively and collectively. Continuing education and distance education for nurses are a process, which inspires, encourages, and supports nurses to begin and continue on that journey decisively and confidently.

7. Curriculum Development

"It is a tool in the hands of the artist (the teacher) to mold his material (the pupils) to his ideal (objective) in his studio (the school)".

—Cunningham

Objectives
After completing this unit, you will be able to:
- State the meaning and definition of curriculum
- Mention the determinants of curriculum
- Explain the nature and elements of curriculum
- Explain curriculum planning
- Explain the process and steps of curriculum development
- Describe the various curriculum models and framework
- Formulate philosophy and objectives
- Explain the selection and organization of learning experiences
- Understand master and individual rotation plan
- Explain the process of curriculum change
- Understand the importance of transcripts and credit system.

Introduction

We plan before we proceed into any activities. Planning is deciding in advance what to do, when to do, how to do, whom to do, and where to do. The success of any activity depends upon the proper and timely planning. Likewise, we plan educational program too. We make blueprint before we build a house. Same way, we have to prepare a blueprint before we start any educational program. The blueprint for any educational program is known as curriculum. In education, curriculum is an important component for teaching-learning process. It includes all the planned experience provided by the school to assist the pupils in attaining the designated learning outcome to the best of their abilities. The dictionary meaning of the word curriculum is a "course, especially the course of study at a university". The word "curriculum" can be used to mean two things. In one meaning "curriculum" is what actually happens during a course—the lectures, demonstrations, and field visits, etc. The other meaning is the written description of what happens. There are various factors involved in the curriculum development and it involves series of steps.

Today, nursing education faces a great transformation as faculty adapts curricula to prepare graduates at all levels for an increasingly complex workforce. This chapter provides an introduction to curriculum and the curriculum development process.

Meaning and Definition

A curriculum is the formulation and implementation of educational proposals to be taught and learned within a school or other institution and for which that institution accepts responsibility at three levels, its rationale, its actual implementation, and its effects.

Curriculum is a body of prescribed educative experience, under supervision, designed to provide an individual with the best possible training and experience to fit him for the society of which he is a part or to qualify him for a trade of a profession.

A curriculum is a systematic arrangement of sum total of selected experiences planned by a school for a defined group of students to attain the aims of a particular educational program—the Florence Nightingale International Foundation.

Bevis (1989) defined curriculum as "those transactions and interactions that take place between students and teachers and among students with the intent that learning take place".

Ronald C Doll (1996) defined curriculum as the "formal and informal content and process by which learners gain knowledge and understanding, develop skills, alter attitudes, appreciations, and values under the auspices of that school".

A composite of the entire range of experiences the learner undergoes under the guidance of the school (Lambertsen, Eleanor: Education for Nursing Leadership).

Glatthorn and colleagues (2006) defined curriculum as "the plans made for guiding learning, usually represented in retrievable documents of several levels of generality".

Stenhouse (1975) defined curriculum as "an attempt to communicate the essential principles and features of an educational proposal in such a form that it is open to critical scrutiny and capable of effective translation into practice".

The Secondary Education Commission Report (1925–1953) states that the "curriculum includes all the totality of experiences that a pupil receives through the manifold activities that go on in the school, in the classroom, library, laboratory, workshop, playground, and in the numerous informal contacts between teachers and pupils".

Bell (1973) defined curriculum as "the offering of socially valued knowledge, skills, and attitudes that made available to students through a variety of arrangements during the time they are at school, college, or university".

"Curriculum is all the learning, which is planned and guided by the school whether it is carried on in groups or individually, inside or outside the school"—Kerr, 1968.

A curriculum is all the educational opportunities encountered by students as a direct result of their involvement with an educational institution. It is the content and composition of the preprimary program, including all daily activities, transitions, and routines, which impact on the child's physical, social, emotional, and intellectual development. It is also a document, which describes a structured series of learning objectives and outcomes for a given subject matter area and it includes a specification of what should be learned, how it should be taught, and the plan for implementing/assessing the learning. Curriculum also refers to a series or sets of intended learning learnt by individuals as a consequence of education.

Concepts of Curriculum

Concept means idea or notion about a particular thing. The concept of curriculum is not static due to its dynamic nature. The concept will keep on change. The traditional concept of the curriculum represented the mastery over the subjects, certain type of knowledge and skills. Passing of the examination was the goal. The traditional curriculum did not consider the needs of the individuals and the individual differences. It mainly tested the memory of the learner and not the values of learning and the learned.

The newer concepts of curriculum accept the education as a dynamic process. Education helps the learner not only learning the concepts, but also it guides and helps the learner to live in the present world making necessary adaptations, solving problems of life, and being creative in planning and progression toward his own future. The teaching learning experiences provided in the school and colleges and the textbooks are helpful in this process.

The modern curriculum aims to promote the all-round development of the individual. It helps him to identify and realize his inner potentials to achieve the goals of his life. This emphasizes the totality of experiences gained inside and outside the educational institution. Modern curriculum is practical and is related to the community life.

It is also one of the balanced one that means it includes all the activities that will cater to the needs of the individual and the society. It keeps up the students needs met in the fast changing society.

In general, curricula respond to:
- What educational purposes should the college seek to attain?
- What educational experiences can be provided that is likely to attain these purposes?
- How can these educational experiences be effectively organized?
- How can we determine whether and to what extent these purposes are being attained?

Three Facets of Curriculum

The facets of curriculum as mentioned in Figure 7.1 include:
1. Goals and purposes of education
2. Process of curriculum
3. Evaluation of products.

Determinants of Curriculum

There are many determinants of curriculum, which may be enumerated in the following ways:
- Political ideology of a nation
- Sociological considerations
- Philosophy of education
- National goals and aspirations
- Religious doctrinaire
- Cultural factors
- Technological and scientific advancements

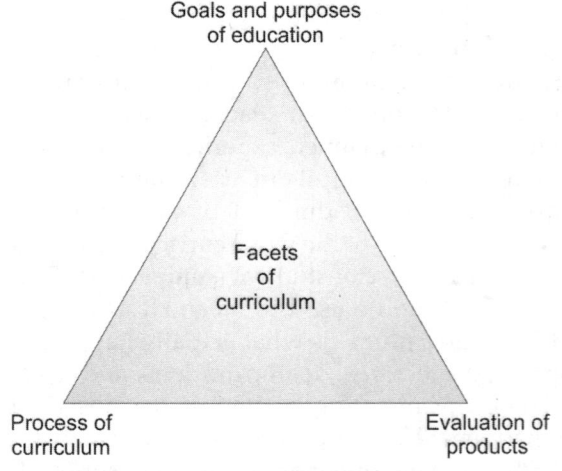

Fig. 7.1: Three facets of curriculum.

- Psychological foundations
- Economic planning
- Need for modernization, etc.

Philosophical Determinants of Curriculum

Philosophy is not only a powerful determinant of aims of education, but it is also equally a strong deciding factor of content of education. The aims speak of "why of education"? content speaks of "what of education"?, and the methods speak of "how of education"?

So, when educational aims are determined by philosophy, the next question that would arise is: "what should be the content of education that should be imparted to the students in order to realize the aims of education"?

> **The characteristics of curriculum, that is determined by the philosophical foundations of education, are as follows:**
> - It aims at the all-round development of the individual.
> - It is based on the philosophy of the nation. It reflects the ideals and aspirations of the people.
> - It inculcates the desired ideals of life in the youngsters.
> - It helps in the development of proper philosophy of life.
> - It is in accordance with the aspiration level of the individual.
> - It enables the learners to learn the desirable cultural values, intellectual virtues, and social norms including moral doctrinaire.
> - It helps in the development of personal and national character.

Philosophical principles serving as determinants of curriculum are:
- Child centeredness
- Need centeredness
- Activity centeredness.

Child centeredness: The naturalistic philosophical movement made curriculum, child centered. It was Jean-Jacques Rousseau, for the first time in the educational history of mankind subordinated curriculum to the child. Froebel, another pioneer, felt that curriculum should be centered on the nature of the child. Prior to that, curriculum had been either subject centered or teacher centered. It was narrowly conceived and single tracked. It was neither productive nor creative. It was mostly bookish and teacher tailored. In child-centered curriculum, the child is the center of the educative process. Hence, the curriculum, the methods of teaching, and the whole of school environment become the child centered and child oriented.

Need centeredness: The principle of need centeredness of curriculum gives the recognition of the interests of children in the process of education. It was due to the impact of pragmatic philosophy of education. It emphasized the importance of building the curriculum around the needs of children. Curriculum should not only reflect the present interests of children, but should also involve larger interests of the human race.

Activity centeredness: In the past, curriculum was considered as the subject matter curriculum. According to Sir TP Nunn, the famous British educational philosopher, the curriculum should be thought of in terms of activities and experiences rather than pieces of "knowledge to be acquired and facts to be stored".

Education is to be imparted by means of educational activities and experiences organized by the pupils themselves, which demand the active participation of the students. Under this principle, subjects are to be studied not as branches of knowledge but as creative and activizing activities.

The project curriculum and the basic curriculum are the examples of the activity-centered curricula. The principle of activity centeredness in curriculum is the contribution of Prof John Dewey, William Kilpatrick, HH Horne, and other pragmatic educational philosophers of the West and those like Mahatma Gandhi of the East.

Sociological Determinants of Curriculum

As the sociological approach to education demands that we should bear in mind the needs, requirements, imperatives, and aspirations of the community for which the curriculum is being prepared, the curriculum should be dynamic, flexible, and revisable to be progressive with the changing times. Sociological approach considers not only the needs of the society, but it also recognizes the needs of the children. It not only takes into its cognizance the needs of the pupils at the present times, but also their future needs as citizens and adult members of the society.

Hence, the following may be considered as the sociological determinants of content of education:
- Needs of the society
- Cultural imperatives of the community
- Values of the nation
- Faiths, beliefs, and attitudes of the people and so on.

> **The characteristics of the curriculum, that is determined by sociological foundations of education, are as follows:**
> - It is framed in such a way as to realize the social aims of education.
> - It makes education an effective media of social control.
> - It keeps in mind the social changes and reflects the social needs of the community.
> - It is dynamic, flexible, and progressive.
> - It transmits the ideals and values that the society upholds and considers to be inherited by the new generation.
> - It is related to social interests and problems of the society.
> - It enables the youngsters to participate efficiently in social life.
> - It inculcates in them respect for different vocations and professions and creates dignity of labor in their hearts.
> - It develops desirable social attitudes in the educands.
> - It aids them in promoting the social progress.
> - It is so framed as to develop each individual to the optimum possible level.
> - It aims at educating for the vacation and vocation.
> - It is functional and socially utilitarian.

The following principles of curriculum construction may be taken as those contributed by sociological foundations of education:
- Integratedness
- Life-centeredness
- Social-utilitarianism.

Integratedness
All knowledge is considered as unitary. Subject matter boundaries are artificial boundaries created for the convenience of piecemeal learning. Logical integration of different activities and subjects, to become a meaningful whole, is being increasingly felt as a dire educational need.

Life-centeredness
Education is of life, for life, and by life. Life-centered curricula and community-centered curricula only reveal nothing but the socialized curricula. Socialized curriculum is that in which, the curriculum is vitally and organically related to the life of the community. It attempts to initiate in the hearts of the pupils and the art of social living. School is considered as the replica of the society. Life-centered curriculum enables the students to become socially efficient, economically sufficient, intellectually alert, physically fit, professionally proficient, and culturally competent person. The socialized curricula view education as the investment on human resources, which will be duly capitalized for development of national resources in the long run. The "Areas-or-Living Curricula" may be considered as belonging to socialized curricula in which, curriculum is organized around classified activities of life, like good parenthood, good home-membership, good citizenship, one-world membership, and the like.

Social-utilitarianism
All education is considered to have transference effect. The curriculum provided in educational institutions will have greater positive transference when there is identity of learning and life situations. Hence, there is an imperative need for the curriculum to be lifelike.

Approaches of Curriculum

Knowledge Approach
In this, curriculum is considered to be belonging to various segments of knowledge called the subjects. Subjects are selected in such a way as to transmit the desirable knowledge to the younger generation as it is not possible to transmit encyclopedic knowledge to them because of too many specialized branches of knowledge that developed during the history of mankind. Sometimes, certain disciplines are brought together to form broad-field curricula or integrated curricula. Sometimes, individual subjects are selected as the subjects of study.

Activity Approach
In this, subjects are pushed into background and activities are selected to form curriculum. The students engage themselves in different activities and acquire knowledge of different subjects incidentally and as byproducts of their activities. Here, the teachers assume the role of consultants or directors of activities and students assume active role. Education becomes learner-centered in contrast to the earlier, which remained purely teacher-centered.

Living Approach
This is life-centered education. According to this, living is learning. Students learn as they live their learning experiences. They learn to the extent they accept what they have lived and retain what they have accepted.

Nature of Nursing Curriculum

The nursing curriculum -
- Is ongoing and flexible, meeting the constantly changing the needs of the society.
- Has societal orientation.
- Is oriented to life situations.
- Is oriented and alive to the needs of the learners.
- Has a blending of ideal and realistic approaches.
- Is dependent on the philosophy and objectives of the respective educational programs.

The nursing curriculum is oriented toward health needs of the individual and society, to meet primary healthcare needs, and focused on national health policy.

Types of Curriculum/Patterns of Curriculum Organization

There are various patterns adopted by curricularists in organizing the curriculum by giving importance to a particular idea or aspect as the focus of the curriculum organization. The different patterns are:

The **subject-centered curriculum** is organized according to how essential knowledge has been developed in the various subject areas with the explosion of knowledge and specialization in each field and the subject divisions and sophistications in each area. According to this organization, a hierarchy of subjects as per their value and mental disciplines is done. The limitations are no place for learner's interest or needs, passive learning by the learner, teacher's transfer of knowledge from text to the learner, and no scope for learner's inspiration and less importance to attitudes, values, and social reality.

The **broad-field curriculum** combines several specific areas into larger fields/areas. The pattern of curriculum permits greater integration of subject matter. It would facilitate more functional organization of knowledge. It permits a broader coverage.

The **child-centered curriculum** shifts the importance from subject to the child. Here, the child/student's interests and needs are considered while framing the curriculum. The curriculum is organized around human impulses to socialize, the impulse to construct, inquire and experiment, and to create artistically. The whole focus is laid on the learner.

The **experience centered/activity-centered curriculum** encourages children/student to use problem-solving skills and methods. Skills and knowledge are acquired as they are needed and subject matter from many fields is used according to the requirements of the tasks. It is centered on the interests of the students. It serves both the purposes for learning and application of what they learnt. The limitation is that it is difficult in transforming/channeling the experiences into organized knowledge.

The **official curriculum** includes the stated curriculum framework with philosophy and mission; recognized list of outcomes, competencies, and objectives for the program and individual courses; course outlines; and syllabi.

The **legitimate curriculum** is the one agreed on by the faculty members either implicitly or explicitly. These written documents are distributed to other faculty members, students, curriculum committee members, and accrediting agencies to document what is taught.

The **illegitimate curriculum** is one known and actively taught by faculty yet not evaluated because descriptors of the behaviors are lacking. Such behaviors include "caring, compassion, power, and its use".

The **operational curriculum** consists of "what is actually taught by the teacher and how its importance is communicated to the student". This curriculum includes knowledge, skills, and attitudes emphasized by faculty in the classroom and clinical settings.

The **hidden curriculum** consists of values and beliefs taught through verbal and nonverbal communication by the faculty. Faculty may be unaware of what is taught through their expression, priorities, and interactions with students, but students are very aware of hidden agendas, which may have a more lasting impact than the written curriculum. The hidden curriculum includes the way faculty interacts with students, the teaching methods used, and the priorities set.

The **null curriculum** represents content and behaviors that are not taught. Faculty need to recognize what is not being taught and focus on the reasons for ignoring those content and behavior areas. Examples include content or skills that faculty think they are teaching but are not, such as critical thinking. As faculty review curricula, all components and relationships need to be evaluated.

The **core curriculum** is a concept born out of necessity to "tame the knowledge explosion" and show the teachers and the learners what are the essential knowledge and skills that the learners should acquire during the course. This type of curriculum develops integration, serves the needs of the students, and promotes active learning and relates to life and learning. In a way, it is an epitome of all patterns of curriculum. Core means all the essential things required for all the subjects.

The Indian Institutes of Technology (IITs) identify three components in their credit-based curricula:
- Hardcore component: Every student must attend and must pass this component.
- Softcore component: Every student must attend this and may pass this component.
- Optional component: Every student can choose optional subjects of personal choice that may attend and may pass.

The curriculum introduced by Gandhiji was child centered, i.e. the development of head, heart, and hand and the approach to the curriculum was craft centered.

Elements of Curriculum

It includes:
- Philosophy and objectives of the educational program
- Selection of learning experiences
- Organization of learning experiences
- Program of evaluation.

Philosophy and Objectives of the Educational Program

An educational institution will have a philosophy, which will be formulated by the management of that institution. The top-level management consists of the managing director, chairman, principal, and other administrative members. It also includes other representatives from the university, community, etc. They formulate a statement of philosophy based on their beliefs and values considering the factors and determinants of curriculum. Such a philosophy serves as a framework within which the organization, school or college, or educational program can function with a purpose and objective. The general philosophy further expressed or simplified into many objectives. Figure 7.2 depicts the relationship between the elements of curriculum.

Selection of Learning Experiences

Learning refers to a more or less permanent change in behavior. A learning experience is something in which the student actively participates and thus results in change of behavior. It is deciding on the content of the curriculum. The learning experiences may be direct or indirect experiences, which are provided in various settings such as in the classroom, clinical area, community, field trip, etc. Selection of learning experience is discussed in the later portion of this chapter.

Organization of Learning Experiences

After selecting the learning experiences, it has to be effectively organized so as to promote efficient learning of the students. While organizing the principles of continuity, sequence, integration, and correlation should be followed. A well-organized curriculum does not omit any of the learning experiences and also it avoids any repetition.

Evaluation of the Curriculum

Evaluation is the term used to describe the process of finding out whether what was expected, desired, or aimed at has been achieved. A curriculum is constructed on some basic principles, which serve as criteria for evaluation. The effectiveness of any curriculum is evaluated on the basis of its utility. The results of evaluation in turn help for improvement and revision of curriculum. It is done by the evaluation of student's performance, teacher's performance, and the evaluation of the objectives. The techniques and tools of evaluation are discussed in the later chapter.

Forces and Issues Influencing Curriculum Development

Issues External to Nursing Profession

- Health issues
- Trend pattern:
  - Global violence
  - The demographic revolutions
  - Globalization and the rise of global economy
  - Technological explosion
  - Environmental changes
  - Natural and man-made disasters.
- Issues in higher education.

Issues Specific to Nursing Profession

- Context of nursing care delivery
- Nursing shortage
- Competencies required and demands of the future.

According to Loretta E Heidgerken (1965), the factors influencing the curriculum development in nursing are:
- Philosophy of nursing education
- Educational psychology
- Society
- Student
- Life activities
- Knowledge.

Factors influencing curriculum

In 2002, Lenburg challenged nurses and nurse educators to consider the following changes that affect the profession and curriculum:
- Rapid knowledge expansion and use of changing information technology
- Necessity for evidence-based practice
- Sociodemographic, cultural, economic, and political influences on health care and education
- Consumer-oriented society and impact on health care and education
- Ethics and bioethical issues, dilemmas, biotechnology, and biogenetic advances
- Shortage of qualified nurses, educators, and other healthcare personnel
- Increasing professional and personal responsibility and accountability; required continuing competency
- Diversity, flexibility, mobility, and delivery of education; changing methods for learning and assessment of competence for practice
- Increasing reality of terrorism in various forms.

Other Issues Involved in Curriculum Construction and Implementation

- **Reason for formulating the curriculum:** This is the aims of education. The educator and the learner must be clear about the aims of education, so that right efforts are made.
- **The beneficiaries of the curriculum:** The beneficiary is the learner. The curriculum should be according to the needs of the learner.
- **Content of the curriculum:** It is the subject taught in the curriculum.

Table 7.1 explains the changing trends in curriculum construction.

The Paradigm Shift in Curriculum

Control versus freedom: In general education, there has been a shift from traditional didactic methods of teaching toward more progressive forms of education, particularly that of student-centered learning. In nursing, there is a growing recognition of the importance of student-

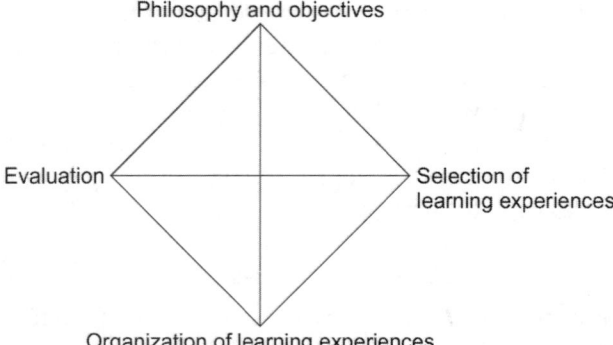

Fig. 7.2: Elements of curriculum.

Table 7.1: Trends in curriculum construction.

From	To
Imposition of adults preferences, values, etc. on students	Goals directed by the student's interests, needs, and capacities as well as the demands of the society
Disregard of individual	Respect for the personality of the individual
More formal, academic, and less social	All-round and social
Provision for mass education	Provision for individualized education
Subject matter curriculum	Broad based, integrated curriculum, irrespective of subject matter boundaries
Curriculum revision by subjects and by individuals	Curriculum revision by adequate group of specialists and as a whole
Measurement by the mere subject matter tests and examinations	Measurement by tests corresponding to the advances made in curriculum.

centered learning and also the need to encourage the student's independence in learning.

Process versus product: Education is moving away from the products of learning. There is a focus toward more of a "process" approach, which views learning experiences as being important variables in the learning process. In nursing also, the patient care revolves around the "nursing process" approach.

Part versus whole: Education is currently moving from collections of separate subjects in curricula toward a more integrated approach, involving the breakdown of the traditional subject boundaries. In nursing, the integrated curriculum is formed and also wherever necessary, the principles of integration and correlation are strengthened.

Institutions versus community: Education is not only the responsibility of the educational institution. It is also the responsibility of the community and in large the societal responsibility.

Models of Curriculum

The term curriculum model refers to an educational system that combines theory with practice. A curriculum model has a theory and knowledge base that reflects a philosophical orientation and is supported, in varying degrees, by child development research and educational evaluation. The practical application of a curriculum model includes guidelines on how to setup the physical environment, structure the activities, interaction with students and their families, and support staff members in their initial training and ongoing implementation of the program. Curriculum models are essential in determining

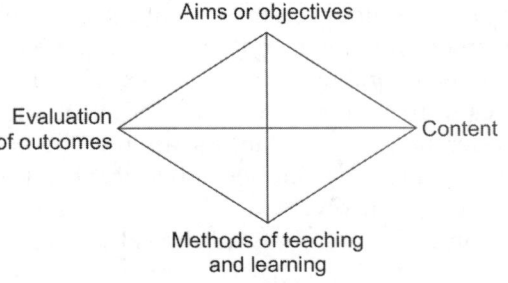

Fig. 7.3: Basic curriculum model.

program content and in training and supervising staff to implement high-quality programs. In order to provide a collegiate program of the highest quality, it is necessary to adopt an appropriate curriculum model. Figure 7.3 shows the basic curriculum model.

Curriculum models are:
- Targeted to the needs and characteristics of a particular group of learners
- Based on a body of theory about teaching and learning
- Used to outline approaches, methods, and procedures for implementation and evaluation.

Curriculum models adopted based on the:
- Nature of profession
- Scientific method used
- Needs of society.

Model 1: The Product Model or Behavioral Objectives

This model is usually ascribed to Ralph Tyler. He viewed education as "a process of changing the behavior patterns of people, using behavior in the broad sense to include thinking and feeling as well as overaction". He identifies four fundamental questions to be answered in developing a curriculum:
- What educational purposes should the school seek to attain?
- How can learning experiences be selected that are likely to be useful in attaining these objectives?
- How can learning experiences be organized for effective instruction?
- How can the effectiveness of learning experiences be evaluated?

Any curriculum consists of four main components:
1. Objectives
2. Content
3. Method
4. Evaluation.

The emphasis of this model is on the achievement of objectives by the student. It is an output model. Tyler stressed the importance of stating objectives in terms of student behaviors: "any statement of the objectives of the school should be a statement of changes to take place in students". This emphasis on student behaviors was taken up by other proponents of the model and led to a move, to limit behavioral objectives to observable, measurable changes in behavior, leaving no room for such things as "understanding" or "appreciation". The behavioral objectives model has influenced education throughout the world. Such objectives were almost universally applied in both classroom and clinical settings.

Implementing a Behavioral Objectives Model

Education Outcome
This is the end result of an educational program.

Educational Aim
An aim is a broad, general statement of goal direction. The educational aim is the most important part of the goal system, since all the other objectives are derived from it. The general goals are subdivided into immediate, intermediate, and long-term goals and in nursing, it is likely that teachers will need to state goals for the learner.

Specific Behavioral Objectives
Also termed as instructional objectives or terminal objectives, these are highly specific statements that describe the changes in behavior that constitute learning. They must always contain a verb that indicates exactly what the learner must do in order to achieve the objective and this verb should describe an observable action, so that achievement can be measured. The following sequence is suggested when formulating educational goals for nursing:
- Formulate the educational aims, ensuring that there is some indication of the worthwhileness of achieving them.
- Formulate the secondary level goals, which will break down the material into manageable sections for study.
- Formulate specific behavioral objectives from the secondary level goals.
- Formulate any experiential objectives from the secondary level goals.

Learner's Observable Behavior
Unless the learner's behavior is observable, it is impossible to assess whether or not an objective has been achieved. Take the objective which states: "the learner will understand the structure of bone". How will the nurse teacher know that the learner has achieved this objective? It is not possible to measure understanding as such, but it can be inferred from certain behaviors. Instead "describe in writing the structure of bone". The word describe is the action verb, which indicates the learner's observable behavior. It is important to select verbs that are as unambiguous as possible and which do not rely on the interpretation of the individual who is reading them.

Conditions under which Achievement will be Demonstrated
It can be an aid to clarity in an objective. Conditions are usually such things as time constraints, use of materials, or special situations.

Standard or Criterion of Performance
Note the example of an objective mentioned below:

The student will establish an IV line using aseptic technique within single prick without danger or discomfort to the patient.

The objective cannot be achieved simply by starting an IV line; it must be done according to the criteria that are with single prick and without danger or discomfort to the patient. This objective contains all three components, the action verb "establish" the condition "using aseptic technique and single prick" and the criterion of "without danger or discomfort to the patient". Criteria and standards are useful whenever, there is doubt as to the level of performance is required in an objective.

Levels of Objective
In order to perform her role adequately, the nurse needs a variety of behaviors. The behavior components arise from knowledge, attitude, and skill component. This is otherwise known as cognitive, affective, and psychomotor domain (Taxonomy of Educational Objectives). Table 7.2 explains the viewpoints of proponents and opponents of behavioral objectives model.

Mode 2: The Process Model of Curriculum
One of the major critics of the behavioral objectives model was the late Lawrence Stenhouse, who formulated an alternative approach known as the "process" model. He saw the use of behavioral objectives acting as a filter that distorted knowledge in schools. The minimum requirements for a curriculum are that it should offer:

In planning:
- Principles for the selection of content—what is to be learned and taught?
- Principles for the development of teaching strategy—how it is to be learned and taught?
- Principles for making of decision about sequence
- Principles on which to diagnose the strengths and weaknesses of individual students.

In empirical study:
- Principles on which to study and evaluate the progress of students.
- Principles on which to study and evaluate the progress of teachers.

Table 7.2: Viewpoints of proponents and opponents of behavioral objectives model.

Proponents	Opponents
They provide the student with clear direction as to what must be learned	It narrows the learning field
Their use encourages the teacher to examine his goals more carefully	They are difficult to formulate for higher level outcomes and hence, encourage trivialization of learning by focusing on lower level outcomes
It is relatively easy to assess student's achievement, as behavior is observable	They are very difficult to formulate for affective domain
They can aid self-instruction	They ignore unanticipated outcomes of instruction
They are accessible to public scrutiny	It only emphasis on the learning of factual information rather than scientific inquiry
They offer a rational system for curriculum planning	They encourage conformity rather than diversity
Students on the whole tend to welcome the clarity that behavioral objectives bring to learning	They are extremely time-consuming to formulate and require continuous updating
They provide a basis for comparison between similar courses in different institutions	It is impossible to state objectives for every learning outcome, even if this was desirable
They offer a system for evaluating the performance of the teacher	Their use reflects a training approach rather than an educational one

- Guidance as to the feasibility of implementing the curriculum in varying school contexts, pupil contexts, environments, and peer group situations.
- Information about the variability of effects in differing contexts and on different pupils and an understanding of the causes of the variation.

In relation to justification: In general, writing the aim of the curriculum will justify for what it is being established, which is also accessible for critical scrutiny. Stenhouse believed that it was possible to organize the curriculum without having to specify in advance the behavioral changes that should occur in students; he argued that the purpose of education was to make student outcomes unpredictable.

The role of assessment in a process curriculum is very different from that in a product model, being of critic rather marker. The teacher is cast in the role of critical appraiser of the student's work, with the emphasis on developing self-appraisal in the student. The worthwhile activity in which teacher and student are engaged has standards and criteria inherent in it and the task of appraisal is that of improving student's capacity to work to such criteria by critical reaction to work done. In this sense, assessment is about the teaching of self-assessment.

Subject-based Process Model

Curriculum Content

Content is selected to exemplify the key concepts, criteria, and procedures, which best represent the structure of a body of knowledge. It is assumed that within knowledge, there are number of distinct types of rational judgment. For example, a moral judgment is not validated in the same way as a mathematical theorem, nor a historical explanation in the same way as a theological proposition. Hirst (1975) has suggested that all knowledge and understanding are located in a number of domains and has proposed that mathematics, physical sciences, knowledge of persons, literature, the fine arts, religion, and philosophy as all having distinctive "ways of thinking".

Learning Outcomes (Ends)

Specifying key concepts, criteria, and procedures as learning outcomes would distort the curriculum. This is because they are problematic within a subject. They should, therefore, become the focus of speculation not the object of mastery. The purpose of the curriculum is to help the learner to think like and see the world as does a historian, a mathematician, an industrial designer, etc. In studying a body of socially prescribed knowledge the student is concerned with the "predatory pursuit of truth". The curriculum is never deliberately vocational and the "truth" may not be of any practical use at all.

Learning Activities (Means to Ends)

It is up to the teacher to devise learning activities for the students, but these should be worthwhile processes in themselves rather than means toward specific learning objectives. These activities will have a wide range of worthwhile cognitive content (unlike games) and they should be designed to illuminate the kinds of rational thinking and judgment that are peculiar to a particular body of knowledge or discipline.

Assessment

The subject-based process model of curriculum cannot be directed toward an examination without loss of quality. In assessment of the student's work, the teacher is an appraiser or critic not a marker. Assessment is about the teaching of self-assessment.

Main Application

There is implicit acceptance of the Stenhouse model in the design of many humanities courses, although most would not accept the abolition of formal examinations in their patterns of assessment.

Objective-based Process Model

Curriculum Content

Content is usually selected on a vocational basis and is concerned with what the learner "needs to know" in order to carry out certain tasks in the workplace.

Table 7.3: Revised Bloom's Taxonomy for cognitive domain.

Sl. No.	Taxonomic levels-Cognitive domain	Verbs used
1.	Remembering: Recalling previously learned information	Defines, describes, identifies, knows, labels, lists, matches, names, outlines, recalls, recognizes, reproduces, selects, and states
2.	Understanding: Comprehending the meaning, translation, interpolation, and interpretation of instructions and problems	Comprehends, converts, defends, distinguishes, estimates, explains, extends, generalizes, gives an example, infers, interprets, paraphrases, predicts, rewrites, summarizes, and translates
3.	Applying: Using a concept in a new situation	Applies, changes, computes, constructs, demonstrates, discovers, manipulates, modifies, operates, predicts, prepares, produces, relates, shows, solves, and uses
4.	Analyzing: Separates material or concepts into component parts, so that its organizational structure may be understood	Analyzes, breaks down, compares, contrasts, diagrams, deconstructs, differentiates, discriminates, distinguishes, identifies, illustrates, infers, outlines, relates, selects, and separates
5.	Evaluating: Make judgments about the value of ideas or materials	Appraises, compares, concludes, contrasts, criticizes, critiques, defends, describes, discriminates, evaluates, explains, interprets, justifies, relates, summarizes, and supports
6.	Creating: Put parts together to form a whole, with emphasis on creating a new meaning or structure	Categorizes, combines, compiles, composes, creates, devises, designs, explains, generates, modifies, organizes, plans, rearranges, reconstructs, relates, reorganizes, revises, rewrites, summarizes, tells, and writes

Learning Outcomes (Ends)

Learning outcomes are specified in terms of what the learners will be capable of doing at the end of the course of instruction. Objectives are written with increasing levels of specificity (Davies, 1975) and by doing so, broad aims and goals are "operationalized". Key concepts, criteria, and procedures are also specified.

Learning Activities (Means to Ends)

By employing hierarchies of objectives, notably Bloom's Taxonomy (Table 7.3), learning activities can be designed to match the appropriate objectives, e.g. comprehending, applying, analyzing, and so on, starting with lower order objectives and moving to increasing levels of complexity. It is up to the teacher to devise learning outcomes together with appropriate learning activities for the students. For this reason, the objectives model is often associated with an authoritarian view of learning, which is instrumental and concerned with techniques.

Assessment

This model of curriculum would claim to lend itself to an objective model of assessment where learning outcomes having been clearly specified can be easily tested. The failure of students to achieve a given set of objectives is seen as the responsibility of the curriculum planner and the teacher. In its purest form, the curriculum is first put through a testing process with a sample of "typical" students. Modifications are then made to the objectives and to the teaching methods as a result of this process of feedback. In some extreme examples of the objectives model, students work at their own pace and are required to achieve "mastery" of one set of objectives before they move on to the next.

Main Application

The objectives model is usually associated with curriculum design in the field of vocational training. It has been pointed out elsewhere that the "reproductive" end of the skills schema is often associated with the "knowledge, comprehension, and application", which are essential prerequisites for higher order problem-solving activities. It follows, therefore, that a careful analysis of existing curricula in higher education will often reveal "training" elements that would benefit from the careful planning required to implement the objectives model.

Table 7.4 explains the various aspects of product and process model of curriculum and helps us to understand its implications in relation to education.

Table 7.4: Comparison between key concepts of product and process models of curriculum.

Product model	Process model
• An output model, i.e. emphasis is on the achievement of behavioral objectives; the product of education	• An input model, i.e. emphasis is on learning experiences; the process of education
• Curriculum activities are seen as means to an end, i.e. achievement of terminal objectives	• Curriculum activities are seen as being worthwhile in themselves
• Learning is seen as a change in observable behavior	• Acknowledges that much learning is not observable
• Teaching is geared to producing predictable outcomes	• Teaching is geared to encourage unpredictable outcomes
• Teacher specifies content in terms of the student's achievement of behavioral objectives	• Teacher specifies content but cannot know in advance what the student will do with that content
• Evaluation is done by assessing the student's achievement of behavioral objectives	• Evaluation is done by critical appraisal of the student's work, using the criteria intrinsic to the discipline concerned; includes self-assessment by the student

Model 3: Expressive Model

Curriculum Content

Content is usually selected on the basis of providing the student with some worthwhile learning activities, usually of an exploratory or problem-solving nature.

Learning Outcomes (Ends)

An expressive "objective" describes an educational encounter. It does specify the behavior the student is to acquire. In the eyes of the curriculum planner, it is often the unanticipated results, which are really important. Eisner has clarified his definition as follows:

"........ an expressive objective is the outcome of an encounter or learning activity, which has been planned (by the teacher) to provide the student with an opportunity to personalize learning. It is precisely because of the richness of these encounters or activities and the unique character of the outcome that the expressive objective becomes so difficult to describe in advance". He goes on to say "I believe that a large percentage of teachers from kindergarten through college tend to think of objectives in these terms".

Learning Activities (Means to Ends)

An expressive objective provides the teacher and learner with an invitation to explore issues that are of particular interest to the inquirer. Engagement, meaning intrinsic student motivation is a fundamental criterion used by teachers to select learning activities. However, it is acknowledged that students may need knowledge and skills previously acquired in an instructional context (see objectives model) in order to be able to explore the issues/problems raised by expressive objectives.

Assessment

In their purest form, expressive objectives are a reflection of the aims and values of an education, which believes in molding student's behavior, often in idiosyncratic ways. Engagement, intellectual, and emotional immersion are seen as a better indicator of educational value than an achievement test. It is the educational journey and not its outcome that provides self-assessment through intrinsic rewards to the learner. In practice, however, most tutors are not in a position to abandon formal assessment and the awarding of grades.

Main Application

The expressive model is usually associated with curriculum design in the field of art and design.

Model 4: Problem-centered Model

The starting point for learning is a problem, a query, and a puzzle that the learner wishes to solve. The content knowledge in this model arises from the work on the problem.

Outcomes (Ends)

Learning outcomes cannot be identified with high levels of specificity because the students are responsible for searching out the knowledge they need in order to approach the problem. However, usually it is the teacher who will have set the problem in the first place and he/she has a pretty good idea of the general learning needs of the students and the resources required to help them clarify the issues. Students are typically expected to work on one subproblem at a time in small teams using experiential learning methods. It, therefore, follows that both interpersonal (team skills) and intrapersonal (reflective skills) are explicitly expressed as an important component of the learning outcomes.

Learning Activities (Means to Ends)

An important element in the rationale for a problem-based curriculum is that, assuming good planning and facilitating skills on the part of tutors, students are motivated, and adopt deep approaches to learning. Training in "learning how to learn" and group learning skills often form part of the learning activities undertaken at the start of problem-based learning modules. However, research has shown that skills of this kind, including problem-solving skills, are best acquired through reflecting on real experiences rather than starting with abstract conceptions.

Assessment

This model of curriculum would claim high quality learning, but a smaller coverage of "content" is compared with more traditional lecture-based methods. Problem-based curricula demand more than knowledge acquisition. Assessment is, therefore, a mixture of tutor marked assignments, peer group assessment of team skills, and self-assessment of intrapersonal skills.

Main Application

The problem-based model is usually associated with vocational courses in health sciences, architecture, engineering, business studies, and education. Apart from its positive effect on the quality of student learning, reasons for introducing the model vary from a desire to familiarize students with typical problems faced by a profession, to a holistic way of introducing students to a "new" curriculum before moving to more traditional teaching and learning methods.

Model 5: The Cultural Analysis Model of Curriculum

This model has been developed by Denis Lawton. This model proposes a curriculum planned on the technique of cultural analysis. Culture is defined as the whole way of life of a society and the purpose of education is "to make available to the next generation what we regard as the most important aspects of culture". Cultural analysis is the process by which a selection is made from the culture and in terms of curriculum planning. Lawton suggests cultural analysis will ask:
- What kind of society already exists?
- In what ways is it developing?
- How do its members appear to want it to develop?
- What kinds of values and principles will be involved in deciding on 3 and on the educational means of achieving 3?

Lawton offers a five stage model for this analysis:

Stage 1. Cultural invariants: This examines all the aspects that human societies have in common, such as economic and moral aspects, beliefs, and other systems.

Stage 2. Cultural variables: Involves analyzing the difference between cultures in each of the systems.

Stage 3. Selection from the culture: This stage consists of comparing the cultural analysis of the systems with the existing school curriculum.

Stage 4. Psychological questions and theories: This stage is not in direct continuity with the previous stages, but is seen as an important consideration for any curriculum development.

Stage 5. Curriculum organization: In this final stage, the curriculum can now be planned on the basis of the cultural analysis carried out in the previous stages, bearing in mind the important psychological question and theories that influence learning and instruction.

Model 6: Other Models and Approaches to the Curriculum

One approach to curriculum planning is Beattie's fourfold model of the curriculum. He suggests that there are four fundamental approaches to the task of planning a curriculum for nursing, each with its own particular strengths and weaknesses:

- **The curriculum as a map of key subjects:** As the name implies, this approach consists of mapping out the key subjects in the nursing curriculum, preferably integrating them by means of themes such as "the human lifespan" to avoid the danger of an isolated collection of topics.
- **The curriculum as a schedule of basic skills:** This approach emphasizes the explicit specification of basic skills of nursing, these skills being selected from recent empirical research into nursing practice. A behavioral objectives approach can be appropriate here, provided that it is not used dogmatically for all aspects of teaching, particularly in relation to the knowledge base for clinical practice.
- **The curriculum as a portfolio of meaningful personal experiences:** This approach puts the student at the center of things by organizing the curriculum around their interests and experiences. This is done by using a variety of experiential techniques such as action research, critical incidents, role play, and the like. There will be a degree of tension between the unpredictability consequent upon student autonomy and the need to ensure sufficient opportunity to cover key areas.
- **The curriculum as an agenda of important cultural issues**: This approach avoids giving detailed subject matter, focusing on controversial issues and political dilemmas in nursing and health care. These issues are chosen because they are open to debate and have no right answer, thereby stimulating discussion and enquiry, e.g. "nurse power or patient power".

Beattie suggests that there are three ways of combining the fourfold framework. The first one he calls the "eclectic curriculum", in which the four approaches are mixed together in some sort of combination. The main problem with this is that the more traditional approaches tend to dominate, leaving only the marginal inclusion of student-centered ideas. Another way is to negotiate each of the key areas with the consumers, the "negotiated curriculum". The third way Beattie calls the "dialectical curriculum", in which the curriculum designer "goes out to do battle", as it were, to engage in a deliberate, principles and committed struggle to combat, challenge, and contest the dominant codes of curriculum.

He further stressed that the curriculum planners in nursing should move from simple-minded, "single model" approaches to complex, multifaceted strategies.

Greaves Curriculum Model for Nursing

Another approach to nursing curricula is that of "Greaves" curriculum model for nursing. The model is based upon the behavioral objectives model referred to earlier and consists of a 4 × 4 matrix.

	Objectives	Content	Methods	Evaluation
Assessment	–	–	–	–
Planning				
Implementation				
Evaluation				

The vertical dimension contains the four components of the rational curriculum model, i.e. objectives, content, methods, and evaluation and the horizontal dimension contains the four elements of the nursing process, i.e. assessment, planning, implementation, and evaluation. This gives sixteen cells in all, each one relating specific aspects of the nursing process to specific aspects of the curriculum process. Hence, curriculum objectives can be defined in relation to each of the four stages of the nursing process, as curriculum content, methods, and evaluation. This curriculum matrix serves as a conceptual framework for planning a nursing curriculum and is firmly based in the nursing process model of care.

Curriculum Planning

Curriculum development is known by varied names as curriculum building, curriculum making, curriculum planning, and curriculum construction. If it is the process of improving the existing curriculum, it is called as curriculum reconstruction or curriculum rebuilding. Curriculum planning is the collective responsibility of the school or college, statutory body, and the significant others. Curriculum is planned at the various levels. In the institutional level, the curriculum committee takes up the responsibility in planning curriculum. It is an ongoing activity. While planning the curriculum, the model of educational process is considered.

The curriculum in nursing does not exist in isolation, but reflects the changing nature of society and its emerging themes. If the curriculum is to be of use to its customers, then it must incorporate the beliefs, values, and developments both of society at large and of the nursing profession itself.

Curriculum planning is a complex activity involving the interplay of ideas from the curriculum field and other related disciplines. However, the ultimate purpose of curriculum planning is to describe the learning opportunities available to students. Curriculum planning involves decisions about both content and the process. It involves many people and levels of operation and is a continuous process.

Characteristics of a Good Curriculum

- Reflects the philosophy of nation
- Represents the culture of the people
- Considers the political situation and demands of the contemporary society
- Based on the culture
- Neither be too broad as to be evasive nor be too narrow without allowing any flexibility
- Will be based on practical experience of the people
- Will be relevant to the society
- Will be comprehensive taking into consideration the needs of the society
- Taking into consideration the level of development of the learners, their nature, and learning readiness
- Have built-in mechanism for evaluation and feedback at every stage—designing, transaction, and implementation
- Provides room for reconstructing experiential aspects
- Will prepare the learners for immediate and long-term future
- Will consider cognitive, affective, and psychomotor domain.

Drawbacks in Curriculum Construction

The defects in designing the curriculum are:
- Remoteness—not related to the needs of immediate future
- Not relevant
- Not adequate
- Not related to practical life—too much of theory
- Rigidity not allowing for updating or enriching
- Obsolescence—outdated, irrelevant, and not considering the recent trends
- Incomplete—not being comprehensive
- No room for interval criticism
- Failure to suggest implementation strategies.

The components of curriculum are:
- Aims or objectives
- Contents
- Methods of teaching and learning
- Evaluation of outcomes.

Sequence in Planning a Curriculum

Planning
Curriculum overall goals
Objectives
Learning experiences
Evaluation

↓

Planning various courses
Goals-Objectives
Learning experiences
Evaluation

↓

Unit planning
Objectives
Learning experiences
Evaluation

↓

Lesson planning
Objectives
Learning experiences
Evaluation

Stages of Curriculum Planning

The Directive Stage

This initial stage lays the foundations for all other stages by identifying the beliefs, knowledge, and concepts that form the basis of the curriculum. This is done by the systematic gathering of information from the literature and also by the exploration of common beliefs about the nature of nursing. This leads to a statement of the philosophy of the curriculum, which in turn serves to influence each successive stage of the curriculum process. This stage lays down a theoretical framework for the selection and sequencing of the content.

The Formative Stage

The overall design of the curriculum takes shape and this design should reflect the philosophy described in stage one. Objectives will be written for specific levels within the course as well as for overall course objectives. Content mapping is used to select content elements for each aspect of the course and also gives staff and students an indication of the sequencing of topics.

The Functional Stage

This is the stage in which the curriculum begins to assume a more practical form. The variety of teaching methods and learning experiences are decided to include both classroom and clinical teaching. The methods of evaluation are also decided:
- Evaluation for continued learning. This is evaluation that provides feedback for students to improve their learning.
- Evaluation for grading. Examinations designed for grading should not be viewed as a learning activity.
- Evaluation for curriculum revision. This involves assessment of the total curriculum package and constitutes stage four.

The Evaluative Stage

When the curriculum is fully implemented and is thus a summative evaluation. There are three aspects to this:
1. Input evaluation: What the students bring to the course, such as mathematical abilities, problem solving abilities, and so on.
2. Throughput evaluation: All the tests and activities that students undergo as they progress through the course.
3. Output evaluation: Achievement of the characteristics identified in the directive stage.

Principles of Curriculum Construction

The Principle of Flexibility

Curriculum should be flexible and not so rigid. Schools must be able to make necessary adjustments based on the local needs and conditions.

The Principle of Sensitivity

Curriculum should be constructed in such a way that it will be sensitive to the feeling of the students, community, and those of the nation.

The Principle of Need-basedness

Curriculum should take into its cognizance the needs of children, community, and those of the nation.

The Principle of Individual Differences

The individual differences among students must also be taken care or by the framers of curriculum. They should develop graded curriculum to cater to the different mental levels of the students—the dullards, the average, and the gifted.

Other Principles of Curriculum Construction

In addition, there are other principles of curriculum construction, which are self-evident. They are listed below:
- The principle of social-utilitarianism
- The principle of child-centeredness
- The principle of pupil-tailoring
- The principle of goal-orientedness
- The principle of integration
- The principle of interest-centeredness
- The principle of activity-centeredness
- The principle of life-centeredness.

Phases in the Curriculum Development

The phases in the curriculum development as mentioned in Figure 7.4 are:
- Developmental phase
- Implementation phase
- Evaluation phase.

Developmental Phase

As curriculum and education are interlocked, curriculum should be so planned as to equip the teachers and learners in bringing the desirable changes in the behavior. Prior to constructing a curriculum, we should consider certain factors. They are:
- Factors relating to the learners:
  - Health
  - Family
  - Vocation
  - Religion and culture

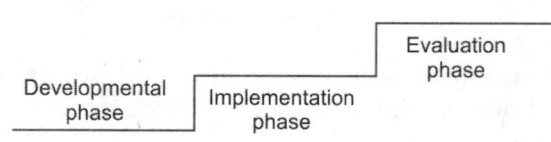

Fig. 7.4: Phases in the curriculum development.

- Employment opportunities
- Social civic and economic aspects
- Psychological aspects and so on.
- Factors related to the teachers:
  - Educational qualification
  - Level of preparation
  - Employment opportunities
  - Social, civic, and economic aspects
  - Psychological aspects.
- Factors related to the subjects:
  - Subject content
  - Hours for theory and practicals
  - Learning experiences
  - Audio-visual aids
  - Methods of teaching
  - Evaluation.
- Factors related to the environment:
  - Physical environment
  - Needs of the society
  - National aspirations and needs
  - Culture and changes in values
  - Problems of the society
  - Social changes
  - Technological changes
  - Economic changes
  - Political changes
  - Manpower need
  - Employment opportunities.
- Resources available:
  - Financial resources
  - Human resources
  - Material resources
  - Government regulations and policies.

Collect the data regarding all the factors and based on the available data, formulate the objectives.

Objectives may be formed in relation to:
- Selection of learning experiences
- Teaching methods
- Audio-visual aids
- Scheme of evaluation.

Based on the objectives, the educators should decide on the learning experiences, i.e. instructional methods and media and evaluation program for the intended curriculum.

Implementation Phase

In this phase, the educators have to implement the planned program, provide appropriate learning experiences of theory and practicals by using various teaching methods and media.

Evaluation Phase

The educators have to use various evaluation techniques to evaluate the effectiveness of learning experiences, teaching-learning methods, and the audio-visual aids used. This helps us to analyze how far we have achieved the objectives.

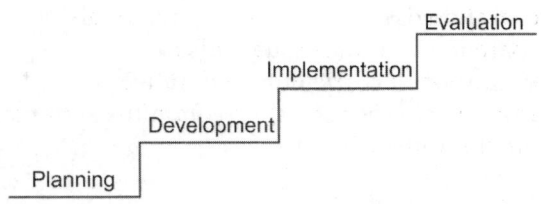

Fig. 7.5: Steps in curriculum construction.

Steps in Curriculum Construction

The steps in curriculum construction as mentioned in Figure 7.5 are:
- Planning
- Development
- Implementation
- Evaluation.

Planning

It is the first step in curriculum construction. It involves:
- Investigation and analysis of existing situation to determine needs and purpose of establishing the nursing education program.
- Statement of philosophy and objectives of the program.
- Identification of members such as nurse educators, administrators, leaders, practitioners, representatives from public, regulatory bodies, etc. who can influence and who should be involved in curriculum construction.
- Making decisions regarding:
  - Student recruitment, eligibility criteria
  - Type of educational program to be established in meeting the demands of the society and primary healthcare
  - Duration of the program
  - Staffing requirements
  - Selection of learning experiences
  - Sequencing and placement of learning experiences.
- Distributing the available instructional time.
- Selection of teaching-learning methods and materials.
- Development of evaluation plan.
- Planning for student guidance and counseling services.
- Planning for student's participation in student's health services program.

Development

This step involves:
- Organization and sequencing of theoretical, clinical, and community learning experiences.
- Planning and arranging for student rotation plans for clinical and community experiences.

- Preparation of teaching-learning materials.
- Preparation of audio-visual aids.
- Constitution of curriculum committee.
- Formation of other standing committees for management of the curriculum.

Implementation

This step involves:
- Actual conduction of teaching-learning activities related to theoretical, clinical, and community components.
- Refinement of teaching-learning methods.
- Assessment of student performance.
- Organizing student guidance and counseling services and other health services.
- Conduction of curriculum committee meetings.
- Periodical revision of curriculum implementation.

Evaluation

This is the final step and it involves:
- Evaluation of students in terms of:
  - Knowledge
  - Skill
  - Attitude.
- Teaching-learning process
- Effective use of audio-visual methods
- Student activities undertaken in the community and institutional settings.

System Approach to Curriculum Construction

The input-process-output model of a system also brings out another dimension of the system approach. In order to use the system approach, the curriculum designer has to go through the following stages:

Selection of Aims, Goals, and Objectives

A curriculum is essentially a planned educational program. Objectives are derived from goals. The goals may be ultimate, mediate, and proximate goals.

In nursing, the ultimate goal deals with the outcomes of 4 years of college program. It describes the end products of education spread over a period of time. It is usually expressed in terms of changes in knowledge, attitude, feelings, and action. Mediate aims may refer to a stage of education or a particular content area, e.g. child health nursing, nursing education, etc. The proximate aims are also called specific objectives. These deals with classroom level behavior. It is otherwise known as behavioral objectives.

Selection of Learning Experience

It is based on the needs of the student and the goals and objectives guide us to select appropriate learning experiences for the students. It is discussed in detail in the following text.

Selection of Content

Selection of subject matter:
- Criteria: Relevance, importance, and priority
- Scope: Amount, depth of coverage, and concentration
- Sequence: Hierarchy and progression of complexity continuity (in learning), balance, and evaluation
- Content: Relevancy, organization, and completeness
- Process (how well was designed)
- Participants (effects on faculty, students, and staff)
- Outcomes (effect on real world).

Organization and Integration of Learning

The below mentioned factors are considered in organizing learning experiences:
- Nature of the learners
- Needs of the learners
- Cognitive development
- Linguistic development
- Psychosocial development
- Moral/affective development
- Professional/vocational focus
- Best teaching methods available
- Faculty development
- Resources (facilities, budget).

Evaluation

It includes the methods used to evaluate the achievement of goals and objectives. It also includes the evaluation of input, process, and the output.

Curriculum Design

A curriculum is a written document that delineates the organization of content, scope, and arrangement of an educational program. It specifies the learning activities designed to achieve specific educational goals (Bevis, 1989). Curriculum frameworks provide faculty with a means of conceptualizing and organizing the knowledge, skills, values, and beliefs critical to the delivery of a coherent curriculum, which facilitates the achievement of the desired outcomes (Boland, 1998).

The curriculum of a school or college of nursing typically includes an organizational or conceptual framework, philosophy and mission statements, a list of outcomes, competencies, or objectives for the program and individual courses, course outlines and syllabi, educational activities, and evaluation methods (Dillard and Laidig, 1998). Furthermore, most curricula specify essential nursing content and application in clinical practice.

The curricula of all nursing programs are based on the Tyler curriculum development model published in 1950. According to this model, a curriculum should include (Bevis, 1987):
- A philosophy
- A conceptual framework
- Behaviorally defined measurable objectives
- Learning activities
- Measurable criteria for evaluation.

Bevis (1989a; 1989b) stated that the incorporation of the Tyler model within nursing curricula began in the 1950s and continued throughout the 1960s and 1970s. Eventually, the Tyler model became the only model for use in developing nursing curriculum for all levels of nursing education (i.e. diploma, associate degree, and baccalaureate degree).

Impact of the Indian Nursing Council on Nursing Curricula

In India, individually and collectively, the Indian Nursing Council sets rules and requirements regarding nursing educational programs and curricula. These rules and regulation typically specify content areas that must be covered, minimum hours that must be spent by all students in clinical settings, and competencies or skills that all students must possess at the completion of the nursing programs.

Conceptual or Organizing Frameworks

The conceptual framework of a nursing program must be an outgrowth of the philosophy of the faculty and must reflect the faculty's philosophical beliefs about person, health, nursing, society, and environment.

The conceptual or organizational framework serves several purposes. It allows faculty to determine what knowledge is important to nursing and how that knowledge should be defined, categorized, and linked with other knowledge (Boland, 1998). Conceptual frameworks provide faculty with a defined cohesive, logical curriculum that outlines learning experience that will help achieve the desired educational outcomes (Dillard and Laidig, 1998).

According to Bevis (1989a), a conceptual framework is an interrelated system of premises that provide guidelines or ground rules for making all curricular decisions objectives, content, implementation, and evaluation, the conceptual framework...... is the conceptualization, articulation of concepts, facts, propositions, postulates, theories, phenomenon, and variables relevant to a specific nursing educational system.

Boland (1998) stated that there are two approaches to determine the organizational framework for the curriculum. Faculty may choose to select a single, specific nursing theory or model on which to build the framework, or they may choose a more eclectic approach, selecting concepts from multiple theories or models. Boland (1998) explained that use of a single theory to develop the conceptual framework will provide a single image with a defined vocabulary shared by both learners and teachers. However, use of a single theory or conceptual model has limitations and poses challenges. One commonly encountered challenge is how to make theoretical explanations of reality understandable for beginning nursing students. Furthermore, the language of the theory and the definitions of the central concepts may be too abstract to be helpful.

To avoid being constrained by a single nursing theory or model, many faculty members choose an eclectic approach. A criticism of using this approach is that it impedes the development of a body of knowledge that is uniquely nursing. The advantage to an eclectic approach is the ability to borrow concepts and definitions that best fit the faculty's beliefs and values.

The framework may contain additional concepts or threads, such as caring, self-care, growth and development, nursing process, and adaptation and may use age or developmental levels to influence designation of major content areas. It may use acute/chronic concepts, the health/illness continuum, practice settings, or the nursing process as the chief organizer. In addition, process threads are usually present throughout the curriculum. These may include the nursing process, problem-solving, interpersonal relationships, communication, research, change, and teaching. Finally, the framework may be primarily process-oriented or content-oriented.

Nursing and nursing education would benefit from an internally consistent core framework that represents more clearly what nursing is and does, while being flexible and adaptable enough to allow for creativity among schools that serve diverse populations in diverse regions in a dramatically changing healthcare environment. This framework:
- Identifies historically significant and currently relevant concepts unique to and inherent in nursing, as well as important concepts shared with other disciplines.
- Provides logical and progressive support and structure that enhance growth and provides for the measurement of outcomes.
- Allows for and is defendant on the inclusion of faculty beliefs unique to them, their institution, region, population, and healthcare system.
- Supports the integration and synthesis of curricular concepts into one whole, which is greater than the sum of its parts.
- Is dynamically stable enough to allow for revision and change with minimum curricular disruption, which is perhaps most important.

Characteristics of Curriculum Framework

The perceived characteristics of the envisaged curriculum framework would include the following:
- Reflects the Indian heritage, acts as an instrument in the realization of national goals, and fulfills aspirations of people.
- Responds to the latest developments in the field of education.
- Establishes integration of theory and practice of education.
- Provides multiple educational experiences to teachers.
- Enables teachers to experiment with new ideas.
- Ensures inseparability of preservices and in-service education of teachers.
- Sets achievable goals for various stages of teacher education.
- Provides for use of communication technology.

The cornerstones in nursing curriculum framework are:
- Nursing knowledge
- Nursing skills
- Nursing values
- Nursing meanings
- Nursing experience.

Descriptively, these cornerstones form the foundation for nursing and nursing education. Nursing knowledge is discipline specific and includes patterns of knowing that are unique to the discipline and help establish disciplinary boundaries. It encompasses not only information that is epistemologically significant to nursing, but includes information from related disciplines that may influence nursing practice.

Nursing Knowledge

Nursing knowledge is influenced by formal education and the ongoing development of nursing skills, values, meanings, and experience. In addition, it is influenced continually by the knowledge, skills, values, meanings, and experience of others, including peers, patients, families, and other healthcare providers. Concepts of nursing knowledge include areas relevant to the provision of care and the advancement of the profession.

Skills

Skills are deliberate acts or activities in the cognitive and psychomotor domain that operationalize nursing knowledge, values, meanings, and experience.

Nursing skills are selected, implemented, and evaluated for with or on behalf of those for whom we care. Implementation of skills requires reasoning that reflects nursing knowledge, values, meanings, and experience. The selection, implementation, and evaluation of nursing skills require the intentional application of specific nursing knowledge, values, meanings, and experience.

Values

Values are enduring beliefs, attributes, or ideals that establish moral boundaries of what is right and wrong in thought, judgment, character, attitude, and behavior and that form a foundation for decision-making throughout life. Values reflect individual, family, social, cultural, and religious influences, as well as personal choice.

Values provide a sense of individuality as well as a sense of common identity with those who share the same or similar values. Values that are shared collectively by individuals within a particular profession reflect the values deemed important for that profession and are operationalized in the form of professional standards and practices (Kozier et al, 1997). Values identified within the nursing profession such as honesty, integrity, and ethics guide the behavior of nurses and directly influence patient care.

Meanings

Meanings define the context, purpose, and intent of language. The language and associated meanings in nursing are derived from nursing knowledge, skills, values, and experience and are shared among nurses. Nursing language applies unique meanings to existing words, as well as to new phenomena.

Experience

Experience commonly refers to longevity or length of time in a position. Nursing experience refers to the unique and active process of defining, refining, and changing.

Experience, as defined by change, is the one thing nursing faculty cannot provide. They can plan the clinical experience and schedule the time, but ultimately it is up to the students to actively become intellectually engaged and involved and ultimately evolve through experiential learning, knowing, and understanding.

The ABC of Curriculum Organization

Bhatia explains the ABC of curriculum organization as articulation, balance, and continuity.

Articulation

It is the horizontal coordination or correlation between subjects. For example, all the relevant subjects are placed together, so that learning becomes easier. All basic sciences are placed together in the 1st year BSc(N) syllabus. The concepts studied and discussed are related to each other and the students can easily correlate the concepts for their practical application. The concepts of anatomy and physiology are related to each other.

Balance

There is a need while designing the curriculum for an appropriate balance. Appropriate weightage should be given to each and every aspect of the curriculum.

Continuity

In organizing content, there should be continuity. There is a link in contents from class to class, grade to grade like vertical continuity. It should also have a continuity horizontally, i.e. continuity between different units. The problem of curriculum organization includes two major dimensions—the content and the learning experiences. The different problems involved in the organization of curriculum are:
- Establishing sequence
- Determining the focus
- Integration of content and skills
- Logical and psychological requirements
- Varieties in modes of learning
- Continuity
- Balance.

Establishing Sequence

According to Smith, Stanley, and Shore, four basic principles are involved in sequencing the curriculum:
1. **From simple to complex**: The content is organized from the simple components to the complex components by creating an interrelationship between each other.
2. **Expository order**: It starts with simple specific concepts to the whole material organization.
3. **From whole to part**: It starts with whole and goes to individual parts.
4. **Chronological**: Here, the content or subject matter is organized in a time sequence either from earlier to later or from later to earlier.

Determining the Focus

The problem of lack of focus in curriculum organization is the major drawback. It is also important to understand whether it should be organized by subjects, topics, or by units. The focus should be on the following:
- The units, topics of the subject
- The core ideas of the topic as focusing centers
- Core ideas can be used as coverage
- Focusing centers as the threads for either a vertical or horizontal integration.

Integration of Content and Skills

Learning becomes more effective when the facts and principles from the field are related to one another. This means seeing relationships between experiences or knowledge. The integration could be horizontal or vertical.

Logical and Psychological Requirements

In the process of organization of curriculum, it should preserve both logic of the subject matter and psychological sequence of learning experiences. We need to decide the logical sequence depending on the content. In psychological requirements, it depends upon the student's reaction, interests, and ways of looking at the subjects. For more effective organization, both of them are need to be considered.

Variety in Modes of Learning

All learn effectively by some method. Some learn more effectively by some methods. So, the wider range of or variety in the modes of learning helps for better learning of the content. The content organization should provide wider scope for it.

Conceptual Framework for Curriculum Design

A framework involves the various elements and its interrelationship. The conceptual framework for curriculum design involves the various curriculum elements and its interrelationship. The following questions may help and give a direction to arrive at the design:
- What is a curriculum?
- What should be included in it?
- What are the important elements in it?
- What is the relationship between various elements?
- What kind of organizational problems creep in?
- How the theoretical design and practical implementation are related?
- What is the sequence of design?

The different components of curriculum can be derived by raising some questions like: what to teach, how to teach, how to evaluate, etc. Then consider the major factors, which form the basis for curriculum. They are:
- Learners and their cognitive level
- Learning process
- Social and cultural demands
- Content of the disciplines.

The steps in curriculum organization are:
- Diagnosis of needs
- Formulation of objectives
- Selection of content
- Organization of content
- Selection of learning experiences
- Organization of learning experiences
- Determination of what to evaluate and the procedures of evaluation.

General Plan for Curriculum

It includes:
- Philosophy and objectives
- Total duration of the program

- Total available hours for theory, practical, clinical and community settings, and cocurricular activities.
- Definition of different courses of study:
  - Theory and practicals
  - Course outline for each course of study
  - Guideline for practicals
  - Master rotation plan and individual course plan
  - Guidelines for cocurricular activities.
- Instructional methods and media for theory, practicals, and laboratory work.
- Scheme of evaluation:
  - Concurrent evaluation
  - Terminal evaluation
  - Uses of results.

Formulation of Philosophy and Objectives

The words "aims, goals, purposes, and objectives" are often used interchangeably in relation to the educational objectives of a school program.

Educational Objectives

Aims can broadly be defined as a general statement, which attempts to give both shape and direction to a set of more detailed intentions for the future.

Educational outcome is the end result of an educational experience and is most general of all terms essential with goal. General goals are subdivided into immediate and long-term goals. Long-term goals are end goals attained by the end of the program or after one has qualified.

Immediate goals are specific for a lesson or unit.

Classification of Objectives

Objectives are classified into three types by Guilbert:

They are general objectives, intermediary objectives, and specific or instructional objectives. General objectives are corresponding to the functions of the learner after completion of the education. Intermediate objectives are arrived at by breaking down the professional functions into component activities, which together indicate the nature of those functions.

Specific or instructional objectives are corresponding or derived from precise professional task whose results are observable and measurable against given criteria.

According to Heidgerken

Central Objectives

It is the core of the unit. It is the central learning product desired and gives clarity, design, meaning, and unity to learning activities determined by objectives. It is the ultimate aim to be achieved.

Contributing Objectives

They are those which help in the attainment of the central objectives. It is dependent on certain understanding, skills, attitudes, and appreciation, which are known as contributory.

Tangible and Intangible Objectives

Objectives in the area of knowledge and skill are highly tangible. Learning outcomes in these areas are easily identified and capable of most direct measurement. The least tangible objectives are in the realms of attitudes, interests, and values; those objectives dealing with understanding, aspects of thinking are of intermediate tangibility.

Sequence for Formulating Objectives

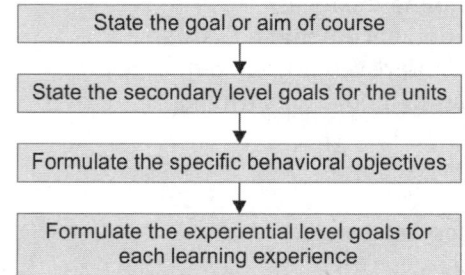

Objectives may be stated as:

Teacher-centered Objectives

They are the activities that the teacher has to do. For example, to demonstrate, to discuss, etc. But these are not the ultimate purpose of the educational program. Any statement of educational objective should specify the desired changes expected in student's behavior.

Subject Matter-centered Objectives

These are objectives stated in the form of topics, concepts, and generalizations. It may be as listing topics and content those are to be dealt with, in the course. These are not a satisfactory form of stating objectives because they do not specify what the students are expected to do with these elements.

Behavior-centered Objectives

Objectives sometimes are stated in the form of generalized pattern of behavior, which may not indicate the area of life or content to which the behavior applies, e.g. objectives stated to develop appreciation, to develop critical thinking, etc.

These are highly generalized objectives and cannot be achieved satisfactorily. It is necessary to specify more definitely the content and the area to which the problem applies.

Learner-centered Objectives

These types of objectives specify what the learner is to do in terms of desired outcome of learning. Learner-centered objectives are an excellent guide to teachers for selection of learning activities, for bringing out desired changes, behavior of learners, and to evaluate the outcomes of learning.

Criteria for the selection and statement of objectives:
- Objectives should be stated in terms of desired changes in behavior.
- The desired changes in behavior should be consistent with the educational philosophy of the curriculum.
- Objectives should be attainable and practical.
- Objectives should be related to the needs and level of learner.
- Objectives should serve as a direction for the teacher and the student.
- Objectives should help in developing the evaluation devices to measure whether the objectives are attained.
- Objectives should be easily understood by the teacher and the learner.
- Each statement has to have only one objective.
- Objectives should be measurable.

Selection of Learning Experiences

Meaning and Definition

An experience is the lesson one learns as a result of or from his/her interaction with people in various and varied situations and/or with the environment.

Learning has been defined as any relatively permanent change in behavior that results as a result of practice or experience.

Learning experiences may be defined as deliberately planned experiences in selected situations where students actively participate, interact, and which result in desirable changes of behavior in the students.

Thus, selection of learning situations together with corresponding learning activities will comprise the learning experiences.

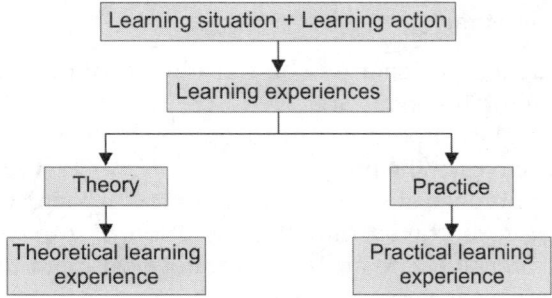

Principles in Selection of Learning Experiences

- Selection should be based on the educational objectives.
- Learning activities should be in relation to real-life situations where the students are expected to practice after being qualified.
- Selection of learning experiences should be done in such a manner that there should be an integration between theory and practice.
- The learning experiences should provide for and assist the students in effective experimental learning.
- Learning experiences should develop the student's logical and analytical thinking.
- While selecting the learning experiences, the focus should be:
  - Community oriented
  - Oriented to meet the health needs and demands of the society
  - Oriented to primary prevention
  - Oriented to nursing care practices of various levels such as primary, secondary, and tertiary levels
  - Oriented to values in nursing.

Criteria for Selection of Learning Experiences

- It should be consistent with the philosophy of the educational institution and lead to the achievement of the ultimate goal of the program.
- It should be varied and flexible, so as to meet the demands of the learners.
- It should provide for sufficient opportunity for self-activity of the student.
- It should provide for the development of higher mental functions such as independent thinking, decision-making, sound judgment, intellectual resourcefulness, and creative and critical thinking.
- It should be based on the needs of the learner.
- It is arranged in a manner that provides continuity, correlation, and integration of theory and practice.
- It should provide for planned evaluation by the teachers and students.

Organization of Learning Experiences

This involves two steps:
1. Grouping of learning experiences
2. Placement of selected learning experiences covering sequencing and integration.

Grouping of learning experiences under subject headings:
Once the learning experiences are selected according to the criteria, it should be organized in such a way that the student will receive maximum benefit. The practice of grouping them under subject heading is one method of organization.

Learning experiences pertaining to learning of various subjects like Anatomy, Physiology, Microbiology, Community Health Nursing, Medical Surgical Nursing, and Fundamentals of Nursing, etc. are grouped under the concerned subject.

The subjects may be again grouped under major headings:

Basic sciences applied to nursing: Anatomy, Physiology, and Microbiology.

Behavioral sciences applied to nursing: Psychology, Sociology.

Nursing: Fundamentals of Nursing, Medical-surgical Nursing, Community Health Nursing, Maternal and Child Health Nursing, and Mental Health Nursing.

Placement

The following are the criteria, which can serve as guide for effective organization of the subject matter and the learning experiences in the curriculum.

Continuity: It refers to the relationship existing between different levels of the same subject or skills.

Sequence: It means placement of learning experiences in such a manner that the students will proceed from simple to complex, concrete to abstract, and from normal to abnormal. Learning of anatomy and physiology in 1st year will help to understand the pathology, which is an altered physiology.

Integration: This means a state of wholeness, harmony, and relatedness. It is blending things together into a harmonious whole. The learning experiences are offered, so that a student can integrate all learning experiences in solving the problems of varied situations.

Correlation: It is also related to the integration. It is bringing together all relevant and related experiences in order to make learning easier.

Teaching System

The teaching of various subjects in the curriculum may be organized in different ways. They are:
- The teaching block
- Partial block system
- Study day system
- Daily classes.

The Teaching Block

For each course or subject, there is a prescribed theory hours. While planning for a course, we have to plan for both theory and practicals. In teaching block, only the subject content or theory is taken for a prescribed period. It is so planned that it is spread at intervals throughout the curriculum. During this, the students are withdrawn from the clinical posting, so that students can concentrate on the learning of subject matter. All the students in the whole class can attend. It makes the planning of curriculum easier.

Partial Block System

In partial block system, the students may be in the teaching block each morning or afternoon for two or three hours per day during the week of their experience. The remaining time they can be in the ward or community area. If this system is followed, daily theoretical instructions are required to spread over a greater length of period to cover the courses of study.

Study Day System

One day in a week can be completely planned for theory classes for students. Thus, in this system, daily classes are not conducted. The advantage is that the students are free from clinical responsibilities for a full day and it is easier to organize the teaching.

Daily Classes

The classes for students are held daily, regularly each day. The students will be in the field in the morning and attend the classes in the afternoon or vice versa.

Planning of Clinical Experience

The planning of clinical experience is the function of the faculty. It should be based on the objectives. It is planned in such a manner that it will meet the needs of the learner at a particular stage in a course and we should make sure that the right clinical experience is provided at the right time. This job is made easier by preparation of the clinical rotation plan. It is must to prepare a separate clinical rotation plan for each clinical area. Rotation means regular, successive, and/or recurrent posting of various groups of nursing students belonging to different classes in specific nursing fields that is different hospital wards, operation theater, labor room, outpatient departments, and community health fields, etc. Rotation plan is a plan which gives the details of rotation of various groups of students into the different areas of hospital for specified period of time.

The factors, which are to be considered for planning a clinical rotation plan, are:
- The plan should be based on the philosophy and objectives of the program.
- The number of students to be posted in each clinical area to be taken into consideration. For example, in intensive care areas, we cannot post more than 3 students at a given point of time.
- The number of departments or wards or clinical areas to be considered.
- The size of the department, bed occupancy, and workload of the particular area are also considered.
- The duration of clinical experience in each area is taken into account.

- Number of supervisory faculty members available in each area to guide and supervise the students is important.
- Consider the Indian Nursing Council/University requirements in relation to clinical experience.

Basic Principles in Planning Clinical Rotation

- It must be in accordance with the total curriculum plan.
- Theoretical instructions should precede as closely as possible the clinical experience.
- The supervisory faculty members are well prepared and be available with the students to provide adequate guidance.
- Selection of areas of experience should proceed from simple to complex.
- The clinical teaching staff should be involved whenever, feasible and must be familiar with the rotation plan. A copy of the rotation plan should be available in each area.
- First year students should be given maximum supervision by clinical supervisors and qualified nursing staff.
- Each student should be rotated in all the areas without missing any area. If for any reason, if she misses any of the area, it should be compensated by planning separately for her.
- Overcrowding in any clinical area with different groups or students should be avoided.
- All the students should complete the assignments and requirements of particular clinical area within that area. They should not carry over any of the assignments and it should be completed before they leave the area.
- The rotation plan must be made in advance.
- Continuity of service, where considered essential, must be maintained.

Master Rotation Plan

The master rotation plan is an overall plan of rotation of all students in a particular educational institution showing the placement of the students belonging to various groups/classes in clinical nursing as well as community nursing fields denoting the duration of such placement together with placement of theoretical teaching block/periods.

It is prepared in advance for the whole year, so that it gives a complete and clear picture about student's clinical and field placement during an academic session.

This plan must include the period of vacation, teaching block, and preparation time/week for examination, examination weeks, etc.

Also, the master rotation plan for each year, i.e. I, II, III, and IV year can be prepared separately and then put up in a combined chart, so that all teachers are aware of the student placement.

Advantages

- Availability of advance plan helps to plan for various curricular and cocurricular activities.
- It informs all the faculty members of the student placement in various clinical and community areas and also the theory hours, so as to enable them to work cooperatively.
- Students are aware of their academic program in advance. This helps them to prepare themselves for working in various settings.
- Evaluation of the program is more effective.
- Nursing service staff members and faculty members are in a position to make tentative advance plans for their vacation, etc. without disturbing the teaching-learning activities.

Individual Rotation Plan

Individual rotation plan is made to make sure that each student in a particular block posting undergoes experience in each area. For example, in four weeks of posting, where the student needs to gain experience in ward management, dietary service, laundry, and record keeping, etc. a plan can be made keeping the individual student's plan of rotation during this four weeks period. It is usually the practice to post two or three students in an area instead of a single student. The objectives of the clinical posting are discussed with the students to gain maximum benefit and also the student should maintain a log book of daily experience in the area of posting.

Curriculum Implementation

The objective of a curriculum is not only to mold the student to a particular shape, status, or career, but to facilitate the process of growth and development according to his/her nature or interest and aptitude.

A curriculum must be implemented if it is to make any desired impact on students. Unless it is implemented, it cannot be evaluated for betterment. A curriculum can be implemented either slowly or rapidly.

Planning Implementation

Apart from curriculum planning in general terms, it is essential that we need to plan the implementation of a curriculum. Planning process addresses the needs and changes necessary and requisite resource for carrying out intended actions. Implementation planning should focus on the factors:

- People
- Program
- Process.

The curriculum design is the basic skeleton upon which the flesh and blood of curriculum transactional process can be built. In the educational system, the planned input (learning material) and process (learning strategies) are organized to cater to the needs of the students.

Curriculum transaction strategies are the teaching methods used to transform the content of the curriculum using these methods.

Resources for Curriculum Transaction

There are various resources used for curriculum transaction. It can be classified as print-based and nonprint-based resources.

Print-based Resources
- Reference book and manuals
- Textbooks
- Periodicals professional magazines and journals collections
- Instructional materials.

Nonprint-based Resources
It includes audio-visual equipment such as computers, television, etc. Apart from the material resources, there are other resources also which can be effectively utilized for instructional purposes. These may be teacher himself, his students, and the environment within which instructional activities are carried out.

Print-based Resources—Textbook

Characteristics of Good Textbook
The characteristics can be discussed under the three main headings:

The Author

The persons who have long experience of teaching the subject and possessing the requisite qualifications should be allowed to become the authors. They should have interest in writing the textbooks.

Mechanical Features

Textbooks should have attractive binding and printing. The quality of papers and type of letters used should be fine and appealing. They must have capturing photographs, figures, and diagrams.

Subject Matter
- Subject matter should cover the whole syllabus.
- There must be proper selection and organization of subject matter.
- Subject matter should be arranged systematically and should be developed in psychological sequence.
- It should fulfill the aims and objectives of the science of teaching.
- Subject matter should be fully illustrated with pictures and sketches.
- It should serve as a guide for demonstrations and individual experiments.
- Subject matter should be written in very simple, clear, and lucid language.
- Each chapter should begin with an introduction and end with a summary.
- Content should be arranged under main headings and subheadings.
- The book should contain a detailed table of contents in the beginning and an index at the end.
- For each lesson, problem (solved and unsolved) and assignments should be given.
- It should mention proper use of teaching aids.
- It should be reasonably priced.
- It should cover the syllabus.
- The facts should be modern and comprehensive.
- It should link science with practical life.
- The content should contain not only the established facts, but also the problems which are being researched and thereby, arousing the interest in the pupils in those problems.

Development of Textbooks

Structure is important for any textbooks. Structure refers to the way ideas are connected together in logical organizational patterns.

Simple listing: A listing of items or ideas where the order of presentation of the item is not significant.

Conclusion/evidence: A special case of simple listing consisting of a proposition and a list of reasons serving as evidence for that fact.

Comparison/contrast: A description of similarities and differences between two or more things.

Temporal sequence: A sequential relationship between items or events considered in terms of the passage of time.

Cause-effect: An interaction between at least two ideas or event, one considered a cause or reason and the other effect or result and problem-solution similar to the cause-effect pattern in that two factors interact, one citing a problem and the other a solution to that problem.

Research has shown that better organized text and text that makes the organization clear to the reader (for example, through the use of signaling) increases the likelihood of the reader's understanding, remembering, and applying the concepts learned from the text. Information in the text that point out aspects or structure has been called "signaling".

Another characteristic of text that influences learning outcomes is local coherence, also called cohesion by linguists. Local coherence is achieved by several kinds of simple linguistic links or ties that connect ideas together within and between sentences. The links are reference, conjunction, or connectives (e.g. and, or, but, because, and however). Repeated references that help to carry meaning across sentence boundaries can decrease reading time and increases recall of text as an integrated unit.

Another aspect of content that affects learning outcomes is the proportion of important to unimportant information, or main ideas to details.

Curriculum Change/Innovation/Revision

Any curriculum should be oriented in the context of comprehensive national health policy, manpower, development policies, and plans that reflect the rational and appropriate deployment of all health personnel in accord with the changes and trends in health care. Change is constant and an ongoing phenomenon in all spheres of life. Everything is subject to change in this world, except the word "change". Change is inevitable and it indicates growth. It is one of the laws of nature. Anything which does not change will lag behind. Change in education is important according to the recent trend in the development of science and technology. These changes in science and technology bring changes in the humanity and in their lifestyles. It is important as well as inevitable in bringing change in the curriculum. Nursing curriculum is oriented toward the care of human life and the problems of human beings are changing. Innovation is the bringing in of something new. Curriculum innovation may be classified on a number of dimensions of change.

Dimensions	Range
Rate	Rapid.....Slow
Scale	Large.....Small
Degree	Fundamental...Superficial
Continuity	Revolutionary....Evolutionary
Direction	Linear.....Cyclical

Innovation implies a new idea or practice, but it is also a process by which these are adopted. Hoyle sees innovation as a continuum, from inventions through adoption. Invention is the creation of something new, whereas adoption involves accepting an innovation that was devised by an outside agency. Most innovations are modification of existing ideas and adoption of other people's ideas. Innovation can be introduced in any component of the curriculum and in more than one at any given time.

The educational program of the nurses must keep pace with the ever increasing needs for better nursing care to individuals, families, and communities at the most peripheral levels too. We must periodically revise the curriculum, if we care about people and nurses to be prepared to carry out the several roles necessary to help people keep them healthy. It is important that as many members of the nursing profession as possible participate in this process, so that it will be as realistic and as practical as we can make it and so that we move into implementing the changes as quickly and smoothly as possible after they are decided.

Why should the curriculum change?

The curriculum should change for the following reasons:
- International trends in health care
- Changes in policies and healthcare delivery systems made by the Government of India
- To emphasize the preventive and promotive aspects of health care
- International demand for nurses
- Globalization
- Changing trends in disease pattern.

Factors Influencing Change, Revision, and Innovation

Innovation requires time, finance, and energy if it is to be done well. The head of the institution plays the vital role in bringing the curriculum change and innovation. The style of decision-making by the head and the other curriculum committee members in relation to curriculum change and innovation is also important. The four styles of decision are as follows:

1. **Tell decision:** The head makes the decision herself, either because it is so important or so trivial.
2. **Sell decision:** The head knows that there is only one course of action, so she tries to persuade others so that it will have a chance of success.
3. **Consult decision:** The head gets opinions from all staff concerned, but takes the final responsibility for making the decision herself.
4. **Share decision:** The head allows other staff to share the decision-making process and accepts the joint decision.

The first two styles may lead to the appearance of mutual consent among the staff, but this may be superficial if they feel the decision has been imposed unilaterally. The third style is one of the most common, since it has clear lines of responsibility. It follows the "management is there to manage" philosophy and also maintains the notion of effective leadership and management as being largely due to personality variables. The fourth style is often thought of as being democratic, with most issues and decisions being put to a vote. However, this is open to abuse if factions develop outside of the meetings in order to block or prevent innovation. Another problem is that consensus often implies some kind of neutral, middle ground, or compromise and this may not foster creative innovation.

Innovation is much more likely to occur in an institution where there is little hierarchical authority evident, where autonomy is emphasized and where morale is high. Organizational health is related to the climate of the institution. The below mentioned organizational factors influence the curriculum change and innovation. They are:

- Goal focus: Goals are clear to members and relatively well accepted by them.
- Communication adequacy: Information is well-distributed.
- Optimal power utilization: Influence is fairly equally distributed, so that the influence of subordinates can be felt at high levels.
- Resource utilization: These are used effectively, particularly personnel resources.
- Cohesiveness: There is a sense of identity between members.
- Morale: There is a feeling of well-being among members rather than dissatisfaction.
- Innovativeness: Moves are made toward new goals and new procedures are invented.
- Autonomy: The organization is relatively autonomous and independent of outside influences.
- Adaptation: Structure is constantly adapting to meet new demands.
- Problem-solving adequacy: The effective system copes well with problems.

Continuum of Climates

Open: The head of the institution is hard working, flexible, and prepared to make rules and criticize when necessary; monitoring is not too close and staff's needs are seen as important. Staff morale is high and relationships are good.

Autonomous: The head is less obvious than in the open styles, allowing staff more autonomy but providing less positive leadership. Staff's social needs are less well cared for, but teachers feel a sense of accomplishments of tasks.

Controlled: The head makes the staff work hard and is authoritarian, with little scope for staff satisfaction socially. Staff responds to this and gain task achievement satisfaction.

Familiar: The head gives very little leadership, but creates a happy atmosphere for staff. Morale is low because they lack direction.

Paternal: The head has little influence over the staff, who see her as interfering rather than leading. There is not much achievement even though staff gets on with the job and the head's approach to social needs is seen as insincere.

Closed: The head is distant and aloof, giving no leadership, and taking no personal interest in the staff as people. There is little job satisfaction.

Guidelines for Change and Innovation

The innovation is made by powerful bodies such as INC and the innovation is aimed mainly at the structure of education.

Innovations are more likely to be accepted if the changes are generated from within the organization, rather than by outsiders, particularly if it follows a curriculum analysis. Innovation ideas are also likely to be acceptable if it involves a reduction in workload, or an emphasis toward something that the teacher desires.

Group discussion is vital, if the innovation is to be accepted and sufficient time must be allowed for this. Opportunity for teachers to put their point of view and for questions to be asked is essential step in the innovative process.

Resistance to change can arise out of peer group norms; it is interesting to see that new nurse teachers, when they leave the teacher training institution, are keen to make innovations, but within a year or so of being in the "real world" most of this was evaporated.

Guidelines to implement change as follows:

- Once curriculum revision or change is done, provide crash courses to reorient teachers in order to orient to changes in the curriculum.
- Convene a small corps of nursing leaders who have demonstrated leadership ability at different levels in the health system, to act as a catalyst group, and initiate, plan, inform, motivate, support, and monitor the implementation of change.
- Try to work with those supportive forces within the organization, rather than against those who are resistant to change.
- Aim to produce a self-motivated team of workers who get power from within themselves.
- Work with the "healthy parts" of the system, i.e. those who have the motivation and resource to be able to improve, rather than on lost causes.
- Ensure that the people who are working for change have the freedom authority to implement the proposed changes.
- Try to obtain involvement of key personnel in the change program, but make this realistic and appropriate.
- Establish a system of continuing education to ensure that those engaged in teaching and practice keep their knowledge and skills updated in pace with changed curriculum.
- Identify the additional competencies to be developed by the faculty members in order to implement the curriculum.

- Strengthen the institution to provide necessary facilities and resources essential to implement the change.
- Encourage the positive attitude on the part of administrators toward these changes as the key to the development of nursing profession.
- Protect team members from undue stress and pressure. Successful manager of change and innovation requires a combination of personal qualities and expertise. She needs to have good interpersonal skills in order to manage the staff and minimize anxiety. She needs to feel secure enough. Allow staff to be involved in some of the decisions about change and be prepared to question assumptions when difficulties arise. Management of change requires vision and belief in oneself, but at the same time the manager must keep her feet on the ground, if she is to put her ideas into practice. It is extremely important that the manager of change should avoid getting enmeshed in the finer details of the system; her role is to be able to have a "birds-eye" view of the whole thing to ensure a holistic outcome.

Steps in Curriculum Revision

Re-examine philosophy, goals, and functions: This must be done to make sure that our goals and the functions for which we are preparing nurses are still in line with recent trends and with the health policies and health systems of the country. It is essential for nurses to know this to understand their implications for nursing. While revising the philosophy, the future of nursing education, the moral, ethical and religious background, characteristics of the people to be served, and our belief about the learning process that is how people learn should be considered. While stating the objectives, it should come from the needs of the society, statement of experts, teaching-learning principles, student's needs, and the statement of philosophy.

Choose an appropriate curriculum design: This is an important step and will affect the success of the whole course. This will include making decisions on the separate subjects to be taught, their order and relationship, and the content of each subject and how it is taught.

Evaluation

As we proceed, we will need to test it to decide if it fits or is consistent with the philosophy, goals, and objectives, which we have stated in the beginning. It is hard to carry out, since it is a challenging task for us and so is often neglected in planning curriculum. If we are not very careful to check at each stage, keeping our beliefs and goals constantly in mind, we will find that the final result is unfruitful one.

Phases of Curriculum Change

There are three phases in the curriculum change. They are:
1. Planning
2. Implementation
3. Evaluation.

Any innovation in curriculum needs planning and a conscious effort to implement the change and evaluation of the effectiveness of change. A change or innovation can be introduced in any component of the curriculum, since total change of curriculum may not be necessary.

The Planning Phase

The followings are the broad categories of curriculum change:
- Introduction of a whole new degree program or specialized stream at the undergraduate level.
- Introduction of a whole new (coursework) degree program at the postgraduate level.
- Introduction of a new subject, or deletion of an existing subject.
- Change in the language taught to undergraduate students.
- Change to or within an elective subject, such as a change in the choice of language.

Much of the academic discussion is concerned with the changes in teaching culture and philosophy that accompany a wholesale move away from traditional (subject-based, knowledge-centered, and teaching-focused) approaches, when institutions turn to alternative (student-based, competence-centered, and learning-focused) approaches that stress the educator's role as a facilitator of learning, rather than a transmitter of knowledge.

Change Processes

Ewell (1997) suggests that most curriculum changes are implemented as piecemeal and in fact, "without a deep understanding about what collegiate learning really means and the specific circumstances and strategies that are likely to promote it". Ideally, according to Lachiver and Tardif (2002), curriculum change is managed in a logical five-step process:
1. An analysis of the current offerings and context
2. The expression of key program aims in a mission statement
3. A prioritization of resources and development strategies
4. The implementation of the targeted curricula change
5. The establishment of monitoring tools and processes.

The following are the factors affecting curriculum change:
- Influential or outspoken individuals
- Financial pressures, including resource availability

- Staff availability or workload
- Employer viewpoints
- Current or prospective students viewpoints
- Student's abilities or limitations, or intake considerations
- Pedagogical argument, or academic merit
- University or government requirement or regulation
- Professional accreditation needs, or syllabi set by professional bodies.
- Academic "fashion", including the desire to remain in step with other institutions.

Factors Influencing Decisions about Curriculum

Influential or Outspoken Individuals

- The first factor initiating change is strong leadership accepted by the academic staff. The key characteristic of such leadership is to have the capacity to attract other academic staff to rally behind principled educational objectives that are supported within the environment.
- The second factor is sharing and accepting the need for change, a point that is often stimulated by noting the discrepancies between the current output and what is desired by employers.
- The extent of a curricular change, whether wide-scale or minor, is a third factor.
- Finally, because many academic staff holds embedded teaching and professional practices, the degree of flexibility for departmental staff is seen as the final factor.

Decisions that affect whole departments and degree programs are often taken by a relatively small core of senior staff. Of course, these staff usually has a considerable depth of experience and is typically the one who are in tune with policies and politics, but it is also possible for decisions to be unduly influenced by staff with strong opinions. Watson (1994) suggests that key individuals have so much influence because of a lack of alternatives.

Financial Pressures

Clearly, there are powerful budgetary forces that influence our decisions. If change in curriculum increases the budget, it may fail to attract the administrator and the provider of the courses. If faculty members are paid according to the demand created in addition as per the new curriculum, it will gain the support of them and introducing and implementing change is also easy. If students are need to pay extra in order to fulfill the demand created by the change in the curriculum, they may resist the change.

Staffing Issues, Including Workload

It is likely that a staff might be asked at short notice to teach the subject, or the theory course, because a colleague has resigned, or a position that has been advertised has not been filled. Staff shortages can mean that we narrow the range of subjects offered. Any additional workload or increased workload will be resisted by the faculty members, which needs to be compensated.

Employer and Industry (Hospital) Viewpoints

While the professional bodies ultimately reflect employer and industry (hospital) expectations, these pressures are also sometimes directly exerted. Many departments and schools have an industry advisory committee to allow a timely flow of such advice and suggestions. The success or otherwise of such committees is heavily dependent upon the energy and time that the industry (hospital) representatives are able to bring to the task. There is much anecdotal evidence that employers have strong opinions about the curriculum, usually requesting more emphasis on transferable skills (such as communication, social, analytical, and critical-thinking skills) in graduates, while feeling that these requests are not heard.

Students Viewpoints

Students often assert that they are not customers; nevertheless, the customer is the one spending the money and can sway decisions. Student opinion is informed by the mass media and by the opinions of parents (also often derived from the media). However, on the whole, student demands appear to be a limited influence on curricula. Students' choice continues to be determined primarily by personal interest.

Students Abilities

In an ideal world, programs would be dictated by our desires to create graduates of the highest possible caliber and we were capable of sourcing the correct raw material in sufficient quantity, perhaps we could achieve that goal. Unfortunately, the exigencies of filling quotas for students mean that the weaker students in our intakes sometimes do not meet our expectations in terms of required skills, or in breadth of knowledge in other ways.

Pedagogical Argument, Academic Merit

Many changes are proposed in curriculum because they are an indisputably "good thing". One would find it hard to argue, for example, that the introduction of laboratory classes into subject that had previously been based solely upon lectures and tutorials was not a "good thing". Similarly, we imagine that most faculties would accept without question that third-year or fourth-year project-based subjects are indispensable for students. For some decisions, the relevance of academic merit is unclear. The numbers of students admitted into a course, their eligibility experience of the faculty members, etc. are some of the factors influencing academic merit. An example where pedagogy is relevant, but only somewhat, is whether certain subjects should be core or elective. An example where pedagogy is arguably irrelevant, although opinions are certainly strong, is choice of a tool for teaching in a database subject or nursing skill.

University and Government Regulation

Another source of pressure is university administration's insistence on internal, national, and international benchmarking. At a more immediate level, failure rates are compared between government regulation and policy changes, which is a further significant factor.

National and International Accreditation Bodies

Discussion of Henkel and Kogan (1999) note that many issues are common in curriculum debates, irrespective of discipline, for example:
- Maintenance of academic standards
- Balance between academic and vocational objectives
- Transferable skills development
- Effective use of resources.

They observe that curriculum change is predominantly incremental. Jones (2002) lists five conditions that promote and sustain changes in the curriculum:
- Mutual trust among stakeholders
- Committed and consistent leadership
- Proceeding with a nonthreatening, incremental pace of change
- Professional development for academic staff
- The use of purposeful incentives.

The planning strategy that is most useful is to provide for feedback prior to total faculty consideration. Feedback is provided by task groups called alter groups (as in alter ego). These critiquing groups provide checks and balances, so that the creators of an idea or task can have the benefit of objective feedback.

The basic planning strategy suggested here is the generation of more than one alternative for every phase of or task in curriculum building. Faculties working together for curriculum change need to develop ground rules that facilitate change and promote healthy group relationships. It is possible to achieve both ends.

The following list suggests ground rules that groups might like to consider for curriculum change communications. Each group should evolve its own list and add to it as it is used.
- Try to have no surprises. Let everyone know in advance plans that are underway.
- Provide as much informational input as possible.
- Make conflicts explicit and legitimate.
- Identify high investment areas (areas of high feelings) and elicit the help of a neutral facilitator either from within the group or from a source unrelated to the problem or issue itself. This enables all factions to struggle or fight "fair" since a facilitator will ensure each participants rights.
- Make risks legitimate and failure salvageable and acceptable.
- Make change in the middle of a trial run acceptable.
- Then if a plan being instituted is not working, alterations in the plan can be made without violating the group's preconceived notion that a trial run has to be run all the way through.
- Try to make it necessary to analyze failure.
- Agree to respond to each others contributions to the group, comments, needs, and behaviors.
- Delay decision-making of final decisions. Make tentative decisions, take a consensus, decide on a trial basis, or accept something as a "provisional" or "working copy".

For change to occur, certain conditions must be provided. The change agent seeks in collaboration with others to establish these conditions, so that planned change can proceed. These conditions are as follows:

Key organizational people must support and participate in the change. In school curriculum change, directors, department chairmen, deans, curriculum coordinators, and key power people must support the idea of planned change.

The curriculum needs to be managed differently. There needs to be a balance between institutional objectives and that of academic staff. Changes are driven by individuals, politics, and fashion more than they are driven by academic merit and external curricula.

Implementation

It involves the actual provision of teaching and learning experiences to the students and the role of teachers in implementation of curriculum. Curriculum implementation is discussed in detail in the beginning of this chapter.

Curriculum Evaluation

Evaluation is the process through which teachers judge the quality of work—their own or their students'. There are two types of evaluative strategies:
1. Formative evaluations, which involve a continual stream of reflection and feedback and allow the educator or student to continually adjust and improve their work while it is ongoing.
2. Traditionally, teachers have emphasized summative evaluations, where feedback is gathered only after instruction has been completed. Both strategies

are necessary to provide for effective curriculum assessment and student education.

Assessment provides a way to measure students' demonstration of learning. It helps us answer the questions: "How much did they learn?" and "How well did they learn it?" and "How well did we teach it?".

According to Applegate (1998), it is defined as the process of delineating, obtaining, and providing information useful for making decisions and judgments about a program of learning. The function of curriculum design is to provide a systematic plan for the achievement of desired outcomes. The faculty must set the standards to measure the intended outcomes versus actual outcomes. She should also choose an evaluation model and evaluate the individual courses as well as the total program\curriculum.

Evaluation (feedback) dictates the road ahead because past events cannot be changed. Evaluation should not come at the end of things, but rather at the beginning and continue throughout any process. The essence of process itself, the secret ingredient that makes an entity a process, is feedback sought or unsought, intentional or accidental, preprogrammed or random.

The philosophy connected to the conceptual framework, the conceptual framework connected to the outcomes, and the outcomes connected to the evaluation bring appropriate input for the curriculum evaluation and make it more purposeful and meaningful.

Any evaluation not so connected will have little relevance to the curriculum and therefore, will be of limited use to faculty and students. Most sources tie evaluation directly to objectives, which is the most common and useful way to proceed with curriculum evaluation. However, this is so only if the objectives are directly related to the setting, student, and knowledge aspects of the conceptual framework.

Curriculum evaluation precedes curriculum change, planning for change, and setting goals and establishing programs. To have evaluation that is programmed for optimal service to the curriculum, baseline assessments must be made.

There are basically two kinds of evaluations—formative and summative. Formative evaluation is taken during the operation of the process or the curriculum. It is used to determine how to reach the goals better and helps to focus on things that must be done to achieve goals. Formative evaluation is usually frequent and is done periodically throughout the time the students are in the curriculum.

Formative evaluation can be done on students and their learning and behavioral changes and on all of the other factors that must be evaluated that contribute to student learning. The primary reason for the existence of formative evaluation is to furnish feedback to the system while the system is in operation and ongoing, so that changes can be made which correct the system to achieve the goals.

Summative evaluation is taken at the end of a period of operation or learning to determine if the goals were achieved. It is a general assessment of the extent and degree to which the desired outcomes or goals have been attained. Summative evaluation comes periodically at the completion of activities, courses, or a curriculum time span such as quarter or semester. Both of these types of evaluation are used for student and curriculum evaluation.

Evaluation of student learning is used for curricular evaluation in that student learning is the purpose of the curriculum. Whether or not students learn what they are supposed to learn is the key to all evaluation. For curriculum evaluation purposes, all the factors facilitating or impeding student learning are examined as follows:

Setting Factors

Materials

- Textbooks, learning resources (including library and audiovisual), practice paraphernalia, and other learning materials such as models equipment, dolls, beds, etc.
- Reality practice resources, agencies, patients, nurses, ancillary workers, etc.
- Conducive physical environment.

Knowledge Base

- Goals
- Content
- Learning activities.

Student

- Entrance characteristics and behaviors
- Interim achievement
- Exit behaviors
- Achievement tests
- State board/University policies.

Evaluation of all these factors, formatively and summatively, provides a thorough curriculum evaluation program. Each of these factors must be evaluated using the program objectives and the student behavioral objectives.

Some of the methods for curriculum evaluation are listed here. Student discussions, organized scheduled student discussion groups containing fifteen to twenty five students, and two or more teachers provide opportunities for students to give direct feedback about strengths and weaknesses in relation to meeting their needs as individual learners and as a group of learners.

Teacher rap sessions, organized scheduled times for faculty to discuss problems, practices, strengths, and weaknesses of the developing curriculum are necessary to provide a constant source of feedback useful for guiding the direction of curriculum change. The same kinds of programs for faculty can be devised as just described for students.

Prepare a performance checklist. A set of definitive program objectives can be further reduced to course and task objectives, so that the steps necessary to attain desired graduate behaviors reflect the requisite progressive levels of attainment. From such a sequential list, one can easily evolve behavioral checklists for determining mastery of specific learning levels. Such a list enables the teacher and student to define, develop, and evaluate true growth of the individual student. Specific behavioral objectives can be utilized as performance criteria.

Homemade data collection instruments, homemade questionnaires are a valuable source of data for the curriculum evaluator. Much of the data provided by evaluation will be quantitative (numerical) and much will be qualitative (descriptive). Qualitative data appear to be more subjective than quantitative data, but both are somewhat subjective. Some sources that are descriptive include:
- Opinions of teachers
- Opinions of students
- Evidence in changes in attitudes and level of commitment
- Changes in values
- The kind quality and quantity of recommendation for changes from teachers, students, and employers
- Compliance with group decisions
- Group morale and perseverance
- Faculty attrition and the reason for it
- Students for that attrition. These clues or evidence about the curriculum will enable faculty to evaluate and describe what is perceived of happening.

Purposes of Curriculum Evaluation
- To make decisions about individuals and about the curriculum
- To plan for placement, promotion, and graduation
- To make decisions about the value or worth of the program of study and the activities implemented to realize the expected outcomes.

Characteristics of Evaluation
- Evaluation is goal oriented
- It is ongoing process
- It is based on some norms and standards
- It is based on the values and valuing of the evaluator
- It is comprehensive
- It is a diagnostic tool.

Doll (1992) identified seven characteristics of evaluation that are useful in guiding faculty efforts in the appraisal of curricula. They are:
- The presence of values and valuing
- Evaluation is goal oriented
- Incorporation of norms (standards)
- Comprehensiveness
- Continuity
- Diagnostic worth, validity, and reliability
- Integration of findings.

Curriculum Evaluation Model
Stufflebeam's educational decision model (1983) addresses the four elements:

Context	Intended ends	Setting, mission, community, philosophy, internal and external forces, and beliefs of faculty
Inputs	Intended means	Resources, support systems, learner, program plan, and curriculum organization
Process	Actual means	Implementation, teaching learning strategies, learning materials, teaching-learning transactions, efficiency, and effectiveness
Product	Actual ends	Learner outcomes and satisfaction, course evaluation

Curriculum Evaluation
It is the process of determining the outcomes of student learning as a result of participating in a program or plan of learning. It involves establishing outcomes and verifying the extent to which these have been obtained.

Program Evaluation
It encompasses a broader view of the educational program and examines competent parts, including faculty, students, fiscal effectiveness, and curriculum and instructional outcomes. Program reviews typically are conducted by the faculty as a self-study and are undertaken to respond to accreditation reviews by state, education, and professional accrediting bodies.

The Evaluation Process

Determine the Purpose of Evaluation
The purpose of the evaluation is identified to facilitate learning, to diagnose problem, to make decisions, to improve teaching learning, to improve AV aids, to motivate, to promote placement services, to plan for remedial services, and to judge effectiveness.

Fix up the Time Limit
The evaluation is of two types: they are the formative evaluation and the summative evaluation. Formative

evaluation is done with the frequent interval and the summative evaluation is done at the end of an activity or instruction, course, or program.

Determine when to Evaluate

It is the time or period during which evaluation is done. In both formative and summative evaluation, the educational administrators should decide the appropriate timing at which the evaluations are done.

Select the Evaluator(s)

It is based on the purpose. Most of the time, formative evaluation will be done only by the internal evaluator. The summative evaluation is done by both internal and external evaluator. The advantage of using internal evaluators includes their familiarity with the context of the evaluation, experience with the standards, cost-effectiveness, and potential for less obtrusive evaluation. The findings of the evaluation can be used immediately. Disadvantages are bias, control of evaluation, and reluctance to share controversial findings. External evaluators are those not directly involved in the events being evaluated. They do not have a bias, are not involved in organizational politics, very experienced, and do not have a stake in the results.

Select an Evaluation Design/Framework or Model

- CIPP—Context, Input, Process, and Product model.
- Client-centered models (Stake's, 1967)—countenance model focuses on the goals and observed effects of the program being evaluated in terms of anecdotes, transactions, and outcomes.

Anecdotes are existing conditions that may affect may affect the outcome; transactions are all educational experiences and interactions and outcomes are the abilities, achievements, attitudes, and aspirations of students that result from the educational experience.

- Assessment models can be developed by an institution and implemented and the results are used by the participants for course, curriculum, and program improvement. Each department can identify the purposes, determine the time frame, develop tool, collect data, analyze and interpret data, and utilize the findings.

Select an Evaluation Tool

The tools may be questionnaire, interview, observation schedules, rating scales, checklists, attitude scales, self-report, journal diary, anecdotal notes, etc. The instrument should be reliable, valid, appropriate, cost-effective, easy to use, and time efficient.

Collect Data

It includes who will collect data, source of collection of data, amount of data, and timing of data collection. Formal and informal (spontaneous comments by the students) data collection is also done.

Interpret Data

Norm-referenced Interpretation

It refers to interpreting data in terms of the norms of a group of individuals who are being evaluated. The scores of the group form a basis for comparing each individual with the other. It helps the evaluator to compare and rank the students among their own group as well as with the other group. The disadvantage is that it mainly focuses on comparison and it may create a sense of competitiveness among students and minimizing assisting students toward mastery of specified content areas.

Criterion-referenced Interpretation

The results are judged against pre-established criteria and reflect the degree of criteria attainment.

The advantages of criterion-referenced interpretation include emphasis on mastery and the potential for all learners to achieve, increased learner motivation, sharing and collaborating among students, and ability to give clear progress reports to learners. Disadvantages are inability to compare students with each other or with other groups, thus assigning grades that reflect differentiation among students.

Report the Findings

Who receives the findings: The evaluator must know to whom the data should be reported. The evaluator should remove the unneeded background information after the report is completed. The evaluator should consider the recipient also. Give only needed information.

When to report findings: Timing of the report is also crucial. It should be reported when information is needed.

How to report findings: It can be reported either verbally or written form and formal and informal. Informal may include talking with the students about his or her performance in a clinical experience, without a structured evaluation.

Use the Findings

The finding of an evaluation is used to assign grades, revise instruction, course, curricular or programs, and demonstrate program effectiveness.

Consider the Costs of Evaluation

Task analysis is taking a big job and breaking it down into small bits that are of a size and nature to be handled. Focusing on the job to be handled offers some reassurance that at least some part of the job, which can be successfully achieved. Success breeds success and the reinforcement of completing one small bit of the total task motivates and energizes the group for the next job.

Level of Curriculum Approval

In the college level:

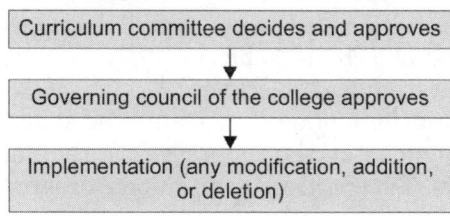

University level:

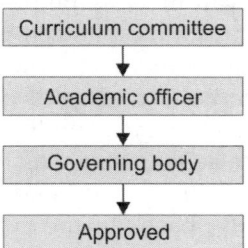

Curriculum committee membership: Elected chairperson from faculty, representatives of alumni, employers of graduates, consumers, representatives from various departments such as social work, nutrition, psychology, family studies, ethics, law, and medicine.

Functions of the curriculum committee

- Initiate curriculum development or revision on its own or undertake on request by the administrator.
- Provide information to the faculty about the progress and seek continued input from the faculty.
- Give ample time for discussion of curricular matters at faculty level.
- When the committee decides, the final product curriculum is brought to the faculty for a final discussion and for vote of approval or disapproval.
- If the faculty does not approve the proposed curriculum, it is returned to the committee.
- If it is accepted at the faculty level, it is forwarded to the next appropriate level for approval.

Faculty Role in Curriculum Development

- Responsible for planning, developing, implementing, evaluating, and revising the curriculum. Also responsible for teaching, guiding, and evaluating students and mentoring faculty.
- Modifies the content, objective, and teaching methods in the courses in which he or she teaches in response to changes in the discipline and practice.
- Self-governance includes the right to develop policies and procedures that affect student's and faculty's conduct and curriculum.
- Curriculum implementation. Check it is implemented properly.
- Actively involve in the development of policies and procedures that affect curriculum.
- Advise the management on issues affecting nursing education.
- Participate and support administrative actions.
- Ensure that the content and learning experiences are appropriately selected toward educational outcomes.
- Collect and analyze relevant information pertaining to the need for curriculum development and revision.
- Develop strategies to facilitate the exchange of ideas and decision-making relevant to curriculum development and revisions.
- Actively participate in curriculum research.
- Involve in curriculum evaluation.

Summary

- Curriculum (plural curricula) is the set of courses and their content offered at a school or university. As an idea, curriculum stems from the Latin word for race course, referring to the course of deeds and experiences through which children grow and mature in becoming adults.
- Three facets of curriculum are goals and purposes of education, process of curriculum, and evaluation of products.
- The curriculum collectively describes the teaching, learning, and assessment materials available for a given course of study. Any curriculum includes the philosophy of the program, total duration, learning experiences, teaching methods, and materials including AV aids and a program of evaluation.
- Elements of curriculum are philosophy of the educational program, objectives of the educational program, duration of the educational program including theory and practical, learning experiences, instructional methods, and materials and program of evaluation.
- According to Loretta E Heidgerken (1965), the factors influencing the curriculum development in nursing are philosophy of nursing education, educational

- psychology, society, student, life activities, and knowledge.
- There are three phases in the curriculum development. They are developmental phase, implementation phase, and evaluation phase.
- While developing a curriculum, the educators have to remember the factors related to the learners, teachers, subject matter, environment, and other resources including financial resources.
- The nature of nursing curriculum is health oriented and it focuses on the national health policy and primary healthcare demands. The steps in curriculum construction are planning, development, implementation, and evaluation.
- Selection of learning experiences is one of the important aspects of the curriculum. The learning experiences are grouped under the subject headings and the principles of sequence and integration are followed in organization of learning experiences. Learning experiences may be defined as deliberately planned experiences in selected situations where students actively participate and interact, which result in desirable changes of behavior in the students.
- There are various teaching systems such as teaching block, partial block system, study day system, and daily classes. Any one of this can be followed in the nursing education system.
- Master rotation plan and individual rotation plans are made in advance, so that it gives complete picture about the student's placement and teaching-learning activities.
- The curriculum should be constructed in such a way that the purpose and educational objectives of the program should be achieved. The educational objective should be stated in clear, unambiguous, and behavioral terms. The students and teachers of the particular educational programs should have a clear perception of the expected results. The teaching-learning activities and learning experiences related to theory and practical components should be in conformity with the educational objectives of the program.
- The curriculum should be constructed in such a way that the purpose and educational objectives of the program should be achieved.
- The words "aims", "goals", "purposes", and "objectives" are often used interchangeably in relation to the educational objectives of a school program. There are general objectives, intermediary objectives, and specific or instructional objectives. The objectives may also be stated as teacher-centered objectives, learner-centered objectives, subject-centered objectives, and behavior-centered objectives.
- The educational objective should be stated in clear, unambiguous, and behavioral terms. The students and teachers of the particular educational programs should have a clear perception of the expected results.
- There are various resources used for curriculum transaction. It can be classified as print-based and nonprint-based resources.
- Any curriculum should be oriented in the context of comprehensive national health policy, manpower development policies, and plans that reflect the rational and appropriate deployment of all health personnel in accord with the changes and trends in health care.
- There are three phases in the curriculum change. They are planning, implementation, and evaluation. Curriculum evaluation is defined as the process of delineating, obtaining, and providing information useful for making decisions and judgments about a program of learning.

8. Teacher Preparation

"Mediocre teacher tells; Good teacher explains, Superior teacher illustrates; Exceptional teacher inspires".

"If you educate a boy, you educate one individual, If you educate a girl, you educate a teacher, If you educate a teacher, you educate a community".

Objectives

After completing this unit, you will be able to:
- Understand the qualities of a teacher
- Explain the duties, functions and responsibilities of a teacher
- Enumerate the characteristics of a teacher
- Appreciate the roles of a teacher
- Understand the skills of a teacher
- Describe teacher education and certification in India
- Explain professional education and development of teacher education and training
- Explain evaluation of teacher.

Introduction

The teacher is a dynamic force of the school. A college without teacher is just like a body without the soul, a skeleton without flesh and blood, and a shadow without substance. As social engineers, the teachers can socialize and humanize the young by their qualities. A teacher is an acknowledged guide or helper in processes of learning.

In education, teachers facilitate student learning, often in a school or academy or perhaps in another environment such as outdoors. A teacher who teaches on an individual basis may be described as a tutor. In Hinduism, the spiritual teacher is known as a guru. There are many sayings on the teacher like "Guru devo bhava" (Guru is God), which reflects the esteem associated with a guru's role.

Two extreme views of teaching often prevailed in the past. According to the first view, teaching is a charisma and so, only charismatic people can teach. The followers of this view believe that teachers are born rather than they are prepared through training. The other extreme view is that anyone who loves children or youth and has a command over subject matters can teach and can teach well too. Both of these views had been contested strongly in the past and the issue has been settled to a great extent (if not at a theoretical level, at least at practical level). Now teaching is an activity which has enough ingredients to be considered as a profession, if not a profession like medicine or law, at least a semi-profession. Therefore, teachers are those professionals who have the legitimate right to practice their profession of teaching.

Concepts of Teacher

"A teacher is the image of Brahma".
—Manu

"The true teacher is he who can immediately come down to the level of the student, transfer his soul to the student's soul and see through and understand through his mind. Such a teacher can really teach and none else".
—Swami Vivekananda

"The teacher's place in society is of vital importance. He acts as the pivot for the transmission of intellectual traditions and technical skills from generation to generation and helps to keep the lamp of civilization burning".
— Dr S Radhakrishnan

"A teacher can never truly teach unless he is still learning himself. A lamp can never light another lamp unless it continues to burn its own flame. The teacher who has come to the end of his subject, who has no living traffic with his knowledge, but merely repeats his lessons to his students, can only load their minds. He cannot quicken them".
—Tagore

"Every teacher and educationist of experience knows that even the best curriculum and the most perfect syllabus remain dead unless quickened into life by the right method of teaching and the right kind of teachers."
—Secondary Education Commission

Essential Qualities of a Teacher

Teacher as a Role Model
Role models are people who set good examples by the words they speak and by the actions they take. Students tend to copy the behavior and mannerism of the teachers. The teacher's entire personality is a reflection on the minds of the students. If the teacher is honest, leads a balanced and disciplined life, the children adopt these virtues as an ideal conduct unconsciously. The ideal teacher is one who through his thoughts, words and deeds, gives an impression of an honest upright life which can serve as a model for the students to copy, follow, and emulate.

Teacher's Character
If the teacher becomes an embodiment of right conduct in thought, word and deed, the students by their association will learn virtue and develop manly qualities. They can be humanized and can live and act like normal human beings. They can become thoughtful, concerned, and courageous.

Teacher's Personality
Every teacher must have a good personality. Radiant, pleasing and impressive personal appearance, refinement, pleasant manners, industry, enthusiasm, drive, initiative, open mindedness, etc. are some of the essential traits of an ideal teacher. External appearance has a psychological effect upon the students. By attractive appearance, he/she can win the love and affection of his/her students and can command respect. He/she should be frank, tolerant, kind, fair, and straightforward so that, he/she can stimulate learning.

Personality Traits
The following are some of the personality traits. A teacher must possess:
- Self-confidence and self-respect
- Good appearance
- Healthy and energetic
- Good intellect
- High character
- Sense of humor
- Optimistic
- Democratic
- Fair and just
- Sympathy and empathy
- Punctuality
- Enthusiasm
- Industriousness
- Sociability.

Personal Values
Some of the personal values a teacher must possess are:

- Love
- Dialog
- Brotherhood
- Forgiveness
- Repentance
- Sharing
- Service
- Team spirit
- Responsibility
- Accountability
- Sympathy
- Justice
- Hospitality
- Nonviolence
- Dutifulness
- Patience
- Courtesy
- Thrift
- Magnanimity
- Sportsman
- Loyalty
- Gratitude
- Tolerance
- Freedom
- Determination
- Coordination

Teacher's Mental Health
We speak of education as a lamp lighting another lamp, one life making another life, and a spirit speaking to another spirit. We can achieve this objective, if the teachers have good mental health. Students develop interest in those subjects, which are taught by pleasing and genial teachers. The teacher makes the emotional atmosphere in the classroom. If she has a good mental health, she can create love, interest, and enthusiasm for learning and a taste in the subject she teaches.

Teacher's Physical Health
A teacher should possess a sound body along with a sound mind. She should have a sound physical health, physical energy, vitality and she should be free from physical defects. This will make her alert, cheerful, happy, dynamic and enthusiastic. She can maintain emotional stability.

Teacher's Social Adjustment
Sociability is another important quality of a teacher. She should have a sound social philosophy and she should make her best contribution to the society. She should know how to adjust herself to the social surroundings in which she lives. She should not be quiet, retreating and introverted. She should be free from worry, anxiety and thinking and feeling about herself. She should mix well in society to have a large body of friends. Normal social life outside the school will go a long way to give her happy social adjustments. A teacher must possess the following social values. They are:

- Discipline
- Respect for elders
- Faithfulness
- Responsibility
- Dedication
- Punctuality
- Ambition
- Confidence
- Cleanliness
- Good manners

Contd...

Contd...

• Devotion	• Creativity
• Sense of competition	• Patience
• Knowledge	• Positive approach
• Fortitude	• Innovation
• Self-reliance	• Courage
• Sincerity	• Intelligence
• Affection	• Truthfulness
• Obedience	• Regularity
• Patriotism	• Self-evaluation
• Honesty	• Hopefulness

Teacher's Professional Efficiency

The teacher must possess a strong sense of vocation and true devotion toward teaching. He should have a genuine love for his calling. For his professional efficiency, he should have knowledge of psychology, educational philosophy, aims, contents, methods and materials of instruction, and skill and interest in teaching. He must possess a fair knowledge of current affairs about his own country and other countries of the world.

Teacher's Academic Achievements

A teacher should possess knowledge on the fundamentals of the subjects he teaches. He should have a sound academic and cultural background.

Teacher's Professional Training

The teacher must have the required professional training, without which he will commit serious pedagogical blunders. Prof Montague in his book, "Education and Human Relations", asserts that, "No one should ever be permitted to become a teacher of the young unless by temperament, attitudes and training, he is fitted to do so".

Teacher's Accountability

Lessinger advocates that each student has a right to be educated in order to become a productive citizen of a country. The parents have a right to know the progress of education of their children. Teachers, being the "educational or human engineers" are accountable for the progress of the student they teach. Because of this, the National Policy on Education, 1986, in India, has made this concept very popular.

Professional Ethics of a Teacher

Teachers, who consider their job as a profession, work only for pay cheque. Their work is considered useful for their own sake, since, they have occupied a professional chair and tried for their own good, at the cost of others. But our cultural heritage proves that true teachers are those who consider their job as honorable. Such teachers work with a sense of self-fulfillment and self-realization.

Prof George Herbert Palmer once rightly said, "If Harvard does not pay me to teach, I would gladly pay Harvard for the privilege of teaching". This should be the professional value of an Indian teacher. An ideal teacher should not work with pecuniary motives, but with a sense of education and for the cause of education.

Toward Students

It shall be the teachers' primary duty to understand the students, to be just, courteous, to promote a spirit of enquiry, fellowship and joy in them, not to do or say anything that would undermine their personality, not to exploit them for personal interests and to set before them a high standard of character, discipline and personality.

Young children need sensitive handling. They need to be looked after by teachers who understand their instincts, learning needs and tendencies along with their capacities and abilities. Teachers make the pupils learn and in the process, help in the development of body, mind, and soul. Teacher can create a joyful environment in the learning center; this would be a delight to any observer, sense of satisfaction to the teacher and a gratifying experience for the learner. Learners must feel secure and assured in the learning environment. This sense of security and assurance is possible only when teachers bestow genuine love and affection for each and every child. It is teachers' commitment to the learner which leads to total development of the child.

Teacher's job is not confined only to imparting knowledge to the learner within the classrooms or the school premises. His accountability is toward the community individually as well as collectively. In a heterogeneous society children come from different backgrounds and strata of society. Their problems are different. They need to be looked after depending upon their specific situations.

Resource mobilization from the community ensuring greater interaction amongst learners, community, and the school is also the responsibility of the teacher. Only a teacher committed to the society can develop a sense of belonging amongst its members. The teachers will have to understand the local community context, participate in its activities and assure that he/she is one amongst them and is willing to be of assistance whenever needed. In the event of natural calamities, drought, floods, fire, etc. the school can no longer remain aloof.

Toward Profession

It shall be the teachers' primary duty to be sincere and honest to their work and to go thoroughly prepared to the class, to endeavor to maintain their efficiency by study and other means; not to do or say anything which may lower their prestige in the eyes of their students.

Teaching is considered as the noblest profession in India and also outside India. The nation has a long tradition of imparting knowledge and wisdom in its own indigenous approach. In past, teachers were most respected citizens of the society, revered by every strata of the populace. The conditions now are different. Teachers are considered employees like others working in different sectors. They have their professional organizations and also trade unions like others and these rarely focus on professional issues.

One of the demands that often emerges is to give a professional status to the teaching profession like medicine, engineering and law.

Toward Society

It shall be the teachers' primary duty to set an example in citizenship, to endeavor to promote the public good, to uphold the dignity of their calling on all occasions, to size up the demands and aspirations of the society, to be dynamic leaders when required and to be ideal followers when desired.

Commitment to Basic Values

Value inculcation, development of values and value education are issues that invite consistent debate in the educational system. Educational policies categorically state that value inculcation is one of the major responsibilities of the educational systems. Value systems could have variations and diversities from community to community and person to person. However, it is certain that the communities everywhere expect the teachers to follow value based approach in their own personal life. There are several justifications for the same. Teachers are the role models and shall remain so in future as well. Further, because of their learning and also the traditions of teaching they are most suited to lead a value-based life. Teachers have accepted this responsibility on their own and majority of the teachers are conscious of the fact that, if their conduct has any blemishes, they would be much more embarrassed than anyone else.

Duties of a Teacher

Safety and Security of Students

- Tell students about purpose of education
- Build one to one relationship with students
- Take-up personality development programs
- Know everything about students
- Make students aware of realities of life
- Inspire students to face problems with braveness
- Apprise students about probable dangers and hazards in and around campus.

Teaching

- Planning
- Preparation
- Presentation
- Evaluation
- Giving feedbacks
- Diagnosis
- Remediation
- Enrichment.

Promotion of Creative Teaching

- Planning
- Testing
- Revising
- Innovation in education.

Teaching as a Pleasurable Activity

- Lecturing
- Working with small groups
- Designing instructional units
- Love for subject matter
- Organizing students.

All such activities can provide deepest satisfaction in teaching and from the act of applying their craft.

Functions of Teacher as an Instructor

Informing the learner of the objectives:
- Presenting stimuli
- Increasing learners' attention
- Helping the learner recall what he or she has previously learnt
- Providing conditions that will evoke performance
- Determining sequences of learning
- Prompting and guiding the learning.

Teaching as Social Service

- It is like nursing
- It contributes to the lives of others
- Decision to teach is deeper than a love for subject matter
- People have attraction to the life of teacher.

Maintaining Teacher's Diary

Teacher's diary is a sort of record of his day-to-day activities. It may show him what he has done, what he is doing and what he plans to do in the future. The teacher's diary is his helpful guide. It will enable him to keep a personal contact with his work, maintaining an active interest in his activities and remind him of his shortcomings, drawbacks, etc. The worth of a diary lies in the regularity with which it is filled and the use to which it is put and also the inspiration which it may give to the teacher to be on his track and not to miss his aim and scheduled targets.

Extracurricular Activities

- Personal guidance
- Career counseling
- Community service.

Conduct of College Activities

- Planning
- Organizing
- Guiding
- Supervising
- Evaluating.

Other Duties

- Recording
- Reporting
- Building relations.

Teacher's Role in Society

Dr Radhakrishnan said that the teacher is like the candle which lights others in consuming itself.

A teacher is a member of society. He lives and works in society. A teacher plays his role toward society in two ways:
1. Inside the school by preparing students for effective citizens
2. Outside the school by assuming the role of a social worker and an agent of social change.

Broad Classification of a Teacher's Role

- Teacher as an agent of social change
- Teacher's role in community welfare
- Teacher's role in elimination of social tensions and conflict
- Teacher's role in international understanding
- Teacher's role in pupil development.

Teacher's Multifarious Role in Pupil Development

- **Confident**: A teacher is expected to win the confidence of the students so as to develop trust.
- **Democrat**: Teacher should follow the democratic values so as to inculcate the same to the students.
- **Detective**: He should be skilled enough to detect the shortcomings of the students.
- **Ego supporter**: He should take all steps to build up and maintain a healthy strong ego and self-concept among students.
- **Equalizer**: He should be impartial and try to develop an egalitarian society.
- **Facilitator of learning**: He works to facilitate better learning in students.
- **Friend and Philosopher**: He must act as a friend and philosopher for the students.
- **Group leader**: He should develop all leadership skills so as to lead the student groups.
- **Guidance counselor and helper**: He provides academic career and personal guidance to the students.
- **Initiator**: He should explore the technology to the best advantage of the students and the progress of education. He should play the role of an educational innovator.
- **Role model**: He should act as a role model for the students.
- **Evaluator**: He should evaluate the students' progress in an impartial manner and inform the students.
- **Moral educator**: He should inculcate the moral values and attitudes among the students.
- **Parent surrogate**: He can play the role of ideal parents by treating students with affection and care.
- **Rationalist**: He should set an example of a rationalist by basing his action on reason.
- **Problem solver**: He should be able to settle the disputes among students in an objective manner.
- **Reformer**: He should focus his work to bring desirable changes among students so as to reform them.
- **Resource person**: He is expected to serve as a resource person for his students as he possesses knowledge of the subject matter and skills better than his pupils.
- **Secularist**: He should play the role of a secularist by having an open mind on the beliefs of students.
- **Upholder of the norms and values**: He must present the norms and values of society in a dignified manner.

Major Functions and Responsibilities of a Teacher

The main functions are:
- Character development
- Effective teaching and learning
- Curriculum development and implementation
- Adjusting individual differences
- Classroom management
- Evaluation of pupil performance
- Developing good family and community relationships
- Total school effectiveness
- Professional growth and ethics.

Character Development

Teacher creates an atmosphere which helps the student to build his character and develops respect for the rights, privileges, and opinions of others. He sets a standard for the students and also helps them to keep up the standard. He helps them to develop a socially appropriate behavior. He directs discussion and develops understanding on moral and ethical values and issues and also to follow them. He encourages each pupil's thinking and action.

Technique of Teaching (Effective Teaching)

He first of all formulates the objectives of teaching and plans well ahead for teaching. He prepares adequately before he takes class. He selects suitable learning materials, AV aids, teaching methods so as to facilitate learning among students. He also constantly evaluates the teaching-learning methods, AV aids used, and student's progress to improve the performance of himself. He is creative enough to attract and maintain interest and attention so that, teaching is done in a receptive environment. He develops desirable work and study skills and habits. He also reports pupil's achievement and progress to parents. He helps the students with poor performance to facilitate learning.

Curriculum Development and Implementation

Teacher helps in the development, implementation and evaluation of curricula. He also participates in the curriculum revision and innovation to make the subject useful for the students and also to meet the changing needs of the society. She serves as a member of the curriculum committee and brings the problems related to curriculum implementation and also helps to choose the alternative methods of curriculum implementation.

Adjusting Individual Differences

He understands the importance of individual differences and follows various techniques to ensure that all students learned equally. He applies the basic knowledge of educational psychology in promoting learning among students. He develops in each pupil a sense of personal growth and value. He maintains discipline by being consistently friendly, fair, and firm.

Classroom Management

He assigns responsibility to pupils for the care and housekeeping of the physical environment of the classroom. He maintains discipline in the classrooms. He inculcates the responsibility of maintaining a healthy environment in the classroom as well as in the school premises among students. He also takes care of all records and registers pertaining to the classroom management.

Evaluating and Reporting Pupil's Performance

He conducts periodic tests to measure the level of students' learning. He also periodically evaluates the assignments, reports, and other work submitted by the students. He also informs the parents about the progress of their own children during parent-teacher meeting and by progress reports.

Developing Good Family and Community Relations

This envisages:
- Participating in parent-teacher and similar activities
- Participating in community affairs.

Making himself available to parents at scheduled times to discuss pupil progress and behavior. He shows a helpful, sympathetic and understanding attitude toward parents and their children's academic problems. Establishing and maintaining a good relationship with parents and reporting of pupil progress, problems and needs.

Total College Effectiveness

It includes:
- Accepting responsibility for the discipline of the pupil throughout the college.
- Cooperating with all coworkers and exchanging ideas in order to improve and provide a variety of approach on the teaching situation.
- Executing all required college regulations and assignments on time.
- Taking positive steps for developing and maintaining faculty and students' morale.
- Contributing constructively to committees, faculty meetings and other college system groups.

New Demands of the Role of Teacher

- There is the explosion of the knowledge and radical changes are occurring in the content areas of all disciplines—humanities, science subjects, and social science.
- The teacher has to keep in view new concepts like individualized instruction, micro-teaching, and programmed learning, teaching machines and team teaching, etc.
- The teacher has to make proper use of the mass media like television, computer, and internet.
- The present teacher is supposed to have a broad view of the subjects he teaches. He cannot afford to teach his subjects in isolation.
- A teacher must adequately familiarize himself with concepts like "work experience", "socially useful productive work" and "community service", etc. as these have become an integral part of the educative process.
- The present teacher is expected to be update and conscious of various explosions—explosion of knowledge, explosion of population, explosion of frustrations, explosions of expectations and explosion of technology, etc.

Some Salient Attributes of an Effective Teacher

Temperance

Can there be a good teacher who lacks self-control in speech and behavior or who is easily irritated? Can there be any effective teaching, if the teacher gets easily provoked by small untimely questions or observations made by some students simply because it was unwanted?

Will the students like a teacher who condemns them using filthy language or manifests emotional outburst on their slight mistake or mischief? Can a teacher command respect of his students if he himself does not respect their sentiments? Will a teacher, exhibiting excessive sensitiveness or irritability while reacting to students' remarks or his colleagues' viewpoints that are totally different from his own issue, be able to gain their confidence and respect? To what extent an impulsive teacher can really cope with sensitive issues pertaining to the learning milieu of an institution? Will a principal or colleagues appreciate a teacher who always displays reactive disposition in meetings, seminars and other school improvement programs? Getting easily annoyed on minor opposition, not agreeing to changes made by others in scheduling home examinations, refusing to adapt to the changing realities in learning environments and inflicting unwanted punishment or disincentives for minor errors of omission or commission on the part of students, etc. are not the characteristics of an effective teacher. Temperament of a well-balanced and adjusted teacher is habitually moderated whenever situations exude provocation, irritability, reaction, emotional response, or excessive sensitivity. Not swayed by impatience, intolerance and personal whims such a teacher does not spoil human relationships with the students, colleagues and the principal in the college situation and with the community outside. Temperance is indeed the most crucial human attribute that a teacher must develop in order to improve his teaching effectiveness.

Empathy

Empathy is the capacity or willingness of a person to participate in the feelings and ideas of others. Concern and fellow feeling mark the characteristics of an empathic person. Expressing one's concern without passing judgment, and in a manner that the child is accepted, is another attribute of empathy. Irrespective of child's behavior or academic inadequacies, acceptance of the child is unconditional because one loves the child and wants to help, care and improve him. This sort of unconditional love and caring makes them feel better about themselves. A teacher, who exhibits and shows empathy toward those wards who deserve care, encouragement, relief, attention, help or guidance, does not only help improve the learners' achievement but also help him become more acceptable, compassionate, concerned and the most sought for teacher in the class, and that is what is needed of a good teacher.

Academic Aristocracy

Academic aristocracy, therefore, refers to the privileged class of such teachers who can really govern the affairs or re-instate the lost prestige of the teaching profession. Effective teaching is, indeed, the result of being effective teachers. A highly qualified subject specialist does not necessarily make a good teacher capable of producing good students if he does not acquire academic acumen, the first requisite of academic aristocracy, which demands from a teacher mental keenness, penetration, discernment and insight into the professional requirements of the subject of teaching. Teaching is an art which not only requires subject expertise but also the knowledge of how children learn and learn with pleasure.

As a person, the teacher must learn to survive and thrive for which he needs to build a strong base of personal potency which rests on a strong identity built on a genuine feeling of self-worth, a satisfied integral person, peace, joy, happiness and satisfaction he has to find within his own being.

Effective communication is another attribute of academic aristocracy. One of the common attributes of successful teacher is that they will all be accomplished communicators. However, proficient a teacher in his subject is, he cannot be an effective teacher unless he possesses well-developed verbal and nonverbal communication skills which help him support effective modes of communication between teacher-student, student-teacher, and student-student.

Thus, a teacher with the academic acumen of being a good learner, an effective communicator and an upright person who does not sacrifice his academic pride, pursuit of excellence and intellectual dishonesty at the altar of his conscience and professional or personal gains deserves to be an academic aristocrat.

Commitment

Another human dimension which is reflected in the characteristics of an effective teacher is his professional commitment. There are two types of teachers—those who make teaching as a living by adopting teaching as a career and those who make teaching as their life style. The latter type go on searching more effective means of teaching and try to learn as much as they can about their environment, about others and about themselves. They adopt teaching as a mission.

Developing Self-esteem

There is a strong linkage between personal and professional dimension of being a teacher. Unless the teacher himself is a fully satisfied and a well-adjusted person, he cannot be a successful functional teacher. Therefore, the first responsibility of a teacher or would-be teacher is having high regard for himself, that is, high self-esteem. Researches have shown that teachers with higher self-esteem are more flexible in their thinking, more willing to learn and more effective in making their students learn.

Being Interesting and Interested

Most of the teachers who inspire their students have varied personal professional qualities. A close look at them indicates that they are interesting people and are interested in students. Passion for life-long learning, pursuit of new knowledge and taking risks are their common attributes. They help students to inquire, explore, examine, question, reason and solve their own problems. They have the knack of making education entertaining and entertainment education (Marshall, 1991).

Choosing a Mentor

A new teacher can get the help of another teacher whom he admires. Even experienced teachers can take advantage of special mentors. Teachers without mentors burn out more easily and develop lower level of self-esteem. (Joyce B Weil et al., 1992).

Making Teaching Meaningful

When the subject is made relevant to life and students are made to feel driven to learn, it becomes meaningful for everyone. It is for the students to know why they study a particular subject or lesson and what benefit they would derive for which the good teachers infuse their students with desire to learn. Creative teachers select variety of media relevant to intended outcomes.

Controlling While Caring

Over-caring teachers create disorder in the class while those who expect over-demanding discipline stifle freedom and initiative of their students. What is needed is to promote self-discipline and encourage teachers and students to multiply respect and care for each other.

Developing Cultural Sensitivity

Ours is a pluricultural nation composed of various religions, ethnic groups, castes, customs, ethos, beliefs, and lifestyles forming different subcultures having freedom to express their ideals. It is the moral responsibility of a passionately committed teacher to cultivate cultural sensitivity and appreciate cultural diversity and teach the same to his students and others.

Humor

It hardly needs any mention that when students feel bored or disinterested or their attention is diverted due to internal fantasies or external stimuli, very little learning can take place. One major premise that learning is fun, if conveyed and practiced in the classroom, it can definitely help in minimizing students' distractions or disinterestedness. To detract him from fantasies and make him interested in learning is the job of the teacher. And for this, playfulness and sense of humor are the most powerful devices to help them accomplish this task. Play and laughter keep them alive and connected with what is happening around. Teachers, who can really appreciate the value of humor, tolerate laughter and fun in the classrooms, invite them and encourage them to stay, are the ones whom the students like and are interested in than those who remain serious, grim, and humorless.

Ethics

What is expected of a teacher is that he should neither himself violate the morality and approved professional standards nor allow his students and others in the profession to ignore moral principles or practices. How far he observes and reinforces professional ethics can be judged in the light of different roles he performs during his teaching tenure. A teacher who himself lacks ethical values cannot cultivate the same among his students.

Reflection

Reflection is an extremely important and a very complex and demanding process. A reflective teacher means that he should be an independent thinker who knows how to reason, think for himself, combine logic with intuition, and being introspective about phenomena within his internal world and the world outside. Developing inquisitiveness by encouraging pupils' questions, asking why and wherefore of things and happenings are important attributes of reflection.

A reflective person is a voracious reader and must know a lot outside his field of study. He has to be aware of the societal trends, economic events, political changes, current media, art, literature, etc. Examining one's own behavior and its impact on others is also the requisite of a reflective person. Confronting problems, which are the outcomes of his actions are to be owned and confessed by him rather than blaming others. This is the sign of reflective thinking. Ross (1989) defines reflective teaching as a way of thinking and learning that requires a special transformation of knowledge, skills and attitudes. Sparks and Colton (1991) states technical reflection which refers to the kind of thinking

the teachers use in making pedagogical decisions about learning, content selection, teaching methods, and learning needs of students. Action plan for becoming reflective envisages:
- Developing conviction that contemplation activity is worth one's time and energy
- Making or reserving time and the right place for daily reflection
- Trying to evaluate the effectiveness of such reflections to one's personal and professional life.

Thus, for becoming a good professional teacher, one has to be a good person. Teacher-pupil relationship, understanding their problems, adjustment needs and wishes for caring, moral support and motivation for higher achievement can only be taken care of by using personal humanitarian approach.

Essential Qualities and Characteristics of Effective Teacher

- Qualities relating to professional requirements
- Qualities relating to character and personality
- Qualities relating to human relationships
- Qualities relating to professional education and training.

Qualities Relating to Professional Requirements

Love of the Profession

The teacher should feel proud of his profession and to realize the importance of the profession. He should develop zeal toward his profession.

Love for Students

Respect for the individuality of each child. The secret of education lies in respecting the pupil. A student wants to be heard. His opinion should not be brushed aside merely because he is a student.

Knowledge of the Child Psychology and Educational Psychology

Knowledge of psychology goes a long way in providing that basic orientation toward problems of education and child development without which there would be considerable waste of time, energy and human resources.

Mastery of the Subject Matter

He must be master of his subject. Any weakness on his part will lower his prestige in the eyes of his student.

Preparation

A well-prepared lesson helps to overcome the feelings of nervousness and insecurity. However able and experienced is the teacher, he could never do without his preliminary preparation.

Skill in Questioning

The success of a class teacher in the class also depends on the art of questioning. With the help of right type of questions a wise teacher can lead the students from dark and unknown regions to known and bright ones.

Thirst for Knowledge and Experimental Spirit

A teacher must refresh himself by constant reading not only about his subjects but books which touch life at every point. He should attend seminars, workshops, refresher courses, etc. to update his knowledge.

Interest in Cocurricular Activities

Cocurricular activities are equally important as the academic subjects and such a teacher can hardly afford to be indifferent to this aspect of school life.

Punctuality

A good teacher will make it a point to be punctual in his work. Following the teachers coming late, the students may also develop in themselves this very habit.

Professional Ethics

A good teacher will believe in professional ethics and adhere to it.

Use of Teaching Technology

Various teaching aids bring clarity and vividness. It is a great asset to the teacher to narrate stories and anecdotes which appeal to children at different ages and attainment levels, abstract words and phrases can be made clear by illustrations.

Knowledge of the Aims of Education

An effective teacher will have the knowledge of the aims of education.

Judicious Use of Praise and Blame

Praise and blame are the two important weapons in the armory of the teacher and these should be used very judiciously.

Awareness of Departmental Rules and Regulations

He must be aware of departmental rules and regulations and he must follow it in order to avoid confusion and facilitate smooth functioning.

Qualities Relating to Character and Personality

Character and Personality of the Teacher

A teacher teaches not only by "what he says and does" but very largely by "what he is". Students are imitative in nature. They imitate the teacher.

Patience

Teacher has to deal with a large number of students having low and high power of understanding. He may have to repeat his lessons many times for the sake of the less intelligent. Some students, by nature, pick up lessons very slowly and a teacher should possess the required patience to make them understand gradually. Good habits are not formed overnight. It requires time and patience to inculcate virtues in the students.

Emotional Stability

The unhappy, frustrated, dissatisfied teachers cannot help their pupils to become happy, well-adjusted young ones.

Good Vitality

The teacher should possess good health condition and keep himself fit.

Good Memory

A teacher with a poor memory is ridiculous. It becomes easier for a teacher having good memory to correlate many things. A good creative memory is one of the qualities that differentiates a good teacher from the mediocre.

Good Voice

The voice of a teacher should be clear, moderately pitched and well-modulated. A thin low voice develops dullness and monotony in the class. A very high-pitched voice or shrill must be avoided. It distracts the minds of the students and does not appeal to their esthetic sense. Plenty of variety must be introduced in the voice.

Just and Impartial

A teacher should be impartial to all the students. He should be fair in his dealings.

Humor and Laughter

A teacher should never make the mistake of laughing at the pupils. He should laugh with them and should also see that they laugh with him and not at him.

True to his Commands

Less commands should be given to the students and when given, they must be stuck to, otherwise they question their effectiveness.

Qualities Relating to Human Relationships

Cooperative Attitude

A teacher must cooperate with his colleagues, head of the institution, parents and all others engaged in the welfare of children and other tasks.

Democratic Attitude

A teacher cannot afford to be an autocrat. A teacher who is to show the way of democracy to the students must develop in himself a democratic attitude. His role is of friend, philosopher and guide not of a policeman.

Political Neutrality

The students should not be exploited for political purposes. The programs of the various political parties must be placed before them in their true perspective.

Religious Tolerance

The minds of the young should not be poisoned through narrow mindedness and bigotry.

Self-analysis on the Part of the Teacher

She should try to find out own shortcomings and try to remove them.

Qualifications Relating to Teaching

Indian Nursing Council and the university have prescribed the syllabus and the qualifications required to be a teacher in Nursing. The government and departments of the states have prescribed minimum academic and training qualifications for different categories of teachers.

Acronym of a Teacher

T stands for	Tact, Tolerance, Truth
E stands for	Efficiency, Enthusiasm, Ethics and Etiquette
A stands for	Adaptability, Affection, Alertness
C stands for	Character, Clarity, Constructiveness, Creativity
H stands for	Hard work, Humility, Honesty, Humor, Human relations
E stands for	Eagerness, Efficiency, and Emotional stability
R stands for	Rationality, Relationship, and Resourcefulness

The teacher should be an integration of all these.

Acronym of a Humanistic Teacher

T - Temperance
E - Empathy
A - Academic aristocracy
C - Commitment
H - Humor
E - Ethics
R - Reflection

The Qualities of a Good Teacher

A teacher should be a gatherer of knowledge: a reader, researcher and compiler. A passion for knowledge needs to be a part of the person, who is going to sow the seed of such passions in children. It is infectious. A teacher is an enthusiast whose vitality and energy will be a source of inspiration.

A teacher needs to be a thinker who reflects on issues. A thinker is not one who knows it all. A thinker is one, who is willing to look up widely and look at various aspects of an issue, one who listens to various arguments, who will accept more than one possibility and suspend judgment. A good teacher has no fear of accepting many solutions or coming to the conclusion that some problems need time to resolve, at other times solutions are not perfect and sometimes there are no solutions.

A teacher should be a facilitator, whose focus is on the child's learning rather than his/her teaching. To be truly child centered the point of view has to be the child's not the teacher's to understand needs, feelings, limitations, fears of the child, to have the patience to explain why certain things need to be done to be flexible with schedules by reading moods, fatigue, boredom levels, and interest factor, and to use materials and methods that are exciting. An authoritarian teacher, who sets all parameters and teaches the child to be dependent on him, is creating a slave to other people's thoughts. The child is denied the opportunity to greatness which is his/her birthright.

A good teacher should be a fun teacher who does methods and manners with imagination, humor and the absurd. He is one who fosters creativity by allowing children to delve into imagined worlds and come up with impossible possibilities to sharpen the lateral parts of their brains.

A teacher needs to be a champion of autonomy. After initial hand holding the goal of all learning must be independence. A teacher needs to encourage the ability to think freely and cogently, to provide the confidence to build courage to have independent thoughts, to take risks in hypotheses and imagination and to foster esteem. Conversely, to train the child to listen to others, to be calm in conflict, to stand up for his/her conviction and argue a point coherently, to take turns without strife, to agree to disagree and to resolve amicably.

A teacher is an empathizer, who has compassion for the child's struggles and anxieties. It needs a conscious emotional effort. Empathy then flows and one can see the child as a sensitive and lost little soul, who needs reassurance, steps, guidance, support and praise to prosper. A teacher is a counselor, who is willing to invest quality time and interest in the child through caring and advice. Approachability is a quality that the teacher must cultivate with warmth and patience. Children are not commodities to be produced in a factory. They are little people with souls and minds, families and friends, difficulties and anxieties. They need to be talked to and more importantly listened to.

No teaching is as effective as silent teaching by example. A teacher is a role model. Children need both men and women as role models. Children are observant and intelligent beings, who pick up nuances of language, flickers of facial expressions, moods, body language and messages found in the eyes. Underestimating their sharpness is a gross error that both teachers and parents commit. Children pick up positives and negatives from adults. Their developing minds are constantly seeking truths, boundaries, values. Therefore, corruption of all kinds by example, are read and imbibed effortlessly, because what is wrong is easier to do than what is right and sometimes more fun. Therefore the misdeeds of a teacher, more than any other adult, will influence children the most, in their growing years.

Similarly, integrity, honesty and diligence are values that will be picked up by just observing, whether it is coming to class on time, marking work and giving feedback, owning up to mistakes, standing for justice in resolving conflicts, or demonstrating priorities.

A teacher should be community contributor in terms of looking at the larger picture of whole community's benefit and improvement. This comes through in word and deed. Awareness of world problems, discussions and debates with children about social and political issues that need a larger perspective when done at impressionable ages, effortlessly build better citizens than all the social studies examinations. Working for the community becomes the best example.

Teachers have the highest influence and power over children. To the child a good teacher is like a God, who can do no wrong. Whether it is academic inputs, healthy gender and social relationships, balanced view of success, coping with failures, establishing priorities or negotiating acceptable standards, a good teacher empowers the child, creating a gigantic personality by breathing life into unmolded clay.

Values and Qualities of Behavior

To be a role model for students, the teacher should imbibe and practice the following values and qualities of behavior. The list, however, is not exhaustive and may be further extended:

- Commitment to task
- Dedication to profession
- Punctuality
- Regularity
- Modesty
- Compassion
- Appreciating students' feelings
- Appreciating students' ideas

- Nondiscrimination among students on any ground
- Fairness
- Integrity
- Tolerance
- Quest for knowledge and acquiring it at depth
- Obedience to authority and regulations
- Self-discipline
- Open-mindedness
- Sense of responsibility
- Spirit of enquiry
- Cordiality in relationship with co-professionals
- Concern for students, particularly the challenged ones
- Gender sensitivity
- Sympathy
- Empathy
- Optimism
- Cheerfulness
- Respectfulness
- Truthfulness
- Patriotism
- Concern for environment
- Personal hygiene.

Self-knowledge involves knowledge of personal strengths, weaknesses, and limits, as well as opportunities for change. It is the essential foundation for personal learning and change. Personal learning involves remaining open to seeking and accepting constructive feedback, including nonverbal feedback, from others (e.g. peers, administrators, students), and willingness to use this feedback for improvement (e.g. enhancing strengths, modifying or eliminating ineffective behaviors).

Compassion and empathy mean showing genuine care and concern for the well-being of others regardless of life circumstances or station, and relating to others genuinely, constructively, respectfully, and supportively, not demeaning or hurting them.

Approachability and inclusivity involve being warm, welcoming, and gracious toward others, reaching out to others, and inviting their participation. This competency encourages the sharing of diverse perspectives.

Collegiality means being able to initiate and sustain effective relationships with peers and others in the organization, demonstrate tact and diplomacy when relating to others, leverage professional and personal networks in positive and constructive ways, and build rapport within the group.

Integrity and trustworthiness involve adhering to an ethical code and acting in ways consistent with that code, being direct and truthful in an appropriate and sensitive way, being accountable for our actions, and respecting confidences.

Composure means being in control of oneself; managing one's emotions and responses in ways that reduce, rather than increase tension and conflict; handling difficult circumstances and "going with the flow" and focusing on the facts and problem-solving, rather than lashing out at or blaming others.

Patience and persistence involve the ability to balance desire for action with need to assess and analyze before judging or deciding. Individuals displaying this competency take time to listen to others; tolerate others' need to process before proceeding; are able to see a plan or project through to completion, even when encountering obstacles; and are willing to take charge and push to get things done, when necessary and appropriate.

Organization and efficiency mean being able to easily access resources (e.g. information, files, people), organize time and workflow in an effective and efficient manner, prioritize tasks appropriately and complete them in a timely and effective fashion, delegate appropriately and let go of unimportant tasks, and avoid wasting resources. Organizational savvy is related to understanding the policies and protocols of the institution, navigating organizational systems to achieve goals, adopting a pragmatic view of the political realities of organizational life, and maximizing our effectiveness within the organization.

Perspective and vision involve being optimistic, future oriented, and willing to embrace change, thinking in terms of possibilities and alternatives, being open to learning new perspectives and developing a broader view of various issues and problems, and thinking globally while acting locally.

World-life balance concerns knowing how to balance work and personal needs and priorities, set appropriate boundaries, and maintain general health and well-being (e.g. diet, exercise, rest and sleep, recreation).

Lombardo and Eichinger (2004) identify a number of "stallers and stoppers" that can inhibit one's effectiveness, reduce one's satisfaction and success in the workplace, and in worst case scenarios, derail one's careers. These include an inability to adapt to change, unwillingness to be open to and tolerant of differences, excessive ambition and self-promotion, arrogance and insensitivity, betrayal of trust unethical behavior, resistance to new learning, poor impulse control (e.g. quick to anger, overly emotional, defensive), professional jealousy, lack of teamwork, poor follow through, and political naiveté and missteps (Lombardo and Eichinger, 2004).

Being committed to our own development and devoting time to learning, growing, and acquiring or enhancing the competencies outlined above will enhance one's success as nurse educators and individuals.

Teaching Skills and Teacher Competency

Teaching as an Interactive Process

Teaching is an interactive process, involving four aspects: Teacher-student, learning process and learning situation.

The teacher creates the learning situation; the process is the interaction between the student and the teacher.

A to Z of Teaching Competencies

A   Alert
B   Brevity, brisk, brilliant, bright
C   Clarity and cooperative
D   Devotion and discovery
E   Enthusiasm and evaluation
F   Feedback
G   Goal setting
H   Honesty, hard work and humor
I   Involvement
J   Judicious
K   Knowledge
L   Linking learning
M   Motivation
N   Need-based
O   Objectivity
P   Practice
Q   Quick and quality
R   Relationship
S   Stimulation
T   Tolerance
U   Unbiased
V   Variety
W   Warmth and wisdom
X   X-ray like
Y   Youthful, and
Z   Zeal

Technical Skills of Teaching

- Stimulation
- Set induction
- Silence and nonverbal cues
- Reinforcing students' participation
- Fluency
- Questioning
- Illustration and use of visuals
- Lecturing
- Reinforcement
- Communication.

Desirable Teaching Skills for Different Stages of a Lesson

- Teaching skills at the planning stage
  - Writing instructional objectives
  - Selecting the content
  - Organizing the content
  - Selection of audio-visual aids.
- Introductory stage skills
  - Create set induction
  - Preparing the minds of the students
  - Introducing the lessons
- Presentation stage skills
  - Questioning skills
  - Structuring classroom questions
  - Fluency in asking questions
  - Probing questions
  - Question delivery and distribution
  - Higher order questions
  - Divergent questions
  - Management of answers.
- Presentation skills
  - Pacing of the lesson
  - Lecturing
  - Illustrating with examples
  - Demonstrating
  - Explaining
  - Discussing.
- Audio-visual aids skills
  - Using teaching aids
  - Using blackboard
  - Using maps
  - Stimulus variation
  - Silence and nonverbal cues
  - Reinforcement.
- Managerial skills
  - Promoting pupil involvement and participation
  - Recognizing attending behavior
  - Class management.
- Closing stage skill
  - Planned recapitulation
  - Evaluating pupil progress
  - Diagnosing learning difficulties of the pupil and taking remedial measures
  - Giving assignments.

Who, Whom, Why, Where, How and When of teaching

It includes:
- Who is to teach? The teacher
- Whom to teach? The student
- Why to teach? Aim of education
- Where to teach? School
- What to teach? Content or knowledge
- How to teach?
  Teaching and learning methods
- When to teach?
- Time of teaching (age appropriate and need based).

Teacher Education and Training

Teachers play a crucial role in the development of the nation. Effective teachers are life-long learners. Teaching techniques of teachers are influenced by the techniques through which they were taught during their school days. Some individuals are born teachers and do not need much training for learning skills of teaching. Their sincerity paves the path for self-learning and some times, such self-made teachers have been found more effective than formally trained teachers. However, in case of majority, teacher learning is facilitated by training programs delivered before entry into teaching profession and also while continuing in teaching profession. They need appropriate knowledge and skills, personal characteristics, professional prospects and motivation if they are to meet the expectations placed on them (Delores 1996).

Significance, Meaning and Functions of Teacher Education

The Education Commission (1964–66) said, "A sound program of professional education of teachers is essential for the qualitative improvement of education. Investment in teacher education can yield very rich dividends because the financial resources required are small when measured against the resulting improvements in the education of millions".

Definition

- According to the Dictionary of education—CV Good (1973), teacher education is defined as "all formal and informal activities and experiences that help to qualify a person to assume the responsibility as a member of the educational profession or to discharge his responsibility most effectively".
- According to the Encyclopedia of Educational Research (1941), Walter S Monroe defines teacher education as "the total education experiences which contribute to the preparation of a person but the term is completely employed to designate the program for the courses and other experiences offered by an educational institute for the announced purposes of preparing persons for teaching and other educational service and for contributing to their growth in competency for such service". Such teacher education programs are offered in teacher colleges, normal schools colleges and universities.

Objectives

- To develop prospective teacher educators with necessary skills and competencies.
- To impart the latest knowledge of the relevant disciplines.
- To upgrade their knowledge and develop a critical awareness.
- To develop the capacity of elaboration, examination, interpretation and communication of ideas.
- To enable them to undertake meaningful educational research for improving the condition of education and society.
- To develop among them the desire for life-long learning for removing anachronism from them.

Functions and Objectives of Teacher Education

Walker W (1967) stated that the function of teacher education is to produce good teachers.

BO Smith in "Teachers for the Real World" (1969) states that "if a student is to be prepared for the evolving world, then an essential attribute of effective teacher is awareness of the realities of the world."

Learning to Be (1972, UNESCO) has stated, "pedagogical training must be geared to knowing and respecting the multiple aspects of human personality".

It has emphasized that, "what once was an art—the art of teaching—is now a science, built on firm foundations, and linked to psychology, anthropology, cybernetics, linguistics and many other disciplines".

About the professional educational status of teacher, the International Encyclopedia of Teaching and Teacher Education (1987) has observed, "enjoying the same social status and prestige as all those who eminently serve society, today's or tomorrow's teacher must be a professional, whose educational program and level should be more and more comparable with the physician's education".

Concepts of Teacher Education

- Education as a liberating consciousness:
  In this, we can be freed from the thoughts, values, systems, and structures that hinder authentic development.
- Education must not alienate learners from their roots:
  In this, education enables us to discover and develop liberating elements which creates a more meaningful human life and appreciates our culture.
- Education must attune us to diverse process at work and teach us the meaning of responsible consumption and caring:
  In this, we are asked to appreciate, share and nurture the life giving resources and processes.
- Education is human conversation with life:
  This implies about the needs, problems, pains, joys, dreams, and hopes of people and the world, a huge classroom where life is a continuing process of education.

Education must teach a "new value orientation" to motivate and inspire the new generation in the understanding of and reverence for life. Figure 8.1 explains the value of teacher education.

In short, education must encourage the values of compassion, the capacity to feel for others, to feel what it is like, to grow under different or difficult circumstances, and to appreciate the human person, irrespective of sex, creed, color, or social status. The education of teachers has to be considered as an integral part of the system of education (Fig. 8.2). It has to focus its attention on the

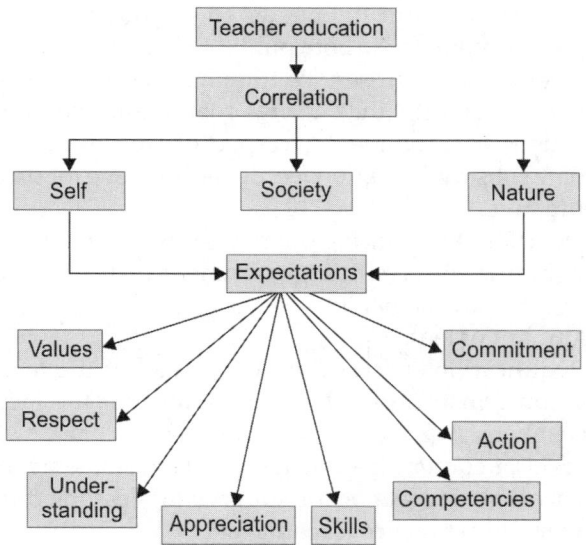

Fig. 8.1: Values of teacher education.

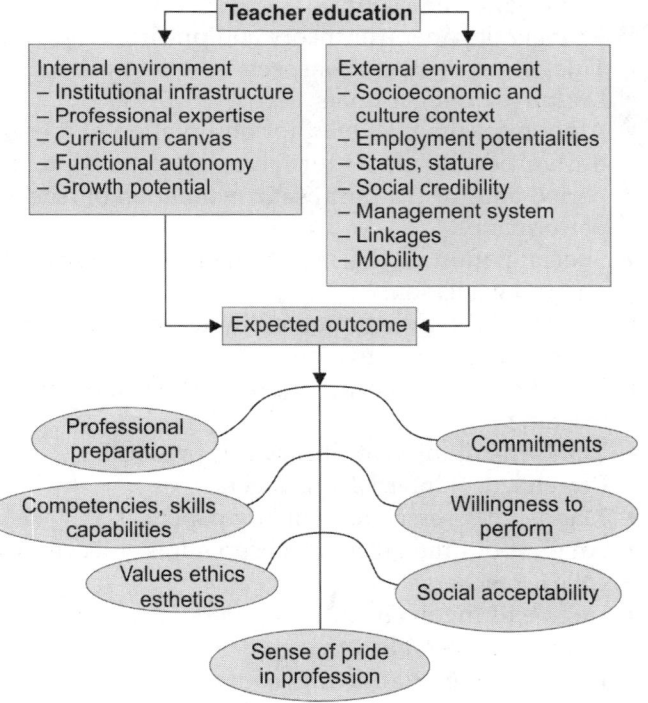

Fig. 8.2: Outcomes of teacher education.

new role of teacher educator. Hence, education is a potent instrumentation for bringing about the desired changes in the society and teacher are to play a crucial role in this noble venture, Human rights can be achieved and sustained mostly through education and training. That's why our Vedic sages have rightly sung:

"Sarve Bhavantu Sukhinah,
Sarve Shantu Niramayah,
Sarve Bhadrani Pashyanthu
Maa Kaschid *Dukhabhagabhavet.*"

This literally means:
Let all be happy,
Let all be free from diseases,
Let all see the auspicious things,
Let nobody suffer from grief.

Types of Teacher Education
- Continuous education
- In-service education.

Continuous Education
According to the commission on teacher education in USA, "continued teachers education means much more than making up defects in preparation. It means continuous growth in the capacity to teach. It means a broadened understanding of human development and human living, i.e. growth in one's capacity to work with others, with classroom teachers and principals in a variety of activities, with the administration, with parents and community leaders and with children age group."

In-service Education
This is self-explanatory. It refers to the education, a teacher receives when he has entered in the teaching profession after he has had his education or training in a teaching institute or college. It includes all the fields, i.e. the refresher courses, etc. that he receives at different institutions.

Functions
- Better understanding of the students
- Building confidence
- Learning methodology of teaching
- Building a favorable attitude
- Familiarizing with school organization
- Creating social insight
- Improving standards
- Training for democracy.

The following are the main functions and objectives of teacher education.

Better understanding of the student: Understanding the student psychology helps him to deal with the students and their problems scientifically so as to help them to overcome and also facilitate learning.

Building confidence: Undertaking training to be an effective teacher builds confidence in the teacher to face the class with confidence and tackle many odd situations that arises during teaching.

Methodology of teaching: Through training, the teacher becomes familiar with the methodology of teaching. Since he has the knowledge, he develops passion for it and does it whole heartedly.

Building a favorable attitude: Training makes the teacher to build strong and favorable attitude toward the teaching profession.

Familiarizing with the latest in education: As the trend in education changes, the teacher training program also aims to incorporate the changes in the educational system. So teacher trainees are educated and informed about the trend in the latest education.

Familiarizing with school organization: During the course of teaching, the teacher trainees are familiarized with the organization and administration of the school.

Creating social insight: They are trained not only in the academic aspects, but also about the community living.

Improving standards: A trained teacher can be a great help in improving the quality of education and also in checking wastage.

Training for democracy: Lastly, training is a must to produce teachers who can teach with zeal and zest and can strengthen the democratic set up of the community. Training is required not only with the sole aim of making one a good teacher but also making him a good citizen.

Selection of Teacher Educators

Factors to be considered in the selection of teacher educators:
- Good physique
- Linguistic ability and communication skills
- A fair degree of general mental ability
- General awareness of the world
- A positive outlook on life
- The capacity for good human relations
- Recruitment
- Internship
- Right tools for evaluation of pupil
- Process and selection of pupil.

Problems in Teacher Education

- Economic problems
- Social problems
- Problems of cultural and social reconstruction
- Crises of morality and values
- Isolation of teacher education
- Expanding scope of teacher education
- Evolving culture specific pedagogy
- Lack of research and innovation.

Variations in Aspects of Teacher Training

The below-mentioned points are some of the variations in aspects of Teacher Training in general stream. Some of them are applicable in nursing too.

Preservice training needs to be improved and differently regulated in both public and private institution while systems for in-service training require expansion and major reform that allows for greater flexibility. Variations are prominent in respect of aspects like:
- State subsidy for tuition fee, degree of scope for private initiative.
- Scope for self-financing programs by examining bodies including universities, government institutions and private managements.
- Amount of fees.
- Qualifications necessary for the head of the teacher training institution/department and for the faculty members.
- Level of content knowledge of a faculty member for teaching a subject or for supervising lessons during internship/practice teaching, etc.

Some of the aspects on which universities inside a State/UT also vary include:
- Total marks for a course.
- Number of papers for theory and practical.
- Titles of papers and the aspects covered by them.
- Lesson planning formats.
- Amount of time devoted for observation of a lesson delivered during internship/practice teaching period and for the purpose of evaluation of teaching performance.
- Specialization of the faculty member required for observing a lesson.
- Types of records maintained by teacher trainees for their practical examination.
- Number and categories of practical work other than teaching.
- Marks distribution for theory and practical.
- Percentage of internal assessment.
- Manner of assessment of theory papers.
- Amount of time given for observation of teaching of college teachers.
- Degree of involvement of teachers in supervision of teacher trainees, etc.

Figure 8.3 explains the components of teacher development.

Other Critical Concerns in Teacher Education

The factors and forces influencing teacher education are many. They are:
- Gradual change-over from conventional programs of teacher education to integrated courses to ensure greater professionalism.
- Increased duration of teacher education programs to accommodate for proper assimilation of emerging professional inputs.
- Stage-specific theoretical and practical components, transactional strategies and evaluation.

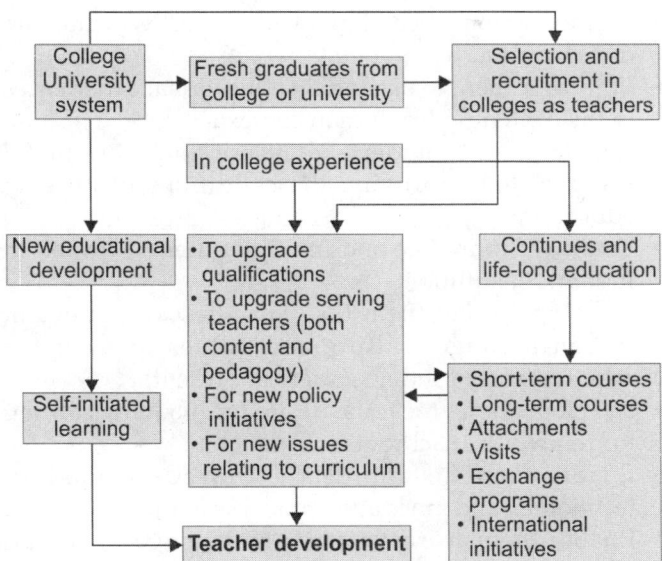

Fig. 8.3: Components of teacher development.

- Plans and programs of teacher education to respond to the expected role performance of teacher.
- Flexible and pragmatic approach to plans and programs of teacher education.
- Proper planning and orientation of education of teacher educators.
- Develop capability to provide for both pre-service and in-service education.
- Undertake research and experiments with innovative educational ideas.
- Act as a resource center for education for a specific area.
- Offer counseling and guidance services.
- Organize need-based programs for educational administrators, planners, curriculum designers, evaluators, etc.
- Impart training for other areas of education, like physical education and special education.
- Act as a link between the college and the university system.

Teacher Educator

There seems to be a broad consensus that the teacher educators are:
- Those concerned with the teaching of academic knowledge and skills relevant to specific subjects in the college curriculum.
- Those concerned with theoretical issues, related to learning and teaching, e.g. child development, sociology, psychology, philosophy, etc.
- Those concerned with more strictly professional knowledge and the skills of the teacher.
- Those concerned with the organization and administration of programs of teacher education.

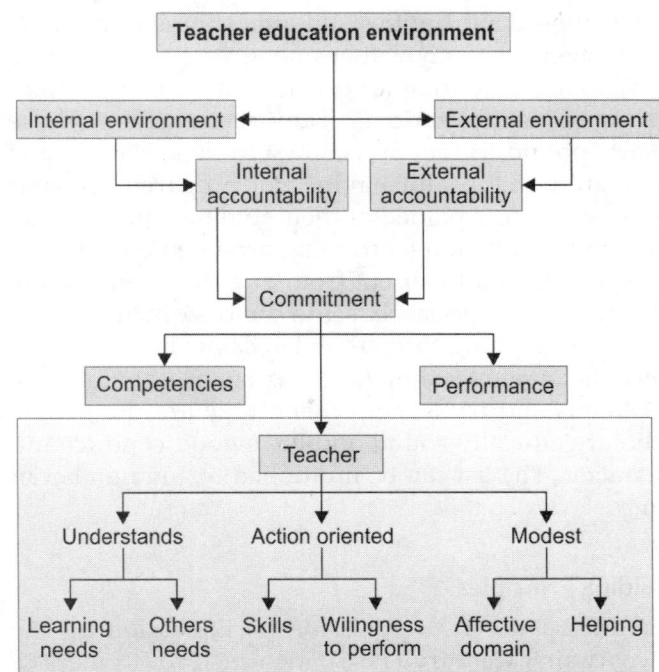

Fig. 8.4: Teacher education environment.

Whereas the first three groups relate more directly to the institutions where teachers are prepared, the fourth suggests the inclusion of educational personnel involved from outside the institutions as well. Refer Figure 8.4 for teacher education environment.

A teacher educator has two main responsibilities, viz. "(i) preparation of good teachers for the colleges, and (ii) development of knowledge and generation of appropriate ideas relevant to teacher preparation and other related processes" (Mehrotra 1990). "A teacher educator is a person who trains and educates would be trainers in the first instance but he or she may also be a head teacher, an inspector or a senior teacher who takes charge of the professional activities of would be teachers, teachers in service and teachers on probation."

The Program of Action of the National Policy, 1986 lists out the following measures to increase teachers' accountability:
- Introducing reforms in the system of selection of teachers.
- Improving the living and working/service conditions of teachers.
- Creating an effective machinery for removal of grievances
- Involving teachers in planning and management of education.
- Motivating teachers' associations in upholding the dignity of teachers and their professional pride.
- Preparing a code of professional ethics for teachers and ensuring that teachers perform their duties in accordance with the acceptable norms.

- Creating opportunities and atmosphere to promote autonomy and innovation among teachers.

Who are accountable teachers and what are their behavior manifestations? They are teachers whose hearts pound, if they have to go to their classes late; they are unhappy for having not prepared for their classes; they are pained at their students' poor result; they think of making surrogate arrangements in case they are obliged to absent from duty for some reason; they try to take special classes to complete their syllabus instead of rushing through the syllabus in the regular periods available; they take cognizance of students, problems and try to help them; they are the people who are ethically sound and have good conduct and character. The list can be multiplied to any number of times.

Guiding Principles

The International Commission on Education for the Twenty first Century (1996), identified four pillars of education, namely:
- Learning to know
- Learning to do
- Learning to live together
- Learner to be, in a way, suggests that the product of the education system shall have to learn, develop and master the techniques and strategies for peaceful and harmonious coexistence with others and to enable the students to acquire these types of learning; teacher education curriculum shall have to be given a new orientation with an emphasis on self-learning and reflection. The development of a teacher as a reflective practitioner shall have to be accepted as the goal of teacher education.

The objectives for the education of teacher educators are as follows:
- Develop in prospective teacher educators necessary skills and competencies needed for preparation of teachers.
- Impart the latest knowledge of the relevant disciplines.
- Upgrade their knowledge of Indian society and education in comparative perspective.
- Relate education and the national needs and develop a critical awareness about Indian realities.
- Enable them to develop new pedagogy relevant to India's needs especially for the poor, destitutes, oppressed, and the underprivileged groups.
- Understand the needs and problems of teachers, teacher education institutions, and the community.
- Enable them to understand the relationship between Indian culture, modern science, health and nursing.
- Develop the capacity of elaboration, examination, interpretation and communication of ideas.
- Promote among them the global perspective of nursing development.
- Empower them to use Indian educational experiences in the contemporary Indian context.
- Enable them to undertake meaningful educational research for improving the conditions of nursing education.
- Empower to imbibe and impart values enshrined in Indian Constitution.
- Develop among them the capacities to reinterpret Indian heritage, culture and values to meet the requirements of Indian society at present.
- Develop among them the desire for life-long learning for removing anachronism from them.
- Enable them to appreciate and adopt modern technology and innovative practices in Indian context.
- Enable them to reconstruct knowledge in Indian context.

Teacher preparation is critical to every system of education. Teacher education policies emerge from national policies on education and health. These are based upon the critical ingredients which broadly include social, cultural and economic aspects apart from factors like diversities, pluralities, and regional variations. An effective program of teacher preparation can be designed only on the basis of appropriate and adequate understanding of its implication for teachers and institutions. It should have an inbuilt capacity to respond to the changes and emerging demands of the society and the community.

Teacher education has to respond to its identified external environment also. It is the people and the society, who judge its totality on the basis of some well-known parameters like:

Relevance as understood by learners, parents, managements, and society.

Credibility as accorded by employment potentialities and levels of affective domain of individuals.

Utility as perceived by the learner for activities in future. Acceptability by all concerned.

Renewal of capacity to respond to changes and aspirations, i.e. an inbuilt capacity for renewal and upgradation.

Teacher education must prepare professionals, who have the capacity to visualize correlation in education. The entire education process is an effort to prepare an individual capable of establishing correlation between self-society and nature.

Curriculum for Teacher Preparation

The crux of the entire process of teacher education lies in its curriculum, design, structure, organization and transaction modes, as well as the extent of its appropriateness. A professional preparation program such as teacher education has to be sensitive to changing field conditions and be flexible enough to accommodate, absorb, delete or perhaps do all these to some extent, in relation to changing field needs. Obviously, this requires continuous effort in all aspects of curriculum.

The major efforts in teacher education curriculum are articulated in terms of the following:
- Conceptual considerations
- Curriculum framework
- Modes of transactions
- Practice component
- Evaluation component
- Innovative efforts.

Conceptual Considerations

The main considerations about conceptualization center around generating a valid knowledge base which is sound in terms of its field relevance, comprehensiveness and feasibility in implementation. Such a base has to comprise conceptual articulations on field practices and experience and processes and the complexities involved in them. Constructing a relevant knowledge base of teacher education involves much more than consolidating the field experience of teachers inside and outside classrooms or instructional situations.

Teacher education curriculum must comprise components that enable both entrant teachers and working teachers to become competent to discharge their functions. In this, the curriculum of teacher education is different in nature from that of other "academic" courses. As in other professional education programs, the teacher education curriculum has to have a knowledge base which is sensitive to the needs of field applications and comprise meaningful, conceptual blending of the theoretical understanding available in several cognate disciplines. It need not a mere admixture of concepts and principles from other disciplines but a distinct "gestalt" emerging from the "conceptual blending", making it sufficiently specialized. Teacher preparation program, on the other hand, introduce a person to the profession by providing a proper context in which he will have to function.

The first and foremost consideration in designing a curriculum is deciding "what" the knowledge component should be. Construction of a relevant knowledge base in teacher education involves a complex intellectual exercise demanding superior academic training and specialization. Its content needs to be drawn heavily from disciplines cognate to education, namely, psychology, sociology, philosophy, etc. The knowledge component drawn from each of these disciplines is, no doubt, relevant to teacher education. However, it must be recognized that these knowledge components represent the respective perspectives with which educational processes and situations can be understood and appreciated.

Curriculum is the most explicit path through which novice teachers are prepared to perform the professional role of teaching and so teacher education program is not only a formality of a required certification but it empowers the young people to play their role as professionals so that they can enter into a teaching profession with confidence and with required competence. Teachers as professionals require some exclusive body of knowledge and skills that provide them expertise to practice. The task of teacher education program is to provide this very exclusive body of knowledge and skills. However, teaching is not only a profession but it is a unique profession. A rich literature is available which highlights the unique nature of teaching. Teaching is in fact a complex, creative and morally laden activity. It has characteristics both of a science and that of an art. So, any model for teacher preparation program, if only confined to technical/mechanical approach, based on apprentice model of skill development leads only toward an uninspired and lifeless teaching and so in the words of Carr such an approach can do more harm than any help to teaching and therefore, in any teacher preparation program a balance between its twin nature of science and art is to be maintained. Perhaps this very realization is reflected in the form of different components of teacher preparation program like:
- Foundation courses and practicals
- Subject specific content-cum-methodology courses
- Teaching practice and practicum.

Some Emerging Concerns

The recent National Curriculum Framework (NCF-2005) has advocated the need for creating constructivist-learning environment in educational institutions and for this, it visualized some basic changes in the role of a teacher. In the constructivist paradigm the role of a teacher has shifted from an information provider or an instructor to a facilitator and a guide, who can create such an environment where learners themselves create their knowledge. In this paradigm, the concept of learning as well as its assessment has drastically changed. The role of a teacher is not now confined to that of curriculum transactor but she has to be actively involved in the process of curriculum development, which includes development of the learning resources and curriculum evaluation.

In nursing profession too, the teacher education program that is preparation at master's level has undergone many changes. The Indian Nursing Council has recently revised the curriculum for MSc (N) Program to meet the demands of the society and to prepare productive members for profession.

At the global level, a new world order has emerged during the last few years. Education is no more a merit goods but it has become a salable and purchasable commodity. As a result of this a large number of private institutions came into existence and mushrooming of privately run education institutions has taken place throughout the country. The democratic ideal of equality is greatly threatened whereas relevance and quality concerns occupy the front seats. Development in the area of ICT has also put some new challenges for teachers. Teachers in the present era are no longer the only source of knowledge but many other or even better sources of information are available before the learners. In the present age of globalized world human survival is also threatened by a number of sources which includes terrorism, pollution of various kinds. To save the future generation from such an alarming situation teacher has to act as an agent of change. He should be caring, creative, and reflective.

Modes of Transactions

Framework (1988) recognizes the problem of transacting curriculum effectively. Teacher education courses at all stages are generally of such a nature that they tend to include too many areas of knowledge and several activities. In actual operation, therefore, the programs often lose focus, coherence, and do not lead to a very integrated view of what is presented in terms of content knowledge, skills and their applications.

Practice Component

The framework includes three major components, viz. theory, practice and internship. It gave up terms like "educational psychology" and preferred to use, instead, terms like "learner: nature and development". The framework provides equal weightage in terms of time to both theory and practice. A part of the practice dimension, compulsory internship as a requirement for certification has been suggested. These have been accommodated by extending the total duration of teacher education to 2 years.

Evaluation Component

Evaluation of any program gives us the feedback of how worthy and effective a program is in achieving its purposes. The curriculum framework for the teacher education program also has to be evaluated for its effectiveness and these findings have to be utilized for further improvement. Evaluation includes all the dimensions of teacher education program and its components. A well-planned and implemented evaluation program usually brings good results for the betterment.

Innovative Efforts

Innovation can be initiated by anybody at any level. It is always good if an individual institution who offers teacher education program initiates it. Innovation can be adopted in planning, organizing, implementation and evaluation. It can be adopted in the methods of teaching, AV aids, research and human resource development, etc. An innovation should be useful, applicable, acceptable, practical, and cost-effective.

Functions of Teacher Education Institutions

Observation of High Quality Teaching

It is imperative for the teacher education institution to provide adequate opportunities to the trainees to observe the teaching of experienced and reputed teachers. This may be arranged in one of the cooperating schools. In addition, demonstration lessons by the teacher educators and screening of video-recordings of samples of "good" teaching must be arranged in the training institution. The observation should be followed by detailed discussion on the strong as well as weak points of the "teaching" observed by the trainees. The trainees maybe encouraged to recall the positive and memorable aspects of the work of their own teachers.

Practicing Teaching in Simulated Situations

After discussing "teaching skills and competencies" and "microteaching" in theory classes, the teacher educators should demonstrate the use of different teaching skills in simulated situations. There should be proper coordination among teacher educators regarding the selection of teaching skills to be demonstrated by them so as to ensure that all the skills are demonstrated by the teacher educators and practiced by the trainees.

Practicing Blackboard Writing

Writing on the blackboard or whiteboard continues to be an important teaching skill, which requires sufficient practice. This aspect of teacher's work assumes greater importance in view of the fact that the quality of handwriting is not emphasized these days in schools. Besides simple writing, the prospective teachers should also be made to practice making diagrams, sketches, etc. on the board.

Learning to Prepare and use Teaching Aids/Materials

The teacher education institutions may organize a workshop to provide training to the student teachers to prepare teaching aids like charts, models, and to use display boards, etc. Besides, they should also learn to use technological aids like OHP, audio cassette recorder and player, VCP, etc.

Learning to Operate Computers

To promote use of computers as an instructional aid, all the trainees must be provided computer training so as to enable them to use it for teaching and learning, both online and offline.

Criticism or Discussion Lessons

After practicing different teaching skills in simulated situations and other essential skills like writing on boards, preparation of teaching aids and learning of computer operations, the trainees should be prepared to deliver full lessons in the subjects of their specialization. Such lessons shall be supervised by the concerned teacher educator and observed by other teacher trainees. The discussion that follows the lesson delivery provides an opportunity to the trainee to have the benefit of the comments and suggestions of the teacher educators and also of their peers.

Preparation for Conducting Action Research and Case Study

To prepare the trainees for this role, the teacher educators should first discuss the concept, objectives, importance, scope and methodology of action research and case study. Thereafter, the trainees may prepare outline of some project, which they may present in a workshop for discussion in the presence of some outside experts.

Preparation for Student Counseling

The preparation for student counseling shall have to be preceded by a detailed discussion on the educational and psychological problems of students, methods of their identification, concept, services and methodology of different types of counseling. If possible, the teacher educators may conduct a mock counseling session with a student or with a volunteer trainee. The video films of a counseling session conducted by a professional counselor may be shown to the trainee teachers. The mock counseling sessions or screening of films should be followed by a thorough discussion on the content and methodology of the "counseling" activity.

The Twelve Roles of the Teacher

A good teacher is more than a lecturer—the twelve roles of the teacher:

The Information Provider

1. **The lecturer:** A traditional responsibility of the teacher is to pass on to students the information, knowledge and understanding in a topic appropriate at the stage of their studies. This leads to the traditional role of the teacher as one of provider of information in the lecture context. The lecture remains as one of the most widely used instructional methods. It can be a cost-effective method of providing new information not found in standard texts, of relating the information to the local curriculum and context of medical practice and of providing the lecturer's personal overview or structure of the field of knowledge for the student.
2. **The clinical or practical teacher:** The clinical setting, whether in the hospital or in the community, is a powerful context for the transmission, by the clinical teacher, of information directly relevant to the practice of nursing. Good clinical teachers can share with the student their thoughts as a "reflective practitioner", helping to illuminate, for the student, the process of clinical decision-making.

The Role Model

3. **The on-the-job role model:** The importance of the teacher as a role model is well documented. The teacher as a clinician should model or exemplify what should be learned. Students learn not just from what their teachers say but from what they do in their clinical practice and the knowledge, skills, and attitudes they exhibit.
4. **The role model as a teacher:** Teachers serve as role models not only when they teach students while they perform their duties as nurses, but also when they fulfill their role as teachers in the classroom, whether it is in the lecture theater or the small discussion or tutorial group. A good teacher, who is also a nurse can describe in a lecture to a class of students, their approach to the clinical problem being discussed in a way that captures the importance of the subject and the choices available. The teacher has a unique opportunity to share some of the magic of the subject with the students.

The Facilitator

5. **The learning facilitator:** The move to a more student-centered view of learning has required a fundamental shift in the role of the teacher. No longer is the teacher seen predominantly as a dispenser of information, but rather as a facilitator or manager of the students' learning. The introduction of problem-based learning with a consequent fundamental change in the student-teacher relationship has highlighted this change in the role of the teacher from one of information provider to one of facilitator.
6. **The mentor:** The role of mentor is a further role for the teacher. The mentor is usually not the member of staff, who is responsible for the teaching or assessment of the student and is therefore "offline" in terms of relationship with the student. Mentorship is less about reviewing the students' performance in a subject or an examination and more about a wider view of issues relating to the student.

The Assessor

7. **The student assessor:** The assessment of the student's competence is one of the most important tasks facing the teacher. Most teachers have something to contribute to the assessment process. Examining does represent a distinct and potentially separate role for the teacher. Thus, it is possible for someone to be an "expert teacher" but not an expert examiner. All institutions now need teachers with a special knowledge and understanding of assessment issues.

8. **The curriculum assessor:** The teacher has a responsibility not only to plan and implement educational programs and to assess the students' learning, but also to assess the course and curriculum delivered. Monitoring and evaluating the effectiveness of the teaching of courses and curricula is now recognized as an integral part of the educational process. Evaluation can also be interpreted as an integral part of the professional role of teachers, recognizing teachers' own responsibility for monitoring their own performance.

The Planner

9. **The curriculum planner:** Curriculum planning is an important role for the teacher. Most nursing schools and postgraduate bodies have education committees charged with the responsibility for planning and implementing the curriculum within their institution. Teachers employed by the school and members of the postgraduate institution may be expected to make a contribution to curriculum planning. Curriculum planning presents a significant challenge for the teacher, and both time and expertise is required, if the job is to be undertaken properly.

10. **The course planner:** The best curriculum in the world will be ineffective, if the courses which it comprises have little or no relationship to the curriculum that is in place. Once the principles which underpin the curriculum of the institution have been agreed, detailed planning is then required at the level of the individual course or phase of the curriculum.

The Resource Developer

11. **The resource material creator:** An increased need for learning resource materials is implicit in many of the developments in education. The new technologies have greatly expanded the formats of learning materials to which the student may have access and make it much easier for the student to take more responsibility for their own education. The role of the teacher as resource creator offers exciting possibilities. At least some teachers possess the array of skills necessary to select, adapt or produce materials for use within the institution.

12. **The study guide producer:** The production of study guides is a further role for the nursing teacher. Study guides suitably prepared in electronic or print form can be seen as the students' personal tutor available 24 hours a day and designed to assist the students with their learning. Study guides tell the students what they should learn—the expected learning outcomes for the course, how they might acquire the competences necessary—the learning opportunities available, and whether they have learned it—the students assessing their own competence.

Multiple Roles of the Teacher

While each of the twelve roles has been described separately, in reality they are often interconnected and closely related one to another. Indeed a teacher may take on simultaneously several roles. However, a good teacher need not be competent in all twelve roles. It would be unusual to find, and unreasonable to expect, one individual to have all the required competencies. Human resource planning should involve matching teachers with the roles for which they have the greatest aptitude. This has implications for the appointment of staff and for staff training.

Where there are insufficient numbers of appropriately trained existing staff to meet a role requirement, staff must be reassigned to the role, where this is possible, and the necessary training provided. Alternatively if this is not possible or deemed desirable, additional staff need to be recruited for the specific purpose of fulfilling the role identified. A "role profile" needs to be negotiated and agreed with staff at the time of their appointment and this should be reviewed on a regular basis.

The role model framework is of use in:
- The assessment of the needs for staff to implement a curriculum.
- The appointment and promotion of teachers to meet educational needs within the institution.
- The organization of staff development activities.
- The allocation of teaching responsibilities to staff.
- Teacher evaluation by staff and students.
- Self-assessment by teachers of their optimum role.
- Construction by a teacher of a "teaching" portfolio.

Professionalization: Concepts and Characteristics

Professionalization is the process of upgrading a social-service-oriented occupation to make it more autonomous, more development-oriented as well as more accountable. Since teacher education is a component of teaching and teaching is essentially a social-service-oriented profession and also because there exists a synergic relationship between teaching and teacher education, both of these need to become professionalized. .

Lieberman's (1986) seven indicators of a profession are as follows:
1. A unique, definite and essential social service.
2. An emphasis on intellectual techniques in performing this service.
3. A long period of specialized training.
4. A broad range of autonomy for both the individual practitioner and for the occupational group as a whole.
5. An acceptance by the practitioner of broad personal responsibilities for judgments made and acts performed within the scope of professional autonomy.
6. An emphasis upon the service rendered rather than the economic gain to practitioners.
7. A comprehensive self-governing organization of practitioners.

As early as 1915, Flexner proposed the following six criteria of a profession:
1. A strong intellectual component or base.
2. Great personal responsibility.
3. Has to be acquired—though theory-based, its techniques can be learnt.
4. Practice-oriented.
5. Strongly organized internally.
6. Motivated by a strong sense of altruism.

Why Professionalize Teacher Education

There are quite a few reasons why teacher education should be transformed into a professional activity:
- Teacher education is a component of teaching and if teaching undergoes changes, teacher education should respond to these changes in terms of theoretical development and practice.
- Both teaching and teacher education have largely overlapping knowledge bases and since their knowledge bases are dynamic, a teacher's and a teacher educator's knowledge base, unless made up-to-date from time to time, becomes outdated.
- Like other disciplines, teacher education is expected to respond to new concerns and issues in a professional rather than a lackadaisical manner.
- The teacher's roles being multiple and prone to change with changes in stakeholders' expectations of education, teacher education would be failing in its duty, if it did not prepare teachers who can perform professionally in keeping with "professional" norms and standards.
- Education deals with a very sensitive area of human relations in that children's education is a matter of high stakes for most parents and they are eager to provide the best possible education to their children so that they (i.e. children) can start their career with an advantage over others.
- Collegiate education touches the life of people; being a basic input to living life with dignity, it makes a qualitative impact on their lives. Education as a fundamental right can make maximum qualitative impact on the citizens' life, if it is manned by professionally competent teachers for which teacher education across all stages must become professional.
- The challenges resulting from globalization and liberalization of education can be best responded to only if education, in general, and teacher education, in particular, become professionalized and both teachers and teacher educators develop a professional mindset.

Who is a Professional Teacher Educator

Thornley (1999) is of the view that a professional teacher educator:
- Accepts teacher learning as an ongoing growth requiring time.
- Allows a high degree of autonomy.
- Recognizes the relationship and interaction of theoretical base to practice.
- Recognizes the complexity of the work of teachers.
- Recognizes unique needs and circumstances of teachers within the contexts of their classrooms and their lives.
- Promotes learning through active engagement and interaction.
- Recognizes the importance of reflection and the ability to be self-critical.

This list of the molar attributes of a professional teacher educator could be the basis of working out more specific behavioral attributes which may read as follows:

A professional teacher educator:
- Plans work on weekly-basis, term-basis and session-basis, and strives for upgrading one's professional knowledge base.
- Reflects on one's performance, especially day-to-day classroom teaching and strives for improving its effectiveness.
- Conducts and supports research, especially action research to improve teacher education and the functioning of the institution and its program(s).
- Takes active part in mid-session and session-end reviews of teacher education program(s) in the institution and tries to improve these through constructive criticism.
- Functions as a responsible member of the faculty, develops concern for colleagues' personal welfare and professional development.
- Ensures one's professional development and supports it for others through participation in professional development activities.

- Shares the vision and goals of the institution, especially those related to education and teacher education and strives for their attainment.
- Accepts one's students and supports and promotes their personal as well as professional development.
- Examines alternative ways and develops innovative techniques for curriculum development, its transaction and evaluation.
- Illustrates through personal example what it means to be a self-regulated learner as well as a self-regulated professional.
- Maintains and promotes a culture of inquiry in one's classroom and institution.
- Takes decisions as a professional in situations characterized by uncertainty and ambiguity.

Once the teacher is committed to transform oneself as a professional and devotes one's efforts to this end, these attributes may cease to appear as unattainable.

Kaplan (1996), proposing a plan of action for teacher educators to enable the profession to give its befitting response to the challenges it now faces, advocated that:
- Quality standards for teachers, teacher educators and teacher education institutions should be formulated and adhered to.
- Teacher educators should think of ways in which inter-professional collaboration can enhance the quality of the nation's teaching force.
- Teacher education should investigate the ways in which improved teaching results in better and more learning by all students.
- Teacher education profession must identify best practices and institutionalize them.

Profession and Professional Education

Any man or woman, who has prepared for exacting service by thorough and disciplined scholarship and training, and who lives and works in the spirit of professional standard, may well be recognized as a member of a profession.

Professional education is the process by which men and women prepare for exacting and responsible service in the professional spirit. The term may be restricted to preparation for fields requiring well-informed and disciplined insight and skill of a high order. Less exacting preparation may be designated as vocational or technical education.

The Responsibilities of Professional Education

The professional man has the responsibility to contribute toward the welfare of the society in which he lives. He must devote his moral energies and intellectual powers to solving current and long range problems. The professional education should bring intelligence and patriotism, thus helps to promote peace and order in the society. A professional man should have purpose and philosophy for his work and life. If a person lacks in such purpose and philosophy, the total effect may be great internal stress and even social deterioration.

Fundamentals of Professional Education

The foundation of professional education should be not only technical skill, but also a sense of social responsibility, an appreciation of social and human values and relationships, and disciplined power to see realities without prejudice or blind commitment. While professional men largely set the pattern of national life, that pattern is much influenced by their earlier intellectual and moral experiences, especially their professional training. The standards and motives of professional practice in the coming years are largely being made in the professional schools of today. An increased sense of social responsibility in the professions cannot be brought about in the man by trying to re-educate mature professional men. It requires a changing of professional education in method and spirit, so that young men entering the professions shall be living and working in the spirit of the new, democratic India.

One of the primary needs is that the professional man shall see the whole problem with which he deals, not merely its technical phases. All technical education should transmit technical understanding, skill and method, not as an isolated discipline, but in its total human and social setting. Failure to do that is largely responsible for failure of modern civilization to produce social peace and harmony.

The problem of professional teaching is one of content as well as of method. If the professional student has acquired wisely selected basic knowledge and the professional way of thinking and working with representative increments of particular knowledge, then he can himself acquire the particular knowledge he especially needs from time to time. If he has mastered the art of using fundamental knowledge to get particular knowledge, the amount of particular knowledge he must accumulate is greatly reduced, and time is made available for the teaching of fundamentals. The converse is not true. If his time is spent in cramming his mind with facts, that very process may make him less competent to work with fundamentals. Every practitioner of professional stature knows that human and social problems are inherent, in all major professional questions and must be dealt with if such questions are to be handled on a professional level.

When and only when problems are thus fully dealt with, is the student in facing a problem forced to ask the truly professional question, "What, all things considered, should be done?", only then can a professional man accept moral responsibility for his own professional conduct, and determine for himself what values his technical competence will serve, instead of leaving this to be determined by others. General human motive and purpose need to be so much a part of professional training that to the student they will be one and inseparable.

Professional development plays an essential role in successful education reform. Professional development serves as the bridge between where prospective and experienced educators are now and where they will need to be to meet the new challenges of guiding all students in achieving higher standards of learning and development.

High-quality professional development as envisioned here refers to rigorous and relevant content, strategies, and organizational supports that ensure the preparation and career-long development of teachers and others whose competence, expectations and actions influence the teaching and learning environment. Both pre- and in-service professional development require partnerships among colleges, higher education institutions and other appropriate entities to promote inclusive learning communities of everyone, who impacts students and their learning. Those within and outside colleges need to work together to bring to bear the ideas, commitment and other resources that will be necessary to address important and complex educational issues in a variety of settings and for a diverse student body.

Equitable access for all educators to such professional development opportunities is imperative. Moreover, professional development works best when it is part of a system wide effort to improve and integrate the recruitment, selection, preparation, initial licensing, induction, ongoing development and support, and advanced certification of educators.

High-quality professional development should incorporate all of the principles stated below. Adequately addressing each of these principles is necessary for a full realization of the potential of individuals, school communities and institutions to improve and excel.

The mission of professional development is to prepare and support educators to help all students achieve high standards of learning and development.

Professional Development

- Focuses on teachers as central to student learning, yet includes all other members of the school/college community.
- Focuses on individual, collegial, and organizational improvement.
- Respects and nurtures the intellectual and leadership capacity of teachers, principals and others in the school/college community.
- Reflects best available research and practice in teaching-learning and leadership.
- Enables teachers to develop further expertise in subject content, teaching strategies, uses of technologies, and other essential elements in teaching to high standards.
- Promotes continuous inquiry and improvement embedded in the daily life of schools/colleges.
- Is planned collaboratively by those who will participate in and facilitate that development.
- Requires substantial time and other resources.
- Is driven by a coherent long-term plan.
- Is evaluated ultimately on the basis of its impact on teacher effectiveness and student learning, and this assessment guides subsequent professional development efforts.

Teachers' professional development refers to the process that encourages and enables them to acquire the set of knowledge, skills, values and behaviors which are essential for them to perform their various expected professional roles in the classroom, school and society. Professional development involves what Schon (1983) called, "reflection-in-action" as well as "reflection-on-action". While reflection-on-action would involve thinking about one's teaching before as well as after the real act of teaching, unlike reflection-in-action, reflection-on-action is a pre- as well as a post-factum assessment of one's professional activities.

Professional development evokes the image of a long-term and nonlinear process. Its success depends crucially on teachers' willing participation in the process as reflection cannot be done by proxy.

Various activities meant for teachers' professional development should be such that they not only invite teachers' reflection but are also able to sustain it through collaborative work. Professional development programs should enable teachers to improve their classroom instruction and their role in school and community, besides enabling them to update their knowledge base.

School education of most Indian teachers was based on the traditional "hydraulic theory", according to which knowledge, like fluids, flows from a higher level to a lower level, from the teacher to the students. This has been completely refuted by the "constructivist theory" of learning, according to which each learner, through peer interaction, actively constructs knowledge through valid representations. Figure 8.5 explains the components of teacher development.

Principles and Techniques of Professional Development

Professional development is the process through which teacher educators acquire new professional knowledge, skills, attitudes, and values that can help them improve their performance and enable them to contribute to making teacher education more professionally rooted.

According to Kwakman (2003), a review of professional development literature based on the cognitive psychological perspective reveals three theoretical learning principles for teachers which are as follows:

Cognition is situated in nature. This is the most basic principle and it implies that learning and knowing are integrated and take place in the everyday world of teachers' activities.

Like any other learning, a teacher's learning is both individual as well as social in nature. This principle implies that teacher learning is both culturally as well as contextually bound and is collaborative in nature.

Sustained learning is essential for teachers to ensure their professional development. This implies that all on-the-job teachers learning can be viewed as professional learning.

"Stallers and stoppers" for professional people

Lombardo and Eichinger (2004), identified a number of "stallers and stoppers" that can inhibit our effectiveness, reduce our satisfaction and success in the workplace, and in worst case scenarios, derail our careers. These include:
- An inability to adapt to change
- Unwillingness to be open to and tolerant of differences
- Excessive ambition and self-promotion
- Arrogance and insensitivity
- Betrayal of trust
- Unethical behavior
- Resistance to new learning
- Poor impulse control (e.g. quick to anger, overly emotional, defensive)
- Professional jealousy
- Lack of teamwork
- Poor follow through
- Political naiveté and mis-steps (Lombardo. Eiplainger, 2004).

Being committed to one's own development and devoting time to learning, growing, and acquiring or enhancing the competencies outlined above will enhance one's success as nurse educators and individuals. It also will ensure that teachers are serving as appropriate and effective role models for the students, who will learn as much from what teachers do, by watching them in action and by interacting with them, as the will from all the knowledge and skills help them learn.

Professional Development Activities for Teacher Educators

Because all teacher educators are basically teachers, therefore, what holds good for professional development of teachers is equally valid for teacher educators. The only differences between professional development activities for teachers and those for teacher educators are those related to level and work contexts. According to Kwakman (2003), all professional learning activities related to teachers and teacher educators can be classified into five categories. These are as under.

Reading

This is a core activity because keeping up with the latest developments in teacher education related to its knowledge base and practice is the foremost duty of all conscientious teacher educators. These activities would include studying literature related to one's subject matter as well as teacher education. In addition to studying literature related to one's subject matter and teacher education, reading activities would include reading professional journals including research—dedicated journals, studying teaching manuals, policy documents and, of course, newspapers with special focus on items on education and teacher education.

Reflecting

Reflection is considered to be another center-stage activity for professional development. It helps us to become self-critical through introspection. Critical reflection can help us improve our professional practice and take clear-headed decisions for resolving problems that are characterized by ambiguity and uncertainty and that suggest multiple solutions. Reflection is a tremendous asset in re-examining theoretical bases of our actions and for reinventing our practice from time to time. Day-to-day classroom teaching, supervising students during the practice of teaching, post-teaching discussions to analyze students' performance and to provide feedback to them, assessment of students' participation and performance in various activities and tutorials, maintaining one's professional development journal, etc. are some of the many occasions to develop and use critical reflection to bolster one's professional development. Reflection and reading can help one self-regulate one's professional development. The knowledge and skills that teacher educators evolve, through reflection, become transferable both in time and space. This can help teacher educators transcend the in-service professional development paradigm.

Collaborating

Undertaking joint work like coordination, organization and conduct of various activities related to teacher education programs, preparing lessons, team teaching, working in committees, developing innovative techniques in consultation with others are major examples of collaborative activities that promote professional development.

Experimenting

Just as school going children differ in their types and levels of intelligence, learning styles, attitudes and values, students, who enroll themselves in a teacher education program also differ from others. In order to enable these

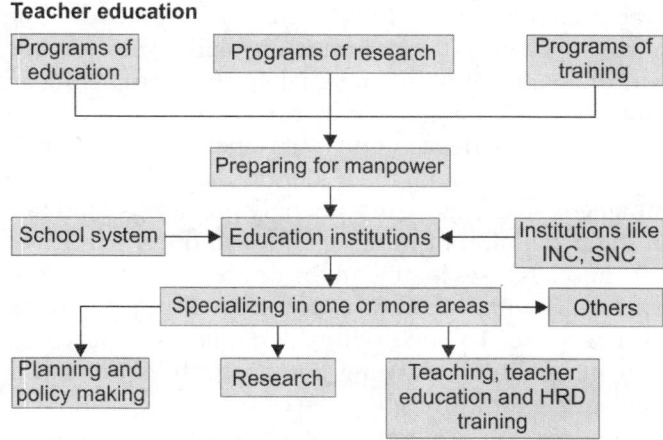

Fig. 8.5: Components of teacher development.

students to use learner-centered techniques for practice teaching, it is necessary that teacher educators too must use learner-centered techniques in their classrooms. This would need experimentation.

A professional activity other than the above is the fifth category proposed by Kwakman. Typical examples of these activities are informal counseling of students, management related activities, extracurricular activities, spontaneous and unplanned student-teacher classroom interaction, etc. In brief, all nonroutine activities would fall under this category. Refer Figure 8.5 for components of Teacher Development.

Qualities Required of a Professional Person

- Self-knowledge involves knowledge of personal strengths, weaknesses, and limits, as well as opportunities for change. It is the essential foundation for personal learning and change.
- Personal learning involves remaining open to seeking and accepting constructive feedback, including nonverbal feedback, from others (e.g. peers, administrators, students), and willingness to use this feedback for improvement (e.g. enhancing strengths, modifying or eliminating ineffective behaviors).
- Compassion and empathy mean showing genuine care and concern for the well-being of others regardless of life circumstances or station, and relating to others genuinely, constructively, respectfully, and supportively, not demeaning or hurting them.
- Approachability and inclusivity involve being warm, welcoming, and gracious toward others, reaching out to others, and inviting their participation. This competency encourages the sharing of diverse perspectives.
- Collegiality means being able to initiate and sustain effective relationships with peers and others in the organization, demonstrate tact and diplomacy when relating to others, leverage professional and personal networks in positive and constructive ways, and build rapport within the group.
- Integrity and trustworthiness involve adhering to an ethical code and acting in ways consistent with that code, being direct and truthful in an appropriate and sensitive way, being accountable for our actions, and respecting confidences.
- Composure means being in control of ourselves; managing our emotions and responses in ways that reduce, rather than increase, tension and conflict; handling difficult circumstances and "going with the flow" and focusing on the facts and problem-solving, rather than lashing out at or blaming others.
- Patience and persistence involve the ability to balance desire for action with need to assess and analyze before judging or deciding. Individuals displaying this competency take time to listen to others; tolerate others' need to process before proceeding; are able to see a plan or project through to completion, even when encountering obstacles; and are willing to take charge and push to get things done, when necessary and appropriate.
- Organization and efficiency mean being able to easily access resources (e.g. information, files, people), organize time and work flow in an effective and efficient manner, prioritize tasks appropriately and complete them in a timely and effective fashion, delegate appropriately and let go unimportant tasks, and avoid wasting resources.
- Organizational savvy is related to understanding the policies and protocols of the institution, navigating organizational systems to achieve goals, adopting a pragmatic view of the political realities of organizational life, and maximizing our effectiveness within the organization.
- Perspective and vision involve being optimistic, future-oriented, and willing to embrace change, thinking in terms of possibilities and alternatives, being open to learning new perspectives and developing a broader view of various issues and problems, and thinking globally while acting locally.
- Work-life balance concerns knowing how to balance work and personal needs and priorities, set appropriate boundaries, and maintain general health and well-being (e.g. diet, exercise, rest sleep and recreation).

Organizing Professional Aspects of Teacher Education

Healthcare is a field which undergoes continuous changes and the evolution of newer methods and techniques in patient care is inevitable. Healthcare industry should adapt to evolving scientific knowledge, technological developments, and societal needs. Nursing practice is at the core of this dynamic healthcare system which has to rapidly update according to the changes. Nurses are providing direct and indirect patient care. Though nursing education and practice go hand in hand, the practice areas adapt to changes very quickly than nursing education. It requires the nurse educators and clinical practitioners work together to facilitate the process. The role of nurse educators is to prepare the students to develop the necessary knowledge, attitude and skills to serve in the profession. The nurse educator has to undertake the profession of nursing and the profession of education. It mandates the preparation of nurse educators in the practice of teaching as well as the nursing profession. Academic nurse educators must be prepared to serve as educators, researchers, and have experience in a clinical specialty area. To serve effectively in the role of academic nurse educator, nurses need pedagogical preparation in curriculum development, teaching strategies, and evaluation methods.

The nursing profession embraces the vital goal of preparing faculty to be expert practitioners, skilled in knowledge generation and knowledge translation in the science of nursing practice and care delivery (American Association of Colleges of Nursing [AACN], 2008; Benner, Sutphen, Leonard, & Day, 2010; Institute of Medicine [IOM], 2011). The nurse educators have the obligation to prepare the next generation of nurses to provide safe, quality care to changing populations in a variety of health care settings. It is imperative that the profession achieve excellence in the educational preparation of nurse educators and advance the science of nursing education (Booth, Emerson, Hackney, & Souter, 2016; Valiga, 2017). The National League for Nursing believes that it is critical that graduate programs in nursing, including master's and research and practice doctorates, prepare graduates with the knowledge, attitudes, and skills to teach, to provide leadership for transforming education and healthcare systems, and to conduct and translate research in nursing education.

The National League for Nursing (2013) advocates for all doctoral nursing programs, including both research and practice doctorates, to "prepare graduates with the knowledge and skills to teach, to provide leadership for transforming education and healthcare systems, and to conduct or translate research in nursing education"

There are minimum qualifications set in the development of nurse educators. In the Indian scenario, the basic level for entry into teaching is the BSc(N). One can work as a clinical instructor/tutor in college or school after successful completion of the undergraduate degree course in nursing. To be a successful nurse educator, one needs to know the teaching learning principles, methods of evaluation despite knowing the profession of nursing. The nurse educator needs advanced academic preparation as well as the clinical area of practice. The nurse educator will lack in nursing skill if they join the educational institution immediately after completing an undergraduate degree in nursing. The reality of clinical practice is experienced only after one assumes the role of staff nurse. Though the undergraduate curriculum in nursing is so extensive this not only prepares a graduate in the profession of nursing and also on principles of education. Nurses joining in the educational institutions as a faculty without clinical experience will be a drawback for everyone. To cope with the demands of teaching as well as clinical learning personally to equip self is challenging for the teacher.

The MSc (N) program is designed to assist students to develop a broad understanding of fundamental principles, concepts, trends and issues related to education and nursing education. It also helps students to develop skills in teaching and evaluation, curriculum development and implementation. Students who enter postgraduate nursing education with a few years of clinical experience will have an advantage of correlating theory with practice. Their background on clinical experience as well as their maturity level will help them to cope with the demand for nursing education. Effective teaching requires a specialized skill set related to curriculum, teaching strategies, evaluation methods and an ability to engage in research and scholarly activities.

The preparation of professional teacher depends on many factors which include the personal factors of the candidate, institutional factors, examination, societal factors and the curriculum for the nurse educators.

Personal factors include the candidates' interest, intelligence, knowledge, attitude towards the nursing profession, desire to learn and grow in the profession, passion for learning and professional acumen.

The institutional factors include the climate, vision and mission, availability of facilities including qualified faculty members, commitment towards curriculum implementation.

Examination factors include the methods of examination in testing the ability of the candidates and the examination reforms.

Societal factors include the demand for the program, value for the education, cost of pursuing a program, job opportunities, scope for further development and the health and educational policies.

Curriculum factors include the objectives, content of the curriculum, distribution of hours for the theory and practical learning and methods of evaluation. The Indian Nursing Council has prescribed syllabus for the undergraduate and the postgraduate nursing education which the university has to adopt. The syllabus undergoes periodic revision as and when the need arises.

More number of nurse educators enroll themselves for the doctoral program in nursing. Though the doctoral program offered here is not a clinical doctorate, the trend is a welcoming one, since the educators are undertaking a research activity. As newer courses are introduced like Nurse Practitioner in Critical Care (NPCC), the clinical doctorate will emerge in the near future.

Need for Evaluation of Teachers

In order to understand clearly the increasing need of teacher evaluation today, let us first try to understand the significant and varied roles teachers play and the meaning and concept of teacher evaluation.

Teacher's Role

One can find that today, as never before, teachers are dangerously overloaded. Their traditional functions of instruction, socialization, evaluation, and classroom management are not regarded as sufficient to make them effective. Present time poses challenges that were never faced by traditional teachers. They are facing a flux in the educational scenario which contains innumerable and complex situations.

We very often find an ever-changing composition in today's classrooms. There are unstable home and community conditions for students from all social classes, poverty, and hunger, and the classroom becomes a mirror of society's varied problems. Teachers are greatly accountable to parents, administrators and students, and due to this there is an increased sense of pressure on teachers. A teacher needs to exhibit leadership traits, and innumerable managerial functions have been added to his every changing role. He/she manages resources, curriculum, cocurricular activities, examination, innovation and changes, time, conflicts, etc. A teacher has to solve various behavioral and social problems in the classroom before he can actually start teaching. Such changes in situation call for effective teachers. What was traditionally regarded as effective may not be relevant in today's circumstances.

Today's teachers are facing situations which their predecessors did not face. Therefore, they have to resort to effective handling of the various competencies in an organizational context which may be different from the one that teacher had to deal with a few decades ago. Evaluation of a teacher's performance, therefore, becomes significant, particularly to identify the strengths and weaknesses of the system.

The need for appraisal of teacher effectiveness becomes also significant in the context of the resources that society allocates to education. Teachers are aware that they are being constantly evaluated, be it in an informal or unsystematic manner, by students, parents, colleagues, superiors and the community at large. However, no systematic, formal procedure of evaluation in relation to their key functional areas appears to have been evolved.

Meaning and Concept of Performance Appraisal

Theorists and practitioners have defined performance appraisal or evaluation in a variety of ways. Performance appraisal is defined as a systematic and periodic evaluation of the worth of an individual to an organization, usually, made by a superior or someone in a position to observe his performance. Still another dimension to this definition is that performance appraisal is a systematic evaluation of an individual with respect to his performance on the job and his potential for development. Performance appraisal involves a systematic, periodic and as far as humanly possible, an impartial rating of an employee's excellence in matters pertaining to his present job and to his potentialities for further development.

Stoner and Freeman (1992) have stated that two major purposes of a formal systematic appraisal are:
- To get the individuals know formally how their current performance is being rated. For example, current rating of a teacher's performance becomes very significant in keeping his multifarious functions in mind.
- To locate individual who need additional training. For example, teachers as essential components of classrooms need to develop on a continuous basis.

By a system of appraisal, their strengths and weaknesses can be identified. Evaluation can reassure teachers that they are doing good and valued jobs, give security and status to well-functioning teachers, spread innovative educational ideas, and reassure that teachers are successfully contributing to society. It also helps to ensure that in-service training and development of teachers match the needs of individual teacher and colleges. It also relates to access to in-service training, career management, guidance, counseling, and training for teachers experiencing performance difficulty.

Need for Teacher Evaluation

The quality of educational experience depends ultimately on the quality of the people who provide them. Teachers comprise a major force in the educational institution. The quality of teachers has, therefore, a direct bearing on the quality of education imparted in the classrooms. The reason for a management's intention to introduce formal appraisal procedures seems to arise from the growth of concern for public accountability. Public interest in education is strong and definitely legitimate. It has to be satisfied under all circumstances. Teacher evaluation has the purpose of letting interested groups know how well, and in what ways, teachers contribute to their students and to society; however, most teachers remain quite tense and apprehensive when it comes to their evaluation. It is something, they would rather avoid. But evaluation being an inescapable feature of the human resources development, plan has to be viewed in the right perspective. Today a teacher can turn evaluation process to his advantage with regard to evaluation and accountability. He must realize that evaluation process offers opportunities for improvement of teaching performance.

Evaluation can bring about renewal of motivation, more effective classroom teaching, improved relationships with pupils and colleagues, more sharing of ideas and problems, and a general improvement in the atmosphere. A well-conducted teacher evaluation gives an opportunity to teachers to get their contributions appreciated. There exists a strong feeling among teachers that appraisal process offers them the opportunity to discuss and reflect, on a one-to-one basis, their individual concerns. The introduction of an appraisal system gives teachers an opportunity to talk about their own performance and the constraints upon it.

Appraisal process can increase the sense of belonging to an educational institution, especially if the process is two-way. A teacher can feel that he has a contribution to make toward the policy-making of the institution.

Information about staff-feelings, achievements, strengths and difficulties, constraints and problems can mean increased sensitivity to working atmosphere and improvement in decision-making and communication. Training needs of the staff become more clearly apparent and this has implications for provision of resources and in-service initiatives. Teacher training programs could benefit from well-documented evaluation reports of successful teachers.

It is felt that a performance appraisal system helps each teacher to understand more about his role and become clear about his functions. The confusion and uncertainties a teacher faces about his job when faced alone, can reduce a teacher's sense of confidence. Evaluation can decrease a teacher's sense of powerlessness and can increase his sense of efficacy. Such systems can be powerful instruments in creating a positive and healthy climate in colleges, motivating them to give their best. The major benefits which result from teacher-evaluation are given below:

For a competent and good teacher:
- To enhance job satisfaction
- To enhance motivation
- To share ideas and expertise
- To support new initiatives and staff development
- To raise or restore self-esteem.

For teachers in difficulty:
- To offer support
- To offer counseling
- To help improve performance.

For the school/college:
- To help pupils through supporting their teachers
- To build a whole school approach; and to identify in-service and staff development needs and plan programs.

For teacher training institutions:
To develop a sound "knowledge base" from evaluation reports.

Student Evaluation of Teacher

The time has come when positive efforts have to be made to involve students directly in the process of teacher evaluation. Pupils' perspectives on teachers go a long way in making teacher-evaluation more objective and worthwhile. Apart from indicating this extent of effectiveness or otherwise of teacher, student evaluation of teachers provides feedback on how teachers can be effective.

Need for Student Evaluation of Teachers

Students have a right and a responsibility to evaluate how well the teacher contributed to the student's ability to master the content, how well the faculty member presented the material in a manner that was understood by the student, yet challenged the student to think and to continue with the process of learning the content, how the faculty member's feedback helped the student in directing his or her energy toward success in the course, and how the faculty member interacted with the student to enhance overall learning and interest in the topic. These are questions only students can answer and the data should be used to guide teachers in making changes in the teaching strategies so that the student responses are favorable in future years.

They also postulate that there needs to be overlap in areas evaluated between that of the peer and that of the student. Areas such as punctuality, preparation for the situation at hand, respect for the audience, and ability to respond to questions can be assessed by peers and students. Evaluation programs that include these items in instruments or formats completed by both peers and students enhance the validity of the data received. When there is inconsistency between the two, actions should be taken to either gather more data or examine the instruments themselves and the context of the evaluation.

If we collect evidence more thoroughly from students, we could get better clues about what and how to improve. Students are good sources of information about their teachers because they know their own situation well, have observed a number of motivation in the classroom, opportunity for learning, degree of rapport and communication developed between teacher and student and classroom equity. The availability of a large number of students as reporters provides high reliability for evaluating many types of teacher performances. Students' report data, often obtained through questionnaires are relatively expensive in terms of time and personnel. Finally, student evaluation of teachers can be justified on the grounds of students as consumers and stakeholders of good teaching.

Tools for Teacher Evaluation by Students

Survey Form

Students can rate their teacher using these forms; the general format of survey forms is to have a number of items or statements about the teacher and class or pupil presented with a scale to indicate the student rating. Some forms have space for open-ended questions but they are difficult to interpret. Surveys with a few items are better than long surveys which try to ask too much. We have to keep in mind that different data sources provide some valuable information to the teacher, not all information. Therefore, long rating forms should be avoided as students get distracted and there are chances of halo effect. Halo effect means that if students find a few characteristics of teacher favorable, they have a tendency to rate them favorably in all. Proper instructions have to be given to students regarding anonymity and to write their own opinion, not what other people think. The survey forms should be distributed to students by a neutral person if possible. The purpose of evaluation should be explained in an honest, positive, and productive climate.

Interviews

Interviews with students can be semi-structured in the form of question-and-answer sessions. They can be conducted by a person who is not the teacher, administrator, principal or a fellow teacher at the school. Student responses can be recorded by the interviewer and a summary report prepared.

Interviews can either be group-interviews or individual interviews. Interviews should involve a large sample of a class rather than the entire group. Group interviews are found to be as valid and reliable as surveys and also cost effective.

Individual interviews permit discussion of more sensitive issues that students in groups might be reluctant to discuss. However, individual interviews turn out to be more expensive in terms of interviewers' time, analysis and presentation of results.

Problems of Student Evaluation of Teachers

Students are still not mature enough, thus their judgment may differ. Students are not subject matter experts; therefore, they might not be able to judge quality and delivery of content taught in the class.

If there exists any kind of friction in the teacher-student relationship, then it may cause problems in assessment. Another problem with student evaluation is that there could be a tendency of some teachers to get high ratings. The possibility arises when one aspect of a teacher's behavior tends to influence student ratings in other aspects. There are chances that the long-term interests of students may get neglected in the process. One common fear that teachers have is that students are too easily influenced by extraneous factors.

Self-evaluation

Self-assessment is an expected part of teacher's professional performance and can provide information useful for planning and teacher improvement. Research tells us that teachers do monitor their own behavior in relation to goals, expectations and outcomes. They are also more likely to act on self-gained data than on information from other sources. Teachers can write a descriptive account, evaluating various aspects of their performance indicating their strengths and weaknesses. The checklist or the rating scale can concentrate on the main tasks and responsibilities of the teacher. The different parts of the job, which has given the teacher the most and least satisfaction, can be focused on. The teacher gets an opportunity to think, reflect and write down the problems and constraints, which come in the way of his/her effective functioning. The different remedial measures which could be taken and the changes which can be brought about in school organization for improving on-the-job performance of teachers can be emphasized.

Teachers get a chance to predict their main targets for the coming year and think about their career advancement. The teacher's performance is evaluated in the classroom, in the community and as a manager. In this process an extensive and detailed set of questions are prepared evaluating all aspects of a teacher's contribution, together with suggesting maximizing potential in the areas of training, further experience, and additional responsibilities. The process also offers much needed opportunities for recognition of valuable contributions and how to help the teacher to develop.

Disadvantages of Self-evaluation

There is a general tendency for weak teachers to over-assess their capabilities while teachers tend to be more conservative while estimating their potential and capacity. Results seem to vary depending on the personality of a teacher. It is seen that confident teachers do not wish to appear overconfident and boastful, while the overconfident ones have no such reservations.

Empirical studies have generally demonstrated that there is a tendency among teachers to give themselves better ratings than ratings given by students, colleagues, and administrators. Most teachers overstate the quality of their own performance relative to others.

Peer Evaluation

Peer evaluation is an evaluation done by colleagues of peers of all teaching related activities for either formative (for development) or summative (for personal decision) purposes. Components of either type of evaluation may include course materials, student evaluations, course portfolios, teaching portfolios, documentation of teaching philosophy, teacher self-assessments, classroom observations, and other activities which may be appropriate to a discipline.

Peer evaluation is a process in which teachers use their own direct knowledge and experience to examine and judge the merit and value of another teacher's practice. The term "peer" means that teachers in both roles are equivalent in assignment, training, experience, perspective, and information about the setting for the practice under evaluation. Teachers, who evaluate peers should not teach at the same school or college and should not be connected with each other socially or professionally. Peer evaluation means, i.e. that a teacher is evaluated by another teacher of similar experience and training, who knows students and school/college conditions of the teacher being assessed. It definitely does not mean using any teacher of any level, having vastly different experience and training or teaching in a different school/college.

> **Who are peer evaluators?**
> The word peer means "a person of equal standing" but in the context of the peer evaluation of teaching, the definition is expanded to include faculty members of the same or different ranks who might also be referred to as colleagues or mentors.

Felder and Irent (2004) suggested that peer evaluations should be done at least twice in a given course by two peers using the same instrument. It is the responsibility of the peers to reconcile their scores and to present in consensus evaluation so that individual bias or preferences are not unduly influencing the outcome. Peers need to evaluate state-of-the-art content, use of evidence-based data in presentation, quality of assessment measures used, consistency of content and the course with the overall curriculum plan, and achievement of defined learning outcomes. Only peers are able to provide this data; students cannot.

Goals of Peer Evaluation

- **Accountability**—in which a judgment is made about the teaching ability of the teacher, which in turn informs the authority about the teacher.
- **Assessment**—in which the teacher's ability are gauged for the purpose of self-correction and improvement.

Guiding Principles of Peer Evaluation

- There must be acceptance of teacher evaluation within the college as an integral part of educational process.
- In the process of evaluation, teacher development will occur only if a constructive approach is followed.
- Collaboration and mutual respect between teacher and evaluator are essential.
- General agreement among concerned parties about the college mission and job assignments must precede implementation of a plan of teacher evaluation.
- Teacher self-appraisal must become a significant part of the process.

Advantages of Peer Evaluation

Peer evaluation has some distinct advantages. Teacher colleagues are familiar with school/college goals, values and problems. They know the subject matter, curriculum, instruction materials. At the same time, they are aware of actual demands, limitations and opportunities that the classroom practitioners face.

Teachers in the same subject area can give highly specific feedback. Peer evaluation removes teacher-teacher isolation. Teachers learn from each other effectively.

As human being, we have access to each other's ideas, information and techniques. In the absence of this kind of evaluation, teachers are unable to learn from colleagues and therefore are not in a strong position to experiment and improve. New ideas become inaccessible to them and they indulge in "safe" and non-risk-taking forms of teaching. A sense of professionalism is strengthened with the idea of shared knowledge. It has been found that one of the main causes of uncertainty among teachers is the absence of positive feedback. Most teachers become isolated in their workplace because they neglect each other. They do not often compliment, support and acknowledge each other's positive efforts.

Peer evaluation offers an opportunity to teachers to plan, design, research, evaluate, and prepare teaching materials together. By joint work on materials, teachers share to a considerable extent, the burden of development required for long-term improvement, thus raising the quality of their work and those attained by their students.

Disadvantages of Peer Evaluation

There are considerable difficulties which exist in peer evaluation of teachers. It is not as easy as it sounds. Reliable procedures have to be devised, they should have credibility to the outside audience and we will have to create a positive culture for peer evaluation. There could be a possibility that the present group of teachers may not be interested to participate in peer evaluation as they may prefer to avoid the responsibility and prefer to leave the task to others. Teachers may also have doubts about their own training and abilities for peer evaluation.

Despite the doubts and reservations which might exist about peer evaluation, most teachers, even the most experienced believe that teachers never stop learning. We all recognize the fact that at times we all need help. Giving and receiving help does not, therefore, imply incompetence. It is a part of the common quest for continuous improvement. It is assumed that improvement in teaching is a collective rather than an individual enterprise and that evaluation and experimentation in concern with colleagues are conditions under which teachers improve.

As a result, teachers are more likely to trust value and legitimize sharing expertise, seeking advice and giving help both inside and outside school, enabling them to become better teachers on the job.

Criteria of Good Peer Evaluation

- Positive approach
- Bottom up growth
- Voluntary participation
- In-depth study
- Professional cooperation
- Respect
- Faculty involvement
- Institutional support
- Utilization of multiple sources and methods.

When there are peer visits to classrooms in the case of peer evaluation, classroom observations have to be made as systematic as possible. They simply cannot be conducted in a haphazard manner according to the whims and fancies of the appraiser.

The following criteria provide the minimal requirements for a fair and systematic observation in teacher evaluation.

The observer should be a neutral outsider or internal member, trained in observation techniques, having established reliability. Observations are taken from a reliable number and timing of visits. Number of visits is evaluation based on the regularity of teacher performance; often this means an adequate number of unannounced visits to the classroom.

Focus of observation is limited to a few major categories of events, and not to a wide-ranging collection of attractive but collusive themes. Recording systems like checklist, narratives, etc. should be systematic and reliable.

Preparation of Nursing Teacher

Defining the nursing faculty role, Boyer (1990) described four types of scholarship in which faculty engage:
1. The scholarship of discovery
2. The scholarship of integration
3. The scholarship of application and
4. The scholarship of teaching.

Scholarship of discovery involves search for new knowledge and research.

Scholarship of integration involves interpretation and synthesis of knowledge across discipline boundaries in a manner that provides a larger context for the knowledge and the development of new insights. Nursing faculty have long integrated knowledge from various disciplines into their practice such as psychology, sociology, etc.

Scholarship of application involves correlating theory into practice, faculty practice in patient care areas, and service to profession of nursing at local, regional, national and international levels. It provides leadership in professional organizations and community or national panels or boards.

Scholarship of teaching involves the ability to communicate the knowledge one possesses to the students, developing innovative curricula, using a variety of teaching methods, and meeting learners' needs, and the teaching is always based on the scholarship of discovery, integration, and practice. Preparation to teach nursing students, preparation for classroom teaching, preparation for clinical teaching, and educational preparation are important.

CNE program, orientation programs, and mentor relationship help in developing the nurse educators. New faculty is assigned to a senior faculty. Orientation program includes the policies and procedures, orientation to instructional strategies and technologies.

Faculty Development

It refers to a planned course of action to develop all faculty, not only those newly appointed, for current and future teaching roles. It is a shared responsibility of the individual, development chair, academic officers and the college itself.

Evaluation of Teaching Performance

It can be done by faculty themselves, administrators, peers, colleagues, and students. It is done to decide on reappointment, merit raises, and awards that recognize and honor excellence in teaching.

Evidence for Teaching Effectiveness

It can be gathered from student evaluations of teaching, peer and colleague observations of teaching and teaching methods, letters from former students, success of graduates in employment, publications of students, teaching awards that recognize and honor excellence in teaching.

Faculty Rights and Responsibilities in Academia

- Core responsibility of faculty is the teaching and learning.
- Evaluation is a major responsibility. Peer evaluation is done for staff development.

- Mentoring of students, newly joined faculty members. According to Lieb's definition mentoring is helping another to reach his or her potential.
- Responsible to expand their service beyond the university and local community.
- Involve in teaching, research, and service.

Competencies of the Nurse Educator

Teaching Competencies

It includes competencies related to curriculum and course development, teaching, using technology in teaching, teaching to learn and evaluating student outcomes.

Competencies Related to Professional Practice

It includes competencies related to relationships with students and colleagues, competencies related to service and faculty governance and competencies related to scholarship.

Summary

- The teacher's place in society is of vital importance. He acts as the pivot for the transmission of intellectual traditions and technical skills from generation to generation and helps to keep the lamp of civilization burning.
- Teachers must possess some essential qualities and personal values. They must fulfill their duties and responsibilities toward students' society and profession.
- India has had its indigenous system of education called the gurukul. The village school in ancient India was called gurukul, as the schooling took place at the home (kul) of the teacher, who was called the guru.
- The Parliament of India through an act set-up in 1995 the National Council for Teacher Education (NCTE) gave it statutory powers for framing regulations and norms for maintaining standards of teacher education in the country. By laying down norms for different teacher education courses the NCTE has tried to regulate standards of teacher education.
- Professional education is the process by which men and women prepare for exacting, responsible service in the professional spirit.
- The professional man has the responsibility to contribute toward the welfare of the society in which he lives. He must devote his moral energies and intellectual powers to solving current and long range problems. The professional education should bring intelligence and patriotism, thus helps to promote peace and order in the society.
- The mission of professional development is to prepare and support educators to help all students achieve high standards of learning and development.
- Teachers' professional development refers to the process that encourages and enables them to acquire the set of knowledge, skills, values and behaviors, which are essential for them to perform their various expected professional roles in the classroom, school, and society.
- CV Good (1973) defines teacher education as "all formal and informal activities and experiences that help to qualify a person to assume the responsibility as a member of the educational profession or to discharge his responsibility most effectively."
- Performance appraisal is defined as a systematic and periodic evaluation of the worth of an individual to an organization, usually, made by a superior or someone in a position to observe his performance.
- Evaluation can bring about renewal of motivation, more effective classroom teaching, improved relationships with pupils and colleagues, more sharing of ideas and problems, and a general improvement in the atmosphere. A well-conducted teacher evaluation gives an opportunity to teachers to get their contributions appreciated.
- Students have a right and a responsibility to evaluate how well the teacher contributed to the student's ability to master the content; how well the faculty member presented the material in a manner that was understood by the student, yet challenged the student to think and to continue with the process of learning the content, how the faculty member's feedback helped the student in directing his or her energy toward success in the course.
- Self-assessment is an expected part of teacher's professional performance and can provide information useful for planning and teacher improvement.
- Peer evaluation is a process in which teachers use their own direct knowledge and experience to examine and judge the merit and value of another teacher's practice.
- Boyer (1990) described four types of scholarship in which faculty engage—the scholarship of discovery, the scholarship of integration, the scholarship of application and the scholarship of teaching.

9. Guidance and Counseling

"When we turn to one another for counsel we reduce the number of our enemies".
—Kahlil Gibran

Objectives
After completing this unit, you will be able to:
- Understand the meaning and concept of guidance and counseling
- Explain the bases of guidance and counseling
- List the need for guidance and counseling
- Enlist the principles of guidance and counseling
- Mention the relationship between guidance and counseling
- Describe the organization of guidance and counseling services
- Enumerate the characteristics and qualities of a good counselor
- Describe group guidance
- Discuss the problems in guidance and counseling
- Enumerate the key dimensions of counseling
- Describe the disciplinary actions.

Introduction

Life is described as a battle for survival or struggle for existence. The struggle for food in order to pacify the hunger is common even in animals, but the human struggle is peculiar in its nature. Because of the knowledge of the human goal, different hungers arise and the struggle to fulfill these hungers is peculiar to human beings. The advancement in science and technology leads any society to grow more and more complex. In such a complex society, an individual has to face many problems for a better adjustment. Guidance and counseling is designed to assist the individual to decide what he should do and how best he should do and how to cope up with the problems one faces in day-to-day life. It does not solve problems for him, but helps to solve those problems by himself.

Guidance or counseling, according to CW Tailor, "assists the individual in the process of self-understanding and self-acceptance, appraisal of his present and possible future socioeconomic environment, and in integrating these two variables by choices and adjustments that facilitate both personal satisfaction and socioeconomic effectiveness".

Meaning and Definition of Guidance

Guidance means to guide, which means to direct or to lead. It is concerned with the best development of the student. In broader sense, guidance is the assistance made available by qualified and trained persons to an individual of any age to help him to manage his own life activities, develop his own point of view, make his own decisions, and carry on his own burdens.

The basic function of guidance is to help individuals who need or seek assistance in varied problem facing situations. The kind and amount of help provided by individuals or groups depend upon their understanding of the concept of guidance.

The term guidance may also be defined as "helping one to see through himself in order that he may see himself through".

Jones (1971) has defined it as "the help given by one person to another in making choices and adjustments in solving problems".

Guidance is both a concept and process. As a concept, guidance is concerned with the optimal development of the individual, educational, vocational, personal, social, moral, physical, etc. both for his own satisfaction and for the benefit of the society. As a process, it includes the gathering of substantive knowledge of the developmental characteristics of an individual.

Significant Guidance Principles and Assumptions

- Every aspect of a person's complex personality pattern constitutes a significant factor of one's total displayed attitudes and forms of behavior.
- Guidance services which are aimed at bringing about desirable adjustment in any particular area

of experience must take into account the all-round development of the individual.
- Although all human beings are similar in many respects, individual differences must be recognized and considered, when providing help or guidance to a particular child, adolescent, or adult.
- The function of guidance is to help a person to formulate and accept stimulating, worthwhile, and attainable goals of behavior and apply these objectives in the conduct of one's affairs.
- Guidance should be regarded as a continuing process of service to an individual from young childhood through adulthood.
- Guidance services should be extended to all persons of all ages who can benefit from it either directly or indirectly.
- Parents and teachers have guidance-oriented responsibilities.
- Proper evaluation of individual to gain knowledge about the individual is must to administer guidance intelligently.
- Accurate cumulative records of progress and achievement should be made accessible to guidance workers.
- Through the administration of well selected standardized tests and other instruments of evaluation, specific data concerning degree of mental capacity, success of achievement, demonstrated interests and other personality characteristics should be accumulated, recorded and utilized for guidance purposes.

Characteristics of Guidance Program

- It is continuous from nursery school to adult education
- It is pervasive
- It is goal oriented
- It is a coordinated effort
- It is student centered.

Meaning and Definition of Counseling

It can mean anything from informal advice that is often given to close friends to formal counseling, undertaken by specially trained professionals. Counseling is a specialized service of guidance and basically an enabling process, designed to help an individual come to terms with her life and grow to greater maturity through learning to take responsibility and to make decisions for himself/herself.

Comier and Hackney (1987) have defined it as the helping relationship that includes:
- Someone seeking help
- Someone willing to give help or who is capable or trained to help
- In a setting that permits help to be given and received.

Counseling is a scientific process of assistance extended by an expert in an individual situation to a needy person.

It is a personal and dynamic relationship that exists between two individuals, a counselor and a counselee, in order to deal with a problem of the latter, with mutual consideration for each other.

Vedanayagam (1988) defines counseling as an accepting and trusting and safe relationship in which client learns to discuss freely what upsets them, to define their goals, to acquire the essential social skills and to develop the courage and self-confidence to implement desired new behavior.

Counseling, according to Perez, is an interactive process conjoining the counselee, who needs assistance and the counselor, who is trained and educated to give this assistance. The counselor initiates, facilitates and maintains the interactive process, and he communicates feelings of spontaneity and warmth, tolerance, respect, and sincerity.

Smith defines counseling as "a process in which the counselor assists the counselee to make interpretation of facts relating to a choice, plan or adjustments, which he needs to make".

According to Wren, counseling is a personal and dynamic relationship between two individuals—an older, more experienced and wiser (counselor) and a younger, less wise (counselee). The latter has a problem for which he seeks the help of the former. The two work together so that the problem may be more clearly defined and the counselee may be helped to a self-determined solution. Table 9.1 briefs the relation between guidance and counseling.

Characteristics of Counseling

- Counseling is a person-to-person relationship
- It involves two individuals—one seeking help and the other, a professionally trained person who can help the first
- A mutual relationship and respect, cooperation and friendliness is established between the two individuals
- Counseling is democratic.

Basis of Guidance and Counseling

Individual

- **Academic growth:** All-round development of the student is the aim of education. For a teacher to teach effectively, besides knowing her subject well, she should know the pupil. A counselor/guidance worker helps the teacher to understand the needs, abilities, and interests of her pupils so that she can help the student to attain the aim of education.

Table 9.1: Relation between guidance and counseling.

Guidance	Counseling
Guidance is a broad and comprehensive process	Counseling is more specific and intense in nature
It is an organized service to identify and develop the potentialities of pupils	It is a specialized service offered to help the individual to solve the problems by them
Information about an individual is collected, recorded and communicated to help them to understand themselves. It forms the basis for counseling services. Pupils are also given information about educational and vocational opportunities	It is a systematic and integrated series of activities carried over a length of period according to the differential needs
It is preventive	It is therapeutic
It can be given by any guidance worker	It is given by specially trained professional
It may be given in any normal set-up	It is given in special set-up
Decision making operates at intellectual level	It operates at emotional level
It may be required by all normal individual	It is required for the individual with problems
Guidance can be given in single meeting	It requires several sessions to grasp the individual's situation in its totality
It is not a profession	It has gained the status of a profession. It is an artistic science and a scientific art
It does not require any special approach on the part of the counselor	It demands an empathetic approach on the part of the counselor, not an emotional involvement

- **Vocational development:** Guidance helps us to develop awareness of self and the world of work and to develop right attitude toward the work.
- **Personal social development:** All people want to be happy. Even the lightest hindrance in the adjustive process tends to cause pain and frustration. Also the individuals differ in their attitudes, abilities, and skills. So the individual's potentialities and capacities vary. The problem of individual is multifactor in origin. These may be related to her health, academics, family, and the environment. Guidance and counseling services help the individual in managing them.

Societal

- **Proper utilization of human resources:** An individual's development in all dimensions helps him not only to satisfy himself in performing a job and also should satisfy the needs of the society. Care is needed for selection of right person for the right job in right place in terms of his abilities, skills, and attitudes.
- **Good citizenship:** A society needs a citizen of honesty, right attitudes, social values, good habits, and social responsibilities to maintain democracy. Guidance and counseling services help a citizen to develop all values.
- **Better family life:** Family is the fundamental unit, a better adjustment within leads to the development of well-adjusted individual. This service helps the individual in building better relationship between pupil and their family members.

Need for Guidance and Counseling

Guidance and counseling have become a great need for pupils for the following reasons:
- Adjustment with one's self as well as with the complex society has become difficult and it brings frustration and conflicts in the individual.
- With the expansion of education, there is an increased demand from the students of any profession which puts them in constant stress.
- The achievement of pupils in some subjects, generally in languages and science, is much below the level of their capacity. This may be on account of poor home environment, lack of clear goals, or difficulties in their studies. Guidance and counseling help them to set clear goals and to cultivate good study habits.
- Education is moving in the direction of specialization with the addition of new information everyday. Students sometimes fail to cope up with the course of studies and new information. Guidance helps them to make the right type of choices and to their future well.
- Students need help not only in their studies but also in their personal and social adjustments. Guidance and counseling extend its hands to the solution of their personal and social problems by training their emotions, developing their interests, and promoting their social efficiency.
- In today's world, there is a wide range of possibilities for a student in terms of occupation. He needs guidance in realistic vocational aspirations, and in making wise vocational choices.
- There are exceptional students in every college like the gifted, the backward, etc. Guidance takes particular care of such children.
- Decision-making is inevitable in an individual's life. Guidance and Counseling services help him to make prompt and wise decisions.

Advantages for the Students

- To understand themselves, i.e. their abilities, aptitudes, interests, personality patterns, their strengths and weaknesses
- To develop their potentialities in the right manner
- To select specialty for their higher education

- To select suitable occupation in the broad field of nursing
- To solve personal and social problems
- To make educational, vocational, and psychological adjustment.

Advantages for the Teachers

- To understand their students, their abilities, interest, strengths and weaknesses, etc.
- To develop their potentialities by detecting maladjustments and solve their problems.
- To improve classroom relationships and emotional climate through emphasis upon democratic procedures.
- To provide education, vocational and psychological guidance.

Advantages for the Administration

- To select candidates at the time of admission.
- To use guidance data in promotional policy and practice.
- To set up and maintain an effective cumulative record system.
- To collect, organize and use occupational information.
- To plan placement and follow-up procedures.
- To identify the areas of the college where improvement is needed.
- To increase the overall efficiency.

Principles of Guidance and Counseling

Holism

It is concerned with the "whole" individual and not just with her intellectual life alone. This process aims at the all-round development of an individual such as physical, mental, social, vocational, spiritual, etc. Problem in one dimension influences the other dimension and so it considers the development of a balanced personality.

> Guidance and counseling program need to be introduced in our colleges and universities to meet the varied needs of the educational system, administration and students in order
> - To help in the total development of the student.
> - To help in the proper choice of courses.
> - To help in the proper choice of careers.
> - To help the students in vocational development.
> - To develop readiness for choices and changes to face new challenges.
> - To minimize the mismatching between education and employment, and help in the efficient use of manpower.
> - To motivate the youth for self-employment.
> - To help fresher establish proper identity.
> - To identify and motivate the students from weaker sections of society.
> - To help the students in their period of turmoil and confusion.
> - To help in checking wastage and stagnation.

Universal Requirement

It is concerned with all, not only with special or problem students. It is required by all individuals at all stages of his development irrespective of age, sex, caste and status, etc.

Evidence

Guidance and counseling services are rendered based on the reliable data, therefore, have adequate data before starting the process. There are so many psychological and nonpsychological tests and various techniques when administered selectively and properly helps to gather information about an individual. It is concerned with student's self-understanding and self-determination. This forms the base for guidance and counseling services.

Individual Difference

It recognizes the existence of individual differences; hence, limitations and problems of each individual are different from one another. Individuals differ in their capacities, skills, intelligence, personality, aptitude, and attitude, and so their problems also vary. A technique which is useful for an individual may not be useful for the other. Guidance and counseling recognizes the uniqueness of the individual.

Student-centeredness

Guidance services should be organized while keeping in view the needs, interests and purposes of the students in the college.

Cause and Effect

It accepts that problems have causes and are inter-related, so a deep knowledge of causes is essential. Counseling services aim at identifying the cause which leads to the present problem so that services can be rendered to the students to alleviate the problem.

Continuous Process

It cannot be restricted to problem solving situation only. The services are not just problem oriented. It is given for the normal students too as it aims for all-round development of the student.

Flexibility

There is no rigid procedure, techniques, and approaches used in this service since it takes into consideration of principle of individual difference. Being flexible without compromising the quality of services will be helpful in achieving the purpose.

Goal Oriented

It is one of the planned activities which is carried out by the counselor and counselee to attain the goal. The goal set should be realistic and attainable one.

Professional Activity

It should be rendered by the trained professional only. It is one of the specialized and helping services which requires training on the part of the counselor.

Growth and Development

Every human being passes through the stages of growth and development, and the problem also varies according to their growth and developmental stage. It is required by all human organisms irrespective of the growth and developmental stage. The counselor has to take into consideration of the developmental stage when they plan for services and it is also not restricted to any particular developmental stage.

Prevention as Well as Cure

Guidance should be organized to deal not only with serious problems after they arise, but also with causes of such problems, in order to prevent them from arising or to prepare the students better to solve the problem.

Organization of Counseling Services

Organization means systematic planning, coordination and conduct of certain activities within the policy framework of the institutions. It is must for any educational organization to organize counseling services so that they can identify the students with problems and help them to solve the problems.

Purposes of Organizing Counseling Services

- To help adolescents with normal developmental problems.
- To help individuals through temporary crisis.
- To identify signs of disturbed/problem behavior at the earliest.
- To refer cases needing specialist treatment.
- To facilitate communication within and between the nursing institutions, home, the communities and the resources.
- To support faculty members who are helping individuals but who themselves want guidance and reassurance.

Objectives of a Counseling Program

- Making help and assistance available to the adolescents regarding their developmental problems.
- Making help available to pupils for coping up with temporary crisis.
- Prompt and early detection of disturbed or deviant behavior in pupils.
- Establishment of referral services.
- Development of effective communication system within the college, hospital, community, and home.
- Effective and appropriate use of resources available.
- Provision of supportive services to counselors.

Types of Counseling Services

Orientation Service

It is meant to help the pupils become fully aware of themselves and the new environment, so that they are oriented to the purpose, history, nature and scope of nursing education and nursing practice.

Appraisal Service

It is meant to gather, record, maintain, and use adequate information about each pupil. The purpose of such service is to help each pupil achieve her optimum potential and for helping her to develop self-insight. The type of information collected includes information about her home, education and occupation of parents, pupil's interest, abilities, aptitude, attitude, health and general behavior pattern. This is collected from the pupil herself, family members, friends, teacher and previous records such as anecdotal record, problem check list, etc. The information collected is recorded in the cumulative record, which is kept confidentially. Only reliable, usable and accurate information should be collected. The record should be clearly maintained with updated information.

Information Service

It is meant to serve the individual and society. Here occupational information is given to the individual. This helps nursing students to prevent unfortunate consequences arising from maladjustments to her job and contributes to her well-being and efficiency. This aids in building good work habits and gives them information about higher training and courses available to them. Career talks, newspapers, employment news, pamphlets, charts, occupational guides, audio-visual materials, etc. are used to convey such message to the nursing students.

Counseling Service

It is the pivot of all services available under the banner guidance and counseling. It aims at developing pupil's self-understanding, self-acceptance, and self-confidence.

> **Issues for Counseling of Nursing Students**
> - The minimum age for the young nursing students is 17 years and they are still in adolescence age group and it is natural to suffer from emotional turmoil.
> - It is conducted as residential program in some of the institutions and demands strict discipline from the students.
> - They are away from their family and home and it may not be possible to visit their home often.
> - As students from different parts of the country study together, also a vast sociocultural background may exist due to different languages, attitude, beliefs, and values. Hence, interpersonal relations with other students may also exist which in turn may lead to frustration and conflict.
> - In the beginning, pupils from low socioeconomic strata of the society, only opted for nursing. Now, it is not so. Pupils from different socioeconomic status choose nursing as their career.
> - Complex learning environment such as classroom, hospital, and community forces them to take extra effort to adjust to the new learning environment.
> - They are expected to play a dual role such as students and nurse when situation arises.
> - They are expected to hide their own values and beliefs and maintain good human relations with the patients and the members of health team.
> - They should face the patients with acute illness, chronic illness, end-stage disease, death and dying, etc. which require emotional balance, balanced personality, and mental maturity.
> - The syllabus and curriculum is very comprehensive and exclusive and thus demands a lot from a student.

Types of Counseling

There are four different types of counseling:
1. Developmental
2. Preventive
3. Facilitative
4. Crisis

- **Developmental counseling** helps individual to achieve personal growth by setting clear goals for future behavior such as developing positive attitudes, values, and morals.
- **Preventive counseling** helps an individual to prepare for future specific concern such as any future failures in the examinations, etc.
- **Facilitative counseling** is also referred to as remedial or adjustive counseling which means to correct a fault or an undesirable behavior.
- **Crisis counseling** helps an individual to overcome any crisis situation such as loss of a family, family conflict, etc. The crisis situation affects the normal behavior of the student. The counselor helps the individual understand the situation and develop new pattern of behavior.

Areas of Counseling

Educational

The educational counseling helps the pupils to get maximum benefit out of education and solve their problems related to education—classroom or clinical and community. It aids him in choosing wisely, in planning intelligently and in pursuing purposefully the curriculum best suited to his needs.

The common educational problems of the pupils are:
- Difficulty in choosing subjects for future study.
- Disillusionment with the chosen subjects.
- Failure in the examination, low marks and substandard performance, etc.
- Fear and anxiety about institution.
- Poor study habits, lack of concentration, lack of interest, and lack of motivation.

The following functions are performed in educational counseling. They are to help pupils:
- To orient themselves to the new purposes and philosophy of nursing education.
- Identify the need of educational planning.
- Make an appraisal of their own abilities and interest.
- Develop study habits most appropriate to study of nursing.
- To orient with clinical field and methods of clinical learning.
- To orient with library and other facilities which are available to them in a college of nursing.
- Choose specialization, according to their needs and interests.
- To give information about higher education.

Vocational

As the individuals differ, so do the occupations. They make different demands from different individuals. This function assists to select an occupation most suited to their abilities, interest and aptitude. It helps them to prepare for it, center it, and progress in it. This function includes helping the students to understand and identify their abilities, values and goals and provides information of occupations such as rewards, conditions of employment, opportunities for advancement, etc. This also provides the information about the financial assistance, scholarships, and fellowships for improving their prospects.

Health and Living Conditions

The services provided are health guidance for physical, mental and social well-being of the students. This also helps to improve the environmental conditions and maintenance of proper sanitation in and around the hostel. The services are aimed to provide satisfactory living conditions along with the balanced diet to the students and promote positive health habits in children.

Personal

Every student faces certain problem about which she may be very anxious. So the counselor provides advice on personal problems. They also face problems of interpersonal relationships with parents, teachers, friends and others. The counselor helps the pupil in developing interpersonal skills and also helps them to accept themselves and others. It aims in developing confidence and alleviate fear and anxiety.

Moral, Religion and Social

Counseling given in this area includes helping the student in developing right ideals and conduct of living. It enables the pupil to inculcate and prioritize their values that would be beneficial to them and to the society.

Leisure

Pupils need opportunities of self-expression in which they can try out their talents and express themselves. They require guidance to make proper use of their potentials and talents. It provides opportunities to develop curricular, cocurricular and extracurricular activities to spend their leisure time more creatively and meaningfully.

Approaches to Counseling

Approach 1: Directive Counseling or Counselor Centered

Basic Assumptions

- Counselor is a professionally trained person, who by his knowledge and experience understands the nature of the problem of the counselee.
- By virtue of the training and the experience, the counselor can help the counselee to solve the problem.

The counselor is very active here. All attention is focused upon a particular problem and possibilities for its solution. The counselee, of course, makes decisions, but the counselor tries to direct the thinking of the pupil by informing and advising. In this approach, counseling tends to be comparatively short and consumes less time as time is not wasted in self-decisions by the individual. This is otherwise known as authoritarian or psychoanalytic approach.

Advantages

- Counselors can create a positive regard toward the clients.
- It tends to be useful for clients, who have difficulty expressing themselves.
- It is less time consuming as the experience of the counselor helps to economize the time by early diagnosing and timely intervention.
- It is the best method for clients who are in crisis.
- The counselor can use various techniques of evaluation and intervention in solving the problem.

Criticisms

- It may give less responsibility to the client and increase the role of the counselor as the trained expert.
- It may not be suitable for clients, who are good in self-analysis and who can decide for themselves.
- Sometimes there is a possibility of ignoring the abilities and skills of the counselee and there is also a risk of dominating the client.

> EG Williamson is the chief exponent of the directive counseling and Carl R Rogers is the chief exponent of nondirective counseling.

Approach 2: Nondirective Approach or Client-centered Counseling

This approach is otherwise known as client-centered or humanistic approach. Carl Rogers suggested this type of counseling.

Basic Assumptions

- Human beings are growth oriented and tend toward self-actualization.
- Every individual exists in a continually changing world of experience of which he is the center.
- Every individual is capable of solving her/his own problems.
- Human beings are intrinsically good and trustworthy.
- The degree to which the counselor is able to create the nurturing relationship by establishing therapeutic relationship will influence the client's possibilities for growth.

The client seeks help of the counselor. The counselor defines the situation, but never suggests answer. He provides an atmosphere for the client to think of probable solutions to his problems. The counselor is very friendly and encourages free expression of the client. The counselor tries to understand the feelings of the client. The counselor by reflecting, clarifying and interpreting these feelings enables the individual to gain insight of his own self.

Advantages

- It is relatively simple to learn and it fosters an open and honest helping relationship.
- It encourages further self-exploration.
- It helps the client to feel reassured that he or she is deeply understood and accepted for his or her feelings.
- It clarifies a client's feelings so that the situations may be viewed more objectively.
- It provides an opportunity for emotional catharsis and bringing relief of pent-up tensions and pressure.
- It encourages the client to move from superficial concerns to deeper and more significant problems.

Criticisms of Client-centered Counseling

- It may give too much responsibility to the client and reduce the role of the counselor as the trained expert.

- Counselors may be unable to create unconditional positive regard because everything is ultimately conditional.
- It does not respond to the difficulties encountered in translating feelings into action.
- It is narrow in its focus on affect and tends to ignore thoughts and behavior.
- It is not useful for clients who are in crisis and require directive intervention.
- It tends to be useful for highly verbal clients and less appropriate for those who have difficulty expressing themselves.
- It is useful for the individuals having tensions or worries. It is more time consuming when compared to directive counseling.

Approach 3: Eclectic Counseling

PC Thorne calls it "Personality counseling". He suggests the following steps:
- Diagnosis of personality maladjustment.
- Securing proper conditions for effective learning.
- Stimulating the client to develop his own resources and assume responsibilities.
- Careful handling of related problems.

The basic components of counseling are:
- **The scientific acumen**: To select proper tools and devices to collect cumulative data about the individual and his environment.
- **The technical ability**: To put together and examine the vast amount of data related to the individual and his environment.
- **The professional competence**: To understand the significance of this data in relation to the problems of the individual.
- **The artistic skill**: To communicate the interpretations to the counselee in a manner acceptable to him.

Basic Assumptions

- It is based on the fact that all individuals differ from one another and their problem too varies.
- No single approach can be helpful to solve the problems.

Eclectism refers to selection and orderly combination of best features from diverse sources into a harmonious whole. An eclectic counselor is thus at times a nondirective counselor who operates on the premises that it is the individual's responsibility to determine his own way of life and choose his own goals. However, at times the counselor is directive when she recognizes that many young people are not ready to assume full responsibility and thus takes the initiative and provides necessary directions. She believes that counseling is the joint venture and it is the joint responsibility of both the individual and the counselor.

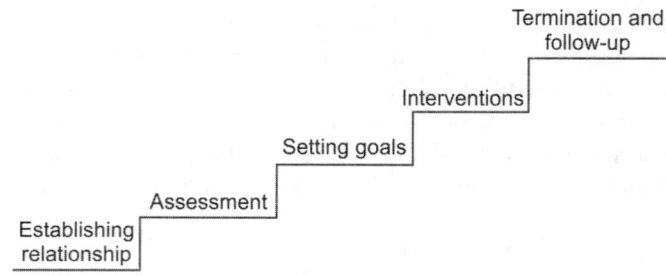

Fig. 9.1: Phases of counseling.

Phases of Counseling

The phases of counseling as depicted in Figure 9.1 are as follows:
- Establishing relationship
- Assessment
- Setting goals
- Interventions
- Termination and follow-up.

Establishing Relationship

It is the important phase in the counseling process as it affects the progress of the process. Each counselee–counselor relationship is unique and it is influenced by the factors such as respect, trust and a sense of psychological comfort. The common skills required in establishing relationship are:
- Introducing counselor to the counselee
- Listening attentively to what the counselee says
- Addressing the counselee by name
- Ensuring physical comfort
- Observing nonverbal cues
- Encouraging open communication

It takes several sessions for the counselor and counselee to establish good relationship.

Assessment

It is the phase in which individuals are encouraged to talk about their problems. Counselor asks information, seeks his views, observes and helps the counselee to clearly state his problem. In this data collection phase, the counselor requires specific skills such as observation, skill in enquiry, making associations among facts, recording, making educated guesses, etc.

Setting Goals

Goals are set based on educated guesses made in assessment phase. The aim is to provide direction to the individual and the counselor. Setting goals may be of two types:
1. Immediate
2. Ultimate.

Sometimes the individual may find it difficult to set goals or some counselor may resist goal setting. The process of goal setting is cooperatively done by both and it requires the skills of drawing inferences, differentiation and teaching individuals to think realistically. The goals fixed are not permanent and it can be changed based on the new information or when new insight is developed.

Intervention

The intervention used will depend upon the approach used by the counselor, the problem and the individual. Hence, the choice of intervention is a process of adaptation and the counselor should be prepared to change the intervention when the selected intervention is not working. The counseling skills needed are skill in handling the interventions, knowledge of its effects, and the ability to read the client's reactions. The interventions are also planned with the consultation of the counselee.

Termination and Follow-up

The successful termination of the counseling process depends upon the planned activities followed in each phase. It must be done without destroying the accomplishments gained and should be done with sensitivity, intention, and fading. It is usual for the individual to have a sense of loss; hence termination should be planned over a few sessions. Follow-up appointments can also be fixed for some time.

Tools and Techniques of Guidance and Counseling

They are:
- **Observation reports**: It is a careful study of the counselee with specific purpose. It can be a participative or nonparticipative observation. By structuring and using rating scale, observation is made easy and accurate.
- **Self-reports**: These are the reports given by the pupil themselves and it may be subjective to some extent. The reliability of the self-report is often questioned.
- **Cumulative records**: It is a method of recording which provides meaningful, significant and comprehensive information about the individual over the years. Besides recording attendance and achievement, it registers pupil's activities, attitude, information about cocurricular and extracurricular activities, etc.
- **Interview**: It is the basic tool of counseling. It is described as conservation with a definite purpose. Interview can be conducted to collect information of the student, family members, friends, etc. By this, the counselor can understand the counselee by direct observation and clarification of doubts. A structured interview gives more reliable and valid data.
- **Individual case conferences**: It gives valuable information about the pupil as it is conducted with a purpose. It helps to analyze the problem behavior in the student, her abilities and shortcomings.
- **Anecdotal records**: It consists of record of important incidents. Care should be taken to record the incident as it has happened. Decisions should not be made on the basis of single anecdote.
- **Problem/interest check list**: It is given to pupils to identify their expressed problems or interest.
- **Rating scales**: These are used to get the assessment of pupil's characteristics/trait such as initiative, responsibility, truthfulness, attitude of cooperation, honesty, etc. either by others or the pupil herself.
- **Sociometry**: It is used to measure the sociability or social distance amongst the members of a group.
- **Psychological tests**: It includes a variety of personality, intelligence, achievement, aptitude tests and projective techniques which are helpful to assess the personality type, intelligence of the student, attitude and aptitude, etc.
- **Parent's views**: It gives information about the parental view of their ward which also may be useful in assessing the students.

Guidance Bureau in Colleges

Guidance is not something that can be separated from the general life of the college. It is a part of every college activity. The important aspects in organizing a guidance bureau in a college are:

Counseling Team

It includes:
- Principal
- Vice-Principal
- College Counselor
- Special subject teachers or HODs
- Medical staff
- Warden
- Parents
- Peer group

They all together can form a committee to render services to the students.

Place for Guidance and Counseling

A separate room should be provided for the counselor to keep records of the students and to conduct interviews without any disturbance and to offer guidance and counseling services.

The specialized services expected of a guidance program in colleges are:
- *Inventory service or data recording service*: This aims at collecting and recording all the pertinent data of a student.

- *Testing service*: This aims to explore the various capacities and shortcomings of a student by administering and interpreting various tests.
- *Information services*: This aims to disseminate educational and vocational information to students.
- *Placement and follow-up services*: This provides help to secure a grade, a place, or a job.

Roles of the Counseling Team Members

Role of the Principal

The principal plays an important role in organizing guidance and counseling services. She is a leader, director, and coordinator of this program. The principal should:

- Recommend to the authorities for the appointment of competent counselor.
- Appoint a guidance committee to study the needs.
- Provide necessary facilities to the guidance worker and staff connected with guidance.
- Provide assistance in planning guidance program in the college.
- Encourage teachers to attend special guidance courses and seminars.
- Inform the parents about the guidance activities available in the college.
- Formulate plans and policies regarding organization of guidance program.

Role of the Teacher

The teacher should:

- Collect information and maintain cumulative record.
- Observe pupils in various situations—in the classroom, in the library, in the clinical area, etc.
- Detect maladjustment of pupils.
- Prepare case histories of problematic students.
- Help the pupils to secure better educational, personal and social adjustments.
- Send information about the pupils to the parents and the principal.
- Help the students in evaluating their own growth.
- To take the help of experts.

Role of the Medical Staff

- To make arrangement for medical examination of each student after a suitable interval.
- To report physical handicaps of students to parents, teachers and to the principal.
- To maintain complete record pertaining to the health of students.
- To develop a program of improving physical health of the pupils.
- To take up follow-up work.

Functions of a Counselor

- Scheduling and conducting interview
- Group guidance
- Individual counseling
- Orientation services
- Data collection
- Contacting outside agencies like parents, guidance bureaus, and employment exchanges
- Placement and follow-up work
- Providing liaison between school, home, and community
- Remedial work.

Qualifications of a Counselor

- MA in Psychology with a course in guidance and counseling.
- Diploma course in guidance and counseling.
- Counselor must have knowledge about personality problems, testing mental hygiene, and counseling techniques.

Skills Required of a Counselor

Personal Skills

Self-awareness and understanding: A person who understands and is aware of self can easily understand the others.

Good health: A counselor requires sound physical and mental health. A healthy person can perform his job well when compared to an unhealthy person.

Open mindedness: A person of open mindedness can receive and accept the other people's values and he will not impose his values on others.

Objectivity: An objective person can stand free from bias and observe accurately.

Trustworthiness: A person who is honest, sincere and keeps confidentiality can only be a reliable person.

Approachability: It is a must. A student should be able to approach the counselor without any fear. His approach should be pleasant and friendly.

Skill in Conducting Interviews

Greeting: A warm and friendly greeting encourages the counselee to feel relaxed thus facilitating the counseling process.

Maintaining eye contact and proper body posture: An attentive and relaxed counselor helps in building proper relationship with the counselee. Maintaining eye contact helps to observe the nonverbal clues from the counselee.

Encouraging participation: A counselor should know the techniques of encouraging the pupil and use it appropriately to gather information from the pupil.

Arrangement of physical environment: A skillful counselor can work in any setting but she needs a conducive environment with comfortable seating arrangement for her efficient work. It not only provides privacy to the counselor and counselee but helps also to establish and maintain good interpersonal relationship and trust thus making work easier.

Problem focus: A counselor should know and help the counselee to focus only on the problem. Beating around the bush will be only of wasting the time and this will not serve the purpose. Since these services are only a short-term service, effective utilization of time is very important. So the counselor should note the verbal and nonverbal cues and help the counselee to focus on the problem.

Identifying an important theme and theme focus: When conversing with the counselee, the counselor can identify the important problem which the student talks it often or having preoccupied with and may be distressed. The counselor directs the individual to focus and talk more about it to assess the problem in depth. This helps both to set goals for future actions.

Goal setting: Counseling assists an individual to attain a goal that the individual and counselor both believe in worth attaining. Once the theme has been identified, the next step is to set a goal that all the future actions are directed to attain the goal. A counselor should assist the individual to set a realistic goal based on the student's abilities and perceptions of her own self.

Maintaining Interaction with the Individual

Restatement: It involves putting the individual's statement into different words to draw the attention or to point out to the individual, what she is finding difficult to verbalize.

Maintaining tension to interview: Sometimes the individual will be apathetic and will not actively participate in the counseling process. The individual can be motivated by asking challenging questions and use of silence and other nonverbal techniques.

Interpretation: It is in the counselor who requires the skill in interpreting the problem and the goal to the students that might give the individual a different view. It should be so presented that the individual feels free to reject, if she so desires.

Managing pauses and silence: Pauses and silence are important techniques in counseling but too long pauses and silence may give a feeling of avoidance or embarrassment to the individual. When used in an appropriate situation, it conveys more meaning.

Other Skills

Communication skills: A counselor requires skills such as listening, writing, use of nonverbal techniques, establishing interpersonal relationships, etc. The prime task for any counselor is to help identifying the problem and goal setting for which good communication skill eases his job.

Diagnostic skills: This involves questioning and assessment strategies to figure out what is going on with a client and formulate a plan for helping the counselee.

Exploration skills: These are used to understand the client's world and collect needed information that will be helpful in later efforts.

Relationship skills: These skills work to build a supportive alliance with clients that is conducive to openness, trust and respect.

Understanding skills: Helps to promote self-awareness and deep level investigations into the nature of presenting concerns and their larger meaning.

Action skills: These help translate identified problem areas. This new understanding helps to turn into sequential steps toward achieving desired goals.

Group process skills: Group process skills are employed in family organizational and consultation settings to resolve conflicts and work toward team objectives.

Evaluation skills: Evaluation skills are used to measure the effects of intervention and if necessary make adjustments.

Group Guidance

Group guidance is any group enterprise or activity in which the primary purpose is to assist each individual in the group to solve his problems and to make his adjustments.

Group instruction means help given to pupils in a group. It is opposed to individual instruction but it may still be individualized instruction. Group tests are tests given to individuals in a group; but the tests are one of the tests of each individual, not of the group.

It refers to the practice of the relationship and activities of counseling in groups or, more simply the counseling of people in groups. It is the process of using group interaction to facilitate deeper self-understanding and self-acceptance.

Characteristics and qualities of good counselor
- A counselor should have keen interest in a wide range of activities.
- He should possess broad and deep knowledge of child psychology.
- He should have superior intellectual ability and judgment.
- He should possess insatiable curiosity and self-learning.
- He must be a man of refined manners.
- He should be sympathetic by nature.
- He should have respect for each other's experience.
- He should be industrious in nature and methodical in work and also have the ability to tolerate pressure.
- He should be well trained in counseling techniques.
- He must be conversant with the administrative, organizational and educational problems in college.
- He must have an identity.
- He should be able to respect and appreciate himself.
- He should accept and open to change.
- He must make choices that shape his lives.
- He feels alive, and his choices are life-oriented.
- He is authentic, sincere and honest.
- He must have a sense of humor.
- He should be willing to admit his own mistakes.
- He must live in the present.
- He should be a man of self-control and stability.
- He should possess high ethical values.
- He must appreciate the influence of culture.
- He should have a sincere interest in the welfare of others.
- He should be deeply involved in their work and derive meaning from it.
- He should be able to maintain healthy boundaries.

Importance
- Through group guidance, information can be given to a large number of students, all at once.
- It is possible for the counselor to obtain general background information about his students and their problems.
- Common problems of the students can be discussed.
- Group guidance is used to orient newly joined pupils to the program of the school/college. They easily acquaint themselves with the traditions, rules, and activities of the school.
- It helps pupils in leadership training.

Principles
- It must always be regarded as a supplement to counseling and not as a substitute for it.
- The nature of the group should be relatively homogeneous in various aspects.
- A project that seems most appropriate to the students should be introduced.
- A person in charge of group guidance should be well versed with this type of work.
- Group guidance should be considered as one of the means, and not the only means of guidance.

Techniques
- Orientation talks
- Group conference
- Field visits
- Career conferences
- Using mass media, etc.

Phases of Activities
- Selection of participants
- Starting the session
- Orientation toward service
- Self-disclosure by members
- Tackling resistance and making common consensus
- Decision making by the group
- Conclusion
- Follow-up.

Problems in Guidance and Counseling

Resistance to Counseling
An individual may not realize that he or she suffers from problem and requires counseling and may not cooperate with the counselor. At the same time, the faculty members also may not realize the importance of counseling process so they just ignore it. The problem can be overcome by gaining cooperation from the individual and the faculty members.

Counseling Individuals of Different Cultures
In this modern world, pupils migrate to the different parts of the world to pursue their studies. It is quite natural to face some adjustment problem when they work in culture, which is not her own. During counseling, the counselor may find it difficult because his own culture is something different from the culture of the students. Because of difference in values, beliefs and customs, the counselor faces problem in counseling. This can be alleviated by understanding the others culture before he starts the counseling process.

Counseling Individuals with Strong Emotions
There are students with strong emotions like fear, anxiety, depression, etc. which may hinder the progress of counseling process. A counselor can remain calm when a student exhibits emotional reaction and if possible help from other medical members can be obtained.

Counselor Burn-out
Any counselor will start his work with great excitement and enthusiasm. But during the course of counseling he feels disappointed and discouraged when he faces resistance in the individual and less progress. All these

may make him less motivated and feel restless, boredom, irritable, fatigue, and lethargic. This problem can be managed by changing the approach, work environment and taking personal care.

Issues Faced by Novice Counselors

Feeling of Inadequacy and Anxiety

Most beginners, irrespective of their training and experience, experience anxiety when they start meeting their clients. Counseling as a profession is full of ambiguities and uncertainties. The counselor must be willing to face and deal with these anxieties. One way to deal with them is to openly discuss these with seniors and fellow counselors.

Being and Self-disclosure

Because of the uncertainty and anxiety associated with the initial encounters with their clients, the beginners tend to be over concerned with what the book says and with the technicalities of how they should proceed. In many instances, the counselors are not being themselves. Probably, it is the desire to be superhuman that drives them to be role fixated.

Tendency Toward Perfectionism

As beginners, counselors want to be more perfect in their profession. It is not possible for the person to know everything. Instead of trying to impress with lack of knowledge, one can always admit the truth and go about searching for satisfactory answers. It takes courage to admit imperfections, but there is a value in being open about them.

Being Honest about Limitations

No counselor can realistically expect to succeed with all clients. It is best to admit that one may not be successful in all the cases. At the same time, the counselor should try to learn the skills, necessary to deal with all kinds of clients by working with diverse groups.

Understanding Silence

Several counselors feel very uncomfortable and even threatened when their clients do not speak. Silence in counseling can have several meanings. Sometimes silence says much more than words. So, when silence occurs, they must be explored to determine what they really mean. Accept silence and pursue its meaning.

Demands from the Clients

Often, the clients make multiple demands. Several novice counselors, in their enthusiasm to be hopeful to the clients, burden themselves with the unrealistic and constant demands. Client may frequently call the counselors when they are at home and expect to talk at length. The best way to unburden these demands is to make it clear in the initial session itself what to expect and what not to expect from counseling. This is often referred to as structuring the counseling relationship.

Clients who Lack Commitment

The clients may not be committed in the counseling process and may be uncooperative. So it is necessary to explain to the clients the goals of therapy without promising what cannot be achieved. They must be told what counseling is about, what the joint responsibilities are and how therapy can help them to get what they want. This helps them to commit and cooperate with the counselor.

Losing Oneself in Clients

The trouble with beginners is that they worry too much about their clients. Sometimes they identify so much with their clients that they lose their own identity. Counselors must learn how to "let clients go" and not carry around their problems until they are seen again. If the counselors lose themselves in clients' problems and confusions, they will be ineffective as help agents. This process of getting emotionally entangled with client issues is called countertransference.

Shaping Responsibility with Client

One of the crucial tasks for the counselors is to find an optimum balance in sharing the responsibility with clients. One mistake that novice counselors make is to assume full responsibility for the course and outcome of therapy. By doing so, the counselors will be taking away from the clients the rightful responsibility to make their own decisions. Sharing of responsibility between the counselor and client must be discussed and sorted out during the initial sessions.

Giving Advice

Many people mistake that giving advice is the same as counseling. Giving advice will make the counselee dependent on the counselor. Counselors help clients to discover their own solutions to their problems. The job of the counselor is to help the client help himself.

Developing a Personal Counseling Style

As far as possible, the beginner should not attempt to mimic someone's therapeutic style. It may be remembered that there is no one "right" way of counseling suitable to all clients under all conditions. Getting stuck to one model inhibits the growth of the counselors. The counselor should attempt to develop a personally distinctive style.

Key Dimensions of Counseling

Individual vs Group

In an individual therapy, the therapist treats one person at a time. The effectiveness of such therapies depends to a great extent upon the therapist–client relationship. In group therapy, several clients are treated at the same time in a group setting. Hence, the interactions and relationship of the group members to one another are important aspects of therapy.

Brief vs Long-term Therapy

Long-term therapies such as classical psychoanalysis involve several sessions a week over a period of years. However, many of the newer forms of therapy, including modified psychoanalytic approaches, are designed to shorten the length of time required.

Supportive vs Depth

The goals of supportive therapies are to reassure the individual, provide needed guidance, and reinforce existing coping mechanisms. Depth therapy is concerned with helping client work through deep conflicts or highly traumatic and painful experiences to achieve better personality integration and more effective coping patterns. Supporting therapy is generally brief, while depth therapy may be either brief or long-term.

Directive vs Nondirective

In directive therapy, the counselor takes an active role asking questions and offering interpretations. In nondirective therapy, the major responsibility is placed on the clients and the counselor may simply try to help the client clarify and understand his or her feelings and values.

Segregated vs Total Push

In segregated procedures, the client sees the counselor periodically in an attempt to work through specific problems, but little attempt may be made to relate therapy to the overall situation. In total push methods, the therapy is directly concerned with other members of the family and often with professional agencies in the community.

Crisis Intervention vs Personal Growth

Crisis intervention therapy is designed to help the client deal with intermediate stress situation, which is approaching or exceeding the limits of his or her capacity to adjust. In personal growth oriented therapy, the primary aim is to help the client to develop increased self-understanding, and realize one's potentialities. Growth-oriented procedure may be used with normal as well as people with adjustment problems.

Inner Control of Behavior vs Outer Control of Behavior

In certain counseling procedures, attempts are made to control environmental variables to bring about behavioral changes, as in the case of using reinforcement. In other procedures, the primary goal is to change the individual's value assumptions in such a way as to foster the inner cognitive control of behavior. Of course sometimes external control may be used to develop inner control.

Disciplinary Problems and Actions

"Experience is a hard teacher because she gives the test first, the lesson afterwards."
—*Vernon Sanders*

Disciplinary problem is any activity or behavior of a student which violates the academic rules and regulations. It is an inappropriate academic conduct of the student against which disciplinary actions can be taken. Disciplinary actions refer to penalties or sanctions imposed for violation of academic regulations against behavior judged as inappropriate for academic conduct.

Types of Disciplinary Actions

- **Disciplinary warnings:** Notice to a student either verbally or in writing that he/she has been in violation of the rules of student conduct or has otherwise failed to satisfy the college's expectations regarding conduct. Such warnings imply that continuation or repetition of the specific conduct involved or other misconduct will result in one of the more serious disciplinary actions.
- **Reprimand:** A verbal or written recognition of a violation of good conduct which admonishes the offender to avoid future infractions. Reprimands are always made in writing. A reprimand indicates to the student that continuation or repetition of the specific conduct involved or other misconduct will result in one of the more serious disciplinary actions.
- **Disciplinary probation:** A disciplinary action which returns the offender to the college community on his or her promise of appropriate future behavior; may include, but is not limited to, ineligibility to participate in extracurricular activities and certain other student privileges. Formal action placing conditions upon the student's continued attendance for violation of the code of student conduct. The action will specify, in writing, the period of probation and any conditions such as limiting the student's participation in extracurricular activities. Disciplinary probation may be for a specified term or for an indefinite period which

may extend to graduation or other termination of the student's enrollment in the college.
- **Dismissal**: Suspension exclusion from the college and college sponsored activities for a specified time. Dismissal may be for a stated or for an indefinite period. The notification dismissing a student will indicate, in writing, the term of the dismissal and any special conditions which must be met before readmission.
- **Restitution**: The college may demand restitution from individual students for destruction or damage of property. Failure to make arrangements for restitution promptly will result in the cancellation of the student's registration and will prevent the student from reregistration.

Ground for Disciplinary Actions

Disciplinary actions that are imposed by the college for the violation of its rules or the laws include the following:
- Dishonesty, such as cheating, plagiarizing or knowingly furnishing false information to the college or to college officials.
- Willful or persistent smoking in any area where smoking has been prohibited and the use or possession of alcoholic beverages.
- Assault, battery or any threat of force of violence upon a student, visitor to the campus, or college personnel. Willful misconduct which results in injury or death to a student, campus visitor or college personnel member, or cutting, defacing, or otherwise harming any real or personal property.
- The use, sale or possession of illegal drugs or substance or any poison.
- Forgery, alteration or misuse of college documents, records or identification.
- Violation of college regulations governing student organizations, the use of college facilities or the time, place and manner of public expression or distribution of materials.
- Unauthorized entry to facilities or unauthorized use of college supplies, equipment, and telephones.
- Possession or use of any firearm, explosive device, dangerous chemical or other deadly weapons while on college property or at college sponsored activities.
- Driving of motorcycles and other off-road vehicles on college property other than the regular roads and parking lots.
- Persistent and serious misconduct where other means of correction have failed to bring about proper conduct.
- Continued disruptive behavior, willful disobedience, habitual profanity or vulgarity, or the open and persistent defiance of the authority or persistent abuse of college personnel.
- Obstruction of pedestrian and/or vehicular traffic while on college property or at college-sponsored activities.

Harassment Including Ragging

Abuse, threats, intimidation, assault, coercion and/or conduct, by physical, verbal, signed, written, photographic or electronic means, which threatens or endangers any person.

> **Presently, there are four state legislations in India that prohibit ragging. These are:**
> 1. The Prohibition of Ragging Act, 1996 (Applicable in the state of Tamil Nadu)
> 2. The Kerala Prohibition of Ragging Act, 1998
> 3. The Maharashtra Prohibition of Ragging Act, 1999
> 4. The Prohibition of Ragging in Educational Institutes Act, 2000 (Applicable in the state of West Bengal).

Theft/Vandalism

Attempted or actual theft, damage, or unauthorized possession or alteration of college property.

Failure to Comply

Failure to comply with directions of college officials and failure to identify oneself to these persons when requested to do so.

Disorderly Conduct

Conduct which is disruptive, lewd or indecent and breaches the peace of the community, regardless of intent.

Stalking

Stalking occurs when a person engages in a course of conduct directed at a specific individual that is likely to cause such individual to have a reasonable fear of harm to his or her physical or emotional health, safety or property. Such conduct may include, but is not limited to: repeatedly engaging in unwanted contact or communication (including, but not limited to, face-to-face communication, telephone calls or messages, electronic mail, written letters, gifts, or threatening or obscene gestures), surveillance, following, trespassing, or vandalism.

Hazing

Hazing is any intentional or reckless act; occurring on or off the college campus; by one person alone or acting with others; directed against a college student; that endangers the mental or physical health or safety of the college student. Specifically, the term "hazing" as defined here includes, but is not limited to physical brutality, such as whipping, beating, striking, branding, electronic shocking, or placement of a harmful substance on the body. Other physical activity, such as sleep deprivation, exposure to the elements, confinement in a small space, physical bondage, "road trips" or taking a student to an outlying area and dropping him/her off, or other activity that subjects the student to an unreasonable risk of harm or that may adversely affect the mental or physical health or safety of the student.

Consumption of food, water, other liquid, alcoholic beverage, drug, or other substance which subjects the student to an unreasonable risk of harm or which otherwise may adversely affect the mental or physical health or safety of the student.

Activity that creates an unreasonable risk of causing severe psychological shock or public humiliation to the student.

Cheating

Cheating is the act of pretending (or helping others to pretend) to have mastered course material through misrepresentation. Examples include:
- Copying from another student's test or assignment.
- Allowing another student to copy from his/her test or assignment.
- Using the textbook, course handouts, or notes during a test without instructor permission.
- Stealing, buying or otherwise obtaining all or part of a test before it is administered.
- Selling or giving away all or part of a test before it is administered.
- Having someone else attend a course or take a test in his/her place.
- Attending a course or taking a test for someone else.
- Failing to follow test-taking procedures, including talking during the test, ignoring starting and stopping times, or other disruptive activity.

Fabrication

Fabrication is the intentional use of invented information. *Examples include*:
- Signing a roll sheet for another student.
- Giving false information to college personnel.
- Answering verbal or written questions in an untruthful manner.
- Inventing data or sources of information for research papers or other assignments.

Management of Disciplinary Problems

Incidents of suspected academic disciplinary violations shall be handled initially at the level at which the incident occurs or at the departmental level. Initial review, decision and action shall remain local, to involve the instructor or academic supervisor and, if desired, consultation with the head of the department. Instructors can freely discuss alleged violations informally with the student. Suspected violations that would result in a penalty should be handled by the instructor in direct communication with the student involved. After discussion with the student involved and their response, the instructor shall conclude, within a reasonable period of time and based on available evidence, whether the suspected violation occurred. Instructors are encouraged to consult at this stage with their department head about the nature of the suspected violations, the nature of the evidence of these violations and the range of penalties under consideration. If the conclusion is that the suspected violation did occur, the instructor shall also choose an appropriate penalty.

The student shall be notified immediately, and in writing, of this decision, the basis for this decision and (when applicable) the penalty imposed. This notification will come from the instructor and/or department/program head depending on the penalty involved.

General Principles

Prior to taking any form of disciplinary action there will be a thorough investigation into any allegation of misconduct or poor performance.

In such cases of alleged misconduct, the students have the right to a fair hearing, with the opportunity to state their case; and the right to be accompanied at such a hearing by a representative of a friend, if desired, before any disciplinary action is taken.

Any disciplinary action taken by the college will be appropriate to the degree of seriousness of the misconduct/unsatisfactory performance and will take account of any mitigating circumstances. Management guidelines on the categorization of the levels of misconduct are held by the head of department.

Procedure for Minor Misconduct

Verbal Warning

Committing minor misconduct will lead to an interview with the student and at this interview the student will have the opportunity to offer an explanation. If it is decided that an offense has occurred, a verbal warning will be given. It will be recorded and placed on the student's file.

First Written Warning

Committing the same or similar misconduct frequently will lead to an interview with the head of department and at this interview the student will have the opportunity to offer an explanation. If it is decided that an offense has occurred, a first written warning will be given to the student (with a copy to the parents if necessary). It will be recorded in the student's file.

Final Written Warning

If the same or similar misconduct is committed again this will lead to an interview with the principal. If it is decided that an offense has occurred a final written warning, which will be recorded, will be issued to the student containing clear notice that a repeat of the misconduct will result in a further disciplinary action.

Further Disciplinary Action

In the event that a student fails to respond to a final written warning or allegedly commits the same misconduct, the student will be subjected to further disciplinary action, which may include suspension, or dismissal.

Procedure for Serious Misconduct

Final Written Warning

Committing serious misconduct will lead to an interview with the principal and at this interview the student will have the opportunity to offer an explanation. If it is decided that an offence has occurred a final written warning, which will be recorded, will be given to the student (with a copy to the parents if appropriate) containing clear notice that repeat of the misconduct will result in further disciplinary action.

Further Disciplinary Action

In the event that a student fails to respond to a final written warning or allegedly commits the same misconduct, the student will be subjected to further disciplinary action, which may include suspension, or dismissal.

Precautionary Suspension

In certain situations, where serious or gross misconduct is suspected, management may need time to carry out a full investigation. In such circumstances the student may be suspended pending a decision.

Disciplinary Warnings

Warnings normally relate to the same or similar misconduct and are not generally transferable between different types of misconduct. Where a number of warnings are called for in respect of different types of misconduct this will entitle management to review the student's overall suitability for continued study and if necessary to issue a final general warning irrespective of the offence. All warnings will clearly state the misconduct concerned with details of any relevant facts, times, dates, events and names and clearly indicate what the eventual outcome will be, if there is no improvement on the student's part or a recurrence takes place.

Preventive Strategies

There are certain strategies and techniques by which we can prevent some unwanted disciplinary problem in students. They are as follows:

Forewarning in the Course Syllabus

In the course syllabus, faculty should express their expectations for the student's behavior in the learning environment. The syllabus is a performance agreement between faculty and students. As such, it is an opportunity to express the ground rules and regulations for engagement. This is the time that faculty should outline behaviors expected of a student. Faculty should keep the discussion positive and indicate the type of behaviors they wish to see from the students. Faculty should also connect these behaviors to the achievement of the learning outcomes established for the course.

Expressing expectations in writing to students from the first day helps the students understand the behaviors faculty expect from the outset. This approach also provides faculty with a guide in case a student acts in a manner that has been indicated as unacceptable. Faculty is in a position to set standards that students must meet. These standards may be both academic and behavioral. The key is that they are clearly expressed and consistently expected of all students.

Reviewing the Institutional Code of Conduct

With expectations clearly outlined in the syllabus, the first class meeting of the semester aims to outline expectations for the course. It is also appropriate to inform students about any policies that the institution has established to guide student conduct. It is recommended that the faculty should briefly address the sections of the institutional student conduct policy that have meaning for the specific learning objectives of the course.

Know Whom to Contact for Consultation

Sooner or later faculty will need to consult with someone regarding student behavior. Students are coming to college more stressed, more financially challenged, more distracted and more over committed than previous generations. The college should designate a person who should be responsible to deal with issues related to student's behavior. Also faculty should know who is responsible for administering the institutional code of conduct.

Know When to Call for Consultation

Just as important as knowing whom to call for consultation, is knowing when to call for consultation and knowing when to refer an unresolved matter to others. When the student's behavior is not with the standards mentioned in the syllabus and student conduct code and if the student is not able to change or refuses to change his behavior, then the faculty should immediately consult with others to identify other ways to work with the student or to make a request for referral services.

Documentation

It is important for faculty to keep notes of student behaviors that have been observed. Faculty may observe behaviors that are not desired but that do not violate the classroom standard that has been set and/or the campus student code. One reason to note these "below the radar" behaviors is that they can escalate to a level that would ultimately violate the classroom standard or the campus standard. The information to document includes time, day, and place where the behavior was observed. It is also important to use descriptive terms and not evaluative statements.

Responding to Student Misconduct

When faculty has reason to believe that a student may be acting inappropriately, there are six steps to use when responding to allegations of misconduct:

1. **Gather and document information:** The information should objectively describe the student's actions and the date, time and others, who were present.
2. **Engage and confront the student about behaviors observed:** At the earliest time possible, meet with the student privately to discuss the behaviors that have been observed. This meeting will inform the student of faculty concerns, allows the student to express his or her perspective of the situation, and provide an opportunity for the student to understand how the behavior affects others and is disrupting to the learning outcomes of the course.
3. **Focus on the behavior:** Faculty should always focus on the behaviors of the student and not to be carried out by other aspects, such as the extent to which one knows or likes the student, or the student academic record. For instance, high achieving students are just as likely to plagiarize as average students. It is important to be consistent in what is expected from students.
4. **Outline the required new behaviors:** The purpose of meeting with the student is to first explore with the student concerns about her or his behavior. Working with student to change any annoying acts provides the greatest opportunity for a collaborative discussion between the student and the faculty. Any administrative violations of the code of conduct should be documented and forwarded to the appropriate administrative office.
5. **Outline consequences of compliance/noncompliance:** Faculty interactions with the student should conclude with the hope that the student will choose to make different choices and will choose to comply with the standards.
6. **Refer unresolved or risky cases to other campus resources:** If, at any time faculty are working with a student and it comes to their attention that the student's misconduct is not being resolved as planned, or if there is evidence that the incidence may escalate in terms of level of disruption or safety to either the faculty or other students, the situation should automatically be referred to other campus resources. Then the procedure for minor and major misconduct will be followed according to the nature of the problem.

Management of Crisis and Referral Services

A crisis is a disturbance caused by a stressful event or a perceived threat. During crisis, the person's usual way of coping becomes ineffective which causes anxiety. The threat, or precipitating event, usually can be identified. It may have occurred weeks or days before the crisis. Precipitating events can be actual or perceived losses, threats of losses or challenges.

Crisis Response

After the precipitating event, the person's anxiety begins to rise, and four phases of a crisis response emerge. In the first phase, the anxiety activates the person's usual methods of coping. If these do not bring relief and support is inadequate, the person progresses to the second phase, which involves more anxiety because coping mechanisms have failed. In the third phase, new coping mechanisms are tried or the threat is redefined so that old ones can work. Resolution of the problem can occur in this phase. However, if resolution does not occur, the person goes on to the fourth phase, in which the continuation of severe or panic levels of anxiety may lead to psychological disorganization. These include the individual's perception of the event, situational supports and coping mechanisms. Successful resolution of the crisis will occur when the person has a realistic view of the event, supports available to help solve the problem, and the presence of effective coping mechanisms.

Types of Crisis

Maturational crises are developmental events requiring role changes. For example, an adolescent boy or girl has to accept the role changes positively because during this period, he or she develops a sense of identity, and also it is a period of confusion and emotional turmoil. The nature and extent of the maturational crisis can be influenced by role models and interpersonal resources.

Situational crises occur when a life event upsets an individual's or group's psychological equilibrium. Examples of situational crises include medical illness, college problems and witnessing a crime.

Situational crises can be accidental, uncommon and unexpected events. For example, fires and floods which disrupt entire communities are situational crises. Man-made disaster also can precipitate situational crisis.

Common crises in educational institutions
- Incidence of ragging
- Suicidal threats
- Fight
- Assault or injuring others
- Damaging the institution's property
- Possessing weapons.

Crisis Intervention

It is a short-term therapy focused on solving the immediate problem. The goal of crisis intervention for the individual or group is to return to precrisis level of functioning.

The counselor should assess the precipitating event or stressor, nature and strength of support systems and coping resources, etc. The individual's support systems are environment, family members, friends and the person himself.

Approaches

Generic approach: It is applied to a high-risk individuals and large groups as quickly as possible. This is used for people with a similar type of crisis. Instructions following an acute stress are sometimes referred to as debriefing. It is used as a therapeutic intervention to help people recall events and clarify traumatic experiences. It helps to vent out the feelings.

Individual approach: It is diagnosis and treatment of specific problem in a specific individual. It helps to restore the psychological safety and corrects the misattributions.

Techniques

Environmental manipulation aims at changing the individual's physical or interpersonal situation in order to remove stress and stressor.

Catharsis is a release of feelings that take place when the individual or group talks about emotionally charged areas. As the feelings about the events are realized, tension is reduced.

Clarification means helping the individual to identify the relationship between events, behaviors and feelings. It helps the individual gain a better understanding of feelings and how they lead to the development of a crisis.

Suggestion is influencing a person to accept an idea or belief. It is a way of influencing the individual or group by pointing out alternatives or new ways of looking at things.

The other methods are reinforcement of behavior, support of defenses and raising self-esteem.

Some of the Common Crisis and its Management

Fight

The principal has to take the necessary steps:
- Ensure the safety of students and staff first.
- Notify security/police.
- Do not let crowd incite participants.
- Disperse onlookers and keep others from congregating in the area.
- When participants are separated, do not allow further visual or verbal contact.
- Document all activities witnessed by staff.
- Deal with event according to institution's discipline policy.
- Notify the parents/guardians of students involved in fight.
- Assess the counseling needs of the students and organize for it.

Assault

- Ensure the safety of students and staff first.
- Notify police.
- Seal off area to preserve evidence and disperse onlookers.
- Arrange for emergency medical services, if victim requires medical attention.
- Do not leave the victim alone.
- Document all activities witnessed by staff.
- Deal with event according to institution's discipline policy.
- Notify parents/guardians.
- Assess the counseling needs of the students and organize for it.

Weapons

- Ensure the safety of students and staff first.
- Notify police.
- Conduct enquiry to collect information regarding type of weapon, safety of persons in the area, state of mind of the suspected person and accessibility of the weapon.
- Separate student/staff member from weapon, if possible.
- Document all activities related to a weapon incident.
- Deal with event according to institution's discipline policy.

Suicide Threat

- Do not leave the student alone.
- Notify the counselor and psychologist.
- Do not allow the student to leave college without parent, guardian or other appropriate adult supervision.
- Arrange for medical services if required.
- Document all activities related to incident.
- Deal with event according to institution's discipline policy.
- Notify parents/guardians.
- Assess the counseling needs of the students and organize for it.

Damaging the Institution's Property

- Ensure the safety of students and staff first.
- Notify police.
- Document all activities related to incident.
- Deal with event according to institution's discipline policy.
- Assess the counseling needs of the students and organize for it.

Postcrisis Intervention Procedures

- Assess the situation to determine the need for postcrisis interventions for staff, students, and families.
- Provide postcrisis briefings for staff, students, and families as appropriate.
- Re-establish routine as quickly as possible.
- **Defusing:** Provide defusing sessions for students and staff as quickly as possible after the emergency. Defusing is brief conversation with individuals or small groups held soon after an incident to help people better understand and cope up with the effects of the incident. Defusing should be conducted by trained individuals.
- **Debriefing:** Conduct Critical-Incident Stress Debriefing (CISD) 3–4 days after the emergency. CISD is a formal group discussion designed to help people understand their reactions to the stress of an event and to give referral information. CISD should only be conducted by trained professionals.
- Arrange for counseling.

Summary

- Guidance or counseling, according to CW Tailor, "assists the individual in the process of self-understanding and self-acceptance, appraisal of his present and possible future socioeconomic environment, and in integrating these two variables by choices and adjustments that facilitate both personal satisfaction and socioeconomic effectiveness".
- The bases of guidance and counseling are individual and societal. There are various approaches to guidance and counseling services such as directive approach, nondirective approach and eclectic approach.
- The areas of counseling are educational, vocational, health and living conditions, personal, moral, religion and social and leisure.
- The phases of counseling are establishing relationship, assessment, setting goals, interventions, termination and follow-up.
- Observation reports, self-reports, anecdotal records, cumulative records, check list, interview, rating scale, etc. are some of the tools used in the guidance and counseling program.
- Counselor requires skills such as personal skills, skill in conducting interview and skill in maintaining interaction with the individual.
- Group guidance is any group enterprise or activity in which the primary purpose is to assist each individual in the group to solve his problems and to make his adjustments.
- Some of the group guidance techniques are orientation talks, group conference, field visits, career conferences and using mass media, etc.
- There are so many problems in counseling. They are resistance to counseling, counseling individuals of different cultures, counseling individuals with strong emotions and counselor burn-out. A novice counselor will also face some of the issues related to counseling.
- Disciplinary actions refer to penalties or sanctions imposed for violation of academic regulations against behavior judged as inappropriate for academic conduct.
- A crisis is a disturbance caused by a stressful event or a perceived threat. During crisis, the person's usual way of coping becomes ineffective which causes anxiety. The threat, or precipitating event, usually can be identified.
- Crises are of two types. They are situational and maturational crisis. The generic approach and the individual approach can be used in crisis intervention.
- Crisis intervention is a short-term therapy focused on solving the immediate problem. The goal of crisis intervention for the individual or group is to return to precrisis level of functioning.
- Postcrisis intervention procedure will help the students and faculty members to resume the routine life.

10. Administration of Nursing Curriculum

"The object of education is to prepare the young to educate themselves throughout their lives".
—Robert Maynard Hutchins

Objectives
After completing this unit, you will be able to:
- Explain the role of curriculum coordinator in administration of nursing curriculum
- Understand the evaluation of educational programs in nursing
- Explain the need for curriculum research in nursing
- Describe the different models of collaboration between education and service.

Introduction

A curriculum is designed to provide a sequence of learning experience that will enable students to achieve desired educational outcomes. Curriculum framework provides faculty with a means of conceptualizing and organizing the knowledge, skills, values and beliefs critical to the delivery of coherent curriculum that facilitates the achievement of the desired curriculum outcomes. Curriculum administration includes curriculum planning, curriculum organization, and curriculum evaluation (Fig. 10.1). In India, the various nursing education programs offered are as mentioned below:

Levels of nursing education
- Diploma in Nursing
- BSc in Nursing
- Post certificate course in Nursing
- Post basic Nursing
- MSc in Nursing
- MPhil in Nursing
- Doctor of Philosophy in Nursing.

Components of the curriculum
- Mission and vision
- Philosophy
- Objectives
- Curriculum design

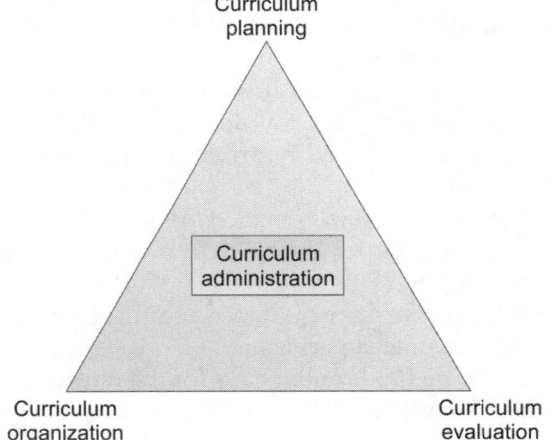

Fig. 10.1: Curriculum administration.

- Organizing framework
- Overall purpose and goal of the program
- End of the program, intermediate, and course objectives.

Curriculum Planning

It is the foremost phase in the process of curriculum administration. It is an essential feature of administrative programs of instruction. In curriculum planning, the following subprocesses are involved:
- Selection of materials
- Organization of content
- Use of instructional materials
- Experimentation
- Appraisal
- Reconstruction

Curriculum Organization

It is a prerequisite of any kind of instructional program. It takes place stagewise, subjectwise, and classwise for

each type of education or course of study. On this basis, the detailed syllabi are prepared, which serve as the basis for writing the textbooks. Curriculum organization is the chief responsibility of the whole educational machinery. The effectiveness of curriculum organization depends on the following:
- Quality of syllabuses prescribed
- Type of handbooks and textbooks prepared
- Adequacy of guidance provided to teachers
- Instructional aids provided and
- Selection of learning experiences, etc.

Curriculum Evaluation

Curriculum planning and organization are not ends in themselves, but they are means to the ends. Hence curriculum evaluation is also the responsibility of the educational institutions.

Evaluation of curriculum, from time to time, is important because it provides the needed feedback for further revision and reformation of the curriculum implemented.

Curriculum evaluation is carried out for:
- Organizing supervisory programs of classroom instruction.
- Providing necessary guidance and direction based on the educational supervision.
- Planning methods and means for the improvement of effective implementation of the evaluated programs.

The details of curriculum administration:

Curriculum personnel	Curriculum administration	Education management
Curriculum planning	Curriculum implementation	Curriculum evaluation Supervision
Objectives content	Syllabus outlines Curriculum guides	Guidance and direction
Grades	Textbooks	Improvement

Curriculum Development

A curriculum is designed to provide a sequence of learning experience that will enable students to achieve desired educational outcomes. Curriculum framework provides faculty with a means of conceptualizing and organizing the knowledge, skills, values, and beliefs critical to the delivery of coherent curriculum that facilitates the achievement of the desired curriculum outcomes.

The purpose of any curriculum development is to meet learner's needs by ensuring that the curriculum meets educational and professional standards and is responsible to the current and future demands of the healthcare system.

Need Assessment

The need for the nursing program is influenced by the:
- Characteristics of nursing shortages and the extent
- Future nursing workforce needs
- Demand
- Specialization in nursing
- Employer's demand
- Employee's views on the types of graduates needed
- Regulatory mechanism
- Finance
- Profession of nursing.

Facilitators of Curriculum Development

- Involvement of the faculty
- Need assessment
- Perceived need.

Designing the Curriculum

Choosing a specific program such as Diploma in Nursing, BSc (N), MSc (N), etc. does not automatically dictate the design of the program's curriculum. It is important for faculty to develop a curriculum structure that will support the type of program desired and the outcomes that are envisioned. The traditional approach to designing curricula offers structured courses in specific sequence. This approach identifies what the student is to learn, when the learning should be. The knowledge of nursing and other support content, nursing skills, critical learning experiences and evaluation methods for assessing learning outcomes are emphasized. These pieces are structured into anyone of a number of curriculum patterns. Two common curriculum patterns are "blocking course content and integrating or threading" course content.

Developing Curriculum Structure

It is structuring the courses in specific sequence. It is done by:
- **Blocking course content:** Blocks of content are structured around particular clinical specialty areas, by client population or body systems, e.g. medical surgical nursing, pediatric nursing, etc. or growth and development, birth, infancy, childhood, and adolescence.
- **Integrating course content:** Faculty identifies concepts considered core to nursing practice and then integrate or "thread" these concepts throughout the curriculum. The concepts are pain, nutrition, personal hygiene, etc. Other concepts are lifespan development, nutrition and pharmacology.

Points to be Remembered in Curriculum Building

- A determination of the desired outcome of the graduates after completing the program.
- Subject-curriculum content.
- Understanding of the culture of nursing's role in society in general and related to health.
- The identification and organization of healthcare problems of the present and the future.
- The identification of teaching-learning strategies to meet the learner needs.

Purposes of Organizing a Curriculum Framework

- To systematically design a mental picture that is meaningful to the faculty and students.
- To provide a blueprint for determining the scope of knowledge.
- To facilitate the sequencing and prioritizing of knowledge.
- To help explain how these ideas or concepts apply to nursing practice.
- To serve as a guide for faculty and students.
- To highlight the purposes they serve, their goals, objectives, content and the methods of instruction and evaluation they promote.

Organizing curriculum frameworks are the educational roadmaps to teaching and learning. As with any roadmap, multiple options are available for arriving at a given destination or outcome.

Guiding Principles for Developing a Curriculum Framework

- The first principle is to choose those concepts that most accurately reflect the faculty's belief about the practice and discipline of nursing. It is generally expressed in philosophy and mission statement of the school. The major four concepts are person, nursing, health, and environment.
- The second principle is to clearly define those concepts.
- The third principle is to explain the linkages between and among the concepts identified.

Outcomes and Competencies in Curriculum Framework

Outcomes are those characteristics student should display at a designated time. Competencies are the behaviors needing to be acquired to develop those characteristics. The outcome is what a student is expected to attain at the end of a program. This is decided based on the changes in healthcare system, value of nursing, philosophy, demand for nurses, health problems, and changes in education system, etc. It also can be viewed as "core characteristics" or those qualities faculty want graduates to display.

The following qualities are essential for a graduate. They are:

- Critical thinker
- Culturally competent
- Knowledgeable coordinator of community resources
- Philosophically aware
- Ethically and legally grounded
- Effective communicator
- Competent provider of healthcare
- Modeler of the professional role, and
- Responsible manager of human, fiscal and material resources.

These essential qualities are then used to guide the development of related outcomes and competencies. Clearly describing the qualities of a professional nurse helps to decide the outcome and competencies. Competency statements are behaviorally anchored and student focused. Competency statements identify the knowledge, skills, and attitudes students need to develop to achieve program outcomes.

Competencies are important to the assessment process as they become the foundation to the design of evaluation tools used in the assessment of student learning. In formulating competency statements one should decide the student [Dip/BSc(N)/MSc(N)] and the level of behaviors and the context in which the behavior is to be exhibited.

Curriculum Enhancement

The implementation of the curriculum involves extensive materials development, numerous reconsiderations of these materials and accompanying pedagogies, and a thorough rethinking of assessment practices, all conducted in a highly collaborative manner by faculty and graduate students.

Specifically, work is focused on ascertaining the curriculum's effectiveness through an examination of learner outcomes and the degree to which they correspond with stated curricular goals, pedagogies, and materials. Much of the initial input for curriculum enhancement comes from the instructors who have put the materials into practice with their students. In addition to teacher feedback, analyses of student performance at each curricular level reveal learner outcomes across the curriculum as well as possible curricular progression.

Role of the Curriculum Coordinator

Primary responsibility for curriculum enhancement lies with the Curriculum Coordinator. He/she is responsible for assuring continued curricular and pedagogical coherence. To accomplish this task, the coordinator works closely with the Departmental Head and with

other coordinators in supervising and coordinating curriculum enhancement efforts. In particular, the coordinator attends to the following components of curriculum enhancement:
- Coordination and preparation of course materials.
- Administration of the departmental placement examination, including supervision and enforcement of proper student placement.
- Organization and coordination of departmental curriculum workshops.
- Attendance at all level coordination meetings.
- Supervision and implementation of instructional technology in order to improve access, pedagogy, and flexibility of instruction within curricular guidelines.
- Dissemination of information to the rest of the department regarding all curriculum enhancement projects.
- Coordination and supervision of curriculum-wide enhancement projects (e.g. oral assessment).
- Clear communication between instructors and coordinators, graduate student teachers and faculty.
- Orientation for first-time graduate student teachers.
- Coordination of faculty class visits.
- Through regular meetings with instructors, the coordinator monitors the effectiveness of materials, pedagogies, and assessment instruments.
- Coordination of assessment procedures. The coordinator coordinates the implementation and scoring of assessment instruments in all sections.
- Class observation. With the assistance of other faculty as part of faculty class visitation program each semester, the coordinator visits and observes other sections in order to provide feedback to instructors, faculty, and graduate students and to gain additional insight into the course's effectiveness at achieving curricular goals.
- Updates and feedback.

Roles of Educational Administrators

Educational administrators are in overall charge of curriculum development. They play the following roles:
- They ensure that educational policies and goals are properly reflected by the curriculum.
- They are also responsible for the realization of the curriculum goals through its effective implementation.
- They see that try-out is made properly and necessary modifications are carried out in it.
- They also take care of proper priorities to be given to different programs at different levels.

Hence their roles related to that of:
- Policy implementation
- Try-out
- Modification
- Evaluation.

Roles of Educational Supervisors

The educational supervisors play the role as:
- Active participants in curriculum development
- Guides of curriculum implementation
- Evaluators of curriculum implementation
- Curriculum reformers.

Roles of Subject Specialists

- Determiners of the curriculum
- Framers of the syllabi
- Writers of the textbooks, and
- Writers of the handbooks.

Role of the Faculty

All faculty members share the responsibility for assuring continued curricular coherence and participate in curriculum enhancement in the following ways:
- Teachers being the classroom implementors of the curriculum developed are now increasingly being involved in curriculum planning to give it a more realistic touch.
- Teachers are the actual implementors of the curriculum in the field. They translate the objectives of curriculum into realities.
- The teachers also play the role of curriculum evaluators. They cooperate with educational administrators and curriculum experts in relating the curriculum being implemented.
- Teachers also play the role of curriculum leaders. As long as curriculum process was centralized, teachers have been kept aloof. Now that decentralized curriculum development process is being carried out, the role of the teachers as curriculum leaders is assuming new dimensions.
- Faculty development. All faculties contribute to curriculum enhancement through their participation in departmental curriculum and pedagogy workshops.
- Course development. Developing new and updating existing courses in-line with the major goals of specific levels of instruction and the curriculum as a whole are important contributions the faculty makes to the quality of the program.
- Participation in curriculum-wide enhancement projects. Faculty also contributes to enhancement projects that span beyond one curricular level (e.g. writing assessment across the curriculum).
- Feedback. Whether in their roles as level coordinators, mentors, or instructors, faculty suggest course or level-specific improvements to the curriculum coordinator.

The teacher is the heart of the curriculum and who should determine in a large measure the actual learning experiences in the classroom and in the clinical learning area. The importance of the teacher must be acknowledged in curriculum planning and he should be allowed a large measure of freedom in planning educational experience for pupils. For the active participation of teachers in the curriculum development, the following points have to be considered:

The teachers are aware of the needs and problems of the students, who are being educated in colleges and schools of nursing. Hence they will be able to understand the knowledge and skills needed by the students for solving their problems and workout varied activities to enable effective learning.

Teachers should be given adequate opportunities to carry out instruction and experimentation in the classroom setting so that they can actively participate in the selection of instructional materials.

Curriculum change should take into consideration the capabilities of the present teachers and it should win the acceptability of the teachers to be effectively implemented.

Role of Graduate Student Teachers

All graduate student teachers participate in enhancing the quality of the undergraduate curriculum in the following ways:
- **Participation in curriculum**: Wide enhancement projects. Graduate student teachers also contribute to enhancement projects that span beyond one curricular level (e.g. writing assessment across the curriculum).
- **Course development**: Developing new and updating existing courses in-line with the major goals of specific levels of instruction and the curriculum as a whole are important contributions graduate student teachers make to the quality of the program.
- **Participation in departmental workshops**: All graduate student teachers contribute to curriculum enhancement through their participation in departmental curriculum and pedagogy workshops.
- **Feedback**: Regardless of their role in the curriculum (e.g. teaching, assisting, observing), they suggest course or level-specific improvements to the curriculum coordinator.

Role of the Professional Organizations

The professional organizations such as Indian Nursing Council and the respective state nursing council take tremendous effort in planning, developing, implementing, evaluating, producing instructional and evaluational material, textbooks, supplementary reading materials and reconstruction of curriculum as and when the necessity arises.

Role of Community

Among the community personnel, the role of the parents in curriculum development deserves special attention, as they are closely related to students who will be influenced by the curriculum developed.

The role of the parents is described as follows:
Some of the well-educated parents are associated with curriculum development and syllabus committees or with the writing of textbooks even if they are not qualified.

During the finalization of the curriculum and syllabus, the outlines are circulated to all educated parents and their opinions are called for, to make necessary modification in the draft syllabi. Some parents are associated in the evaluation committees as the members.

Role of the Students

Students are the clientele for whom the curriculum is developed. They are the most affected by the curriculum. Hence there is dire need to actively involve them in the curriculum development and its implementation as well.

Evaluation of Educational Programs in Nursing

Program Evaluation

It is a process of making judgment about the extent to which a particular educational program achieved its objective and is also measuring the extent to which a program delivered is effective and efficient in fulfilling its intended purpose of its development or creation.

Evaluation of the total program of the college is the collective responsibility of all concerned. The overall evaluation of the college is known as an institutional review of the program.

Evaluation can be carried out by the internal members of an institution or an external agency or those concerned with quality of nursing education such as respective State Nursing Council, Indian Nursing Council, respective university and an accrediting agency. These organizations periodically conduct inspection and evaluate an organization for fulfilling the requirements and maintaining standards to assure quality nursing education for students.

Aims of Program Evaluation

It has the following aims:
- To measure the progress of a program
- To identify any problem and to resolve any conflicts
- To enhance utilization of available resources
- To provide baseline information for future evaluation and planning
- To modify and to make any remedial measures
- To increase the efficiency and effectiveness of the program

- To promote cost effectiveness
- To improve the quality
- To increase the image of an institution.

Components of the Program to be Evaluated
- Philosophy and objectives of the college
- Admission criteria
- Staff welfare activities
- Faculty position
- Curriculum
- Student's performance
- Infrastructural facilities
- Records and its maintenance.

Who will evaluate?
- The consumers
- The stakeholders
- The general public
- The administrators
- The faculty members
- The alumni
- Any specifically appointed committee.

The Program Evaluation Plan
This should consist of the major areas of evaluation and its components, time frame, data to be collected, use of existing data, decision regarding who has to evaluate, and the purpose of evaluation.

Models of Evaluation

Tylerian Model
According to Tyler, the evaluation is a continuous process. With the help of feedback, it is possible to reformulate and redefine objectives; this process of recycling keeps the program and evaluation system dynamic and the program also functions at an optimal level. Tyler has arranged evaluation plan into seven sequential steps. They are to:
- Establish broad goals/objectives
- Classify objectives
- Define objectives in behavioral terms
- Find situations in which achievement of objectives can be seen
- Develop/select measurement techniques
- Collect student performance data
- Compare data with behaviorally stated objectives.

Stufflebeams Context, Input, Process, Product (CIPP) Model
Evaluation is done in the following aspects. They are:
- Context evaluation
- Input evaluation
- Process evaluation
- Product evaluation.

Context Evaluation
It provides the information pertaining to the environment in which the evaluation is being carried out. It is a kind of situation analysis. It starts with diagnosis stage and includes the objectives and operations of the whole system. It involves the following:

Organization structure: The size, complexity, design and the channel of communication, span of control, method of delegation, well-established roles and responsibilities of the individual member, authority, etc. should be evaluated in terms of its influence in the attainment of preestablished goals and objectives and the product.

Mission and goal give direction for any organization and its program. The product depends on the mission and goal. The mission and goal should be reflected in the product if it is rightly conceived. A periodical review of mission and goal helps in checking the product.

Environmental scan: It includes the analysis of the views and perception of the mission and goal and the product by the stakeholders.

Review of policies and procedures: Each organization has its own policies and procedures, which are established to attain the objectives. Evaluation of these policies and procedures and thorough review of this helps in checking the product.

External regulation or forces: It is also essential to consider the governmental policies related to the program, regulatory mechanism such as the respective council or association, university norms in relation to the product outcome.

Input Evaluation
This is the next stage of evaluation. Input evaluation mainly evaluates men, money, material, and policies to implement goals. The input from the following are considered:

Faculty members: It is evaluated in terms of number, qualification, salary structure, their effectiveness, efficiency, and capability in achieving the objectives.

Support staff: They are also evaluated in terms of their number, qualification, effectiveness, efficiency, salary structure, etc. They include the administrative staff and the other nonteaching staff, who are all involved in this program implementation and evaluation.

Students: Number of students admitted, admission criteria, selection methods, and the methods of financing for the students are evaluated.

Material resources: The materials used in the program such as books, study materials, computer, AV aids, teaching materials, etc. are evaluated for their utility value. Library evaluation includes the number of books, recent edition books, journals, access to various e-journals, and facilities in the library to promote learning and other library services. Internet facilities and xeroxing facilities are also evaluated.

Physical facilities: It includes the classroom, rooms for faculty members, space for various laboratories, auditorium, examination hall, playground, working space for administrative staff and other nonteaching staff, etc. and its adequacy, availability, utility, feasibility, furniture facilities, etc. are also considered.

Financial input: Facilities available for students to get loans in paying the program fees and meeting the expenses toward the learning of the course content is taken into consideration.

Counseling services and medical services: It is also the student support services to be provided in any course.

Budget for the college: Money is required to meet the expenses toward the day-to-day maintenance, salary, scholarships, use of technology, infrastructure addition and its maintenance, faculty development, affiliation fees, deposits, and others.

Clinical facilities: Hospital, community, its location, utility, various departments, policies of the hospital and involvement of the staffs in clinical learning of students are also to be evaluated.

Policies: It is the policies established in running the program in regulation of the students, staffs, faculty members and the disciplinary procedures are also included in the input evaluation.

Process Evaluation

This stage mostly focuses on the implementation aspect. It tries to find out the congruence between the planning and factual situation. Process evaluation monitors the strategy adopted to implement the program and gets constant feedback and also identifies the defects in the program. It includes attention to curriculum, student admission, progression, graduation activities, faculty development, and the evaluation of faculty, staff and administrators. It also includes admission policies, entrance examinations and requirements, progression standards for students, supplementary exams, and graduation procedures.

Faculty evaluation: Their service, roles and responsibilities, productivity, workload, contribution, professional development, publication and research work are all evaluated. The faculty members are evaluated based on the following:

- Teaching
- Peer review of teaching
- Classroom visits
- The review of teaching and learning methods
- Teaching awards
- Professional letters of recognition
- Research publications
- Internal and external peer review documents
- Report from class and clinical visits
- Students' papers
- Students' projects, care plans, and assignment papers.

Research/Scholarship: It includes getting scholarship for any research project and grants-in-aid from any funding agency.

Evaluating Service: It is the evaluation of the clinical practice of the faculty members.

Teaching and teaching strategy evaluation
- By students—2–3 times per course
- By peers—2 times by 2 peers/course
- Using self-created portfolio—Each time class taught
- By Administrators—End of semester or year and more often as needed.

Evaluating faculty development: It is the evaluation of the staff development program organized by the institution. The following are evaluated:
- Formal and systematic plan
- Orientation services
- Ongoing support services
- Mentoring programs
- Continuing education programs.

Evaluation of administrators: A formal evaluation of administrators usually occurs at regularly specified intervals. A common plan includes annual review by the administrator's immediate supervisor and a comprehensive evaluation for every 3–5 years. Individuals from six levels are capable of conducting or participating in this review. They are the immediate supervisor, peers within the institution, faculty subordinates, clients served, and the administrator under the review.

Authority, responsibility, decision making style, and interpersonal relationship are the areas to be evaluated.

Evaluation of supporting staff: A periodic evaluation of nonteaching and supporting staff helps to assess their effectiveness and contribution toward success of the program.

Product and Outcome Evaluation

Finally the product evaluation looks into the final product, i.e. whether the curriculum has accomplished the desired objectives. Product evaluation provides data to match with the mission and goal of the program. It also correlates the context, input and process data to the outcome of the program. The final decisions based on all data include program continuation, modification or termination. The following products are evaluated:

Student outcomes: Student learning outcomes, graduation and attrition rates, employment rate, licensing examinations, certification examinations, employment rate, etc.

Employer product utilization and satisfaction: It is the extent to which the graduates possess the skill and knowledge to be employed in an organization.

Alumni employment rates and profile: It gives the idea of long-term employment and the demand for the graduates of any particular organization or for any course in the labor market.

Eisner's Connoisseurship Model

This is one of the qualitative models of evaluation. Unlike quantitative models such as Tylerian model and CIPP model, this model does not collect data. The evaluation mainly narrates, describes, and makes a thorough portrayal of the event or situation. Elliot Eisner stressed that the evaluator must be an educational critic. Eisner says that an educational evaluator should raise certain qualitative questions such as what has happened at a particular point of time on a particular day at a particular event or situation when a new program was introduced, and how the program can be made more effective. The stress is mostly laid on the qualitative aspects of college life. The criticism made should help them with the description, interpretation, and assessment of the situation. He also says that this evaluation refers to referential adequacy and structural corroboration than the scientific validity.

Structural corroboration refers to a continuous enquiry about whether the various parts of a criticism fit together as a consistent whole. Referential adequacy involves checking to see if critical observations and interpretations are empirically grounded allowing cadres to experience the evaluated phenomena in a new and better way.

Criteria for Evaluation of a Program

Whichever program we plan to evaluate, we should bear in mind the following criteria:

Consistency with the objectives: Evaluation should be consistent with the objectives to be achieved through the program.

Comprehensiveness: It shows whether the required tools for evaluation are used or devised suitably to know whether all the aspects related to the program are taken care of. Thus, the suitable instruments of evaluation are very essential to do comprehensive evaluation.

Sufficient diagnostic value: The appropriate strengths and weaknesses of the program should be given through the evaluation. Curriculum framers need to think and plan for various objectives and qualitative and informal methods of appraisal.

Validity: The tool used in evaluation should be valid to bring the accurate results.

Unity of evaluation judgment: The evaluation cannot be conducted at a time. Each part of a single unit has to be considered with respect to the students, the program, learning outcomes, and so on. Each one has to be evaluated then and there and all of them need to be looked at in unity, and final decisions are made.

Continuity: Evaluation should be continuous throughout the year. It should be carried out regularly and continuously to strengthen every dimension of curriculum development.

Curriculum Improvement

Curriculum improvement focuses on two approaches—one in grass roots and the other is top-down approach. In the first one, the teacher and the students are included in the process and with their experience and the feedback they get from interaction they try to improve upon the curriculum. In the top-down approach it may be developed at the top. The personnel involved in implementation may not be involved in curriculum making.

The major ingredients are:
- Personality
- Materials
- Physical environment and facilities
- Defensible ideas
- Support and resistance.

Personality

Mostly curriculum improvement depends on the teachers' personality. In other words the curriculum improvement and professional development of teachers are interdependent. The teacher has to accept the changes brought due to curriculum improvement. They have to be educated and trained to deal with the new curriculum.

Materials

The curriculum improvement also depends on the quality of instructional materials. Material is a means for curriculum improvement. The material has to be prepared carefully.

Physical Environment and Facilities

It is very important to think about facilities to improve the physical environment to have an impact on curriculum improvement.

Defensible Ideas

Basically curriculum improvement is dependent on various changes or ideas that are supplemented with the existing curriculum to improve further. Here the concept of defense indicates the amount of better justification available for a particular idea in curriculum.

Support and Resistance

It is very essential that it needs a support from various levels right from the authority otherwise known as "gate keepers", whose decisions are important and they support for the proposal to come into implementation level. It also requires support from the faculty, students, and significant others.

Curriculum Research in Nursing

Research is the application of scientific method in the study of problems. Research is a systematic attempt to obtain answers to meaningful questions about phenomena or events through the application of scientific procedures. Research in curriculum is a systematic attempt to gain a better understanding of all components of curriculum. It is an application of scientific method to the study of curriculum.

Curriculum inquiry or research is a realm, which enables to think about curriculum problems.

There are some basic elements in curriculum and its implementation. Research in these elements helps one to improve one's curriculum and evaluate it. They are:
- The teacher
- Subject matter
- Learners
- Milieu.

Travers (1969) has pointed out some areas of curriculum research which need consideration by researchers in the field of education. One of these is concerned with the structure of subject matter. In nursing, research can be done in relation to placement, adequacy of content, prescribed theory and practical hours, and its relation to fulfillment of learning objectives.

Another area proposed by Travers (1969) is concerned with the development of techniques for making analysis of the psychological demands placed on the learner by various learning experiences. The development of audio-visual materials and their impact on the learning of subject matter also fall within the area of curriculum research.

Research also can be done in organization of curriculum, adaptation of curriculum to local needs, effects of examination on curriculum organization, analysis of textbooks, concept development on various subjects, effectiveness of various teaching methods, human relation in curriculum development, study habits, duration of college work, revision and modernization of curricula. As technology advances and the dynamics of disease changes and newer diseases emerge, it is necessary to upgrade the curriculum. In order to upgrade, there is a need for systematic curriculum research so that the revision of the curriculum may be worked out as a well-coordinated program of improvement on the basis of the research findings. The preparation of suitable textbooks and other teaching materials is also basic to the success of any attempt at curriculum improvement. Thus, not only does the suitability of the existing textbooks need to be verified, but there also seems to be a need for investigation into the best types of textbooks. The research would also help us in solving the problems that relate to the vocabulary, content, printing, and illustrations of textbooks.

Teacher education and preparation is another area where research is required. Teacher education refers to the total educative process which contributes to the preparation of a person for a teaching job in colleges. The educative process includes the program of courses and other experiences offered by an educational institution and universities offering courses for the purpose of preparing persons for teaching and other educational services and for contributing to their growth in the competency for such service. Thus, research in the areas of syllabi, curriculum and program is essential for qualitative improvement of nursing education.

The research in curriculum needs to be focused on the following issues:
- Whether the designed curriculum is in tune with the philosophy of nursing education.
- How can the curriculum be planned to meet the individual differences of pupils?
- How can the curriculum be related to the needs of developing nation and the manpower requirements of our country?
- How can the curriculum be related to the global needs and demands?
- How can the theory and practice component in the curriculum be correlated?
- What kind of preparation and training is required for teachers to make the curriculum a meaningful experience for pupils?
- What is the relative importance and suitability of each course of study?
- What type of instruction or teaching strategies should be best suitable for implementing the curriculum?
- What are the future needs of the pupils as far as curriculum is concerned?
- What method of evaluation helps in assessing the effectiveness of curriculum in all stages?
- When does the existing curriculum need reformation and changes or revision?
- What is the effective clinical learning environment for the students?

- How can the effective clinical learning environment be provided for the students?

There is a need for curriculum research in nursing because of the changing needs of the society. Nursing is a discipline where the core is the patient that is the human being. The curriculum of nursing education mainly revolves around the care of human being. A well-planned and implemented curriculum ultimately improves the welfare of the society which requires in-depth research in curriculum planning, implementation, and evaluation.

Different Models of Collaboration between Education and Service

Nursing education brings its particular focus to bear on the need to bridge the theory-practice gap. Organizational structures such as lecturer-practitioners, lecturer-clinicians, clinical lectures and joint appointments are discussed to promote theory–practice correlation. A theoretical component is essential if a practice-based discipline, like nursing, is to develop. Nursing only really develops if improvements in patient care become manifest. Patient care requires efficient implementation of nursing actions. Research can serve as a link between theory and practice. Nurse educators and clinicians must come together to work out conjoint approaches on matters of mutual professional interest. Until that happens, graduates of nursing education programs will not be optimally prepared for the realities of practicing their profession, and nursing service administrators will not be able to use the knowledge and skills of graduates optimally to serve patients.

The Basic Principles of Correlation

Theory + Practice = Correlation
Cognitive domain + Psychomotor domain = Affective domain
Curriculum content + Curriculum implementation = Expected behavioral change

An organization which promotes the conjoining of the academic nurses and the practice nurses may bridge the theory practice gap. The benefits are increase in consensus about the value and standards of practice, the use and management of resources and talents from both sides, the development of common set of values and common culture in nursing. The problems are faculty or staff overload, confidence of the faculty in their ability to practice, inability of the practice staff to teach the students, equality in tenure, promotion and rewards for both faculty and practice personnel, etc. The faculty has to perform certain tasks to correlate theory with practice. The faculty prior to the clinical posting of the students and during the clinical training has to do the below mentioned duties.

Preclinical Preparation
- Intellectual training
- Practice in skill laboratory
- Clarity of the purpose of the practicum
- Development of reasoning and critical thinking skills.

During Clinical Training
- Appropriate placement of the students.
- Drawing out what the student knows and help them build-up additional knowledge on clinical situations.
- Helping the student explore, make connections, realize what they know, and how and why it is relevant to this situation.
- Questions to the student cue the student to relevant issues in this situation.
- Pulling the students into discussion and encouraging them to think about the likely clinical symptoms for a particular condition.

Constraints in Reducing the Gap between Theory and Practice

Faculty
- Lack of practical knowledge and experiences
- Inadequate knowledge on student psychology
- Poor understanding of students
- Personal attributes, personal qualities, and personality
- Failure to recognize the importance of correlation
- Inappropriate faculty-student ratio.

Students
- Lack of prerequisite knowledge and skill
- Stress and anxiety
- Physical and mental illness
- Inability to use equipment and technology
- Poor communication skill
- Resistance to active participation.

Time
Inadequate for activity and debriefing.

Resources
- Inadequate clinical facilities
- Poor funds
- Poor library facilities and audio-visual equipment.

Overcoming the Problems

The following are the tips to overcome the problems:
- Make a list of the main aims of clinical education.
- Identify the problems which can arise in clinical learning and also the characteristics of effective clinical experiences that avoid those problems.

- Provide rich clinical experience and ensure various practice opportunities.
- Be with the students.
- Motivate them in performing appropriate action.
- Give feedback.
- Model their own thinking process.
- Have learners work together.
- Collaborate with colleagues.
- Use different educational strategies.
- Be challenging to the students.
- Be emotionally satisfying for the students.
- Stimulate development of alternative perspectives of the problem or issue.
- Be sufficiently varied to prevent boredom.
- Allow for and exploit the potential of the students.
- Use results of clinical nursing research into practice.

Clinical Learning Experience

Learning activities should:
- Clearly relate to the desired objectives, competencies, learning domain, and domain level.
- Be geared to and appropriate for the cognitive, affective or psychomotor development of the students.
- Be challenging so that they move students to higher levels of cognitive and affective development.
- Be emotionally satisfying for the students.
- Stimulate development of alternative perspectives of the problem or issue.
- Be sufficiently varied to prevent boredom.
- Articulate and allow application of some previous learning experiences.
- Provide a foundation for subsequent learning.

Faculty Role

- Manager
- Assessor
- Advocate
- Facilitator
- Guide
- Motivator
- Counselors
- Instructor
- Collaborator
- Coordinator
- Observer
- Feedback giver
- Evaluator
- Coach
- Mentor
- Preceptor
- Critical thinker
- Role model
- Analyzer.

Strategies to Integrate Teaching with Practice

- Problem-based learning
- Clinical correlation map
- Clinical studies assignments
- Clinical presentation/case presentation
- Learning diaries
- Concept mapping
- Inquiry-based learning
- Case-based teaching method/care study
- Simulation
- Drama
- Reflective learning
- Applying social and behavioral science perspectives to clinical practice.

Reflecting on Experience—A Strategy to Correlate

As students realize that the knowledge they have gained from practical experience can be the building blocks of theory and there needs to be a dialog between what is found in practice or in the practical situation and what is expected. Unless the teacher is prepared for such an incident in the process of debriefing students' experiences, the opportunity for clarification may be lost. Without such an exploration with students, simply being in a clinical situation does not indicate that the student has "experienced". Learning is more effective when the students reflect on experiences.

Burnard's (1987) model gives a straightforward set of steps of the cycle of experience-reflection-new experience as follows:
- Practical experience
- Sharing of experience
- Reflection in a group on that experience
- Discussion based on the outcome of reflection; new learning is planned and developed
- Evaluation of learning and planning to apply the learning.

Applying Theory to Practice through Clinical Supervision

Effective mentorship is critical in delivering high quality care, ensuring patient safety, and facilitating positive development of staff. Nurses must use mentorship skills in providing workplace, informal and formal, one-to-one supervision to support workers especially the nursing students in order to facilitate their professional maturity. This will enable support workers to apply theory to practice and encourage them to test new skills in a safe and supportive environment (Miller et al. 2000). A successful mentor will seek to develop staff whilst working alongside with team members in a mentoring and coaching role.

The mentor needs to provide an appropriate learning environment, relevant resources, and the desirable level of structured support and guidance to promote professional growth and development. The individual support worker must interact with the mentor in a manner which suggests they are prepared to learn. They must demonstrate personal motivation and an attitude that is open to acquiring new knowledge. Workplace learning, through structured mentorship, coaching and supervision needs to be recognized by organizations as an important future strategy in bridging the theory to practice gap, motivating support workers, and promoting the application of knowledge to practice (Dewar and Walker, 1999).

Santos and Stuart (2003) advocate that even though organizations invest millions of pounds in training programs they often devote little attention to evaluating the effectiveness of training. There has been a recent cultural shift in continuous professional development away from classroom-based teaching to interactive workplace learning through good mentorship.

Mentorship is not dissimilar to leadership, which Adair (2002) defines as "the art of influencing people to follow a certain course of action, the art of controlling them, directing them and getting the best out of them". Effective leaders are required to use problem-solving processes, communicate well, and demonstrate leadership fairness, competence, and creativity. In comparison, mentors should be dynamic, passionate, have a motivational influence on other people, be solution focused, and seek to inspire others. By demonstrating an effective mentorship style, the nurse will be in a powerful position to influence the successful development of staff, ensuring that professional standards are maintained and enabling the growth of competent practitioners.

Training should not be confined to the classroom and should include practical as well as theoretical elements; there should be good supervision which promotes accountability of the students and also provides feedback in a supportive environment. Supervision ensures the competence of the students and provides pastoral support (Naknikian et al., 2002; Nancarrow and Mackey, 2005).

A study conducted by Coffey (2004) found that responses from support workers to questions regarding the type of training they preferred displayed an overwhelming interest in an "on the job" model of training. In considering a new practice model, we should examine the usefulness of work-based mentorship and supervision as part of training strategies where the one-to-one mentorship relationship is the most important element in clinical instruction.

Much of the available research pertains to the mentorship of qualified professionals such as nurses, social workers, and medical students. There appear to be very few studies which relate directly to the application of theory to practice through supervised practice and mentorship of unqualified support workers.

Models of Collaboration between Education and Practice

With the globalization, nurses are going to face more competition at domestic and international markets. It, therefore, requires nurses with competencies and advanced knowledge to compete in the job market. It is the responsibility of nursing education to cater to this need. The outputs of an institution are graduates, researched knowledge, new skills, and change in value system and attitude of the people and the transmission of sociocultural tradition. For these outputs, the institutions depend upon their curricula, infrastructure facilities, equipment, funds, and qualified and efficient faculty members. With the utilization of these facilities, the institutions carry out their teaching activities and research, and obtain the output. On the other hand, the purpose of the hospital whether Government or private is quality patient care, economic development, services to society and human resources development. For achieving these purposes, hospitals require skilled human resources, infrastructure facilities, equipment, and research and development. If there is an interface between the institution and hospital, this helps both being benefited mutually. The following are some avenues where institution and hospital can have interface for mutual benefit. Institution can utilize hospital for enhancing students' learning and developing their own faculty members.

Educational Institution and Hospital Interface

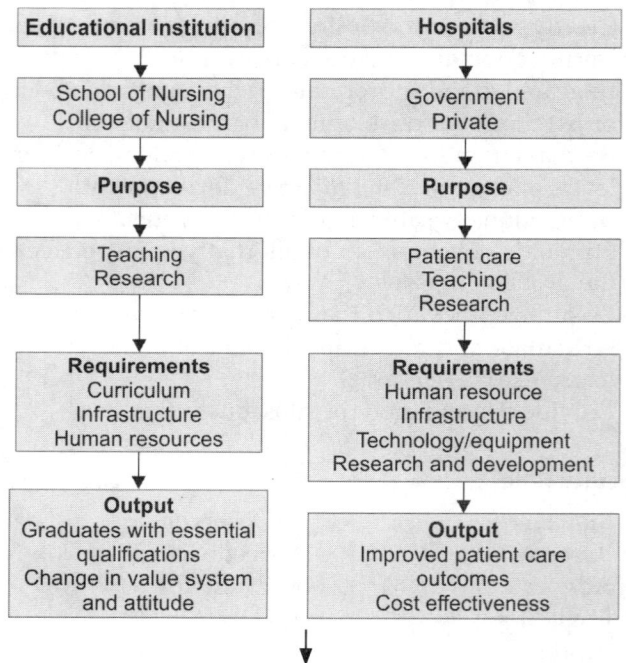

Source: Modified from original model— University-Industry Interface, *University News,* July 24, 1995.

Interfaces

Mobility and Exchange of Faculty
The nurses in the service side can come to various departments of college and schools of nursing and share their experiences with the faculty members and the faculty members can go to the hospitals to gain first-hand experience and also participate in the service of the hospital. This will enable them to make their teaching up-to-date and relevant. The teachers should utilize the opportunity to learn when they go for supervising the students in the clinical area.

Joint Consultancy
Personnel of hospitals should have constant communication with the faculty members and researchers of the college. For their teaching and research also the faculty members should be in constant touch with the needs of the hospitals. Such a communication may be facilitated by the top level managers of the hospitals and heads of the college.

Sharing of Resources
There are many types of equipment, books and other materials in the college of nursing which are underutilized, and due to financial difficulties many such resources are not obtained by the college. Same is in the case of hospitals too. Hospitals may subscribe periodicals and journals and may also have libraries which are not optimally used. If these valuable resources are properly utilized on sharing basis, both hospitals and colleges will be benefited and with the recent development of networking all the hospitals and colleges in the city, state or even the country as a whole can be the members and take advantage of each other's resources.

Curriculum Development
Curriculum upgradation and framing new curricula are regular and necessary activities of a college along with the university and the nursing council. The criterion for this is that curricula should be need-based and useful to the immediate society. Therefore, it is essential that the hospital personnel shall form a part of the committee for framing curriculum. The committee shall only take care of the present needs of the industries but will also have a futuristic perspective in developing curriculum.

Staff Development
Staff development is an important function of the manager irrespective of organizations. It is not mere growth or learning by the staff but the group interaction which enable the staff to develop together. Hospitals and colleges today shall organize such forums and provide such avenues to its staff to learn from each other in their concerned areas. For this, both can organize seminars, conferences or workshops by inviting people from the concerned areas for sharing knowledge and experiences.

Training of Students
The nursing educational institutions, either for all specialties or for few specialty areas, get affiliated with the hospitals for training their students in the clinical areas. The hospitals, therefore, shall adopt some practical aspects of the courses and these courses can be directly related to their own requirements. For training of the students, the faculty and hospital personnel shall have proper planning and the duration and timing be planned out. Moreover, due weightage to such training should be given for promotion and certification of students.

Research and Development Collaboration
The collaboration will help the universities to overcome the resources crunch and generate knowledge by optimizing the use of resources in the research and development laboratories, adapt new and imported technology to meet the global competitiveness, enrich teaching and research in the universities with the back-up or field experience. So, the process of collaboration will bring excellence in hospitals and colleges.

Quality Control and New Technology Adaptation
Liberalization and globalization of market has forced the hospitals to go for quality control and services. Adapting and developing a new technology is very much essential. The nurses must be aware of the current modalities of the treatment of various illnesses and for this, the faculty must be utilized to update the nurses of the current trends.

Sponsorship of Research
The hospitals being the immediate consumers of the nursing students shall sponsor research programs of the colleges and in turn should become accountable in this regard. The hospitals may ask the students to conduct those researches which are useful to them for improving patient care outcomes.

Funding
Funds may be collected from various sources like hospitals, alumni, trusts and sponsors, government and universities and from the colleges, and this can be utilized for research purposes which ultimately improve patient care.

Summary

- A curriculum is designed to provide a sequence of learning experience that will enable students to achieve desired educational outcomes.
- Curriculum framework provides faculty with a means of conceptualizing and organizing the knowledge, skills, values, and beliefs critical to the delivery of coherent curriculum that facilitates the achievement of the desired curriculum outcomes.
- Organizing curriculum frameworks are the educational road maps to teaching and learning. As with any roadmap, multiple options are available for arriving at a given destination or outcome.
- Program evaluation is a process of making judgment about the extent to which a particular educational program has achieved its objective and is also measuring the extent to which a program delivered is effective and efficient in fulfilling its intended purpose if its development or creation.
- Evaluation of the total program of the college is the collective responsibility of all concerned. The overall evaluation of the college is known as an institutional review of the program.
- Context evaluation provides the information pertaining to the environment in which the evaluation is being carried out. It is a kind of situation analysis. It starts with diagnosis stage and includes the objectives and operations of the whole system.
- Input evaluation is the next stage of evaluation. Input evaluation mainly evaluates men, money material, and policies used to implement goals. This stage mostly focuses on the implementation aspect. It tries to find out the congruence between the planning and factual situation. Finally, the product evaluation looks into the final product, i.e. whether the curriculum has accomplished the desired objectives. Product evaluation provides data to match with the mission and goal of the program.
- Curriculum improvement focuses on two approaches—one is grass roots and the other is top-down approach.

11
Management of Nursing Educational Institutions

"A child educated only at school is an uneducated child".
—George Santayana

Objectives
After completing this unit, you will be able to:
- Understand the management of nursing educational institutions
- Explain the development and maintenance of standards and accreditation in nursing education programs
- Understand the role of Nursing Council, Board and University
- Appreciate the role of professional associations and unions.

Introduction

The concept of management is associated with the phenomenon of group activity. Everywhere in a modern society, we find a group of people working in all spheres of human activity. Management is the process of efficiently getting activities completed with and through other people. Educational administration includes the techniques and procedures employed in operating the educational organization in accordance with established policies. It is same in administration of nursing educational institutions. Administration of nursing educational institutions such as college of nursing and school of nursing includes maintenance management and developmental management. It includes the management of man, money, material, activity, and time. It also involves the management functions such as planning, organizing, directing, recruiting, staffing controlling, budgeting, staff development, etc. There are different courses offered in nursing such as ANM, DGNM, BSc(N), Post-basic BSc(N), MSc(N), and MPhil and PhD in nursing. The Indian Nursing Council, State Nursing Council and the University with which an institution is affiliated play a vital role in establishing and maintaining standards in nursing education.

Management of Nursing Educational Institutions

Review of Various Course Requirements

The steps in starting ANM/DGNM/BSc(N)/PBBSc(N)/MSc(N) program.

Steps in Starting Programs

1. The first step is to obtain essentiality certificate/no objection certificate from the concerned State Government. The name of the school/nursing institution along with the name of the Trust/Society with full address shall be mentioned in No Objection certificate/essentiality certificate.
2. The next step is to get recognition from the concerned State Nursing Council which is a mandatory requirement.
3. Then the Indian Nursing Council shall after receipt of the above documents/proposal would then conduct statutory inspection of the recognized training nursing institution to assess the suitability with regard to availability of teaching faculty, clinical and infrastructural facilities.

The following establishments/organizations are eligible to establish/open a nursing institution:
a) Central Government/State Government/Local body;
b) Registered Private or Public Trust;
c) Organizations registered under Societies Registration Act including Missionary Organizations;
d) Companies incorporated under section 8 of Company's Act.

General Requirement for all Programs
- Separate building/block for teaching and hostel
- Open space to facilitate outdoor games for students
- Well-furnished office rooms for principal, faculty and staffs

- Well-furnished classrooms with cross-ventilation, adequate lighting
- Well-furnished hostel rooms with ventilation, lighting, etc.
- Well-furnished nursing laboratories with cots, mannequins, and equipment as per the number of programs and students
- Well-furnished nutrition laboratories with provisions for stove with gas connections, wash basins, working tables and adequate utensils for conducting cooking demonstrations
- Well-furnished library, with ventilation, lighting and provision for cupboards, racks, tables and chairs with latest edition books and journals
- Provision for safe drinking water
- Provision for fire extinguishing
- Toilets—in the teaching block, provision for common toilets for faculty members and staff, separately for male and female; provision for common toilets for students, separately for male and female students
- In the hostel, one toilet and one bathroom for 2-6 students, separately for male and female students
- Garage to park vehicles
- Teacher-student ratio, 1:10.

Clinical Facilities

The eligible organizations /establishments should have their own parent hospital. The minimum requirements for the number and type of beds will vary according to the programs offered like Diploma, UG, PG, Post-basic Diploma in Nursing and Nurse Practitioner Critical Care program. Refer Indian Nursing Council website for the details.

Nursing Programs-Purpose, Requirements, Facility

Auxiliary Nurse Midwifery

Purpose

The auxiliary nurse midwifery (ANM) course is given to prepare the candidates for rendering preventive, promotive, restorative, and emergency healthcare services to individuals and community. Also, they are trained to provide neonatal, midwifery services and child care services at home, clinic, and school. They also have the responsibility to guide trained birth attendants, anganwadi workers and other community health activists and volunteers. They are expected to coordinate and collaborate with other health team members, NGOs and to act as a team member in the healthcare delivery system and participate in all the National Health and Family Welfare programs at community level.

Admission Requirements

12th pass.

The minimum age for admission shall be 17 years and the maximum age for admission shall be 35 years.

Duration

Two years.

Requirements

The school should be located in a Community Health Center (CHC) or a Rural Hospital (RH) having minimum bed strength of 30 and maximum 50 and serving an area with community health programs.

It should be affiliated to a district hospital or a secondary care hospital.

Any hospital with 150 beds with minimum 30–50 obstetrics and gynecology beds, and 100 delivery cases monthly can also open ANM school.

They should also have an affiliation of PHC/CHC for the Community Health Nursing field experience. Existing ANM schools attached to District Hospitals should have PHC annexe (accommodation facility for 20–30 students) for community health field experience.

Physical Facilities

- Staff Room-1
- Faculty Room-1
- Class Room-2
- Nursing Laboratory-1
- Nutrition Laboratory-1
- Library-cum-Study-1
- Audio–visual Aids Room-1
- Provisions for Toilets
- Multipurpose Hall–1

Hostel Facilities

Each training center should have permission for accommodating at least 60 students at a time in the hostel with:
- Furnished double rooms for students
- Kitchen, dining hall, pantry, store room
- Bathing and toilet facilities
- Study room
- Common room and recreation room
- Visitor's room
- The hostel should be adequately furnished with electric and running water facilities and facilities for outdoor and indoor recreation.

Clinical Facility

District hospital or a secondary care hospital with minimum 150 beds can be used.

Teaching Faculty
- Principal—A person with MSc(N) with 3 years of teaching experience or BSc(N) with 5 years of teaching experience.
- Nursing Tutor
- BSc Nursing/Diploma in Nursing Education and Administration/Diploma in Public Health Nursing with 2 years of clinical experience.

Diploma in General Nursing and Midwifery

Purpose

This diploma in general nursing and midwifery (DGNM) course is offered to prepare the students to demonstrate competency in providing preventive, promotive, restorative healthcare to individual, sick or well, using nursing process. They are prepared to function effectively with members of the health team and demonstrate use of ethical values in their personal and professional life. They are expected to show interest in activities of professional organization and recognize the need for undertaking research and participate in continuing education for professional development. They also should demonstrate basic skills in administration and leadership.

Admission Requirements

10+2 class pass with aggregate of 40%.
Age for admission shall be 17–35 years.

Duration

Three years.

Physical Facility

Academic Block
- Classroom/lecture hall-3
- Laboratories
  - Nursing foundation laboratory
  - Community health nursing laboratory
  - Advance nursing skill laboratory
  - Nutrition laboratory
  - OBG and pediatric laboratory
  - Preclinical science laboratory
  - Computer laboratory
- Multipurpose hall
- Common room (male and female)
- AV aids room
- Staff room
- Principal room
- Vice principal room
- Faculty room
- Library
- Toilet facilities.

Hostel Block
- Rooms for students (single or double)
- Toilet facilities (one latrine and one bathroom for 5 students)
- Visitor room
- Reading room
- Store room
- Recreation room
- Dining hall
- Kitchen and store
- Warden room.

Clinical Requirements
- Parent or affiliated hospital with 100–150 beds with the minimum bed occupancy 75%.
- It should have all the specialties with nursing staffing pattern as per INC norm.
- It should be within the radius of 15–30 km, and 1:3 student-patient ratio must be maintained.

Faculty Requirements
- Principal: MSc Nursing with 3 years of teaching experience or BSc Nursing (Basic)/Post-basic with 5 years of teaching experience.
- Vice-Principal: MSc Nursing or BSc Nursing (Basic)/Post-basic with 3 years of teaching experience.
- Tutor: MSc Nursing or BSc Nursing (Basic/Post-basic) or Diploma in Nursing Education and Administration with 2 years of professional experience.

Bachelor of Science in Nursing [BSc(N)]

Purpose

The BSc(N) course is provided to develop the candidates to apply knowledge from physical, biological, and behavioral sciences, medicine including alternative systems and nursing in providing preventive, promotive and restorative nursing care to individuals, families and communities. They should provide nursing care based on nursing process using latest trends and technology. They are expected to practice within the framework of code of ethics and professional conduct, and acceptable standards of practice within the legal boundaries. They should demonstrate leadership and managerial skills in clinical/community health settings so as to promote toward advancement of self and of the profession and conduct need based research studies in various settings and utilize the research findings to improve the quality of care.

Admission Criteria

10+2 pass with aggregate of 45%.
  Minimum age for admission shall be 17 years on or before 31st December of the year of admission.

Duration

Four years.

Physical Facilities

Academic Block

- Classroom/Lecture hall-4
- Laboratories
  - Nursing foundation laboratory
  - Community health nursing laboratory
  - Advance nursing skill laboratory
  - Nutrition laboratory
  - OBG and pediatric laboratory
  - Preclinical science laboratory
  - Computer laboratory
- Multipurpose hall
- Common room (male and female)
- AV aids room.

Administrative Office

- Store room
- Record room
- Staff room
- Principal room
- Vice-principal room
- Faculty room
- Library
- Toilet facilities.

Hostel Block

- Rooms for students (single or double)
- Toilet facilities (one latrine and one bathroom for five students)
- Visitor room
- Reading room
- Sick room
- Store room
- Recreation room
- Dining hall
- Kitchen and store.

Clinical Facilities

A 150 bedded own or affiliated hospital with all specialties which can provide for 1:3 student and patient ratio. The affiliated hospital should be within 15–30 km radius.

If the institution has both BSc and GNM, the hospital should have 240 beds or more.

Faculty Requirements

Professor-cum-Principal

MSc Nursing with total 15 years of experience after MSc(N) with minimum of 12 years of teaching experience. PhD(N) is desirable.

Professor-cum-Vice-Principal

MSc Nursing with total 12 years of experience after MSc(N) with minimum of 10 years of teaching experience. PhD(N) is desirable.

Professor

MSc(N) with 10 years of experience after MSc(N) out of which 7 years should be teaching experience. PhD(N) is desirable.

Reader/Associate Professor

MSc Nursing with total 8 years of experience after MSc(N) with minimum of 5 years of teaching experience. PhD(N) is desirable.

Assistant Professor/Lecturer

MSc Nursing with total 3 years of experience after MSc(N).

Clinical Instructor

MSc(N), PBBSc(N) or BSc(N) with 1 year of experience.

Note: The experience for each level of faculty requirements subject to change as per INC norms and regulations.

Post-basic BSc(N) [PBBSc(N)]

Purpose

This course is offered by the institution to prepare the candidates to provide preventive, promotive, and restorative nursing care using nursing process for patients/clients, families and communities. They should develop competency in applying the concepts and principles from selected areas of nursing, physical, biological and behavioral sciences and demonstrate skills in communication, interpersonal relationship, leadership and managerial skills and skills in teaching. They are expected to practice ethical values in their personal and professional life and participate in research activities and utilize research findings in improving nursing practice. They also should recognize the need for continued learning for their personal and professional development.

Admission Criteria

- 10+2 pass + GNM
- Should be a registered nurse.

Duration

Two years.

Physical Facilities

Two (2) lecture halls in addition to facilities of BSc(N). Proportionately the number and size of the room will increase based on the number of students.

MSc(N)

Purpose

This course is offered to prepare the candidates, who can utilize/apply the concepts, theories and principles of nursing science and demonstrate advance competence in practice of nursing and as a nurse specialist. They are expected to have leadership qualities and function effectively as nurse educator and manager and actively undertake nursing research and to effect change in nursing practice and in the healthcare delivery system. They should have interest in continued learning for personal and professional advancement.

Admission Criteria

Passing of BSc(N)/BSc Hons.(N)/Post-basic BSc(N) with minimum of 55% aggregate marks.

Minimum 1 year of work experience after Basic BSc(N). Minimum 1 year of work experience prior or after Post-basic BSc(N).

Duration

Two years.

Physical Facilities

Two (2) lecture halls and classroom for each specialty for 2 years in addition to facilities of BSc(N). Proportionately the number and size of the room will increase based on the number of students.

Nurse Practitioner in Critical Care

Nurse Practitioner Critical Care Program is intended to prepare registered BSc Nurses to provide advanced nursing care to adults who are critically ill. The nursing care is focused on stabilizing patients' condition, minimizing acute complications, and maximizing restoration of health. These nurse practitioner's (NP's) are required to practice in tertiary care centers. The program consists of various courses of study that are based on strong scientific foundations including evidenced based practice. They may prescribe drugs, medical equipment, and therapies when authorized by the nursing regulatory council/s and state or national laws. The NPCC is prepared and qualified to assume responsibility and accountability for the care of critically ill patients under her care. After successful completion of this program, they are expected to diagnose and treat patients with critical illnesses as well as preventive and promoting care relevant to such illnesses and patients' responses to illness. It is a clinical residency program emphasizing a strong clinical component with 20% of theoretical instruction including skill laboratory and 80% of clinical experience.

Physical and Learning Resources at College/Hospital

- One classroom/conference room at the clinical setting
- Skill laboratory for simulated learning (hospital/college)
- Library and computer facilities with access to online journals
- E-Learning facilities.

Staff Resources

Full time faculty qualified NP in the specialty/MSc in relevant specialty (one faculty for every 5 students)
   Professor-cum-coordinator 1
   Reader/Associate Professor 1
   The above faculty shall perform dual role or a senior nurse with MSc qualification employed in the tertiary center.
   Medical/nursing faculty preceptors.

Eligibility for Admission

Registered BSc nurse with a minimum of 1 year clinical experience, preferably in any critical care setting prior to enrollment.

Number of candidates: 1 candidate for 5 ICU beds.

Duration of the course: 2 years.

Master of Philosophy in Nursing

Purpose

This course is offered to strengthen the research knowledge of the nurses and also to provide basic training required for research in undertaking doctoral work.

Eligibility

Pass with at least 60% marks in MSc Nursing.

Duration

One year.

Doctor of Philosophy in Nursing

Any specialty department or the college can be recognized as a research center by a medical university to offer the program. To recognize as a research center, the concerned university will be inspecting the college or department; once found suitable, by paying the prescribed fee they become eligible.

Post-basic Diploma in Nursing

Purpose
The course is given to train nurses to render quality care to patients and also manage and supervise patient care in clinical and community settings. They also expected to teach nurses, allied health professionals, patients and communities in areas related to their specialty and conduct research.

Admission Criteria
RN and RM with 1 year of clinical experience.

Duration
One year.

Diploma Courses
- Cardiothoracic Nursing
- Critical Care Nursing
- Midwifery Nursing
- Neuroscience Nursing
- Oncology Nursing
- Orthopedic and Rehabilitation Nursing
- Psychiatric Nursing
- Neonatal Nursing
- Operation Room Nursing
- Emergency and Disaster Nursing

The above courses can be started based on the clinical facilities available.

Functions of Education Management Planning

"If you are failing to plan you are planning to fail".

Planning is the basic or primary function of management. In simple words, planning is deciding in advance what to do, when to do it, how to do it and who is to do it. Planning involves determining objectives to be achieved, establishing planning premises, formulating policies, procedures and rules, determining alternative course of action, evaluating the available course of action and selecting the right type of action to achieve the desired results.

Educational planning is defined as the process of preparing a set of decisions for action during a specific period of time directed at achieving organizational goals. In the words of JP Naik, educational planning implies taking of decisions for future action with a view to achieving predetermined objectives through the optimum use of scarce resources.

Features of Educational Planning
- Educational planning is futuristic.
- It is goal-oriented.
- It forms the basis for all other functions.
- It is an intellectual activity.
- It is pervasive.
- It is a continuous process.
- It is flexible.
- It is a group activity.
- It involves choosing among the alternative course of action that may be most suitable for achieving the goals.

Importance of Educational Planning
- Planning helps to formulate the objectives clear and specific, and gives a plan of action to guide the efforts of the organization toward achieving educational goals.
- It helps to ensure optimum utilization of resources, both men and material available within the institution and makes various functions more effective and efficient.
- It seeks to get best advantage of the facilities and helps in saving time, effort, and cost by eliminating all wasteful and unproductive activities.
- It helps in drawing out plans of action for various departments, fostering cooperation and unity of purpose among them.
- Planning establishes and identifies specific goals to be achieved. These goals serve as standards of performance to be accomplished. If the actual performance deviates from the planned one, then necessary corrective steps are taken. Thus, planning provides a base for control.
- Planning provides opportunities for creative thinking and innovation for educational planners.
- A systematic and orderly educational planning acts as a motivating force to the employees to contribute to the goals.

> Time table is one important aspect of planning. The time table is an outline of the day's work, which indicates time of beginning and ending of the college day; time of beginning and ending of each class period, activities period, and work period; subjects and activities offered; days on which each class and each activity met; name of the teacher in charge of each class or activity; and time, length and number of intermissions. A time table is just like a mirror.

Types of Educational Plans

Strategic Planning
This is a long-term planning for 5–10 years. Strategic educational planning takes into consideration the totality of the educational activities.

Operational Planning
It is also called current use plan or short-term planning normally extending to a period of 1–3 years. While strategic plans indicate goals to be achieved in general

terms and formulated by the top level management, operational plans are prepared in specific terms. They take into consideration primarily short-term objectives and are concerned with day-to-day activities.

Standing Plans

Standing plans are meant for repeated use and are meant to meet similar situations recurring again. They are used again and again. They are readily available guides to action. It is used for considerably a longer period of time.

Single Use Plans

These plans have a single use or one time use for accomplishing specific objectives. A single use plan cannot be used over and over again and a new plan has to be devised to achieve new objective.

Steps in Educational Planning

The following are the steps considered in any sound educational plans:
- Setting the goals and objectives
- Generating the alternative course of action
- Analyzing and evaluating the alternatives
- Choosing the best.

Institutional Planning

Institutional planning is a program of development and improvement prepared by an educational institution on the basis of its felt needs and the resources available with a view to improving its programs and practices.

Objectives of Institutional Planning

JP Naik has listed the following objectives of an institutional plan:
- It aims at involving every teacher in the formulation and implementation of plans.
- It aims at allowing freedom to teachers to think of new ideas for the improvement of instruction and other programs in the school.
- It increases involvement and job satisfaction to teachers.
- It aims at proper and effective utilization of resources.
- It aims at providing the local community with an opportunity to help for improvement of the educational institution.
- It aims at imparting realism and concreteness to educational planning.

Scope of Institutional Planning

Institutional Objectives

The institutional administrator, at the beginning of each year, term or semester, will examine the specific objectives of the institution and its programs. These objectives should reflect the overall state of national objectives. They should also be carefully considered, noted, defined, and reflected in the institution's daily programs and functions.

Building Planning

It includes developing the physical infrastructure for existing use and for future expansion.

Program Planning

The administrator has the responsibility in planning program. The administrator prepares a comprehensive program of activities for the institution, bearing in mind the objectives and the general goals of education. A good institutional program plan will ensure continuity, sequence, and integration of the programs. The cocurricular and extracurricular activities must relate to one another.

Resource Planning

The administrator must note that the funds and facilities are limited. He must make plans for ensuring continuous supply of these resources. Such plans include arrangements for students' admissions and placement, staff appointment, development and appropriate allocation, use and accounting of institution's funds. The plans for resource acquisition, use and accounting depend on clear specification of the objectives and programs of the institution, as well as setting up a systematic program of budgeting, accountability, and control.

Work Scheduling

The administrator has to schedule the work for each and every employee of an educational institution. She should decide in advance the various tasks to be performed and who and when should be performed. A proper scheduling of work avoids duplication and ensures the effective utilization of human resources thus helps to achieve the objectives of the institution.

Organizing

"A structural framework of relationships".

Organizing refers to the formal grouping of teachers and activities to facilitate achievement of someone and he has to be made responsible for accomplishing the objectives to achieve the desired results. All this necessitates establishment of authority and responsibility relationships among various categories of personnel working in an educational organization. The organizing function, thus, has two aspects. Basically it is a process and it also results in establishment of a structural framework of relationships.

Steps Involved in Organizing

There are three basic elements of management of organization, namely:
1. Identification and grouping of work
2. Delegation of authority and responsibility
3. Establishment of relationships.

Importance of Organization

A sound organization is the first requisite of sound management. A sound organization has the following advantages:
- A well-defined assignment and grouping of work facilitates better administration and efficiency.
- It facilitates for the expansion and growth.
- It provides ample scope for adoption of new technological developments.
- It helps for the optimum use of human resources.
- It promotes better coordination among employees.
- It stimulates creativity among members and gives freedom for initiative to do the work in a better manner.

Organization Structure

Structure connotes the framework within which people act. It is the internal differentiation and patterning of relationships. In practice, structure is concerned with the pattern or network of relationships between various individuals, positions and roles in the enterprise. It is the process of logically grouping activities, delineating authority and responsibility, and establishing work relationships that will enable both the organization and the individuals to realize their mutual objectives.

Delegation of Authority

As institutions grow in size and complexity, no one person can perform all the tasks or exercise all the authority that is needed to accomplish goals. Delegation of authority denotes the superior vesting part of his powers to his/her subordinates. A single individual, however talented or efficient, cannot accomplish all the tasks by himself. The only way to achieve the desired results is to divide his load of work and to share it with others. In the process of delegation, in an educational institution, the principal divides the work and entrusts a part of the work to others.

Delegation involves:
- Dividing one's work and entrusting a part of it to others,
- Granting authority to perform the assigned work, and
- Ensuring that the subordinates perform the work according to the established standards.

Elements of Delegation

Delegation is defined as the entrustment of work and authority to another person and the creation of obligation or accountability for performance. Thus, authority, responsibility, and accountability are essential elements of delegation.

Authority: Authority is defined as the sum of legitimate rights and powers entrusted to an individual to carry out his/her assigned responsibilities or duties. Authority implies power and right to get the assigned work performed and involves the right to command, act, and make decision, direct and control.

Responsibility: It refers to a duty that is those mental and physical activities which an individual is required to perform by virtue of his membership in the organization. It denotes the obligation for the accomplishment of assigned duty. George R Terry has defined responsibility as the obligation of an individual to carry out assigned activities to the best of his ability. It must be noted that responsibility as an obligation cannot be delegated. The person who delegates continues to be responsible for what he has delegated.

Accountability: It means to be answerable for one's conduct in respect to obligations fulfilled or unfulfilled. Accountability is the obligation to carry out responsibility and exercise authority in terms of established performance standards.

Problems of Delegation

What to Delegate?

The head of the institution should decide what he/she should or should not delegate. The authority and responsibility should not be delegated for making final decisions on planning, organizing, and controlling the activities.

How Much to Delegate?

The authority to be delegated depends upon the nature of the job. While policy matters are decided by the head of the institution, the delegate is given authority to execute the job assigned to him.

How Far Down to Delegate?

As authority and responsibility go together, authority could be delegated to all those who do the work at the operating levels.

Obstacles to Delegation

The obstacles to effective delegation may rest either with the superior or with the subordinate.

The obstacles with the superior are:
- Unfamiliarity with the art of delegation
- Reluctance to delegate
- Attitude toward subordinates
- Fear for subordinates.

The obstacles with the subordinates are:
- Not willing to assume responsibility/take risk
- Lack of self-confidence and initiative and fear of failure
- Lack of incentives
- Lack of required resources.

Prerequisites for Effective Delegation

The success of delegation depends on the personality, skill, and attitude of the person who delegates and to whom it is being delegated.
- The climate of openness, trust, and confidence among employees at all levels to be ensured for effective delegation.
- The superior should not have any feeling of insecurity that by delegating they would be making themselves redundant.
- The superior has to motivate the delegate if they are reluctant to accept any delegation due to lack of confidence.
- Clear definition of responsibility and authority at each position eliminates the scope for confusion.
- The individual who delegates remains responsible for tasks he has delegated; he must ensure that his subordinates do the work.

Human Resource Planning

"Planning for the right kind of people for the right job at the right time".

According to EW Vetter, human resource planning (HRP) is a process by which an organization should move from its current manpower position to its desired manpower position.

Through planning, management strives to have the right number and right kind of people at the right places at the right time, doing things which result in both the organization and the individual receiving maximum long-run benefit.

According to Leon C Megginson, human resource planning is an integrated approach to performing the planning aspects of the personnel function in order to have a sufficient supply of adequately developed and motivated people to perform the duties and tasks required to meet organizational objectives and satisfy the individual needs and goals of organizational members.

Objectives

The important objectives of human resource planning in an organization are:
- To recruit the human resource of required quantity and quality.
- To foresee the employee turnover and make the arrangements for minimizing turnover and filling up of consequent vacancies.
- To meet the needs of the programs of expansion, diversification, etc.
- To foresee the impact of technology on work, existing employees, and future human resource requirements.
- To improve the standards, skill, knowledge, ability, discipline, etc.
- To assess the surplus or shortage of human resources and take measures accordingly.
- To minimize imbalances caused due to nonavailability of human resources of right kind, right number in right time and right place.
- To make the best use of its human resources.
- To estimate the cost of human resources.

According to Wickstram, the HRP consists of the following activities:
- Forecasting manpower requirements
- Making inventory of the present manpower
- Anticipating manpower problems
- Planning the necessary programs.

Human resources in college

Teacher as a resource
Teacher is an important instructional resource. As most of the classroom activities are dominated and controlled by the teacher, his knowledge, skills, experiences, and competencies decide to a large extent, the effectiveness of teaching.

Student as a resource
A student can also help in making instruction joyful, interesting, useful, and effective. In a classroom, there are students with varied personalities, socioeconomic backgrounds, and intellectual abilities. If all these are explored and integrated into a teacher's teaching, teaching certainly becomes very effective.

Human resource planning in educational institutions involves the following:
- Determination of the effective departments—teaching department like Medical Surgical Nursing department, Community Health Nursing department, etc. and non-teaching department like office, library, games, etc.
- Determinations of the work hours of each department.
- Analyzing the need for shifting system.
- Calculation of the teaching workload in each curriculum.
- Determination of reopening date after the summer vacation and the closing date for the summer vacation and number of holidays including Sundays.

- Determination of effective working days.
- Determination of the important events and celebration of the institution such as founder's day, institution day, annual day, sports day, etc.
- Based on the above, number of teachers required for each curriculum department is to be calculated.
- In the same way, number of staff required to carry out the office administrative work of the educational institution is also to be calculated.
- Required qualifications, qualities, and characteristics are to be written; the procedures to be followed in the process of selection are to be framed in the form of recruitment rules, policies, and procedures.
- After framing all the rules, policies and procedures, the type of training, period of training, and matter of training to be given to the selected persons are to be decided.
- The career advancement programs with a view to develop the teaching and nonteaching staff are to be constructed.
- Rules for the compensation for awards, rewards, and punishments are to be made.
- Different activities to be carried out by the teaching staff and nonteaching staff in the course of the business of the educational institutions are to be determined and the same are to be made clear to the staff.

Human Resource Inventory

The purpose of the HRP in the education institution is to assess the present and the future demand and requirement. Usually all the educational institutions maintain the details of each employee. It usually consists of the following:
- Name
- Date of birth
- Father's name/Husband's name
- Marital status
- Post for which he/she is appointed
- Qualification at the time of appointment
- Qualification acquired every year
- Compensation
- Scale of pay
  - Basic pay
  - Promoted scale
  - Personal pay, if any
  - Awards and rewards
  - Any other compensation
- Promotion
  - Date, month and year
  - Promoted position
  - Reasons and grounds for the promotions
- Achievements, if any
- Languages known
- Training given and attended
- Number of papers published
- Punishment given and its details
- Sickness, if any and its details
- Capabilities
- Number of lectures given outside
- Performance rating
- General problems faced by him/her.

This HR inventory will help the organization to select the individual teachers, staff for training and for promotion and transfer. This can provide necessary information to the top management level for decision making purpose at crucial point of time.

Recruitment

"Discovering the sources of manpower for placements".

In an educational institution, the teaching staffs are the primary staff, whereas the administrative staffs are the supporting staff. Both the teaching and nonteaching staffs are to be recruited and placed.

The term recruitment means bringing the applicants to the selection in the educational institution. It forms the first stage in the process which continues with selection and ceases with the placement of the candidate. As Yoder points out "Recruitment is a process to discover the sources of manpower to meet the requirements of the staffing schedule and to employ effective measures for attracting that manpower in adequate numbers to facilitate effective selection of efficient working force".

Factors Affecting Recruitment
- Size of the institution
- Number of departments
- Courses offered
- Specialization offered
- Employment conditions in the community
- Working conditions, salary, and other benefits
- Rate of growth of the institution
- Plan for the future expansion
- Cultural, economic and legal forces, etc.

Steps of Recruitment Process
- Preparation of the recruitment policy and rules.
- Planning and assessment of recruitment programs.
- Demand forecasting.
- Determination of the sources of recruitment.
- Writing job description and person specifications.
- Drafting the application forms and instructions to the candidates.
- Preparation of the advertisement and release in the media.
- Collecting filled up application forms.
- Handing over to the selection department.

Recruitment Policy

This, in general, serves as a guide to thinking and action of those who have to make decision in the course of accomplishment of the educational institution's goal and as such here the recruitment of the teaching and non-teaching staff. Such a policy asserts the objectives of the recruitment and provides a framework of implementation of the recruitment program in the form of procedures.

A good recruitment policy must contain these elements:
- Institution's objectives
- Identification of the recruitment needs
- Preferred sources of recruitment
- Criteria for selection and preferences
- The cost of recruitment and financial implications.

Sources of Recruitment

The sources may be internal and external.

Internal Sources

These include personnel who are already working in the institutions, i.e. its present working force. Whenever any vacancy arises in the institution, somebody within the institution is upgraded, transferred and promoted for the new position.

External Sources

These sources lie outside the institution. They usually include:
- New entrants to the labor force, i.e. the young and fresh graduates.
- The unemployed.
- Retired experienced persons.

Methods or Techniques of Recruitment

Direct Method

In this method, the management of the institution sends recruiters to colleges. In most colleges, recruiting is done in cooperation with the placement office of a college. Sometimes an organization solicits information from the head of the institution and from the professors about students with an outstanding record. Other direct methods include sending recruiters to seminars and setting up exhibits at fairs, etc.

Indirect Method

Indirect methods involve mostly advertising in newspaper, on the radio, in trade and professional journals, technical magazines and brochures. Senior posts are largely filled by such methods when they cannot be filled by promotion within.

Third Party Method

These include the use of commercial or private employment agencies, state agencies, placement offices of colleges and professional associations, recruiting firms, indoctrination seminars for college professors and friends and relatives.

Selection

The selection starts from the point where the recruitment is over or ends. The term recruitment refers to the activity of bringing the adequate number of applicants to the education institutions for the teaching and nonteaching posts. The selection process begins only after an adequate number of applicants has been secured through the recruitment. The selection procedure is concerned with securing relevant information about an applicant. The objective of the selection process is to determine whether an applicant meets the qualifications for a specific job and to choose the applicant who is most likely to perform well in that job.

Selection process starts with the initial screening interview and concludes with the final employment decision. The traditional selection process includes preliminary screening interview, completion of application form, employment tests, comprehensive interview, background investigations, physical examination, and final employment decision to hire.

Steps in Selection Procedure

- Receipt of the application form from the recruitment section
- Screening the applications
- Preliminary interviews
- Asking for additional information
- Tests, if any
- Interviews
- Checking of references
- Provisional selection
- Final selection
- Medical examination, if any
- Placement
- Induction.

Placement

It is the determination of the job to which an accepted candidate is to be assigned, and his assignment to that job. A proper placement of a worker reduces employee turnover, absenteeism and improves morale. The newly selected teachers and office bearers are to be placed on jobs for which they are being selected. After selection, the employee is generally put on a probation period ranging from 1 to 2 years after his employment and may be regularized, provided that during this period his work has been found to be satisfactory.

Induction

The newly selected teachers may not have the full acquaintance with the changing circumstances. They may not be in a position to know fully about the rules and regulations of the educational institution. Everything will be new for them. So there is an absolute necessity to orient them to the changed circumstances. This activity is called induction. So induction is a technique by which a new employee is rehabilitated into the changed surroundings and introduced to the practices, policies, and purposes of the institution. In other words, it is a welcoming process; the idea is to welcome a newcomer, make her feel at home and give her a feeling that her own job, however small, is meaningful and has significance as a part of the total institution.

Objectives of Induction

- It leads to reduction of such anxieties; dispels the irrational fears of present employees and holds colleagues responsible for assisting the newcomer, so that he may feel confident.
- It helps minimize the reality shock, which may be caused by the incompatibility between what the employees expect in their new jobs and the realities they are confronted with.
- It helps to introduce the new employee and the institution to each other, to help them become acquainted and to help them accommodate each other.

Budgeting

"A tool for financial control".

Educational institutions must prepare budgets and use them as tools of financial control. A budget is a detailed plan of operations for some specific future period. It is an estimate prepared in advance of the period to which it is applied. According to Gordon and Shilinglaw, budget may be defined as "predetermined detailed plan of action developed and distributed as a guide to current operations and as a partial basis for the subsequent evaluation of performance." The Institute of Cost and Management Accountants, England, defines a budget as "a financial and/or quantitative statement, prepared prior to a defined period of time, of the policy to be pursued during that period for the purpose of attaining a given objective". Thus, the following are the essentials of a budget:

- It is prepared in advance and it is a plan of actions for the future.
- It is related to a future period and is based on objectives to be attained.
- It is a statement expressed in monetary and/or physical units prepared for the implementation of policy formulated by the management.

Meaning of Budgetary Control

Control means, "Some sort of systematic effort to compare current performance to a predetermined plan of objective, presumably in order to take any remedial action required". According to JA Scott, "it is the system of management control and accounting in which all operations are forecast and as far as possible, planned ahead and the actual results compared with the forecast and planned ones". Thus, the budgetary control involves the following:

- Establishment of budgets
- Continuous comparison of actual with budgets for achievement of targets and placing the responsibility for failure to achieve the budget figures
- Revision of budgets in the light of changed circumstances.

Differences among Budgets, Budgeting and Budgetary Control

- Budgets are the individual objectives of a department, etc.
- Budgeting may be said to be the act of building budgets.
- Budgetary control embraces all and in addition includes the science of planning the budgets themselves and the utilization of such budgets as a tool for the business planning and control.

Budgetary control has become an essential tool of management for controlling costs and maximizing profits.

Advantages of Budgetary Control

- It compels the management to plan for the future.
- It helps to coordinate, integrate and balance the efforts of various departments in the light of the overall objectives of the enterprise. This results in goal congruency and harmony among the departments.
- It improves the quality of communication. The organization's objectives, budget goals and plans, authority and responsibility and procedures to implement plans are clearly written and communicated through budgets to all individuals in the enterprise.
- It helps to optimize the use of the organization's resources, both capital and human.
- It increases the morale and thereby the productivity.
- It develops profit-mindedness and cost-consciousness.
- It permits the management to focus attention on significant matters through budgetary reports. Thus, it facilitates management by exception and thereby saves the management's time and energy.

- It measures efficiency and enables self-evaluation and the progress.

Classification of Budgets

The following are the most common basis of classification:
- According to time
- According to function
- According to flexibility.

Classification According to Time

Long-term budgets: These budgets are designed for a long period generally for a period of 3–10 years. They are concerned with planning of the operations of a firm over a considerably long period of time.

Medium-term budgets: These are budgets for a period of 1–3 years. These normally relate to expansion of activities geographically involving forecast of income, expenditure and profit or loss.

Short-term budgets: They are designed for a period generally not exceeding 12 months.

Current budgets: These budgets cover a very short period, say, a month or a quarter. They are essentially short-term budgets adjusted to current conditions or prevailing circumstances.

Rolling budgets: Some institutions follow the practice of preparing a rolling or progressive budget. There will always be a budget for a year in advance. A new budget is prepared after the end of each month/quarter for a full year ahead. The figures for the month or quarter which are rolled down are dropped and the figures for the next month or quarter are added.

Classification According to Function

Enrollment budget: This budget forecasts total enrollment in terms of quantity, value, course, periods, areas, etc.

Production budget: It is based on enrollment budget. It forecasts quantity of production in terms of materials, periods, areas, etc.

Cost of production budget: This budget forecasts the cost of production. Separate budgets are prepared for different elements of costs such as direct materials budget, direct labor budget, office overhead budget, etc.

Purchase budget: This budget forecasts the quantity and value of purchases required for production. It gives quantity wise, money wise and period wise information about the materials to be purchased.

Personnel budget: This budget anticipates the quantity of personnel required during a period of production activity. This may be further split up between faculty and administrative personnel budgets.

Research budget: This budget is related to the research work to be done.

Capital expenditure budget: This budget provides information regarding the amount or capital that may be required for procurement of capital assets during the budget period.

Cash budget: This budget is a forecast of the cash position by time period for a specific duration of time. It states the estimated amount of cash receipts and the estimation of cash payments and the likely balance of cash in hand at the end of different periods.

Master budget: It is a summary budget incorporating all functional budgets in a capsule form.

Classification According to Flexibility

On the basis of flexibility, budgets can be divided into two categories:
1. Fixed budget
2. Flexible budget

Fixed budget: A budget prepared on the basis of a standard or a fixed level of activity is called a fixed budget. It does not change with the change in the level of activity, e.g. 100 students for a summer course.

Flexible budget: A budget designed in a manner so as to give the budgeted cost of any level of activity is termed as a flexible budget. Here a budget is prepared for different levels of activity, e.g. 100, 200, 300, and 500 students for a summer course or any other course.

Others Types of Budget

Operating budget: The budget shows planned operations for the forthcoming period, including revenues, expenses and related changes in an inventory. It covers in its ambit enrollment budget, production budget, cost of production budget, etc. Operating budget usually consists of two parts:
1. Program budget
2. Responsibility budget

Program budget: It consists of estimated revenues and costs of the major programs that the institution plans to undertake during the forthcoming period. Such a budget can be prepared in respect of each project or course giving details of revenue, costs, and resultant profit in respect of each one of them. However, they are not suitable for exercising control over individuals since various persons may be responsible for individual costs of a project or course with no one of them being responsible for total operation. It is also termed as a project or a product budget.

Responsibility budget: It is a budget which identified the revenues and costs with an individual responsible for their incurrence. Such a budget is an excellent control device since it identifies with the individual only such revenues and costs which are controlled by him.

Enrollment budget: Enrollment and revenue budgets are important budgets as regards to educational institutions. Enrollment budget is a forecast of total enrollment expressed and incorporated in quantities and/or money. It is prepared in relation to the courses offered, types of students, such as national and international, and duration, etc. It is usually done with the analysis of past enrollment with adjustment for current conditions.

Expense budget: Expenses budget in respect of educational institutions can be prepared departmentwise/coursewise/expenditure-classwise, and so on.

Performance Budgeting: Performance budget may be defined as a budget based on functions, activities, and projects. Performance budgeting may be described as a budgeting system where *input* costs are related to the end results, i.e. performance. It involves evaluation of the performance of the organization in the context of both specific as well as overall objectives of the organization.

Discipline

"Self-discipline is the best discipline".

No organization can grow and prosper without discipline and so the case of educational institutions. The educational institutions are the places where the discipline is being taught. Discipline is absolutely necessary with not only the students but also the teaching and other staff members. Maintenance of effective discipline in the educational institutions ensures the most economical and optimum utilization of various resources including human resources. The effective discipline is the basis for growth and development of education, education innovation, research and the better coordination with the meaningful human relations.

Meaning and Definition

Actually the discipline is the practical behavior of a person. But the discipline differs from situation to situation, person to person, and according to the relations. The Webster's dictionary gives three basic meanings of the word "discipline".
1. Discipline is the training that corrects, molds, or perfects the mental faculties or moral character.
2. It is control gained by enforcing obedience, and
3. It is punishment or chastisement.

Need for Disciplinary Measures

Disciplinary measures are absolutely essential:
- To increase the efficiency of the employee—both teaching and nonteaching.
- To maintain peace, prevent anarchy and regulate behavior of people including students.
- To bring the change.
- To convert the static staff to the dynamic staff.
- To move toward the predetermined goal of the educational institutions.
- To promote the teamwork by providing equal treatment.

Aspects of Discipline

There are two aspects of discipline. They are positive and negative.

Positive Aspects

Employees believe in and support discipline and adhere to the rules, regulations and desired standards of behavior. Discipline takes the form of positive support and reinforcement for approved actions and its aim is to help the individual in molding his behavior and developing him in a corrective and supportive manner. This type of approach is called positive approach or constructive discipline or self-discipline. Positive approach takes place by payment of adequate remuneration and incentives, appropriate avenues for career advancement, appreciation of proper performance and reinforcement of approved personnel behavior or actions, etc. which all motivate employees to adhere to certain rules and regulations or exercise self-control and work to the maximum possible extent.

Negative Aspect

Employees sometimes do not believe in and support discipline. As such, they do not adhere to rules, regulations and desired standard of behavior. As such, disciplinary program forces and constraints the employees to obey orders and function in accordance with the set rules. This approach to discipline is called as negative approach or corrective approach or punitive approach. This approach is also called autocratic approach as the subordinates are given no role in formulating the rules and they are not told why they are punished.

Indiscipline

Indiscipline means disorderliness, insubordination and not following the rules and regulations of an organization. The symptoms of indiscipline are change in the normal behavior, absenteeism, apathy, go slow at work, increase in number and severity of grievances, persistent and continuous demand for overtime allowance, lack of concern for performance, etc.

Approaches to Discipline

Human relations approach: The employee is treated as human being and his acts of indiscipline will be dealt from the viewpoint of human values, aspiration, problems, needs, goals, behavior, etc. Under human relations approach, the employee is helped to correct his deviations.

Human resources approach: The employees are treated as a resource and the acts of indiscipline are dealt by considering the failures in the areas of development, maintenance, and utilization of human resources under the human resources approach.

Group discipline approach: The group, as a whole, sets the standards of discipline and punishments for the deviations. The individual employees are awarded punishments for their violation under the group discipline approach.

The leadership approach: Every superior administers the rules of discipline and guides, trains, and controls the subordinates regarding disciplinary rules under the leadership approach.

Judicial approach: In judicial approach, indisciplinary cases are dealt on the basis of legislation and court decisions.

Some of the Disciplinary Procedures

Issuing a letter of charge to the employee: The management can issue the charge-sheet to the employee for his misconduct. It should indicate clearly and precisely the charges of indiscipline or misconduct.

Calling upon him for explanation: Explanation should also be called from the employee who has performed some misconduct.

Consideration of the explanation: The employer has to consider the explanation given by the employee. When the employer is satisfied with the explanation, they may not take any disciplinary action. On the contrary when the management is not satisfied with the explanation, there is a need for serving a show-cause notice.

Serving a show-cause notice: In the show-cause notice, the employer provides another chance to the employee to explain his conduct and rebut the charges made against him.

Holding of a full-fledged enquiry: An enquiry officer will conduct a full-fledged enquiry and he should record his findings in the process of an enquiry. He may also suggest the nature of disciplinary action to be taken. The employee must be given a reasonable opportunity of being heard.

Nature of punishment: It includes dismissal from the service, suspension for some time, demotion, transfer or withdrawing some privileges such as cutting the increments or promotions.

Types of Punishment

Oral warnings: Whenever an employee commits minor omissions, he may be given an oral reprimand by the superior concerned. Repeated warnings may bring down the level of morale of the employee; oral warnings should be used sparingly.

Written warnings: Written warning is given, whenever oral warnings fail to achieve the desired behavior.

Loss of privileges and fines: Sometimes some amount of fine may be charged for the employee and certain privileges, e.g. leave facilities or canteen facilities are cut.

Punitive suspension: Under punitive suspension the employer prohibits the employee from performing the tasks assigned to him and the wages are withheld or withdrawn during the period of such prohibition.

Withholding of increments: This is a major punishment. Under this method, the employer withholds the annual increments of the delinquent employee in a graded scale.

Demotion: Under the kinds of punishment, an employee is reduced to a lower grade from the grade enjoyed by him earlier.

Termination

The employee's services can be terminated in the following forms:

Discharge and Dismissal

When the conduct of an employee is damned to be incompatible with the faithful discharge of his duties and undesirable or against the interests of the employer to continue him in employment, dismissal will be justified. This is an extreme kind of punishment. But in case of discharge, an employer terminates the employment of employee either by giving agreed advance notice or by paying money in lieu of such notice. Though both discharge and dismissal culminate in termination of employment, discharge is regarded as some kind of punishment less severe than that of dismissal. Discharge requires either an advance notice or payment of money in lieu thereof, whereas there is no such requirement in case of dismissal.

Discharge Simpliciter

If termination of the service of an employee may not be on account of his misconduct but may be for certain other reasons which do not cause a slur on him. This is referred to as discharge simpliciter. In such a case, if the employee challenges the employer's bona fides, the employer must prove them.

Follow-up

After taking disciplinary action except for the termination, there should be proper follow-up. The disciplinary action should not make the employee repeat his mistake.

Creating a Climate for Discipline

- Make rules, guidelines, regulations, procedures, etc.
- Prepare the managerial policies.
- Clearly state that to whom each staff has to report.
- Have clear cut duties and responsibilities for each job position.
- Ensure proper and effective supervision.
- Make a proper system of routine activities.
- Keep a record of the important activities to be carried out.
- Establish the standards for each activity.
- View discipline as a corrective measure.
- Maintain consistency in disciplinary actions. Do not institute discipline on routine basis.
- Be clear with the disciplinary actions taken for any misconduct and communicate the same to all.
- Make all such issues in writing in the form of manual and such manuals are to be distributed among the staff.

Public Relations

"A goodwill and mutual understanding between an organization and its publics."

Public relation (PR), in general, is a management function that involves monitoring and evaluating public attitudes and maintaining mutual relations and understanding between an organization and its public. Public could include shareholders, government, consumers, employees, and the media. It is the act of getting along with people we constantly come in touch with. It focuses on two-way communication and fostering of mutually beneficial relationships between an organization and its public. Today, public relations affect all types of organizations. Public relation analyzes the effects of organizational policies and the reactions of the public. The public is a very important part of an organization and is essential for its survival and success.

Today, nursing has the opportunity to shape the future of healthcare. Nurses are creating partnerships with physicians, other healthcare professionals, patients, and family members. Nurses are assuming leadership roles in case management, managed care, and home health. This is a critical period in the history of nursing. We must seize the opportunity to market the nurse's role. We must let the public understand what nursing is all about. Public relation strategy helps the nurses to do this. Nurses also have a public relations responsibility to maintain a positive image in this time of changing healthcare. Nurses can influence the changes and promote their roles by adopting various public relation activities.

Meaning and Definition

The Institute of Public Relation of England defines public relations practice as "the planned and sustained effort to establish and maintain goodwill and mutual understanding between an organization and its publics". As public is more diverse, public relation is essential to communicate with them. The basic components and activities of public relations as mentioned in Table 11.1 explain the importance of public relations. In this connection, public is concerned with many marketing tasks like:

- Building and maintaining image.
- Handling problems and issues smoothly.
- Reinforcing positioning.
- Influencing the public to a position favorable to the service provider, and
- Preparing the public favorably while launching new services.

The Role of Public Relations for Nursing

- Building awareness and a favorable image for nurses and to nursing profession.
- Closely monitoring numerous media channels for public comment about nursing and nursing profession.
- Managing crises that threaten the nurses and the image of nursing profession.
- Building goodwill among patient, family, and the public through community, philanthropic and special programs, and events.

Advantages of Public Relations

Public Relations offer several advantages:

- PR is often considered a highly credible form of promotion.
- A well-structured PR campaign can result in the target market being exposed to more detailed information than they receive with other forms of promotion. That is, media sources often provide more space and time for explanation of a product or service.
- Depending on the media outlet, the concept about the nursing may be picked up by a large number of additional media, thus, spreading a single story to many locations.
- Public relations objectives can be achieved at very low-cost when compared to other promotional efforts.

Table 11.1: The basic components of public relations.

Counseling	Providing advice to management concerning policies, relationships, and communications.
Research	Determining attitudes and behaviors of the public in order to plan public strategies.
Media relations	Working with mass media in seeking publicity.
Publicity	Disseminating planned messages through selected media to promote the image of nursing.
Employee/Member relations	Responding to concerns, informing and motivating other employees or members.
Community relations	Planned activity with a community to maintain an environment that benefits both.
Public affairs	Developing effective involvement in public policy and meeting the public expectations. The term is also used by government agencies to describe their public relations activities and by many corporations as an umbrella term to describe multiple public relations activities.
Government affairs	Relating directly with legislatures and regulatory agencies on behalf of the nurses and nursing profession. Lobbying can be a part of the government affairs program.
Issues management	Identifying and addressing issues of public concern that affect nursing.
Financial relations	Creating and maintaining investor confidence and building good relationships with the financial community
Industry relations	Relating with organization and other healthcare industries and with trade associations.
Development/ Fund-raising	Demonstrating the need for development and encouraging the public to support nursing, primarily through financial contributions.
Special events	Stimulating interest in a person (nurse who has contributed to the nursing profession), or nursing service by means of a focused "happening"; also, activities designed to interact with public and listen to them.
Marketing communications	Combination of activities designed to sell nursing service, or idea, including advertising, collateral materials, publicity, promotion, direct mail, trade shows, and special events.

Disadvantages of Public Relations

First, while public relation uses many of the same channels as advertising, such as newspapers, magazines, radio, TV and Internet, it differs significantly from advertising in that marketers do not have direct control over whether a message is delivered and where it is placed for delivery.

Second, while other promotional messages are carefully crafted and distributed as written through a predetermined placement in a media vehicle, public relation generally conveys information to a member of the news media (e.g. reporter) who then recrafts the information as part of a news story or feature. Thus, the final message may not be precisely what the marketer planned.

Third, while a PR campaign has the potential to yield a high return on promotional expense, it also has the potential to produce the opposite if the news media feels there is little value in running a story pitched (i.e. suggested via communication with the news outlet) by the marketer.

Fourth, with PR there is always a chance that a well-devised news event or release will get "bumped" from planned media coverage because of a more critical breaking news story, such as wars, severe weather or serious crime. Finally, in some areas of the world the impact of traditional news outlets is fading forcing public relations professionals to scramble to find new ways to reach their target markets.

Objectives of Public Relations

Public relations are used to address several broad objectives including building awareness and creating interest.

Providing information: PR can be used to provide customers with more in-depth information through articles, collateral materials, newsletters, and websites. PR delivers information to customers that can help them gain understanding.

Stimulating demand: A positive article in a newspaper, or a TV news show or an advertisement on the Internet, often results in a discernible increase in demand or product sales.

Reinforcing the brand: The public relations function is also involved with brand reinforcement by maintaining positive relationships with key audiences, and thereby aiding in building a strong image. Today it is even more important for companies and brands to build a good image. A strong image helps the company build its business and it can help the company in times of crises as well. Same thing can be applied to educational institutions too.

Public Relations Tools

Print Media

It is the common tool used in public relation such as newspaper, etc.

Press Release

The press release is the most common material provided to media outlets. These documents provide a brief, yet thorough, description of an upcoming activity.

Photographs

There are usually two types of photographs in publicity portrait shots, where people pose for the camera and smile, and candid, where the subjects are doing something.

Case Histories/Studies
Case studies which show a good image of the nurses are shared with the media/investors, community, etc.

Editorials
No money, high credibility, however, no control over message.

Advertorials
Advertisement + Editorial.
Control over message, pay lesser than an advertisement. It is a strategic tool, but should not be used too often.

Interviews/Features
Meeting journalists. Here, there is a room for different interpretations. Even though the media contact will likely rewrite them, possibly including additional quotes or information they research on their own, the press releases should be written well enough. Sometimes a press release will encourage a reporter to do more, such as conduct a full interview with chapter members or write a feature article on an upcoming project.

Brochure
A booklet published by the nurses which contains the profession's background, its ethics, vision, mission, its past, present and future, etc.

Poster and Calendar
Any poster or calendar used to achieve a public relations objective.

Written Speech
The typewritten or printed text of a speech given to achieve a public relations objective.

Internal Newsletters and Publications
It is within the organization to create awareness and to inform the activities to other departments.

Event and Press Support
Special events are acts of news development. The ingredients are time, place, people, and activities. Exhibitions, seminars, and workshops are some of the events, which can be reported.

Letters to the Editor
Submitting these articles does not require a media contact. This also gives an opportunity for any member to submit a letter on their chapter for printing in a local or campus newspaper.

Analysts Brief
One tells about the organization, what it is doing. It is done to influence the consumers, employees, and media.

Conferences and Seminars
Sponsoring conferences and seminars is one method of public relation activity.

Internet
This one medium has helped transform the whole business of marketing and public relations. In a way, it gives any organization, the ability to promote themselves without having to rely solely on other media outlets. Websites and e-mail are the two most common methods to use the Internet for PR purposes.

Website
An organization's website should not only be designed to serve as a resource for members, but it should also present a positive message to nonmembers just "browsing through". Brief descriptions of history, past projects and activities, and long-standing relationships with other organizations may give an outsider a positive impression of the fraternity. Like the newsletter, information for members should not just inform, it should also encourage involvement and develop enthusiasm.

E-mail
Today, this has become the most common method used for communication between fraternity members. It can also be used to promote an organization to fellow students and others, but it should be used carefully.

Audio and visual
This division includes any audio or audio-visual presentation or program, which serves a public relations objective.

Audio Presentation
Any sound-only program, including telephone hot lines and other recorded messages, radio programs, public service announcements and audio news releases help to promote an organization.

Audio-Visual Presentation
Any internal or external audio-visual presentation using still illustrations, with or without sound, using one or more projectors will be helpful.

Film or Video
Any film or video which presents information to an organization's internal audiences achieves the purpose.

The key tools available for PR include:
- Media relations
- Media tours
- Newsletters
- Special events
- Speaking engagements
- Sponsorships
- Employee relations
- Community relations and philanthropy.

Media Relations

Key tools used in media relations include:

Press kits: It includes written information such as news, release, organization background, key spokesperson biographies and other supporting materials that provide information useful to reporters.

Audio or video news releases: These are prerecorded features distributed to news media that may be included within media programming.

Matte release: Some media, especially small local newspapers, may accept articles written by the organization often as filler material when their publication lacks sufficient content. PR professionals submit matte releases through syndicated services (i.e. services that supply content to many media outlets) or directly to targeted media via e-mail or fax.

Website press room: While hard copies of materials are used and preferred by some media, marketers are well served by an online press room that caters to media needs and provides company/organization contact information.

Media Tour

On a media tour, an organization's spokesperson travels to key cities to introduce a service rendered by them by being booked on TV and radio talk shows and conducting interviews with print and Internet reporters or influencers (e.g. bloggers). The spokesperson can be an employee of the organization or someone hired. A media tour may include other kinds of personal appearances in conjunction with special events, such as public appearances, speaking engagements or autograph signing opportunities.

Newsletters

An organization that has captured names and addresses of customers and potential customers can use a newsletter for regular contact with their targeted audience. They can use newsletters to provide content of interest to customers as well as information on services and events of importance. Effective newsletters are sought out and well received by interested audiences.

Special Events

Special events can be designed to reach a specific narrow target audience. As with all PR programs, special event planners must work hard to ensure the program planned conveys the correct message and image to the target audience.

Speaking Engagements

Speaking in university meetings, conferences, graduation ceremonies, etc. provides an opportunity for experts to demonstrate their expertise to potential clients/customers. Nevertheless, the right speaking engagement puts the organization in front of a good target audience and offers networking opportunities for generating customer leads.

Employee Communications

For many larger organizations communicating regularly with employees is important in keeping employees informed of organization's programs, personnel issues, as well as keeping them updated on new ventures and programs. In larger firms, an in-house PR department often works in conjunction with the Human Resources Department to develop employee communications.

Community Relations and Philanthropy

For many institutions fostering good relations with key audiences includes building strong relationships with their regional community. An organization implements programs supportive of the community ranging from supporting local organizations such as schools and institutions (e.g. community activities, parks) to conducting educational workshops (e.g. for teachers, parents) to donating product for community events and charitable fund raisers. The goal is generally to develop a positive relationship with members of the community (i.e. be known as a good neighbor). Some organizations also make an effort to contribute to charitable organizations.

Additional PR Activities

In addition to serving as means for helping to achieve marketing objectives, public relations professionals may undertake additional activities, aimed at maintaining a positive image for an organization. These activities include:

Market Monitoring

Monitoring public comment about an organization and its service is becoming increasingly important especially with the explosion of information channels on the internet. Today monitoring includes watching, what is written and reported in traditional print and broadcast media and also keeping an eye on discussions occurring through various Internet outlets such as forums, chatrooms, blogs and other public messaging areas. Organizations must be prepared to respond quickly to erroneous information and negative opinions about their service as it can spin out of control very quickly through the new technology channels. Failure to correct misinformation can be devastating to an organization's reputation.

Crisis Management

Marketers need to be prepared to respond quickly to negative information about the organization and its service. Today, with the prevalence of the internet and wireless communications, negative information can spread rapidly. Through monitoring, marketers can track the issues and respond in a timely fashion.

Trends in Public Relations

The newer technologies, especially internet is quickly gaining widespread acceptance among internet users and is becoming new media outlets. The important trends in public relations include the following.

Voicing Opinion

Developing websites has long been time-consuming and expensive, and it requires technical competency. But this changed with the evolution of easier-to-use site development applications, which allow for quick creation and convenient updating of site content. Where previously the main objective of a website was for advertising, delivering information, the web now serves as a platform for people to voice their opinions. There are two key applications that fall into this category—blogs and forums.

Blogs

Blogs, short for weblogs, are a phenomenon that shows just how powerful and influential the internet has become as a communication medium. Millions of blogs are now available, and specialized search engines have been developed to search millions of postings. Blogs may be most famous as a tool for discussion, but they are also becoming an important communication tool for public relations. These blogs allow nurses to post messages updating developments and, thus, serve as useful PR tool.

Forums

Web forums are the child of the old internet bulletin board services where people can post their opinion often anonymously. Forums pose both opportunities and threats for those involved in PR. The forums can cause major problems as a breeding ground for rumor and accusation. Public relations personnel must continually monitor forums and respond to misguided comments posted on a web discussion board to help squelch rumors before they can catch fire.

Really Simple Syndication (RSS) Feeds

An important trend for delivering information is through an internet technology known by the acronym RSS (Really Simple Syndication or Rich Site Summary). This technology makes it easy for people to know when new content is posted to a website.

The nature of the technology allows anyone who links to the RSS feed to instantly receive details of the content. Many journalists and other media members are finding this to be a more convenient way to acquire information.

Podcasting

The emergence of the Apple iPod and other digital audio players has significantly altered how people listen to music by allowing easy downloading of desired songs. But the use of audio players is not limited to music downloads; a fast growing application is to deliver other content including programming. Public relations may utilize podcasting to be a quick and easy way to send out audio news releases and other promotional material.

Search Engine Optimization

Publicity is about getting media outlets to mention the name of a product, company or person. For several years internet marketers have recognized the importance of getting their organization and their services listed in the top rankings in search engines. So called efforts at Search Engine Optimization (SEO) involve concerted efforts and specific techniques to attain higher rankings.

Facebook

Facebook is a popular free social networking website that allows registered users to create profiles, upload photos and video, send messages and keep in touch with friends, family, colleagues, and others. This can be a powerful way to communicate with customers and potential customers, allowing them to see one's product or service without having to visit one's premises. This function can be used to promote public relation. Through Facebook, one can create awareness of their brand and advertise about their product.

Twitter

Twitter is an online news and social networking site where people communicate in short messages called tweets. Tweeting is posting short messages for anyone who follows the person on Twitter. Twitter is used to connect people with the same interests. This process of connecting people who are complete strangers can be done with the use of hashtags. Hashtags, which are denoted with the "#" prefix, are added to tweets so members of the community can share in the conversation. A tweet is a post in the twitter. Twitter is also used for branding purposes, bringing information of a brand out to the masses easily. Tweeting about articles and web pages helps drive more traffic to them, ultimately creating the possibility of better rank.

Instagram

Instagram is a social networking app made for sharing photos and videos from a smart phone. Similar to Facebook or Twitter, everyone who creates an Instagram account has a profile and news feed. When one posts a photo or video on Instagram, it will be displayed on his/her profile. It is like a simplified version of Facebook, with an emphasis on mobile use and visual sharing. Just like other social networks, one can interact with other users on Instagram by following them, being followed by them, commenting, liking, tagging and private messaging. Every user profile has a "Followers" and "Following" count, which represents how many people they follow and how many other users follow them. This can be effectively used in public relations.

So how can nursing contribute to these changes? First, no one can do it for us. We must take the risks and inspire others. When we read or see something about nursing, we should respond. Write a letter to an editor or media journalist; express your views and offer positive examples. Remember, the most powerful image builder is how nursing presents itself with clients, peers, and the public. First impressions are very important. Finally, nursing should participate in community and political activities. As nurses assume new roles and contribute to the changing market, the profession will be seen as a necessary and dynamic part of healthcare's evolution. In turn, this will inspire and motivate both current and prospective nurses.

Nurses have a public relations responsibility to maintain a positive image in this time of changing healthcare. Nursing, which is the most populous healthcare profession, is most strongly perceived by how nurses present themselves. All these changes in nursing and how healthcare is practiced can enhance the image of nursing. Nurses can be seen as a positive role model, collaborator, and integral change agent. Nursing should focus on its successes and contributions. Negative images of nursing will then vanish.

Performance Appraisal

"Subjective assessment based on objective measurement".

Definition and Meaning

The performance appraisal is a recent and modern terminology used in every organization to revive the work performance of their employees. It is also otherwise known as behavioral assessment, employee evaluation, personnel review, staff assessment, service rating and fitness report, etc. However, the term performance appraisal or evaluation is most widely used.

According to Heyel, the performance appraisal is "the process of evaluating the performance and qualifications of the employees in terms of other requirements of the job for which he is employed, for purposes of administration including placement, selection for promotions, providing financial rewards and other actions, which require differential treatment among the members of a group as distinguished from actions affecting all members equally". It is a process of estimating or judging the value, excellence, qualities or status of some object, person or thing. According to Hendry, it is the evaluation of work done during specified period against the background of the total work situation. Performance appraisal is assessment of how staff member is doing his job. Employee performance is the product of three underlying factors, that is, ability, motivation, and environment. A defect in any of the three will impair his performance. The objective of the performance appraisal is to encourage and development of employee who will meet the organization's objectives.

Evaluation is a subjective judgment based on objective measurement.
—Gardner

Evaluation is a process of judging the value or something by certain appraisal.
—Goods

Importance of Performance Appraisal

Performance appraisal helps in:
- Determining the training needs of an employee. It serves as a base for coaching and counseling the individual by the superior.
- Providing adequate feedback to each individual for his or her performance.
- Improving or changing behavior toward some effective working habits.
- Providing data to administrators with which they may judge future job assignments and compensation.

Improving the efficiency of an organization by attempting to mobilize the best possible efforts from individuals employed in it.
- Planning for promotions, transfers, and job rotations.
- Maintaining individual and group development by informing the employee of his performance standard.
- Determining increments and provide a reliable index for promotions and transfers to positions of greater responsibility.
- To determine job competence.
- To enhance staff development and motivate personnel toward higher achievement.
- To discover employee's aspirations and to recognize accomplishments.
- To improve communications between managers.

Principles of Performance Appraisal

There are some basic principles that can help to minimize the difficulties associated with performance appraisal which include:
- Objectives of appraisal are informed to all parties.
- Results of appraisal are informed to all persons.
- The appraisal process and tool are developed with input from all levels of employees affected by the job responsibilities.
- In nursing, certain principles must be followed to evaluate subordinate's job performance accurately and fairly as given below.
- Assess performance in relation to behaviorally stated work goals.
- An adequate representative sample of the nurse's job behavior should be observed to provide a basis for evaluation.
- Compare supervisor's evaluation with employee's self-evaluation. The nurse should be given a copy of her job description, performance standards, and performance evaluation form to review before the evaluation conference.
- Involvement of personnel in all phases of evaluative process increases beliefs in the fairness, and accuracy of the evaluation establishes a commitment to the evaluation and increases motivation and utilizes the results.
- Clear and concise role delineation and job descriptions enable employee, employer, and client to know the duties and responsibilities of the job.
- Clear standards and criteria for measuring performance increase the objectivity and validity of evaluation.
- Use of appropriate assessment tools and sufficient evaluative data gathered from varied situations increases the validity of the conclusions in the assessment of work performance.
- Use of self-evaluation process promotes growth and development of the appraiser and contributes to better quality of care.
- Informal and formal assessments that are noted and recorded systematically provide significant input to the evaluation process.
- The evaluator who establishes mutual trust and confidence with the person evaluated and who is familiar with the criteria for evaluation increases the accuracy and usefulness of the evaluation.
- A well-planned performance review session increases the workers' effectiveness and promotes satisfaction.
- Improvement of workers' competence leads to self-improvement strategies with coaching by management.
- An evaluation process that includes reciprocal participation both vertically and horizontally provides an avenue for high level of morale and job satisfaction.

Teaching Evaluation Model

Polifroni Ec (2008) suggested this model.
Teaching and teaching strategy evaluation is done by:
- Students—2 to 3 times per course
- Peers—2 times by 2 peers per course
- Self-created portfolio—each time class taught
- Administrators—end of semester or year and more often as needed.

Performance Appraisal Process

The process of performance appraisal includes:
- Assess institutional and personal needs and set goals
- Develop policies and procedures for performance appraisal
- Establish performance standards, objectives, and time frame
- Communicate these standards to the employees
- Assess the performance
- Compare the actual with the standards
- Discuss periodically the results
- Initiate corrective actions when necessary
- Evaluate the performance.

Components of Comprehensive Appraisal System

It provides an over-reaching framework for the process:
- Clear determination of the abilities required for the position (job description).
- A match of the key requirements for the position with the individual capabilities (match abilities of the employee with job requirements).
- Development of the abilities of the employee (staff development).
- Using a motivational reward system to enhance employee performance.

- Performance attributes of an individual are determined by two elements such as ability and motivation.

Tool for Performance Appraisal

- Free response reports
- Ranking
- Performance checklist
- Rating scale
- Numerical rating scale
- Lettered rating scale
- Graphic rating scale
- Descriptive rating scale
- Forced choice writing
- Behaviorally anchored rating scale (BARS).

Obstacles of effective performance appraisal are:
- Lack of support from top management
- Resistance on the part of evaluators
- Evaluate biases and rating errors, which result in unreliable and invalid ratings
- Lack of clear, objective standards of performance
- Failure to communicate purposes and results in unreliable and invalid ratings
- Lack of suitable appraisal tool.

Problems of performance appraisal:
- Halo effect
- Horn effect
- Central tendency error
- Self-aggrandizing effect rates worker so as to create favorable view of manager.

Alternative Types of Performance Appraisal

To minimize the factors of bias in the performance appraisal, the manager should utilize other methods to perform a fair evaluation of the performance on each employee.

Some of the alternative methods include:
- 360-degree evaluation: It can be obtained by seeking input from approximately four sources—a peer, a physician, a subordinate, and a self-evaluation.
  Once all the input is obtained, the evaluating manager adds his or her input and merges the feedback to develop the final score.
- Management by objectives: In this method, the employee and manager establish performance goals for the upcoming appraisal year.
  Management by objectives may be helpful in defining goal and objective for the next year and providing the manager with a specific set of goals to follow up with the individual at regular intervals.
- Peer review or peer evaluation: Peer evaluation is an evaluation done by colleagues or peers, of all teaching related activities for either formative (for development) or summative (for personnel decision) purposes. Components of either type of evaluation may include course materials, student evaluations, course and teaching portfolios, documentation of teaching philosophy, teacher self-assessments, classroom observations and other activities which may be appropriate to a discipline.

Peer evaluation is a process by which employees of some professional rank and setting evaluate one another job performance against accepted standard.
—O'Loughlin and Kaulbech

Purposes

- It provides feedback to share ideas among nurses.
- It helps to compare the consistency of nurse's performances and its standard.
- It helps to recognize outstanding performance of nursing staff.
- To identify the area and share there is a need of further development.
- It provides personal and professional growth.
- Promote accountability to one's practice.
- To maintain high quality of nursing care.
- To determine pay raises and promotions.

Who are peer evaluators?
The word peer means "a person of equal standing" but in the context of the peer evaluation of teaching the definition is expanded to include faculty members of the same or different ranks, which might also be referred to as colleagues or mentors.

Guiding Principles of Peer Evaluation

- There must be acceptance of teacher evaluation with the college as integral part of educational process.
- In the process of evaluation, teacher development will occur only if a constructive approach is followed.
- Collaboration and mutual respect between teacher and evaluator are essential.
- Teacher self-appraisal must become a significant part of the process.

Types

Peer evaluation can be informal or formal. It may be formative or summative.

Informal Feedback

Nurses frequently observe and judge their colleagues' performance. The feedback may be informally shared among them on an ongoing basis.

Formal Feedback

The evaluation process is fully integrated into the structure of an organization. A formal feedback system should have the job description and clearly defined standards of practice to be measured.

Formative Evaluation

It describes activities that are to provide teachers with information that they can use to improve their teaching. It is intended for their personal use, hence it is less formal.

Summative Evaluation

It describes activities that are conducted to gain information needed to make personnel decisions such as promotion, reappointment, tenure, or comprehensive review of tenured faculty relative to teaching performance. It is more formal in nature.

Characteristics of Peer Review

Peer review should:
- Be collegial
- Be open
- Use multiple sources of data
- Be honest and ethical
- Be formative.

Who will Evaluate?

Some agency: Peer evaluators are selected by lot.

In other: The nurse herself selects for evaluators (one or more evaluators).

In some other agency: All appraisers should work in the same unit as the evaluator.

Appraisers meet together and decide, who will evaluate each aspect of nurse's performance.

Peer Evaluation Process Includes:
- Review of an employee's self-evaluation including short- and long-term goals.
- Review of reference letters, committee work, special project, additional education, performance evaluation from the immediate managers, care plans, charting, observation of the nurse, patient interview, summary of the findings and presentation of the findings, recommendation of the nurse are done and a written review is prepared.
- Once the candidate is evaluated there should be a peer review interview for feedback. All feedback must be well documented on the review material. Rumor reports are not permitted.

Disadvantages

- Peer review can be threatening and time consuming.
- Staff needs to be educated on the process of peer evaluation.
- May cause distrust among colleagues.
- Friendship among the peers can result in inflated evaluation or interpersonal conflict may result in unfair appraisals.

Student Evaluation of the Teacher

Students have a right and responsibility to evaluate, how well the teacher contributed to the student's ability to master the content, how well the faculty member presented the material in a manner that was understood by the student, how the faculty member's feedback helped the student in directing his or her energy toward success in the course, and how the faculty member interacted with the student to enhance overall learning and interest in the topic. These are questions only students can answer and the data should be used to guide teachers in making changes in their teaching strategies so that the student responses are favorable in future years.

Self-evaluation

Self-evaluation is the evaluation of one's job performances.

Self-evaluation is important for nurse leader because knowledge of self will enhance their leadership ability and potential.

The Reasons for Self-evaluation

- Each individual knows himself best and is aware of his strength and weakness and of his efforts to achieve his personal and his organization's goal.
- To gain information for self-improvement, growth and development and the achievement of personal goals in a socially acceptable manner.
- To enhance and improve human relations.

Demerits of Self-evaluation

Individuals do not wish to reveal their weakness and shortcomings on the job, more so as this information may be used against them when administrative decisions are taken.

In general, self-appraisals are inflated as most employees have been unrealistically favorable of their own performances.

Academic Audit

"An educational exercise."

Academic audit is an educational exercise to assess and evaluate the performance of teachers and to have a pragmatic view about what the present status of academic standards is. This helps in measuring the true performance and contributions of every teacher on regular basis as well as to guide him about the areas where further improvement is needed. The ultimate purpose of academic audit is to bring improvement in the performance through techniques of motivation and control.

Objectives of Academic Audit

- To establish a goal-oriented performance appraisal system in educational institutions.
- To remove bias, prejudices, and subjectivism in the method of performance evaluation.
- To bring out a high level of performance evaluation.
- To motivate teacher to contribute extensively for improvement of educational standards and development of academic culture.
- To introduce an invisible but effective mechanism of educational control.

Academic audit is an evaluation system which not only intends to evaluate the performance of teachers but at the same time it throws light on academic culture in an educational institution. It not only tells us to what a teacher has done in an academic year, but at the same time explains how educational institutions and planners have helped the teachers in achieving their desired target. The educational planners can establish an ideal academic audit system after considering the following factors:

- The nature of the institution.
- The type of academic activities and performance of the institution.
- Courses and educational programs conducted by the institution.
- Qualifications and standards of teachers.
- Type of infrastructural facilities available in the institution.
- Various conditions governing the education activity.
- Facilities available for research, extension and development activities in the institution.
- Linkages with other institutions of national repute.
- Facility of retraining and refresher program provided to the teachers.

Advantages of Academic Audit

It can help the educational planners, heads of institutions, and educational policy makers as well as the teachers to understand the strengths and weaknesses of the existing educational system. The academic audit helps in various ways to have a rational performance appraisal of the teacher.

Academic audit as a tool for performance appraisal helps in:
- Regular teaching and educational advancement
- Career advancement
- Professional excellence
- Enhancing quality standards

- Developing socially useful and productive research
- Value generation
- Generating new vistas of knowledge
- Planning social and extension services.

Format for Academic Audit to Teachers

Name :
Age :
Sex :
Name of the department :
Position held :
Previous position :
Date of joining :
Years of experience in present position :

Academic Performance

Workload as per norms	Period/ Week	Actual work done	Remarks
Teaching			
GNM			
BSc(N)			
Post-basic BSc(N)			
MSc(N)			
Clinical Supervision			
GNM			
BSc(N)			
Post-basic BSc(N)			
MSc(N)			
Guidance to research scholars			
Extension activities			

Publications (National/International)

Sl. No.	Title	National/ International	Name of the Journal/ Volume/Issue	Month and year of publication

Research Activities

Independent research activities undertaken
- Completed during the years:
- Continued during the years:
- Project in the primary stage of commencement:

Sl. No.	Nature of enquiry	Area	Scope	State of completion

Number of research projects guided:
- Undergraduate
- Postgraduate
- PhD

Contribution in Administration of Institutions/Departments

Do you help the Administrator in Management of the following Activities?

Areas of work	Nature of work and details
Admission	
Test and evaluation	
Extracurricular activities	
General administration	
Sports	
Laboratory management	
Discipline	
Academic excellence	

Do you help the University in the following Activities?

- Membership of board of examination
- Membership of board of studies
- Membership of standing academic council
- Membership of senate
- Membership of sports, curricular bodies
- Membership of research committee.

Innovative Teaching Techniques

- Do you celebrate special day?
- Do you conduct contests and competitions?
- Do you arrange exhibitions?

Extension Work

- Have you worked for any social organization?
- Are you a member of any social organization?
- Have you delivered guest lecture?
- Have you given key note address at the conferences?

Contribution in Social Activities

Worked and participated in
- Tree plantation   Yes/No
- Social forestry   Yes/No
- Organ donation   Yes/No
- Family planning   Yes/No
- Blood donation   Yes/No

Details of CNE Participated

Sl. No.	Theme and title	Organized by	National/ International	Month and year

Details of Paper Presentation

Sl. No.	Theme and title	Organized by	National/ International	Month and year

Organized Interdepartmental Activities

- Special day celebration
- Quiz
- Essay competitions
- Workshops/seminar
- Exhibitions
- Any other.

Organized Intercollegiate Activities

- Special day celebration
- Quiz
- Essay competitions
- Workshops/seminar
- Exhibitions
- Sports events
- Cultural programs
- Any other.

Organized Inter-university Activities

- Special day celebration
- Quiz
- Essay competitions
- Workshops/seminar
- Exhibitions
- Sports events
- Cultural programs
- Any other.

Membership

Are you a member of professional/academic associations?

Name	Nature of membership	Since when	Activities undertaken

Are you a member of different libraries?

Name	Nature of membership	Since when	Activities undertaken

Are you member of NGO promoting social cause?

Name	Nature of membership	Since when	Activities undertaken

Are you a member of cultural/educational institutions promoting regional, cultural activities and heritage?

Name	Nature of membership	Since when	Activities undertaken

Reading Habits and Journals

- Do you have your personal library?
- Do you prefer to buy books related to your topics of interest?
- Do you subscribe to journals and magazines?

Sl. No.	Nature of journals	Specialty	Nature of subscription

Awards won for your contribution

Name	Award	Purpose or area of excellence	Institution conferring award

Staff Welfare Services

"Staff Welfare Services $\propto$ Productivity".

The welfare measures to the employees do always have the direct relation with the productivity. The educational institutions also provide the various welfare measures to the teaching and nonteaching staff and other staffs in the institution. The welfare measures include:

- Safety measures including first aid
- Lunch rooms
- Rest rooms
- Recreational activities
- Credit societies
- Housing
- Medical and welfare
- Pension
- Gratuity
- Provident fund and the like
- Academic freedom
- Canteen facilities
- Career advancement facilities
- Children education facilities
- Loan facilities
- Foreign tour on study purpose
- Further education facilities
- Housing loan
- Leave facilities
- Leave travel concession
- Medical facilities
- Motor vehicle loan
- Publishing their findings out of research
- Savings schemes
- Transport facilities.

Career Development

Everyone in the world is engaged in some economic activities which will give bread and butter. If such economic activities are having the nature of growth and development, then it is said to be career. As far as the educational institutions are concerned, the main incumbents are the teachers and the administrative staff. Career for the teacher means, the profession and for the administrative staff, it means their post. Career planning is done by the individual as well as the organization.

Career is a sequence of separate but related work activities that provide continuity, order and meaning in a person's life. Career is defined as an individually perceived sequence of attitudes and behaviors associated with work related experiences and activities over the span of the person's life.

- A career path is the sequential pattern of jobs that forms a career.
- Career goals are the future positions one strives to reach as part of a career.
- Career planning is the process by which one selects career goals and the path to these goals.
- Career development is those personal improvements one undertakes to achieve a personal career plan.
- Career management is the process of designing and implementing the goals, plans and strategies to enable the organization to satisfy employee needs while allowing individuals to achieve their career goals.

There are two types of employee mobility in career development actions. They are internal and external mobility.

External mobility refers to movement of an employee from one organization to another seeking better placement based on his skills and the requirements and needs of various organizations. Employees resort to external mobility techniques and the organization resorts to external candidates when the chances of suitable placement on either side or both the sides are non-existent within an organization. An employee prefers internal mobility as long as he is sure of getting suitable placements/employment within the organization. Similarly organizations may resort to internal mobility until they find suitable candidate to different jobs.

Purpose of Internal Mobility

- To improve the effectiveness of the organization
- To maximize the employee efficiency
- To ensure discipline
- To adopt organizational changes.

Types of Internal Mobility

Promotions

Promotion is an advancement of an employee to a better job—better in terms of greater responsibility, more prestige or status, greater skill and especially increased rate of pay or salary. It is the upward reassignment of an individual in an organization's hierarchy, accompanied by increased responsibilities, enhanced status and usually with increased income though not always so. The other one is transfer which is not common in an educational institution.

Faculty Development Programs

Faculty means those qualified individuals to teach a particular branch of Arts and Science. Faculty development refers to all professional development activities that expand and improve both the role and abilities of the faculty and which are planned and arranged by its employers.

Purposes

- Upgrading the competency of those faculties who have been inadequately prepared.
- Upgrading the knowledge and skills of those who have stayed behind.
- Updating knowledge and skill of those who would like to assume new responsibilities or go further in their position.
- Motivating faculty to continue to learn through their own efforts.
- Updating the faculty with current information, trends, and issues.

Steps in Organizing Faculty Development Programs

- Formulate objectives and policies for faculty development program
- Identify the learners' need
- Translate learning needs into objectives for that program
- Identify content, that is, information to be taught
- Select teaching methods
- Select instructional materials
- Develop evaluation strategies and feedback
- Conduct the actual program
- Evaluate the effectiveness
- Incorporate the results into the future program.

Library

"A knowledge store".

A good library contributes effectively to an educational program. It not only opens the door to new knowledge but stimulates critical thinking and helps to develop independence in seeking and obtaining information. An up-to-date, varied selection of books and other library material also encourages and assists the staff in study and research both for self-improvement and for the benefit of the students.

To promote the desire and habit of general reading among students, in addition to the textbooks, which convey only brief and systematic knowledge and information, a well-organized library is a necessity. Library must be made the most attractive place in the college so that students are naturally drawn to it without any compulsion. The function of a library is not only to collect and stack the books but also to bring them to the reader. The fundamental duty of a librarian is to bring books and readers into proper contact.

Location

It should be conveniently located in quiet and attractive surroundings. The library may be separate for nursing college or it may be combined with the other courses, where an institution is running multiple courses. The size will depend on the number of users. In general, it should be large enough to accommodate the students. Adequate ventilation and good lighting, both natural and artificial, are essential.

Furniture and Equipment

It should include:
- Comfortable chairs and table of convenient height
- Metal book shelves or cupboards with glass doors
- Bulletin boards
- Book and newspaper display rack
- Journal display rack with space for back numbers
- Boxes for pamphlets
- Stationery items such as index cards, borrowers cards, labels and registers.

Requisites of a Library

- One or more librarians and assistants to help the librarian
- Library committee to advise
- Policies and specific procedures for library
- Budget for the library.

Librarian

A qualified and skilled librarian(s) is essential to manage the library effectively. They are helped by the library assistants. The functions of a librarian include:
- Maintaining up-to-date record of all books, journals, etc.
- Maintaining all pertinent records and registers such as accession register and others
- Classifying and cataloging all books and journals
- Displaying books and other materials of current interest
- Checking for worn out and sending it for binding
- Participating actively in library committee meetings
- Ordering for books or renewal of journals, etc.
- Timely report to the principal of the issues of importance pertaining to the library
- Organizing and conducting stock verification.

Library Committee

The committee members include the librarian, principal, staff, and student representatives. The functions of the library committee include:
- Preparing the budget and review
- Selection and purchase of new books and journals
- Formulating policies
- Encouraging the use of library
- Determining library requirements
- Implementing disciplinary actions.

Policies

Policies are formulated regarding:
- Hours at which the library will be open
- Holidays
- Beneficiaries
- Reference and issue books
- Period for which the book may be borrowed
- Disciplinary actions for delayed return, loss or damage of the library belongings and properties
- Discarding the outdated books.

Budget

Budget is required for equipping library with:
- Furniture
- Book shelves and racks
- New books and journals
- Stationery items
- Maintenance of library such as electricity, etc.
- Binding of books and back volumes
- Payment of librarian and other persons.

Library Holdings

It usually includes:
- Dictionaries—general, medical and nursing
- Encyclopedias
- Government data and other reports
- Books on basic sciences
- Books on nursing sciences
- Newspapers
- Selected biographical and philosophical books.

Organization of Books

Books are usually arranged as per the classification system adopted in an open shelf for easy access. Reference books may be kept separately. It is good always to classify the books in selected groups for easy maintenance. Each book should be given a specific accession number and the details such as the author name, title, publisher, place, year, cost, etc. should be maintained. For borrowing, a card system can be maintained, which will facilitate checking.

Hostel

"Second home of the pupils".

The hostel is considered as a center of citizenship training and second home of the pupils. Many good qualities of head and heart are developed at the hostel. It is always convenient, if the college is equipped with the hostel in the same campus. In some places the hostel may be located little away from the college campus. Though it is not mandatory for the students to stay in the hostel compulsorily, many students wish to stay in the hostel for better learning and performance.

A hostel should provide a conducive, relaxed atmosphere and environment which will contribute to the total development of the student. It also encourages healthy living by providing opportunities for learning how to live in a group, to share interests and activities and to assume responsibility for her day-to-day living. The hostel should be provided with adequate sanitary facilities.

The hostel should not be treated merely as a place for boarding and lodging of the pupils. It should provide all the opportunities for promoting healthy habits and developing good qualities like fellow feeling, cooperation, mutual help and punctuality. The hostel life should cater to the needs of the future citizens by providing ample opportunities for civic training. The warden should be democratic and work as a philosopher and guide of the inmates. Her sociability, sympathy, understanding, sincerity, broad mindedness and impartiality must win the confidence as well as regard from the students. She must be a woman of character and vision.

The warden should pay frequent visits to the physical, academic and living facilities and ensure proper functioning of various mechanisms and agencies involved in hostel administration. The inmates should be encouraged to share the hostel administration and decision making, so that they will be trained in democratic management and community living.

Physical Infrastructure

- Room for warden
- Office for warden
- Room for staff and housekeeping personnel
- Room for students
- Dining room
- Kitchen
- Pantry
- Store room
- Sick room
- Recreation room
- Reading room
- Visitor's room
- Sanitary annexes
- Washing areas.

Policies for the Hostel

Policies are framed regarding:
- Number of staff to be resident
- Visiting hours for the students
- Mess arrangements for the staffs and students
- Isolation procedures
- Disciplinary actions for any violations.

Student's Room

It should be well equipped with adequate ventilation and lighting. The space for single room is not less than 100 square feet, and for the double room, it should be not less than 150 square feet, i.e. 75 square feet or more for each student. For each student, there should be a cot, shelf to store books and clothings, chair and table, dressing table with mirror. It is good, if they provide separate accommodation for the students on night duty for uninterrupted sleep and rest.

Common Rooms

It should be attractive and furnished with comfortable chairs, sofas, etc. There should be a separate room for students to read. A recreation room should have a television, radio, a record player, table tennis, and other indoor games, etc.

Visitors' Room

It should be situated near the entrance of the hostel and also in proximity to the warden's office for supervision and monitoring.

Pantry

A small pantry with facilities such as a table, sink, storage, water, and washing is helpful for the students to make tea and some hot drinks.

Sick Room

A sick room with adequate facilities such as cot, table, and chair helps in isolating the students during the time of sickness and promotes rest and provides special care to them.

Warden Office

The warden office should be equipped well and also it should have telephone facilities. It should be located near the visitors' area.

Room for Housekeeping Staff

There should be a separate room for housekeeping staff and domestic staff who are nonresident, where they may leave their belongings and where they may rest. It should have toilet facilities.

Store Rooms

There should be adequate storage space for linen, extra furniture and furnishings, and the kitchen supplies. It should have adequate shelves which will protect articles from moisture, insects, vermin, and other hazards.

Laundry

There should be facilities for washing, drying, and ironing of clothes by the students. Drying space should be available for both indoor and outdoor.

Kitchen Premises

Kitchen should be well ventilated, well lit and equipped with cooking facilities. There should be 24 hours water supply, and proper facilities should be ensured for washing and drying all the utensils.

Dining Hall

The dining hall should be large enough to accommodate the students. It should have adjacent handwashing facilities. It should be well ventilated and lit.

Sanitary Annexes

It is constructed at a rate of one bathroom and toilet for every six students. Additional hand washing facilities and mirrors are provided. There should be 24 hours water supply and if not possible there should be a facility for storing water. There should be covered dustbins, which should be emptied periodically.

Indoor Games and Sports

It is good, if hostel is equipped with indoor games such as carom boards, table tennis, etc. and also it should have sports items under the custody of warden for the students to play and enjoy.

Nursing Standards

"A level of excellence".

A standard is a means of determining what something should be. In nursing education, the standard refers to the established criteria for the provision of nursing education. In case of nursing practice, standards are the established criteria for the practice of nursing. Standards are having permanent value. A nursing standard can be a target.

Standard is an established rule as a basis of comparison in measuring or finding capacity, quality context and value of objects in the same category. Standard is a broad statement of quality. It is a definite level of excellence as adequately required, aimed at or possible. Standard is a predetermined baseline condition as level of excellence that comprises a model to be followed and practiced. It is used as a measurement tool.

"A standard is a model of established practice which has general recognition and acceptance among registered professional nurses and is commonly accepted as correct standards of practice are agreed on levels of competence as determined by the ANA and specially nursing organizations" [ANA—1996].

"Standards are defined as authoritative statements that describe a common level of care as performance by which the quality of practice can be determined or measured.

Purpose of Standards

In order to provide a high quality of nursing education, it is necessary that nurse educators develop standard of education and appropriate evaluation tools.
- Standards give direction and provide guidelines
- Standards provide a baseline for evaluating quality of nursing education and thereby quality care
- It helps to plan for the faculty recruitment, development of infrastructure and others
- It aids in curriculum planning, implementation, and evaluation
- It assists in planning for student welfare activities and staff welfare activities
- Standards help improve quality of nursing care, increase effectiveness of care, and improve efficiency
- A standard may help to improve documentation of nursing care
- Standards may help to determine the degree to which standards of nursing care maintained
- Standards help supervisors to guide nursing staff to improve performance
- Standards may help to improve basis for decision-making
- Standards may help justify demands
- Standards may help clarify nurses' area of accountability
- Standards may help nursing to define clearly different levels of care.

Importance of Standards in Nursing

- It is an authoritative statement by which the quality of nursing practice, service, and education can be judged.
- In nursing practice, standards are established criteria for the practice of nursing.
- It is a guideline, a recommended path to safe conduct and aid to professional performance.
- It provides a baseline for evaluating quality of nursing care, increases effectiveness of care, and improves efficiency.
- Standards help supervisors to guide nursing staff to improve performances.
- Standards may help to clarify nurses' area of accountability.
- Standards may help nursing to clearly define different levels of care.
- Standard is a device for quality assurance as quality control.

Characteristics of Standards

- Statement must be broad.
- Must be realistic, acceptable and attainable.
- Standards of nursing care must be developed by members of the nursing profession, preferably nurses practicing at the direct care level with consultation of experts in the domain.
- It should be phrased in positive terms.
- Must be understandable and stated in unambiguous terms.
- Must be reviewed and revised periodically.
- May be directed toward an ideal, i.e. optional standards or only specify the minimal care that must be attained, i.e. minimum standard.
- And one must remember that standards that are workable are objective, acceptable, achievable, and flexible.

Purposes of Standards in Education

The purposes of publishing, circulating, and enforcing nursing standards in education are to:
- Improve the quality of nursing education
- Decrease the cost of nursing education
- Ultimately to improve the patient care.

Classification of Standards

A. Nursing care standards in hospital can be divided into end and mean standards.
   - End standards: The end standards are patient-oriented; they describe the change as desired in a patient's physical status or behavior.
   - Mean standards: The mean standards are nursing-oriented; they describe the activities and behavior designed to achieve end standards.

   End standards require information about the patients. A mean standard calls for information about the nurses' performance.

B. Nursing care standards can be classified according to frame of references, relating to nursing structure, process and outcome.
   - Structure standard: A structural standard involves the set-up of the institution. The philosophy, goals and objectives, structure of the organization,

facilities and equipment and qualifications of employees are some of the components of the structure of the organization. For example, recommended relationship between the nursing department and other departments in a healthy agency are structural standards because they refer to the organizational structure in which nursing is implemented. It includes people, money, equipment, staffing policies, etc. The use of standards based on structure implies that if the structure is adequate, reliable, and desirable, standard will be met and quality care will be given.

- Process standard: Process standards describe the behaviors of the nurse at the desired level of performance. A process standard involves the activities concerned with delivering patient care. These standards measure nursing action involving patient care. The standards are stated in action verbs that are in observable and measurable terms. For example, "the patient demonstrates". The focus is on what was planned, what was done and what was communicated as recorded. In process standard, there is an element of professional judgment, i.e. determining the quality as the degree of skill. It includes nursing care technique, procedures, regimens, and processes.
- Outcome standard: Descriptive statements of desired patient care results are outcome standard because patients' results are outcome of nursing intervention.

An outcome standard measures changes in the patient health status. This change may be due to nursing care, medical care or as a result of variety of services offered to the patient. Outcome standards reflect the effectiveness and results rather than the process of giving care.

Thus, structural standards are agency- or group-oriented and process standards are nurse-oriented whereas outcome standards are patient results-oriented.

Normative standards describe practices considered "good" or "ideal" by some authoritative group. Empirical standards describe practices actually observed in a large number of patient care settings.

Standards for an Educational Institution

- Structure standard
  It includes:
  - The philosophy
  - Goals and objectives
  - Organization structure
  - Men or people
  - Money
  - Material
  - All resources
  - Policies and procedures
  - Job description
  - Personal qualification of the personnel
  - Evaluation procedures
  - Curriculum planning
  - Staff welfare program
  - Budget and other control.
- Process standard
  - Implementation of curriculum
  - Teaching-learning activities
  - Conduction of staff-development program
  - Implementation of evaluation.
- Outcome standard
  - Student satisfaction
  - Results
  - Staff satisfaction
  - Curriculum effectiveness
  - Goal achievement.

Sources of Nursing Standards

- Professional organization or association, e.g. TNAI
- Licensing bodies, e.g. statutory bodies, INC, SNC, etc.
- Universities and Boards, e.g. The TN Dr MGR Medical University.
- Institutions/healthcare agencies, e.g. University Hospitals, Health centers.
- Department of institutions, e.g. Department of Nursing.
- Patient care units, e.g. Specific patients' unit.
- Government units at National, State and local level.
- Individual standards, e.g. personal standards.

Accreditation in Nursing

"A certification of an organization".

Accreditation is formal testament by a recognized group that an institution or program has met established standards. It is the certification of organizations. It provides documented validation of the qualifications of the organization to carry out its stated goals and objectives (Schwirian, PM). It is a process by which a voluntary, nongovernmental agency or organization approves and grants status to institutions or programs that meet predetermined standards or outcomes (Zerwekh, JA). According to Zook and Haggerty, accreditation is "the recognition accorded to an educational institution... by some agency or organization which sets-up standards or requirements that must be compiled with, in order to secure approval".

Selden describes it as "the process whereby an organization or agency recognizes an institution or university program of study as having met certain predetermined qualifications and standards".

Purpose

- To certify to the public that an institution has met established standards.
- To encourage peer review by the faculty and staff of the institution.
- To facilitate the transfer of students from one institution to another.
- To assist prospective students in deciding which institution to attend and join.
- To assist prospective employers in identifying qualified personnel.
- To raise the standards of education for the practice of a profession.

Types

Institutional accreditation: It is accreditation of the institution as a whole, without differentiation among the various curriculums. It looks at the institution as a total operating unit. It focuses attention on the general characteristics of an institution; its objectives, infrastructure, faculty and resources. Of major concern are questions of program integrity, administrative and academic control, quality assurance, availability of resources and supervisory accountability.

Specialized accreditation: It is otherwise known as the program accreditation, where the program run by the institution is accredited with utmost importance. The accreditation bodies are often associations or councils of professions like medicine, nursing, etc. The principal objective is to ensure that the quality of education and training meets the minimum requirements of the profession. The accreditation requirements are clearly defined, and emphasize the infrastructure, the facilities and the personnel required for satisfactory professional preparation. Evaluation is invariably external and conducted by visiting teams comprising of members of the profession. These two types of accreditation are not equivalent; institutional accreditation does not validate a program to the same extent as specialized accreditation. Whereas specialized accreditation usually requires that the program be housed in an accredited institution, institutional accreditation does not require or imply that each curriculum or department within that institution is accredited.

Beneficiaries of Accreditation

The common beneficiaries are:
- Students
- Faculty
- Graduates
- Practicing nurses
- Consumers of nursing services
- Administrators.

Aspects/Areas Reviewed under Accreditation Process

- Administration and governance
- Finance and budget
- Faculty, students and resources
- Program outcomes.

Problems

- As the number of accrediting agencies mushroomed, charges increased, decreased standardization and duplication began.
- Has never defined "quality of education".
- No relationship between accreditation standards and subsequent success of the graduates.
- Discourages innovation and experimentation.
- Evaluating an institution in terms of its own objectives and does not permit meaningful comparisons.
- It is used by special interest groups as a means of achieving or protecting private purposes.

Stages of Accrediting Programs

- Initiation of the process
- Conduction of a self-evaluation study
- Accreditation visit
- Evaluation by the board of review or peer group
- Continuing self-evaluation and ongoing program improvements.

National Assessment and Accreditation Council

National Assessment and Accreditation Council (NAAC) was established by the University Grants Commission (UGC) on 16th September, 1994 for ensuring quality in higher education, in pursuance of the National Policy on Education and the Program of Action (POA), in 1986. It is located at Bangalore. NAAC is entrusted with the task of performance evaluation, assessment and accreditation of universities and colleges in India.

Benefits of Accreditation

- Institution to know its strengths, weaknesses, and opportunities through an informed review process
- Identification of internal areas of planning and resource allocation
- Collegiality on the campus
- Funding agencies look for objective data for performance funding
- Institutions to initiate innovative and modern methods of pedagogy
- New sense of direction and identity for institutions
- The society looks for reliable information on quality education offered

- Employers look for reliable information on the quality of education offered to the prospective recruits
- Intra- and inter-institutional interactions

NAAC assesses and grades institutions of higher education through a three-step process and makes the outcome as objective as possible. Though the methodology and the broad framework of the instrument used for assessment are similar, there is a slight difference in the focus of the instrument depending on the unit of Accreditation, i.e. Affiliated /Constituent colleges/ Autonomous colleges/Universities/Health Science/ Teacher/Physical Education. NAAC can perform the following:
1. Institutional Accreditation
   University: University Central Governance Structure along with all the undergraduate and postgraduate departments.
2. College: Any College—affiliated, constituent or autonomous with all its departments of studies.
3. Department Accreditation: Any department/School/ Center of the University.

The range of Cumulative Grade Point Average with the letter grade and status is given below:

Range of institutional Cumulative Grade Point Average (CGPA)	Letter Grade	Status
3.51–4.00	A++	Accredited
3.26–3.50	A+	Accredited
3.01–3.25	A	Accredited
2.76–3.00	B++	Accredited
2.51–2.75	B+	Accredited
2.01–2.50	B	Accredited
1.51–2.00	C	Accredited
≤1.50	D	Not accredited

Accreditation refers to the certification given by NAAC which is valid for a period of 5 years.

Steps in Assessment

Step 1: Preparation of the self-study report by the institution, its submission to NAAC and in-house analysis of the report by NAAC.

Step 2: Peer team visits to the institution for validation of the self-study report followed by presentation of a comprehensive assessment report to the institution.

Step 3: Grading, certification, and accreditation based on the evaluation report by the peer team.

National Assessment and Accreditation Council has identified the following seven criteria to serve as the basis for its assessment procedures:
- Curricular aspects
- Teaching-learning and evaluation
- Research, innovations, and extension
- Infrastructure and learning resources
- Student support and progression
- Organization and management (Governance and Leadership)
- Institutional values and best practices.

Grading

The assessment is on a four points scale.
- A—Very Good
- B—Good
- C—Satisfactory
- NA—Not Accredited.

If the overall CGPA is more than 1.51, the institution gets the "Accredited status" and any score less than that will lead to "Not accredited" status. The NAAC accreditation is valid for five years.

Indian Nursing Council

The Indian Nursing Council is an autonomous body under the Government of India, Ministry of Health and Family Welfare and was constituted by the Central Government under section 3(1) of the Indian Nursing Council Act, 1947 of parliament in order to establish a uniform standard of training for nurses, midwives, and health visitors. The basic aims, objectives, and functions of Indian Nursing Council are as follows:
- To establish and monitor a uniform standard of nursing education for nurses, midwives, auxiliary nurse midwives, and health visitors by doing inspection of the institutions.
- To recognize the qualifications under section 10(2) (4) of the Indian Nursing Council Act, 1947 for the purpose of registration and employment in India and abroad.
- To give approval for registration of Indian and Foreign Nurses possessing foreign qualification under section 11(2)(a) of the Indian Nursing Council Act, 1947.
- To prescribe the syllabus and regulations for nursing programs.
- Withdrawal of the recognition of qualification under section 14 of the Act in case the institution fails to maintain its standards under Section 14(1)(b) that an institution recognized by a State Council for the training of nurses, midwives, auxiliary nurse midwives, or health visitors does not satisfy the requirements of the council.
- To advise the State Nursing Councils, Examining Boards, State Governments and Central Government in various important items regarding nursing education in the country.

- Recognition of nursing institution as per the act.
- Registration of qualified nursing professionals mentioned above and maintenance of state registers for the purpose of development of inter linkages and reciprocities with corresponding councils in other states of India.
- Monitoring of professional ethics.
- Regulation and surveillance of professional conduct and take action against practice of their professional by quack and check malpractice.

Refer to INC website for further information.

State Nursing Council

The state nursing council is an autonomous statutory registration body for registering qualified nurses, midwives, ANMs, MPHWs, and health visitors. A council has president/vice president, registrar and staff of the council. The functions of the council includes the registration of qualified nursing professionals, regulation of training programs by conducting inspection, checking malpractice and maintaining professional ethics, foreign verification, coordinating with the INC and with various other government departments and universities. The council conducts inspection for the institution, who are conducting the programs such as ANM, MPHW, DGNM, BSc(N), Post-basic BSc(N), MSc(N) and Nurse Practitioner Program. The council ensures that all facilities are available for conducting any of the nursing programs before granting permission. It also conducts the surprise and periodical inspection to identify the deficiencies in that institution. If necessary, it also conducts reinspection to ensure that the deficiencies are rectified. It periodically sends communication to all the educational institutions to inform the issues of importance to nursing and health.

Board-CMAI

CMAI is a registered, nonprofit, charitable organization. CMAI is the health arm of National Council of Churches in India (NCCI). They undertake programs in training, research, community service, institutional consultancy, policy advocacy, interface of theology and medicine, information dissemination and others.

Objectives of CMAI

- Prevention and relief of human suffering irrespective of caste, creed, community, religion, and economic status.
- Promotion of knowledge of the factors governing health.
- Coordination of activities for training doctors, nurses, allied health professionals and others involved in the ministry of healing.
- Implementation of schemes for comprehensive healthcare, family planning, and community welfare.
- Rendering health in calamities and disasters of all kinds.

Functions of the Nursing Examination Board

- To coordinate and bring a uniform standard of nursing education, in accordance with the requirements of the Indian Nursing Council and State Nursing Council.
- To verify the eligibility requirements of the students before each examination.
- To arrange to conduct examination and issue diploma certificates to successful candidates.
- To maintain and enhance the educational standards of Schools of Nursing by arranging continuing education programs/workshops/exhibitions.
- To prepare the calendar of events at the beginning of each academic year.
- To decide the disciplinary action against students/concerned staff in case of malpractice in examinations.
- To nominate members for the panel of examiners for Ist, IInd and IIIrd year of GNM nursing examinations.
- To appoint the examiners before annual and supplementary examination.
- To appoint an auditor to audit the board accounts.

University

Universities are various types. They are:
- Central universities
- State universities
- Deemed universities.

Functions of University

- Regulation of its own colleges and affiliated institutions.
- Conducting inspection and granting permission for admission.
- Conducting examination and announcing the results.
- Conducting graduation.
- Ensuring faculty welfare and development.
- Ensuring student welfare and development.
- Organizing various programs such as book exhibition, job fair, seminars, conferences, intercollege competitions, sport meets, etc.
- A university can have its own colleges to offer various programs or it can have affiliated colleges. It can offer programs or courses related to Arts and Science, Medical and Paramedical, Engineering, Agriculture, etc.

Various Departments of University
- Admission
- Registration
- Academic section
- Examination section
- Research section.

Professional Associations

Meaning and Definition
Generally the association means the combination of the people of same category for their common interest. They will meet as and when the need arises and when their common interest is affected and when their common interest is to be developed. Through the association, the employees and workers solve many problems. Professional body or professional organization, also known as a professional association or professional society, is an organization, usually nonprofit, that exists to further a particular profession, to protect both the public interest and the interests of professionals.

Many professional bodies perform professional certification to indicate a person possesses qualifications in the subject area, and sometimes membership in a professional body is synonymous with certification, but not always. Sometimes membership in a professional body is required for one to be legally able to practice the profession. Many professional bodies also act as learned societies for the academic disciplines underlying their professions.

Associations are organizations of persons with common interests. Merton defined a professional association as, "an organization of practitioners, who judge one another as professionally competent and have united together to perform social functions, which they cannot perform in their separate capacity as individuals". Associations exist in all profession and in all parts of the world. Associations serve their individual members through a variety of services.

Professional associations provide a vehicle for nurses to meet present and future challenges and work toward positive profession related changes that keep pace with societal changes.

As far as the educational institution is concerned the employee associations are formed among the teachers and office staff to promote their own welfare.

Characteristics
- It is relatively permanent
- It is voluntary in nature
- It is an instrument of defense against exploitation
- It is an association of educated persons
- It is for the common purpose.

Principles
- Unity is strength
- Collective bargaining
- Promotion of common interest
- Career advancement
- Opportunity for the self-career development
- Economic security
- Security of service.

Benefits of Belonging to a Professional Association
- Developing leadership skills.
- Recognition through certification. Certification is a formal but voluntary process of demonstrating expertise in particular areas of nursing.
- Legislative lobbying power. Association lobbies the government to influence the laws affecting nursing.
- Other benefits—publications, continuing nursing education, discounts in train, eyeglasses goods and services.
- To negotiate collective bargaining to get the dues in terms of finance and nonfinance.
- To get along with their fellow-workers in a better way and to gain respect in the eyes of their peers.
- To safe guard the common interest of the professionals.
- To promote public relations.

Deciding which Associations to Join
In making decisions about joining an association, nurse should ask several questions.
- What are the purposes of this association?
- Are the association's purposes compatible with my own?
- How many members are there nationally, statewide and locally?
- What activities does the association undertake?
- How active is the local chapter?
- What are the benefits of membership?
- Does the organization lobby for improved healthcare legislation? How successful is it?
- Is membership in this association cost-effective?

Becoming a Productive Association
- Members join as members, attending meetings, volunteering for committees, participation in the association activities.
- Professional associations are the vehicle through which nursing takes collective action to improve healthcare, and nursing membership in professional association is considered essential for true professionals.
- Should be an enlightened one, so that it may be able to guide and direct the association's movement properly.

- Should have a solid foundation, so that it may be strong enough to achieve success in the realization of its objectives.
- Should have clear objectives.
- Should be run by the members for the members.
- Should have honesty and integrity of purpose.
- Should look beyond its own horizon and recognize and fulfill its proper role in the life of the nation and of the community in the midst of which it lives and functions.
- Should have a sense of responsibility.
- It should be democratic.

Whom do Professional Associations Serve

The Public
Professional associations serve public by establishing codes of ethics and standards of practice, socializing new members to these codes and standards and enforcing codes and standards in practice.

The Profession
Professional associations serve the profession by being by being the mechanism through which the collective interests of its members are pressed collectively and focused politically. Collective action means the activities are undertaken on behalf of a group of people, who have common interests. Professional association helps nurses use collective action to push for political responses to benefit consumers of healthcare and members of the profession.

Individual Members
Professional associations serve individual members by providing continuing education and ensuring mechanisms for a professional work place. They work by forming relationships with the public and other professions and by ensuring that the profession's work is properly understood and supported by the public, government officials and other healthcare professionals.

Professional Association Activities

- To communicate information to members through newsletters, journals, etc. The contents include the health and nursing issues, continuing nursing education topics issues of interest to members.
- It formulates code for nurses.

Joining and Using Professional Associations in Nursing

Nurses have the responsibility to join in one or more nursing associations both as an extension of their interest in nursing and to support their fellow nurses.

Types of Associations

- Broad purpose professional association. For example, Trained Nurses Association of India. The purpose of establishment of TNAI is wide and it is discussed later in this chapter.
- Specialty practice association. Nurses, who work in a particular specialty area, can establish an organization, e.g. Association of Nurse Midwives, American Association of Critical Care Nursing, Emergency Nurses Association, and Association of Rehabilitative Nurses.
- Special interest association. For example, National Black Nurses Association, Jamaican Nurses Association, National Hispanic Nurse Association and Transcultural Nursing Society. These were established to serve the interest of the particular group.

List of Some Nursing Organizations (International)

- American Academy of Nursing
- American Nurses Association
- Canadian Nurses Association
- International Council of Nurses
- Japanese Nursing Association
- National League for Nursing
- Royal District Nursing Service
- Sigma Theta Tau
- Space Nursing Society
- United American Nurses
- United States Navy Nurse Corps
- Washington State Nurses Association

The Trained Nurses' Association of India

The association had its beginning in the Association of Nursing Superintendents, which was founded in 1905, at Lucknow. The organization was composed of nine European Nurses holding administrative posts in hospitals. They saw the need to develop nursing as a profession and also to provide a forum where professional nurses could meet and plan to achieve these ends. The movement gathered momentum and soon nurses, other than nursing superintendents, were seeking to share in:

- Upholding in every way the dignity and honor of the nursing profession.
- Promoting a sense of esprit de corps among all nurses.
- Enabling members to take counsel together on matters relating to their profession.

The Association of Nursing Superintendents, therefore, sought the help and cooperation of nurses throughout the country. At the annual conference held in Mumbai in 1908, a decision was taken to establish Trained Nurses' Association. The association was inaugurated in 1909. The two organizations shared the same officers until 1910 when, at the first Trained Nurses' Association (TNA) Conference, held at Banaras (UP), the TNA members elected their own officers.

In 1922, the Association of Nursing Superintendents and Trained Nurses' Association were amalgamated and called the Trained Nurses' Association of India (TNAI).

The association has established within its jurisdiction the following organizations:
- Health Visitors' League (1922).
- Midwives and Auxiliary Nurse-Midwives Association (1925).
- Student Nurses Association (1929–30).

Membership
The membership consists of the following:
- Full members: Fully qualified registered nurses.
- Associate members: Health visitors and midwives and ANMs.
- Affiliate members: Student nurses and members of the affiliated organizations, e.g. Christian nurses' league and catholic nurses' Guild of India.

Functions of TNAI
(Adopted from TNAI official website)
- To enunciate standards of nursing education and implement these through appropriate channels.
- To establish standards and qualifications for nursing practice.
- To enunciate standards of nursing service and implement these through appropriate channels.
- To establish a code of ethical conduct for practitioners.
- To stimulate and promote research designed to enhance.
- To stimulate and promote research designed to enhance the knowledge for evidence-based nursing practice.
- To promote legislation and to speak for nurses in regard to legislative action.
- To promote and protect the economic welfare of nurses.
- To provide professional counseling and placement service for nurses.
- To provide for the continuing professional development of practitioners.
- To represent nurses and serve as their spokesperson with allied national and international organizations, governmental and other bodies and the public.
- To serve as the official representative of the Nurses of India as a member of the International Council of Nurses.
- To promote the general health and welfare of the public through the Association programs, relationships and activities, e.g. disaster management.
- To render care as per the changing needs of the society.

Nurses' Charter
In 1937, the TNAI adopted the Nurses' Charter, which formed the basis for TNAI'S representations to government and other employing authorities on vital matters like upgrading, development and standardization of nursing education (Basic and Post-basic), improvement of living and service conditions for nurses throughout India and registration of qualified nurses. Sustained efforts of the TNAI also brought about the constitution of the Indian Nursing Council and also State Nursing Councils, which established a uniform system of nursing education in the country and nurses qualified from recognized institutions could practice in any part of the country. The Indian Nursing Council Act was passed by an ordinance on December 31, 1947. The council was established in 1949.

Standardization of Nursing Education
In the early days, TNAI assisted in the formulation of basic nursing curricula and, in later years, the association was instrumental in promoting the establishment of degree courses and post-certificate programmers in teaching and administration.

As early as 1933, an Education Committee was appointed. The Committee of Nurses appointed through the TNAI to advise the Bhore Committee (The Health Survey and Planning Committee, 1941–1944) took up again the question of establishing degree courses which were accepted by the government. The colleges of nursing were established in Delhi and Vellore (Tamil Nadu) in 1946. The recent educational activities of the association are conducting educational conferences and workshops. Various conferences and workshops were organized on various nursing topics from time to time by TNAI.

Service Condition for Nurses
The association is officially recognized by the government of India as a service organization. The voice of the association is accepted as the voice of nurses in India, and the resolutions adopted by it and presented to the various authorities, are well received and generally accepted for implementation, sooner or later.

Publications
The publications of the association include the following:
- Handbook of the TNAI (First copy published in 1917). Revised edition published in 1997.
- The Nursing Journal of India, a monthly publication, first published in 1910 and the editor was Miss ME Butcher. The first Indian editor was Miss Asoka Roy.
- A Public Health Nursing Manual by Lilian Bischoff and others which is now available in its revised form of a Community Health Nursing Manual.
- Hindi translation of Basic Principles of Nursing Care by Virginia Henderson.

- Indian Nursing Yearbook was started in 1982.
- Simplified microbiology.
- Nursing Administration and Management (First edition, 2000).
- History and Trends in Nursing in India (First edition, 2001).

There are many books published by the TNAI. Refer to the TNAI website for further details.

Rapport with Government of India

- Government recognition as service association: The association is considered to be on a par with other service organizations.
- Issue of railway concessions: In 1991, railways granted concession to TNAI members and the association was authorized to issue certificates to members for getting concession. Students are given 50% concession for educational trips.

Affiliation with Government Committees and Councils

The contribution of TNAI to the findings of Bhore Committee and Mudaliar Committee as well as to other similar bodies has been considerable. Its views have been considered as the most authentic for the nursing profession in processing the findings of such official committees. TNAI played an important role in the High Power Committee on Nursing and Nursing Profession (Report: 1987). Its link with the INC has given rise to a number of endeavors for the promotion of nursing education and other aspects of the profession.

Affiliation with Other Organizations

It is an associate member of many other associations and societies doing welfare activities in their own fields. These societies are: Indian Red Cross Society, Indian Public Health Association, Association for Social Health, Indian Hospital Association, Federation of Delhi Hospital Welfare Societies, Tuberculosis Association of India, Indian Leprosy Association and National Institute of Public Cooperation and Child Development. These associations and institutions too involve themselves in the activities of TNAI on a reciprocal basis.

The TNAI takes part in the activities of important social organizations devoted to the welfare of women, especially National Council of Women in India, National Federation of Indian Women and All India Women's Conference. The association is invited to all important deliberations of such bodies and effort is made by the TNAI representatives to keep these organizations informed of the problems of practicing nurses.

Affiliation with International Council of Nurses (ICN)

A landmark was TNAI's affiliation with International Council of Nurses (ICN) in 1912. TNAI was among the first eight National Nurses' Associations (NNAs) which joined ICN and was represented first time at its Congress at Cologne. There has been a setback in the continuity of TNAI affiliation with ICN in recent years due to financial constraints. Since May 1995, TNAI stands disaffiliated from the ICN.

Affiliation with Commonwealth Nurses Federation

Around 1974, the TNAI became a member of the Commonwealth Nurses Federation (CNF). The association with CNF has been fruitful in many ways.

Affiliation with Scholarship Funds

In an effort to assist suitable nurses toward advanced nursing education, funds were collected in 1943 from various organizations and individuals for scholarship purposes. The association is the trustee for the administration of funds thus raised. There are now, 10 different funds, 4 of which are for specific courses. One of the ways in which the TNAI carries out its educational objectives and serves the cause of nursing, is by being the trustee for various scholarships:
- Kapadia Memorial Scholarship Fund
- Margaret Jehan Scholarship Fund
- Ajmer Minto Sister's Scholarship Fund
- Lady Linlithgow Scholarship Fund
- Rajkumari Amrit Kaur and Miss Adranvala Scholarship Fund
- Tata Memorial Scholarship Fund
- Lady Minto Nursing Scholarship Fund
- Military Nursing Service Scholarship Fund
- Florence Nightingale Fund for Research in Nursing.

National Conferences

The TNAI now holds its national conferences biennially. Till 1960, the association was having annual conferences at the national level. These became biennial and were held on alternate years to Student Nurses Association conferences. The Student Nurses Association also holds its national conferences biennially. The biennial conferences of TNAI and Student Nurses Association follow each other in consecutive years. On the occasion of the TNAI Biennial conference, both the general body of the TNAI and its house of delegates meet simultaneously.

Continuing Education

From the very beginning, the association has believed in the fundamental right of people to have good health and nurses as health professionals to help people to attain or maintain an optimum level of health. It has believed in continued updating of nursing knowledge and skills through continuing education.

Celebration of International Nurses' Day

The birthday of Florence Nightingale (May 12) is celebrated as International Nurses' Day every year. The TNAI organizes a fitting celebration on this occasion at the headquarters and publicity is given on the life and work of the Lady with the Lamp. Some eminent personalities are associated with these celebrations so that the young nurses can draw benefit and inspiration from their experiences. The information about the nursing profession is propagated through various publicity media.

Welfare Activities

Nurses' welfare fund: As far back as 1938, the TNAI became conscious of the need for some concrete financial aid to nurses who were old, and having spent their lives in the service of others on small salaries, and with little or no pensions, found themselves in difficulty. The fund depends entirely on donations from nurses and those interested in nurses. Many nurses in need have been helped by this fund on numerous occasions. A number of old and handicapped nurses are receiving help on a regular basis.

Staff welfare fund: A memorial fund in the name of late Miss Lakshmi Devi was created for the headquarters' staff in 1970. Reimbursement of a fixed amount in a year for the medical expenses incurred by the staff could be made from this fund. The fund called the "Lakshmi Devi Staff Welfare Fund", has been built-up by monthly contributions from the members of the staff and donations made by TNAI members till the end of 1976. Now it is also constructing old age homes for the nurses.

National Awards

The scheme of national awards for nurses was introduced by the Government of India in 1971 at the suggestion of TNAI. It was initially open only to nurses employed in government institutions. Later on, the government accepted the recommendation of the TNAI for their being open to nurses working in voluntary health service agencies who are rendering service to humanity.

The Nursing Journal of India

The association brings out a monthly magazine, The Nursing Journal of India, as its official organ. The journal, which is published in the first week of every month, is the main link for communication between the members of the association on all important matters.

Summary

- Educational administration includes the techniques and procedures employed in operating the educational organization in accordance with established policies.
- Administration of nursing educational institutions such as college of nursing and school of nursing include maintenance management and developmental management. It includes the management of man, money, material, activity, and time. It also involves the management functions such as planning, organizing, directing, recruiting, staffing controlling, budgeting, staff development, etc.
- There are different courses offered in nursing such as ANM, DGNM, BSc(N), Post-basic BSc(N), MSc(N), and MPhil and PhD in nursing. The Indian Nursing Council, State Nursing Council and the University with which an institution is affiliated play a vital role in establishing and maintaining standards in nursing education.
- Educational planning is defined as the process of preparing a set of decisions for action during a specific period of time directed at achieving organizational goals. In the words of JP Naik, educational planning implies the taking of decisions for future action with a view to achieving predetermined objectives through the optimum use of scarce resources.
- Institutional planning is a program of development and improvement prepared by an educational institution on the basis of its felt needs and the resources available with a view to improving its programs and practices.
- Organizing refers to the formal grouping of teachers and activities to facilitate achievement of someone and who has to be made responsible for accomplishing the objectives to achieve the desired results.
- Human resource planning is an integrated approach to performing the planning aspects of the personnel function in order to have a sufficient supply of adequately developed and motivated people to perform the duties and tasks required to meet organizational objectives and satisfy the individual needs and goals of organizational members.
- Recruitment is a process to discover the sources of manpower to meet the requirements of the staffing schedule and to employ effective measures for attracting that manpower in adequate numbers to facilitate effective selection of efficient working force. It is the determination of the job to which an accepted candidate is to be assigned, and his assignment to that job.
- Budget is defined as a financial and/or quantitative statement, prepared prior to a defined period of time, of the policy to be pursued during that period for the purpose of attaining a given objective.

- The Institute of Public Relation of England defines public relations practice as "the planned and sustained effort to establish and maintain goodwill and mutual understanding between an organization and its publics".
- Performance appraisal is the process of evaluating the performance and qualifications of the employees in terms of other requirements of the job for which he is employed, for purposes of administration including placement, selection for promotions, providing financial rewards and other actions which require differential treatment among the members of a group as distinguished from actions affecting all members equally. It is a process by which employees of some professional rank and setting evaluate one another job performance against accepted standard.
- Self-evaluation is the evaluation of one's job performances. Self-evaluation is important for nurse leaders because knowledge of self will enhance their leadership ability and potential.
- Academic audit is an educational exercise to assess and evaluate the performance of teachers and to have a pragmatic view about what is the present status of academic standards.
- A good library contributes effectively to an educational program. It not only opens the door to new knowledge but stimulates critical thinking and helps to develop independence in seeking and obtaining information.
- A hostel should provide a conducive, relaxed atmosphere and environment which will contribute to the total development of the student. It also encourages healthy living by providing opportunities for learning how to live in a group, to share interests and activities and to assume responsibility for her day-to-day living.
- A standard is a model of established practice which has general recognition and acceptance among registered professional nurses and is commonly accepted as correct standards of practice are agreed on levels of competence as determined by the nursing organizations.
- Associations are organizations of persons with common interests. Merton defined a professional association as "an organization of practitioners, who judge one another as professionally competent and have united together to perform social functions which they cannot perform in their separate capacity as individuals".
- Professional associations provide a vehicle for nurses to meet present and future challenges and work toward positive profession related changes that keep pace with societal changes.

12 Communication and Educational Technology

"The aim of education is the knowledge not of fact, but of values".
—Dean William R Inge

Objectives
After completing this unit, you will be able to:
- Understand the concepts of communication and educational technology
- List the uses of communication technology in education
- Explain various educational technologies used.

Introduction

In the changing world, education is not fulfilled without the integration of information and communication technology. One cannot depend only on the same big blackboards, an overhead projector, etc. in curriculum implementation. Usage of modern technology in the field of education is inevitable in the changing scenario. No one can disagree with the concept of global village and its impact in nursing. The educational and communicational technology aids in teaching and learning. Communication is defined as a process by which an individual, the communicator transmits to modify the behavior of other individuals. Communication is facilitated by the modern technology. The proliferation of information and communication technology has brought profound changes in the availability of information. Educational technology can be conceived as a science of techniques and methods by which educational goals can be realized. It is not primarily concerned with the task of prescribing the goals, although, it does help in specifying the goals and translating them into behavioral terms. The communication technologies not only aim at making educational opportunities more accessible, but also make them extremely attractive to the students. Communication technology can improve the flavor of the message to be conveyed and knowledge to be gained. They motivate and hence involve the students in learning; attract and hold their attention for optimum learning and help them retain knowledge thus gained.

Definition of Educational Technology

According to GOM Leith, "Educational Technology is a systematic application of scientific knowledge about teaching-learning and conditions of learning to improve the efficiency of teaching and training. In the absence of scientifically established principles, educational technology implements techniques of empirical testing to improve learning situations".

According to BC Mathis, "Educational technology refers to the development of a set of systematic methods, practical knowledge for designing, operating and testing schools".

Robert M Gagne defined, "Educational technology can be understood as the development of a set of systematic techniques, and accompanying practical knowledge for designing testing and operating schools as educational systems".

IK Davies has defined the term Educational technology as "it is concerned with the problems of education and training in context, and it is characterized by disciplined and systematic approach to the organization of resources for learning".

Objectives of Educational Technology

- To determine the goals and formulate the objectives in behavioral terms.
- To analyze the characteristics of the learner.
- To organize the content in logical or psychological sequence.
- To mediate between content and resources of presentation.
- To evaluate the learner's performance in terms of achieving educational objectives.
- To provide the feedback among other components for the modification of learners.

Uses of Communication Technology

The following are some of the uses of communication technology to education:

Easy and Wide Accessibility

With the help of terrestrial network transmissions and satellite-based communication, radio and television are able to extend its reach over the entire length and breadth of India. With the telephone and its improved versions, people all over the world can reach each other instantly. Computers, of course, have brought tremendous efficiency within the reach of people. Similarly, videotext technology adds the possibility of having access to more information. This technology can retrieve textual information, figures, and graphics from remote databases, and also allow people to have access to various frames of information on the home television screen connected to a computer database through wireless transmission. There are three main categories of teleconferencing, namely, audio-conferencing, video-conferencing and computer-conferencing. Internet and the World Wide Web provide tremendous opportunity for reaching people worldwide. Electronic mail (e-mail), which is cheap and instantaneous, has become the order of the day. Individualized learning is planned so as to allow for self-paced, mastery learning.

Teaching

Communication technology has strong multiplier effect and it can be tapped for aiding the teaching-learning process. Advanced communication technologies such as videotext, teletext, video-disk, and computers are being used for education in developed countries. Developing countries also in a phased manner started integrating this technology in the field of education. Communication technologies coupled with flexible homework and learning schedules will provide more productive time for education, training, and work.

Specific Uses

The importance of communication technologies in education lies in its student-centeredness. The students can listen to radio to increase their knowledge, watch television to learn new things, and use computers to collect, process and store information. The student takes the help of the videotext and teletext to gather specific information to enrich his/her store of knowledge.

Some Specific Educational Uses of Communication Technology

Course Planning

Computer can help immensely in designing and planning of courses.

Course Management

The computer can store all the data generated in the process of planning and implementing the course. A final analysis of the quality of the course materials or impact of the course is possible since these can be recalled from the computer and necessary improvements can be incorporated to increase the effectiveness of the course.

Student Support Services

Distance education, with the growth and availability of electronic media, has taken a very gigantic leap. A sensible use of the electronic media can give tremendous support to the distance learners. Regular teleconferencing can be a vital student support service using communication technology.

Print Material

Print material is the primary instructional input in the distance education system in almost all distance education institutions. Here too the impact of the modern technology in terms of quality, efficiency, and cost has been extremely beneficial. With laser printing and desktop publishing, the print medium has undergone a second revolution.

Barriers of Communication Technology to Education

Technological Factors

New communication technologies are not free from technical problems. For instance, lack of a regular flow of electricity can make technologies defunct.

Appropriateness

The technology chosen should suit the geographical conditions of the country. Those developing countries which are large and have a difficult geographic terrain need technologies that suit them.

Accessibility

In many countries communication technology is used first for commercial purposes then for educational. Certain constraints such as lack of sufficient memory, lack of interest amongst educators and administrators, lack of sufficient software/courseware, lack of political will, etc. will invariably affect the accessibility of a technology to the educational sectors.

Handling

An electronic device will become redundant, if one does not know to operate it. There are devices which can be operated with simple know-how, but there are some sophisticated devices, which need special efforts and skills to handle them. Since the technologies are changing fast, one finds it difficult to keep oneself up-to-date in handling and maintaining them.

Maintenance

It is quite often that various technologies are imported or adopted from the developed countries without having made adequate arrangements for maintaining them. One such device develops technical problems. The reasons for poor maintenance facilities may be due to lack of expertise, lack of resources, infrastructure, nonavailability of spare parts, or indifferent attitude of users.

Software/Courseware

It is a fact that there is a dearth of relevant software/courseware for educational sectors all over the world. Most of the developing countries depend on the courseware imported from the developed countries. Such courseware may not suit the sociocultural and educational needs of the students. The nonavailability of the relevant courseware hampers the growth and development of the communication technology in the educational sectors.

The teachers are usually not involved in planning and preparing the courseware (There is a difference between software and courseware—software refers to computer programming while courseware refers to all teaching materials that store information, e.g. radio and television programs).

It is very difficult to cover the entire syllabus by one technology—medium. Therefore, other media are required to achieve the educational objectives in their totality, but it is very difficult for many countries to adopt the multimedia approach to teaching-learning.

Educational Factors

Communication technology demands a change in the role of teachers. Teachers, the important component of the educational system, play a crucial role in the adoption of a technology or an innovation. They can mar the success of any media at the institutional and actual operational level. Their attitude toward technology is thus an important determinant.

Adoption of technology needs a lot of resources and every institution cannot afford to have such costly devices.

Human and Administrative Factors

If the students do not have access to the technology being implemented, the situation may cause serious problems. The situation will immediately create two classes of students—the "haves" and the "have-nots", which in turn will cause various human problems.

Economic Factors

The application of any communication technology is a costly affair. The investment runs to several lakhs of rupees. Such a huge investment requirement forces many of them not to use the technology.

Equipment-related Factors

The problems pertaining to the equipment arise mostly with the application of the imported technologies. The equipment, i.e. the hardware is imported from various foreign agencies or from developed countries. Thus, for maintenance the adopting countries will have to rely on the foreign agencies. This dependency causes havoc as the officials of the adopting countries cannot have total control on all the aspects of such technologies.

Limitations of Communication Technology

- Shortage of investment capital
- Ineffective organization and management
- Inadequate policies for the promotion
- Planning, monitoring, and evaluation
- Quantity and quality of services
- Price or cost and affordability
- Instructional design knowledge.

Some of the Educational Technologies Used

Print Media

Print is the principal medium through which students learn. They spend about 90% of their time reading and writing.

Merits of the Print Media

- Print provides relatively permanent instructional material.
- Can be processed whenever one wants to.
- Free from strict time schedules.
- Ensures more and better learning.
- Allows the learners to learn at their own pace in a style been suited to them.
- Learners, who have learnt to read, prefer the use of print medium.

- Uniquely suited to abstract thinking.
- Remains the cheapest educational medium to use.
- It helps develop understanding of complex concepts and processes.
- It develops basic learning skills of reading and writing that helps a learner become more and more autonomous.
- It helps learners to take stock of their learning through interpolated questions.

Limitations of Print Media

- Problem-solving calls for direct action, hence print cannot be a substitute of direct action.
- Effective use of print medium depends upon a reasonably adequate level of literacy among learners.
- Print is effective only, when the reader possesses well-developed cognitive skills for comprehesing the text and evaluating its thought content.
- Reading printed material is much more time consuming than viewing the same content through images, e.g. TV program.
- Print material can provide theoretical information but cannot provide with the skills required.
- The language of the printed lesson is chosen according to the writer's assumption about average readers. Once written, the language of a printed lesson is fixed; it does not change for below-average or weak learners.

Electronic Media

Electronic media comprises of the nonprint media such as television, radio, film, photographs, slides, audiotape, videotape, computer, videodisk, etc. This media has its own merits and certain limitations.

Merits of Electronic Media

- It can simultaneously reach learners at different places.
- It can provide excellent support to the print media because of their versatile capabilities.
- It can make educational experience more comprehensive.
- Some electronic media can record the learner's performance and provide extremely useful feedback.
- The use of electronic media has proved psychologically exciting for students. These media have the power to stimulate interest and appeal to the neoliterate.
- The electronic media achieve learner involvement and participation and thereby facilitate learning.
- It helps to provide a learning atmosphere in which students achieve and participate in the learning process.
- Electronic media have the flexibility of accommodating individual needs and interests, especially through computers.
- Some technological devices like audio cassettes and video cassettes allow the learners the freedom to choose how much information they would like to be exposed to. These technologies also enable them to choose their own convenient time to receive any given information.

Radio/Audio Medium

Since its very inception, the radio has been and is being used to serve a variety of purposes—to inform, to educate, and to entertain people. Continued technological innovations have made radio broadcasting increasingly available to a large number of people throughout the world.

The radio is the cheapest and the most easily accessible of the other three electronic media, i.e. audio cassette, television, and video cassette. It caters to people of different ages and levels of maturity. For instance, while it provides learners with new joys of learning, it can develop their command over vocabulary, promote concentration and critical listening and improve fluency and confidence in speech and discussion. It can be used for formal and informal education.

Strengths of Radio/Audio Medium

- Easy accessibility
- Wide coverage
- Low capital investment and operating cost
- Easy learner-reception
- Effective thought promotion
- Motivative supportive facilities
- Easy production
- Effective-creation/transmission of reality
- Feasible mode of learner-enrichment
- Direct instruction.

Limitations of Radio/Audio Medium

- The radio is not a flexible medium. There is no face-to-face interaction, dialog or discussion between the listener and the speaker/producer.
- The doubts/queries arising in the mind of a learner cannot be attended to immediately. There is no provision for immediate feedback to the learner.
- It may not be an effective medium for all types of course materials, e.g. the subjects which need demonstration or visual illustrations cannot be taught effectively through radio.
- Radio programming demands experienced and creative personnel with both production and academic background.
- The more heterogeneous the audience; the more difficult it is to produce a radio program of common utility or appeal.

- The span of attention of a learner is short and the retention of factual information is generally low.
- The technical staff concerned with the planning and production of radio program often lack adequate knowledge of the relevant pedagogical needs of the learners and their characteristics.

Educational Radio Production Process

The process of an educational radio program demonstrates a flow in its production process right from forming a concept to the final output in the shape of a program. The flow in the process pertaining to production and utilization of educational radio program constitutes the following steps in a broad sense:
- Policy
- Planning
- Preparation
- Preproduction
- Production
- Review
- Teacher notes/Support material
- Transmission
- Feedback and evaluation.

Educational Television

Television constitutes an important medium widely used to disseminate information to its viewers. It has the advantage of the audio as well as the video. Hence, it has a greater appeal than the radio and the print media.

Kinds of Television Broadcasts

Live Broadcast

Under this system, educational events are directly telecast. Immediate transmission of the programs to a large number of audiences is possible through the live telecast.

Recorded Broadcast

Under this system, prerecorded programs are telecast as per the transmission schedule. The existing educational television services in the country depend mainly on the already produced programs. Such programs can be well-planned and evaluated at each developmental stage. Recorded programs could be of a better quality than live broadcasts because all facilities in terms of time, manpower equipment, etc. are exploited for producing these programs.

Closed Circuit Television Broadcast (CCTV)

Under this system, the prerecorded or live programs are transmitted in a closed circuit. It is the link between the studio and a series of classrooms, usually by means of cables installed in an institution to transmit educational programs. The system can link several classrooms or institutions, and allow transmission from any of the classroom studios.

Merits of Television as Educational Tool

Television caters to the masses of people including people living in remote areas.
- Television programs are well-planned and presented, thus providing higher quality of instruction.
- Rapid and continuing change in curricula and instructional methods are made possible through educational television.
- It reduces dependency on teacher.
- Television provides in-service training for teachers to improve their teaching methods and skills.
- It has proved its effectiveness/supremacy in teaching certain subjects such as agriculture, science, geography, oceanography, etc.

Limitations of Television Media

- Television is a one-way communication, and as such it does not provide for interaction.
- Teaching through television is expensive.
- Students differ in their learning speed and style. Hence, it cannot cater to the speed of every learner.

Compact Disks (CDs)

The CDs are considered to be more effective medium than the television broadcast. The reasons are:
- They are more flexible and convenient in their use
- The students have full control over their pace of learning in terms of their time and place of using the CDs
- The replay facility has made it more suitable to individualized learning.

Digital Library

A digital library comprises digital collections, services and infrastructure to support lifelong learning, research, scholarly communication as well as preservation and conservation of recorded knowledge. The digital library is not a single entity and it requires networking technology to connect many entities. All linkages are transparent to end users. Universal access to digital content and information is a goal.

Digital libraries, like traditional ones, will select, acquire, make available and preserve collections. The major difference will be that digital libraries will consist of machine-readable data. This implies that the traditional concept of a collection must be revised to accommodate materials that are accessible electronically.

A digital library is a library in which collections are stored in digital formats and accessible by computers. The digital content may be stored locally or accessed remotely via computer networks. A digital library is a type of information retrieval system. According to Arms (2003), a digital library is a managed collection of information with associated service where the information is stored in digital format and accessible over a network.

Digital content will be of two types—items created and existing primarily in machine readable format and materials converted from the traditional format, e.g. printed texts and pamphlets, images, motion pictures, and recorded sound. Digital library collections contain fixed permanent documents available in the digital format. To satisfy global resources sharing, digital library is able to transfer data within and outside the countries breaking the physical boundaries of data.

Objective of Digital Library

- To capture, store, organize, and distribute information.
- To introduce, provide, and retrospect services.
- To have large digitized databases.
- To provide facility for networking and resources sharing.
- To improve the cost-effectiveness of library operations.
- To provide coherent view of all information within a library in any format.
- To digitize the document for preservation.

The digital library involves the following:

- Organized collection of multimedia and other types of resources.
- Resources are available in computer processable form.
- The function of acquisition, storage, preservation, and retrieval is carried out through the use of digital technology.
- Access to the entire collection is globally available directly or indirectly across a network.
- Supports users in dealing with information objects.
- Helps in the organization and preservation of the above objects via electronic/digital means.

Requirement of Digital Library

Digital library requires well-tested and proven information technologies including the multimedia kit.

Computer technology: Programs, computer languages, data handling, memory, processing, storage, server, UPS, etc.

Audio-video technology: Local area network, wide area network, circuit networks, broadcast networks, telecommunications service like telephone, TV, VCR, DVD, telex, teletext, facsimile, internet, e-mail, videotext, bulletin board, online databases, videophones, and videoconferencing.

Printing and publishing technology: Computer prints, dot matrix printers, laser printers, electronic typewriters, offset litho printers, desktop publishing, pagemakers, electronic publishing, etc.

Natural interaction technology: System software, artificial intelligence, etc.

Operating system: Disk operations, networking, multitasking, etc.

Scanner: Slide scanner, HP scan jet, microfilming scanner, digital camera, barcode scanner, etc.

Services of the Digital Library Shared Cataloging

A librarian and information manager can use the catalog information available in a major university library or a resource center for cataloging new publications added to the library. A document is cataloged only once at the time of entry into the network. Other libraries, which procure that document later need not spend time in cataloging but can download the cataloging information from the network.

Current Awareness Services

List of latest additions to the library, namely books, patents, periodicals, standards, audio-visual material or any other can be put into the internal web for user attention.

Bulletin Board Service

The major bulletin board service available on the internet is known as network news. Net news consists of thousands of individual bulletin boards on topics as diverse as education, hobbies, science, politics, entertainment, and employment opportunities.

The Document Supply/Delivery Services

It will enable a library to request to another library for a copy of document to be transmitted via e-mail or fax.

Digital library and information center can provide following services to its users:

- Remote information services
- Inter-library loan service
- Union catalog
- Internet information sources
- CD-ROM database
- Referral services
- File transfer protocol.

Advantages of Digital Libraries Storage and Preservation

1. Digital information can be copied without error. As a result, preservation in a digital world does not depend on permanent object and keeping it under guard.

2. *Ubiquity*: Another key advantage is ubiquity. Many simultaneous users can access a single electronic copy from many locations. Copies can be delivered with electronic speed, and it would be possible to reformat the material as per the reader preference.
3. *Support wider range of materials*: Digital storage also permits libraries to expand the range of material, they can provide to their users. Digital material can permit access to videotapes and new kinds of multimedia material that are created only on computer and have no equivalent in any traditional format.
4. *Access current information*: For researchers, digital libraries provide access to up-to-date current literature and thereby help them to be aware of current trends.
5. *Others*
   - No physical boundary
   - Round-the-clock availability
   - Multiple accesses
   - Information retrieval
   - Structured approach
   - Wider storage space
   - Added value
   - Distance learning.

Problems of Digital Library Technological Obsolescence

- The major risk to digital object is no physical deterioration, but technological obsolescence of the device—(hardware and software) to read them.
- *Dependence on technologies*: Digital library is dependent on telecommunication and computer system for information utilization and transfer.
- *Technological problems*: As on today, the technology has not percolated to the required level, to make the digital libraries acceptable on par with the conventional libraries with printed documents.
- *Bandwidth*: Digital library will need high band width for transfer of multimedia resources but the bandwidth is decreasing day by day due to its overutilization.
- *Expensive*: The major obstacle to digitalization is that it is very expensive especially to undertake in-house digitalization. Initial cost of establishing digital library is high.
- *Copyright*: It is very easy to copy and replicate digital information. Copyright law gets violated in digital environment more due to lack of control over content access and reproduction of multiple copies of digital information.
- *Pricing in the digital environment*: Pricing of information in the digital world is going to be very complex. Ownership is expected to give way to licensing, pay per use, etc.

Factors of Change to Digital Libraries

The limited buying power of libraries, complex nature of recent document, storage problems, etc. are some of the common factors which are influencing to change to digital mode. Some other factors are:
- Information explosion.
- Searching problem in traditional libraries.
- Low-cost technology when considering the storage capacity and maintenance.
- *Environmental factor*: The uses of digital libraries are the cleanest technologies to fulfill the slogan "Burn a CD-ROM save a tree".
- New generation needs.

Online Teaching and Online Learning

Education and training have gone through a number of radical changes in terms of design and delivery methods over a period of time.

The internet is emerging as a global mass with the potential to transform education. Currently, the online learning has emerged as a new paradigm of learning with the advent of internet as the medium of delivery.

The online training combines the flexibility of distance education and the interactivity of conventional classroom-based education.

Characteristics of Online Teaching and Learning

Instructional Design

One of the most powerful features of the internet is its ability to provide interactivity among geographically-distant people. It has a lot of scope for providing an instructional design that can make the learning much more interesting and easier.

Anytime-anywhere Learning

The online training provides an efficient and cost-effective learning with anytime and anywhere flexibility. Online training offers the possibility to obtain skills without the trouble of commuting and attending training in a classroom. The 24-hour access to course materials allows the learner to learn on his/her own time and pace.

Access to the Best Faculty

More than the convenience, the online learning provides opportunities to interact with best of the faculty, who would otherwise be unavailable. Additionally, it also helps the learner to master the communication skills needed in the cyber world.

Rich Learning Experience

Online courses have the capacity to offer a rich learning experience that takes full advantage of the electronic medium.

Online training is much more learner-centered than conventional classroom training. In online, the learner can read, listen, observe, and interact. Then one can interact with other students and tutors to discuss about what he/she is learning.

Classroom Goes to the Learner

The biggest advantage is that, there is no physical classroom to go, and attend the class on a prefixed schedule. Rather, the learner can attend the online class whenever he/she has time and still participate in all the discussions, which is like a place between the fellow learners and the faculty. Lectures, coursework, assignments, questions, discussion—all take place at the learners' convenience—online. Plus, the learners receive personalized instructor feedback, and share insights and information with fellow online students.

Instructional Model

An outline of learning delivery system can be leveraged in various instructional models and every program or course can have a combination of instructional delivery models. Broadly, these instructional models can be grouped into the following:
- Completely online based
- Online supported
- Post-course online support
- Online resource center

The online supported courses will address the learning needs where the personal contact with the faculty is essential and requires some amount of hands-on training for mastering the skills. The post-course online support is ideal for providing mentoring or handholding of participants, who attended short in-service courses. Table 12.1 shows a model for faculty teaching online.

Content Development

This refers to development and production of learning materials as per the instructional technology and design formulated, based on the learning requirements.

It is recommended that the institutions should develop in-house expertise in learning material development for the online delivery. The institutions should have a facility for in-house development with a small development team to start with. In addition, the faculty needs to be oriented in online content creation as per the process outlined for development.

Learning Delivery System

This refers to creation of the site and various navigation systems, database design, messaging systems and other

Table 12.1: A model for faculty teaching online.

Antecedent conditions	Context	Strategies	Consequences	
Support system	**Online curriculum**	**Collaboration/planning**	**Faculty adjusting to online teaching**	
• Administrative support technology	• Faculty learn new role and new pedagogies	• Faculty development	*Positive*	*Negative*
• Partnerships	• Requires high energy	• Faculty team development	• Flexible	• Social isolation
• Online resources	• Requires creativity	• Faculty mentoring	• Thoughtful responses	• Delayed responses
• Faculty teams	comfortable		• Socially connected	• Lack of spontaneity
Use of technology to teach online	**Online environment**	**Rethinking faculty role/ redesigning course**	**Faculty role changed**	
• Software/hardware	• Portable	• Using critical thinking skills	• Increased faculty workload	
• Course management system	• Convenient	• Using trial and error	• From authority figure to facilitator	
• Technical skills	• Comfortable		• Working with partnerships and teams	
Policies for distance learning	**Adjusting time frames**	**Developing online communication techniques**	**Increased awareness of course**	
• Ownership	• 24/7 environment	• New and effective communication methods	• Increased challenges	
• Compensation	• Available in a timely manner	• Engaging web pages	• Shared learning	
• Workload	• Requires increased communication	• Designing motivating media	• Managing diversity	
		• Using reflective writing	• Community of learners	
		• Maintaining/revising	• Effective way of doing business	
		• Preparing course ahead of time	**Changing relationship with students**	
		• Dealing with new technology Dealing with software	• Miss face-to-face contact	
			• Know students better	
			• Take a different form	

Source: Ryan M, Hodson-Carlton KS, Ali NS. A Model for Faculty Teaching Online: Confirmation of a Dimensional matrix. 2005;44(8):363.

operation systems, including the administrative interface and integrating them together as a learning delivery system.

Delivery Site

The site should reflect the personality of the institution, its programs and services, the type of image it wants to present; and provide sufficient information for all the stakeholders of the site, color, fonts and images are part of the site personality.

The navigation should be simple and user-friendly. All basic information should load fast in the most common browsers and should be reachable in minimum number of clicks. Site content structuring should reflect the structure of the institution. Site navigation and learning navigation should be differentiated and easily accessible. In general, the major facilities offered in the online delivery site can be broadly grouped into two:
1. Learner facility.
2. Administrative facilities.

Some of the features that can be made available in the facilities are listed below:

Learner Facilities

- Online registration
- Create and modify personal info/profile
- Track learning plan progress
- View all enrolled courses from the learning desk
- View/browse courses from the personal learning desk
- View reports on assessment results
- Check their understanding/learning
- Access the online library
- Access the resource center
- Send queries to the faculty for doubt resolution
- Participate in the relevant peer discussion forums
- Take preassessment test
- Take practice tests
- View the learning plan
- Practice exercises
- Take practice assignments, projects, and case study analysis
- Facilities for synchronized discussion with peer and faculty
- Audio and video embedded courses.

Administrative Facilities

- Create and modify user accounts
- Create and modify user role
- Create and update courses
- View and produce reports on course usage
- Track learning plan progress by learner, course and group/batch
- View learners by course, date and curriculum
- List learners by key information
- Create and control access for batches/groups/subgroups.

The important aspect of the online learning is the kind of interactivity, it can provide for the geographically dispersed learners. The faculty needs to be available for an online seminar or answering a student query. Queries on specific courses, tutorials, mentoring, maintaining of various student interactive forums, seminars and conferences, are part of this service. In addition, this will also include updating of resource centers and online library.

Other than learning services, the students need to be provided service on admission and registration, responding to the front office queries, preliminary counseling, admission and registration. There should be a dedicated team/person (depending on the load) to handle this service.

Infrastructure Set-up

This component takes care of the basic infrastructure that is required to deliver online education to its learners and creation of learning materials and infrastructure for the learning service personnel.

Regarding the hosting of online set-up, the institution's own information infrastructure (networking, hardware, and software) can be used or it can even host the online delivery system on a third party's (ISP or who has facility for hosting) infrastructure and subsequently shift the site to own facility.

Ongoing Operations

- Maintenance of various systems, site and other infrastructures.
- Providing services pertaining to learners' queries and other interactive services.
- Management of learning services.

Virtual Campus

Virtual campus offers some interesting features that will enhance learners' learning experience. Its library has a collection of references, including many full text articles. The learner may bookmark selections for later reading. In the campus community network, the learner can talk to other learners and professionals in his field. Another important feature of virtual campus is campus club. The learner can create a club to share information with a group of people sharing a common interest.

Functions of Virtual Campus

- Provides learning resources
- Serves as a student adviser
- Provides information
- Helps in seeking feedback
- Acts as a tutor support.

Limitations of Virtual Campus

The human relations in computer-mediated communities cannot be as intimate, strong and affect laden as in social communities.

The primordial feelings of fear, love and anger cannot be transmitted online, because the participant knows intellectually but more importantly, intuitively that she/he can turn off the machine and avoid the impact of the forces.

Virtual Classroom

In the recent era of globalization, technological advancement has increased dramatically in every sphere including mainstream education. These advances have introduced new educational nomenclature, i.e. "virtual education", "virtual classroom", "virtual universities", "online courses", "electronic" and "cyberspace institution", etc. Profound investments in technology in this decade have given rise to a worldwide explosion of information.

Virtual classroom has taken a lead role in the teaching-learning process. Generically, the virtual classroom is a teaching and learning environment located within a computer mediated communication system. It consists of asset of group communication and work "spaces" and facilities that are constructed in software.

The virtual classsroom, an innovative program brings the university into the homes and workplaces of students through the use of computers. A virtual classroom is defined as a computer accessible online learning environment intended to fulfill many of the learning facilitation roles of a physical classroom. A virtual classroom is a learning environment created in the virtual space.

Virtual schools are of three broad categories, i.e. independent, collaborate and broadcast. According to Russell (2001), independent models can often be referred to as "asynchronous" because they do not rely upon direct communication between teacher and students, as they do not avail of chat or videoconferencing facilities. Synchronous models usually involve more communication and collaboration through videoconferencing and live chats. Broadcast models allow students to access lectures or broadcasts on the internet. All these models offer a wide range of learning flexibility in virtual environments that serve the individual needs of the learner regardless of their age, gender, religion, nationality, or disability. Table 12.2 shows the needs of the virtual learners.

A virtual classroom environment successfully mixes up different media inputs, i.e. (a) face-to-face plus virtual classroom which can vary from adding system use to enrich on-campus courses conducted to traditional means; to distance courses where system use is supplemented by one or two face-to-face meetings, (b) virtual classroom as the sole means of delivery, with the use of print media in the form of textbooks or course notes, and (c) multimedia, i.e. virtual classroom plus video, audio or audiographic media. Thus, there is a move toward multimedia-based interactive learning process and computer assisted instructional system.

Table 12.2: Relationship between the assumptions and the needs of the virtual students.

Assumptions of the adult learners	Needs of the virtual students
As people mature their self-concept moves from that of a dependent personality toward one of a self-directing human being.	Programs-based on the ability to meet the educational needs of nontraditional students.
Adults accumulate a growing reservoir of experience, which is a rich source for learning.	Focus on the learner, rather than the instructor.
Adults' readiness to learn is closely related to the developmental tasks of their social roles.	Cost-effectiveness
Perspectives change as people mature from future application of knowledge to immediacy of application.	Reliable technology that is easy to navigate and transparent (that is user friendly or easy for novice users to learn)
Adults are motivated to learn by internal rather than external factors.	Appropriate levels of information and human interaction.

Unique Features of the Virtual Classroom

- Leverage—the students can learn from a single professor
- Cost savings
- Accessibility
- Convenience
- Flexibility
- Efficiency
- Automated administration

Advantages of Virtual Classroom

For students:
- Saving time, cost factors
- Removes the need to travel to the physical classroom
- Easy access from any computer
- More helpful for the physically challenged
- Can respond to material at their own speed and time
- Facility for instant reviewing
- Less learning time

For teachers:
- The teacher needs not to work from an office or classroom

- Can work as part time. Saves teacher's time because of easy update of the content.
- The changes or updates are instantly accessible to everyone enrolled in the classroom.

Characteristics of Virtual Classroom Learning

Virtual classroom also needs equivalent equipment and tools in the form of network-based software application to allow a group of instructors and students to carry out the learning process. The output of virtual teaching-learning process depends upon the factors like students' motivation for self-learning, subject expertise and communication skills of the teacher, online problem-solving facility, connectivity to e-library, and use of technology-based lightly interactive multimedia, etc.

Basically, there are four principles to be kept in mind for successful teaching in the virtual classroom such as dealing with:
1. Media richness
2. Timely responsiveness
3. Organization
4. Interaction.

In the traditional classroom, a pleasing voice, occasional jokes, dramatic gestures, eye contact with the teacher and the classroom interaction can help to enliven a long lecture. But in virtual classrooms, there is only the computer screen and the printed pages. Even if the multimedia is there, long segments of lecture-type materials are boring. Hence, in order to maintain interest, the instructor should use written language in a skillful way by putting some humor and metaphors. The instructor should deliver small segments of lecture with print/prerecorded materials accompanied with opportunities for students' participation.

Secondly, unlike the traditional classrooms, the students in the virtual classroom will not receive an immediate response to their questions and comments. This can be very frustrating. In this case, in order to encourage the students, the instructor can promote more active participation/interaction and provide the feedback to students, in the virtual classroom more frequently/daily. Thirdly, unless the study materials of online courses/virtual classrooms get organized, students will become very confused. Therefore, the instructor must establish regular rhythms and schedules, based on dividing the course into modules which last a week, a week and half, or two weeks each so that the participants can plan ahead in terms of when they will need to sign online and when work will be due, and so that the group moves through the topics in an orderly manner.

Another strategy is for the instructor to enter the stimulus materials for each week's work on a regular basis, with new material predictably appearing at least twice a week. The most significant determinant of the students' satisfaction in the online courses/virtual classrooms is the amount and quality of interaction between the instructor and the students, and/or among the students. This is not always easy for the instructor. Collaborative learning is encouraged in case of virtual classrooms which emphasize group/cooperative efforts among faculty and students. In this context, knowledge is viewed as a social construct, and therefore, the educational process is facilitated by social interaction in an environment that facilitates peer interaction.

The physical format of the textbook does not easily allow student and teacher to depart from the prescribed path, or to link to new concepts and ideas from other disciplines. The virtual textbooks move the learners beyond content mastery to information seeking and problem-solving skills. This enables the learner to evaluate and synthesize information from diverse sources and understand and apply the difference between facts and opinions, grasp multiple and diverse perspectives and draw insights from these and utilize these within the context of one's own knowledge base and experiences.

The web seems to be more suitable for learning, where the information can be delivered in both linear and nonlinear format. It can be presented via multimedia with text, pictures, video, sound, and animation. Vast amount of information can be searched and downloaded from internet. Traditional classrooms, most teachers make use of a chalkboard for further clarification of a point. But the instructor of a virtual classroom may use the whiteboard to answer questions from students. Such tools allow images to be displayed, manipulated, annotated, and shared between two learners or among a whole group. An important part of the physical class environment is the personal interaction. Allowing all students to "hear" the questions and answers helps everyone to learn and encourages additional questions. In virtual learning environment, list servers can be used to redistribute e-mail messages. Use net newsgroups, computer conferencing and collaborative work spaces may serve for sharing this kind of interactions. Virtual classrooms use videoconferencing, and teleconferencing to make the presentation more attractive and lively. Virtual classrooms are more accessible, flexible and convenient in their approach toward education, students and teachers.

Recent research found that online courses supported critical thinking skills, leadership, communication, problem solving and ethics. Often the students prefer the delivery mode and work at their own pace, and take time to analyze and synthesize the learning materials.

Learning in virtual classroom is not natural and spontaneous rather artificially created. The teacher in the virtual classroom is present in virtual image, not physically. Thus, virtual classroom lacks the human touch. The virtual students seem more frustrated, not only from the technology but from the inability to ask the teacher questions in a face-to-face environment.

For availing the facilities of virtual learning, learner has to be matured, self-motivated, computer literate and well-versed with the components of virtual classroom. Primarily the teacher in the virtual classroom follows the lecture-cum-demonstration method with multimedia use which is suitable for higher level courses. It is not suitable for lab-based and activity oriented courses. There is no scope for testing the entry level behaviors; thus a teacher cannot judge the degree of disparity among students. Also the differences in learning styles and ranging aptitude levels would result in further discrepancy. As more numbers of schools and universities are now operating online, it is becoming increasingly difficult to judge and evaluate the academic virtue and quality of education provided by them. In virtual classroom, the teacher's communication skill is more important than any other competencies, i.e. managerial or interpersonal or liaisoning skills. There is a little scope for the all round personality development of the children. Individual caring, counseling, emotional sharing mentoring, etc. are absent in virtual classrooms with the teacher only present on the audio-visual screens. There is little scope for direct teacher-student intervention and two way communication. The factors, like subject expertise, communication skill, expression through body language, personality, skill of holding students' interest and attention play a very crucial role in virtual learning and the success of the programming course primarily depends on these factors.

The whole system of virtual classroom education is based on technological advancement and operations and any sort of technical fault will create chaos in the education system. Another disadvantage with online courses is that students may encounter problems with software compatibility, connection, connection speed, server unreliability, computer problems, etc. If students encounter problems they may become easily discouraged and dissatisfied with online education. Moreover, the misconception persists that online courses are easier. But in reality, online courses are equal or more challenging than traditional face-to-face courses because the primary responsibility for facilitating learning shifts to the students. Thus, if a student is not motivated and matured enough to be reflective and evaluate his own learning strategies, he/she may not succeed in virtual education. So, the students need to be self-motivated to keep on track. No face-to-face contact with classmates or instructors can lead to feelings of isolation or lack of connectiveness.

E-Learning

E-learning is an emerging educational paradigm where learners identify specifically what they need to learn and access it quickly from a wide variety of educational providers, instead of taking whole courses from local educational institutions on their fixed schedule. Ideally, e-learning is the exact content and delivery method that the learner needs and it is available at the time and place the learner needs it. E-learning helps learners stay on top of today's fast paced education world.

E-learning incorporates Web and internet-based applications as well as CD-ROMS. The learners can learn at own pace. E-learning is delivered straight to the desktop of the learner through an internet or intranet connection.

Advantages of E-Learning
- Content can be stored and reused by others.
- Mobile learning. Learning is possible at anywhere and anytime.
- Personalization and interactivity.

E-Teaching

E-teaching is a teaching and learning approach that combines the best features of traditional in-class instruction with the communication and resource potential available via the web. It is a technique that uses the internet to improve student success by enhancing and extending classroom instruction via the web. Faculty uses internet to post course materials and web-based warm up assignments before class, and students use materials on the web to prepare for each class. The faculty member in turn uses student responses to create an interactive classroom environment that emphasize active learning and cooperative problem solving and decreases the use of traditional lecture.

E-Tutoring

Online tutoring or e-tutoring is the new and emerging technique for live one-on-one tutoring sessions. E-tutoring can be defined as teaching, support, management and assessment of students on programs of study that involve a significant use of online technologies. E-tutoring contains vital differences in terms of time, distance and the specific technologies adopted, and these all have implications for teaching staff. The capacities required can be quite different to face-to-face teaching both in terms of integrating appropriate forms of technology into learning activities and in managing and supporting students' learning online.

E-tutoring provides live, online coaching, homework help and focused exam preparation from the tutors, irrespective of geographical location. Each student is offered personalized learning and individual interaction with a tutor. Tutoring online has been made very simple by recent advances in whiteboard and voice technology. The coaching is live using audio and a shared whiteboard. Every student is evaluated on his or her capability to learn and the tutoring is designed to take care of each student's individual capability. For online tutoring an internet connection, a computer microphone and computer speakers are needed.

Qualities of E-Tutor
- She should be an expert in her subject, IT and soft skills.
- She needs to build rapport, generate enthusiasm and maintain interest.
- She must be proactive to make things happen, be a catalyst to help learners get going on a course.
- She must be patient to understand the needs of the learners.
- She should have the ability to assess the needs of the students by picking up on the hints and reading between the lines.
- She should be able to fix problems before they even arise.

Computer Managed Learning
Computer managed learning (CML) is a learning system that allows the learners to take courses outside of a classroom environment, but within a structured timetable. The learners can study the assigned material on their own and complete a series of computerized unit tests, and final exams. The task of CML is that of using the computer to manage the learning sequence. The computer can define the student's tasks, identify appropriate teaching materials. CML systems are software packages with several common features, including generating tests from banks of questions, marking the test generated, analyzing the results and keeping records of students' marks and progress. CML systems have been used for many years predominantly for summative evaluation.

Advantages of CML
- CML is flexible
- CML is partially self-paced
- Instructor accessibility.

Teleconferencing

A teleconferencing (also known as a video-teleconference) is a set of interactive telecommunication technologies which allow two or more locations to interact via two-way video and audio-transmissions simultaneously.

Teleconferencing is an electronic means which can bring together three or four people in two or more locations to discuss or share the use of two-way and one-way video, both full motion and slow scan, electronic blackboards, facsimile, computer graphics, radio satellite and videotext. But, the most essential part of all forms of teleconferencing is a good quality audio system to help immediate interaction among the participants for information exchange.

Educational teleconferencing can be a valuable medium for education. It involves the use of several media and permits interactive group communication by means of a two-way broadcast. Three main types of teleconferencing are:
1. **Audio-teleconferencing:** Teleconferencing, where the audio medium is used as a two-way communication, is known as audio teleconferencing. It requires a multi-telephone line electronic switch or interconnection device called a "bridge" to which the user can attach a wide variety of data transmission devices and telephones. Audio equipment used with the bridge are the usual handsets, speaker phones, radio telephones and microphone speaker units.
2. **Video-teleconferencing:** This type of teleconferencing is arranged by combining two-way video media. This is now a popular mode in higher education institutions, particularly for academic discussion and even for conduct of interviews, viva-voce examinations. Video-teleconferencing increases the quality of interaction because the teacher/expert and the student can see each other and can share their feeling and experiences.
3. **Computer teleconferencing:** It is the most effective way of teleconferencing. With the adequate facility of suitable hardware, information can be sent and received at the convenience of both the teacher and the student with the use of computers. Computer conferencing can be text-based or full video-based.

Among these three, audio-teleconferencing is the most commonly used technique in educational institutions. The flexibility, low capital and operating costs of audio-teleconferencing make it a means of communication that is of special interest to institutions serving students, who live in small and widely separated communities.

Organization of Teleconference Sessions
The process of teleconferencing consists of four stages:
1. **Planning:** Advanced planning is very important for the success of teleconferencing. This requires the number of students and the duration of each session.
2. **Preparation of materials:** Educational teleconferencing requires the use of printed materials including charts and diagrams.
3. **Preparing the students:** Preparing students for an active participation is a prerequisite for the success of teleconferencing. The student should know in advance about the content to be discussed and the objectives to be achieved.
4. **Conduct the actual session:** The session should be interactive so that all the students can actively participate and learn as much as they can from the conference session.

After the conference is over, the necessary feedback should be obtained from the students. This will also help the students to know their performance.

The sessions can also be recorded so that it could help the students who could not participate in the conference.

Advantages of Teleconferencing

Teleconferencing is very useful when the students are widely scattered.

The system can be adjusted quickly to serve large or small groups.

Access to the instruction in the program can be controlled through a limited number of off-campus centers.

The system provides the facility for immediate feedback to the learners.

Benefits of Teleconferencing

- Expands learning opportunities
- Adds excitement to traditional methods
- Teaches planning and organizational skills
- Teaches public speaking skills
- Improves students' memory retention
- Enhances students' understanding
- Minimal investment
- Time saving.

Limitations of Teleconferencing

- Teleconferencing is a costly technique of instruction.
- It requires efficient telephone and television network throughout the country.
- The chances of technical failure are high.

Multimedia

Multimedia presentations are those that are assembled (or authored) inside the computer and played by it on a monitor or projection screen. Multimedia presentations are, however, assembled outside and played from any device using their own display apparatus.

Application of Multimedia

Multimedia is applicable in all fields, such as, nursing management, education, business, broadcasting, etc. in different forms.

Multimedia Classroom Environment for the Learners

Learner-centered education is about shift or change in educational design from existing traditional to the innovative practice for the betterment of education. Multimedia instructional network system based on information and communication technology is able to fulfill the learner needs and expectations, to attract the learner's attention in the classroom, to involve them in a healthy learning environment. The multimedia classroom environments for the learners are as follows:

Hand Raising

If learners get a doubt they can press the scroll lock key as a help button. The teacher hears a beep sound and gets a hand raise on a learner's computer icon. Then the teacher gets into conservations mode with the learner and clear his doubt, while all the other learners overhear them. Instead of conversation, the teacher and the learner chat through remote messaging board also. The advantage in this case is there is more flexibility in getting the doubt cleared than the conventional class.

File Transfer and File Submit

The teacher can transfer any file or all the learners to the desired location on the learner's machine. Through the file submit function the learner can also submit his work to the teacher electronically. File submitted by the learner gets stored in a particular location of the teacher machine which the teacher can go through anytime.

Net Movie

Through net movie, movie can be played on the teacher machine and broadcasted to all the learners' screens in real time. It resembles as if the movie runs on the learner computers whereas, it is actually running on the teacher machine only, but the screen and the voice get transferred to the learners' machine. This is useful for showing a video content without the help of the projector.

Group and Group Talk

The teacher can divide the learners into groups at will. One learner in the group is selected to work like the teacher and execute functions like broadcast, file transfer, demo and net movie for that group. The selected learner and his computer act like the teacher and teacher-machine for that group. The learner can be divided into multiple voice and message chatting groups. This is an excellent tool for group discussion.

Remote message: The teacher and the learners can communicate with each other by sending messages.

One-to-one voice chat: The teacher can talk with any one logged-in-learner. The other learners won't be disturbed.

Hardware and Software Requirements for Developing Multimedia Educational Tools

A basic multimedia computer requires sound, graphics, a CD-ROM drive and a rather large hard disk. The development of multimedia educational tools requires a combination of the following hardware and software systems:

VCRs, CD-ROM drives, videodisk player, scanners, speakers, audio input devices, color printers, video recorders, mass storage devices, multimedia networks, video editing program, simulation and animation packages, graphics and statistics software, audio editing programs and image enhancement packages.

Constraints in Using Multimedia Computer

- Lack of trained people and necessary skills among the people to use the multimedia system.
- Lack of software to integrate, control, coordinate, manage and adopt the various media for human computer interface.
- Lack of search and pattern recognition, capability for locating information.
- Lack of standardization.
- High-cost to get the multimedia system.

Internet in Education

Internet is an open nonparticipatory computer communication infrastructure that reaches every corner of the globe, carries information on every topic and is available to users round the clock. Technically it is a global collection of interconnected networks. It allows computer users to share equipment, programs and information available in different sites. Hence, it is also known as "Information Superhighway".

The internet works on the Transmission Control Protocol (TCP) and Internet Protocol (IP). These two are collectively called TCP/IP. For sending data into another machine TCP divides the data into little packets and IP puts the destination address on each packets. The internet addresses have two forms—one for the understanding of the user and the other for the machine. Typically, an address on the internet looks like this:

Username@host.subdomain.domain

Where username is the log in name of the user, host is the local network server grouped into domains. The domains are classified as geographic and nongeographic. The following shows the list of domain names in below:

Domain Name in Internet			
Geographical		Nongeographical	
.in	India	.com	Commercial Organization
.au	Australia	.net	Networks
.de	Germany	.gov	Government
.jp	Japan	.mil	Military Networks
.uk	United Kingdom	.edu	Educational Institute
.ca	Canada	.org	Organization

The internet has grown up and evolved as an open system where individuals and organizations can join and become online. There are several bodies that look after the technical standards in terms of technology of the internet.

The common internet service providers in India are BSNL, Airtel, Jio, Vodafone, ACT Fibernet, Hathway, TATA teleservices, etc.

In education, the learners can access and use resources available on the internet. Learning can be done at any time convenient to the user. The timing of the library, interaction with the teacher is not rigid. They can be approached at one's own convenience.

Information disseminated through printed books takes considerable time to be updated. Retrieving information through the internet not only provides access to information instantaneously at low cost, but also provides access to the latest information as updating online courses is much easier and relatively inexpensive. The internet and World Wide Web (WWW) provide opportunity for collaborative learning; makes web based teaching possible and facilitates interactivity for learning.

At present a large number of courses are available online in the web.

As with other form of education, internet-based teaching has distinct advantages and disadvantages.

Advantages of Internet

- The resources are available to any computer on the internet with the proper software.
- No space or time restrictions are present in a virtual course. Time zone differences are consequent.
- Internet resources such as www based materials are distributable across multiple platforms.
- The technology is relatively easy to use.
- Sources are available across the entire internet.
- Web-based materials are easy to update, providing student access to current information.
- The internet provides a student-centered learning environment.
- A variety of learning opportunities can be provided to accommodate learning style differences.
- Students become skilled at using internet resources.

Disadvantages

- Traffic congestion on the internet may become a major issue.
- Courses may focus on the technology rather than the content.
- Web-based course materials may be time consuming for the teacher to develop.
- Faculty members must accept a new teaching paradigm, that of facilitator and manager of learning virtual course, the professor does little professing.
- Although today's students as a whole are more technologically literate than ever before, many are intimidated.

Lack of access may handicap some students, and in distance education lack of access will exclude lower socioeconomic neighborhoods.

Courses with internet components often attract non-student participants, especially on the web.

Internet Services

The internet provides many services: to send and receive mails (e-mail), support for special interest scholarly lists and newsgroups, remote login to a computer (telnet), and the file transfer from remote locations (FTP).

Telnet

One type of utility protocol is telnet, which enables a computer on a network to log on to another computer and read the information stored on it, if it has an account on the other machine. In telnet, the computer of the user is known as the "local" computer and the computer logged on to is known as "remote" or "host" computer. Once the connection is established the instructions given are executed on the remote computer but the effect in the form of information display is on the local computer. The physical distance between the local and remote computers is of no consequence. Users can telnet into a huge database, which is part of the host computer, to do research or even telnet into libraries around the world to get information about a certain document.

File Transfer Protocol

File Transfer Protocol (FTP) is a program used for copying files from one machine in the internet to another. People, who like to share their resources, such as articles, databases and other information put them at FTP sites and in this way they become available to others for viewing and also for downloading. The biggest advantage of FTP is that the information is available in electronic form. Logging on to an FTP server is similar to connecting to a telnet server. FTP is a fast, efficient, and reliable way to transfer information.

Electronic Mail

Electronic mail (e-mail), as the name suggests, is a mailing system which uses various data communication devices as its medium. The e-mail is the ability to compose, send, and receive mail via electronic media. It is a highly popular facility of internet used for message exchange.

The computer on the internet finds paths through the Internet Protocol Address and gets forwarded quite quickly. Today, e-mail is undoubtedly the most widely used service on the internet.

Components of e-Mail

The basic format of any e-mail is:
- The recipient's address
- The sender's return address
- The subject of the message
- The body of the message, and
- Enclosures consisting of one or more file (optional).

The data can be sent in any format in the form of an attachment but the recipient must have the required software to run the attached file.

To send or receive e-mail, you need an electronic mail program or software. All e-mail softwares have similar structures having a message header, body of the message and optional file attachment. The message header has the following:

To	The address to which the message will be sent.
From	This includes the e-mail address of the sender. This is automatically filled in by the e-mail program.
Subject	This is optional, but it is always better to give a subject to your message to help the receiver to decide whether to read or not.
CC	This stands for carbon copy. In a computer environment, it is the addresses of the additional recipients of the message.
BCC	This stands for blind carbon copy. This is similar to that of CC except that the Email address of the recipients specified in this field do not appear in the received message header and the recipients in the To or CC fields will not know that a copy sent to these address.
Attachments	Some e-mail programs keep it separately. This allows the sender to post files of different formats.

Internet Chatting

Internet permits interpersonal chatting through talk program where you can chat with one or more persons in the real time environment.

Developing an Internet Connection

For a basic set-up, three items are necessary:
- An adequate computer with modem
- An installed phone line and
- An internet service provider.

For Establishing an Advanced Internet Connection

Establishing an advanced internet connection in which all computers within the institution are connected to the internet is also not difficult. Again, three conditions must be met.
1. Establish a local area network
2. Purchase an internet router
3. Install an ISDN, DSL, or TI, a large high speed line that can accommodate many users.

Technology and Teachers' Role

Technology has caused a revolution in the way we teach and learn but there can be no real revolution unless the faculty changes how they teach. Geser and Olesch (2000) observes: "what we need is a renaissance of the teacher, a teacher, who is fit for working in a networked learning environment and ready to be the guide on the side instead of the sage on stage". Prensky (2007) observes: "In general students are learning, adopting, and using technology at a much more rapid pace than their teachers and many teachers are highly fearful of the technologies that the students take for granted." Teachers can and should be able to understand and teach where and how new technologies can add value in learning. To do this, teachers must learn and understand about these technologies and make necessary effort in adapting this in the teaching-learning process. Some of the emerging technologies such as Skype, Podcasting with Digital Audio Recording, Moodle (a course management system), Wikis (collaborative encyclopedias) and Blogs are redefining the way teachers teach and students learn. With these emerging technologies, the teacher is no longer the sole dispenser of knowledge and the teacher takes the role of guide and facilitates learning.

Mobile Learning

Mobile learning or m-learning is defined as "using mobile technologies, including mobile phones and handheld devices to enhance the learning process. As "mobile" implies that the technology is wirelessly connected, this means that learners are not restricted to one learning environment and m-learning allows them to access information everywhere and at any time. The fact that many students already own and carry mobiles remains a key factor in their potential for education. Students doing fieldwork are using mobiles to take notes and photographs and send them directly to a course blog, where they receive instructor feedback; colleagues using virtual collaboration tools have access to materials while traveling or otherwise away from their computers.

Wireless Technologies

The term "wireless technologies" is self-explanatory and can be associated to m-learning to some extent. Wireless technology allows the learner to access information at their convenience. One example is bluetooth with which a learner can access internet connection. This technology makes it possible for learners to access almost any internet content and motivates them to learn at their own pace and in an environment that suits them.

Skype

"Skype" is software that allows one to talk to people over the computer. With a fast connection, Skype allows one to talk to people over the computer for free of cost except for the cost for internet usage and connection. If one has a good internet connection (e.g. broadband) he/she can talk to anyone in the world and the reception is very clear. To use this service, users are required to have an internet connection, have downloaded the program and have a microphone and headset. Skype is quite useful for language teachers and learners.

Podcasting

Podcasting is the method of distributing multimedia files, such as audio programs or music videos over the internet for playback on mobile devices and personal computers. Podcasts are digital recordings stored in a music file which can then be uploaded to a computer. Like any file published on the internet, the file can be downloaded to one's own personal media player. The media player can be personal computer, iPod, MP3 player and even mobile phone. For using podcast technology, one needs the correct software such as iTunes for MAC or Windows or Juice for MAC, Windows or Linux. Teachers can create their own podcasts using free audio-recording software or they can refer students to podcasts that are related to the subject they are teaching as supportive information. The education podcast network allows teachers to connect and collaborate via a podcast. They can view podcasts created by academics within their field of expertise. Podcasting enables the participating teachers to share their knowledge, insights, and passions for teaching. Podcasting provides teachers with the flexibility to post important segments of their lectures online, or their interviews with experts, but also allow students to view and create their own podcasts on material covered in class, or in their textbooks.

Wiki

Wiki is sometimes interpreted as the acronym for "what I Know is", which describes the knowledge contribution, storage, and exchange up to some point. The name is based on the Hawaiian term wiki, meaning "quick", "fast" or "to hasten". A wiki is a group of web pages that allows users to add content, as on an internet forum, and also allows others to edit the content. Content displayed on a wiki can be constantly modified, with changes being recorded as the content is updated. Wikis can be used as a general source for class materials and for class communication. Teachers can also post class assignments to a wiki and students can create a portfolio for their peers to review.

Weblogs

A weblog is a website where entries are commonly displayed with possibility to maintain, add or edit content on regular basis. A typical weblog combines text, images and links to other blogs, web pages and other media related to its topic. The ability for readers to leave comments in an interactive format is an important part of many weblogs. Most weblogs are primarily textual, although some focus on art (artlog), photographs (photoblog), sketchblog, videos (vlog), music (MP3 blog), audio (podcasting) and are part of a wider network of social media. Micro blogging is another type of blogging, which consists of weblogs with very short posts.

Weblog allow teacher to communicate with students and parents as the can log daily class activities. The teachers and learners can easily create their weblogs to disseminate and share ideas, study materials, research work/findings or their views on different educational aspects. They can regularly edit their postings on their weblogs and use weblogs to universalize their ideas and achievement for academic world and community. Teachers can also use weblogs as portals to list home assignments, classroom procedures and class work. Students can use the weblog to post their own work and have it commented by their teachers and classmates.

Moodle

Moodle is a virtual learning environment. It is an online space designed to mimic the classroom experience. Moodle is like a virtual classroom and Moodle homepage behaves just like a website does. It must be hosted by an outside source and is not free. There are links to the course calendar, online syllabus, weekly topics, assignment descriptions, discussion forums and so on. A teacher can have control over the entire site. The teacher can monitor student activity, add/delete any of the content, keep track of grades which can be either accessed or hidden from student view. Teachers can post links to the class calendar, links to assignments that need to be completed, an online syllabus, and discussion forums. This gives students ability to find information they may have missed because they were absent from class. Teachers can also create and give tests, monitor students' activity, edit content, and organize grades. Moodle also allows for a class forum where topics relevant to course material can be discussed. A great benefit of having a class forum is that students are given the freedom to gather their thoughts and express themselves without the pressures felt in classroom discussions.

Instant Messaging (IM)

IM is an acronym for Instant Messaging. It is a tool that successfully supports informal communication. A form of IM is SMS technology. IM is a synchronous learning tool which in an e-learning context can provide the student with real time and instant learning opportunities. IM as a real time communication tool can be utilized as a delivery option for hearing impaired students. This allows them to access teachers without a third party to interpret. Learners can also use this to get automated feedback from assignments or questions, freeing the tutor from any additional workload. As such, IM can be used to engage and maintain learner's interest as correspondence occurs in a timely manner.

The above discussed emerging technologies are quite helpful for teachers to foster a learning environment of excitement and interactivity. Meleises (2008) suggests success in the use of ICT in education depends largely on teachers and their level of skill in integrating ICT into the teaching process and in utilizing ICT to provide learner-centered interactive education. Readiness for new technologies is a challenge associated with change. Teachers who resist change may impede or limit their student's learning and skills. Teachers need to apply technologies wisely to real problems. To put into nutshell:

Teachers are required to:
- Have knowledge, skills, and understanding of concepts related to emerging technologies.
- Stay abreast of recurrent and emerging technologies.
- Apply technology-enhanced instructional strategies.
- Identify and locate technology resources.
- Plan for managing technology resources.
- Use technology to support learner-centered teaching.
- Apply technology in assessing student learning.
- Use technology resources to engage in an ongoing professional development.
- Use technology to communicate and collaborate with peers, parents, and the larger community.
- Apply technology to enable and empower learners.
- Facilitate equitable access to technology resources for all learners.
- Attend programs to learn updated knowledge and skills about emerging technologies.
- Research about educational impact of emerging technologies.

Summary

- Educational technology is a systematic application of scientific knowledge about teaching, learning and conditions of learning to improve the efficiency of teaching and training.
- A digital library is a library in which collections are stored in digital formats and accessible by computers. The digital content may be stored locally or accessed remotely via computer networks.
- E-tutoring can be defined as teaching, support, management, and assessment of students on programs of study that involve a significant use of online technologies.
- A teleconferencing (also known as a video-teleconference) is a set of interactive telecommunication technologies which allow two or more locations to interact via two-way video and audio transmissions simultaneously.

- The internet provides many services to send and receive mails (e-mail), support for special interest scholarly lists and newsgroups, remote login to a computer (telnet), and the file transfer from remote locations (FTP).
- The internet works on the Transmission Control Protocol (TCP) and Internet Protocol (IP). These two are collectively called TCP/IP.
- Mobile learning or m-Learning is defined as "using mobile technologies, including mobile phones and handheld devices to enhance the learning process.
- The term "wireless technologies" is self-explanatory and can be associated to m-Learning to some extent. Wireless technology allows the learner to access information at their convenience. One example is bluetooth with which a learner can access internet connection.
- "Skype" is software that allows one to talk to people over the computer. With a fast connection, Skype allows one to talk to people over the computer for free of cost except for the cost for internet usage and connection.
- Podcasting is the method of distributing multimedia files, such as audio programs or music videos over the internet for playback on mobile devices and personal computers. Podcasts are digital recordings stored in a music file which can then be uploaded to a computer.
- Wiki is sometimes interpreted as the acronym for "what I Know is", which describes the knowledge contribution, storage and exchange up to some point. The name is based on the Hawaiian term wiki, meaning "quick", "fast" or "to hasten".
- A weblog is a website where entries are commonly displayed with possibility to maintain, add, or edit content on regular basis.
- Moodle is a virtual learning environment. It is an online space designed to mimic the classroom experience. Moodle is like a virtual classroom and Moodle homepage behaves just like a website does.
- IM is an acronym for Instant Messaging. It is a tool that successfully supports informal communication. A form of IM is SMS technology.

Appendices

Appendix 1: Comparative study of idealism, realism, naturalism and pragmatism.

Subject	Idealism	Realism	Naturalism	Pragmatism
Exponents	Socrates, Plato, Kant, Spinoza, Barkley, Fitche, Schelling, Green, Gentile Hegel, Shankaracharya, Dayanand, Rabindranath Tagore, MK Gandhi, Sri Aurobindo Ghosh, Swami Vivekananda.	Erasmus Rebellias Milton, Lord Montaigue, John Locke, Mulcaster, Bacon, Ratke, Commenius, White head, Bertrand Russell.	Aristotle, Comte, Hobbes, Bacon, Darwin, Lamarck, Huxley, Herbert Spencer, Bernard Shaw, Samual Butler, Rousseau, etc.	CB Pearce, William James, Schiller, John Dewey, Kilpatric and others.
Fundamental principles	1. Idealism insists on God. To achieve God, spiritual education is necessary. 2. Accepts the existence of spiritual world. 3. Spiritual values are supreme and universal. 4. Values are predetermined. 5. Idealism is a complete spiritual view point. 6. It is a monistic concept.	1. Realism believes in individual and social development. 2. It believes in the importance of material world. 3. Cause and effect relationship—Scientific principles are universal and universally accepted. 4. Problems of real-life become ideals and values. 5. Fully scientific attitude. 6. It is a pluralistic concept.	1. Naturalism does not believe in God. Nature is everything. Nothing is beyond it. 2. It believes in matter and importance of material world. 3. Physical and natural principles are supreme and universal. 4. There is no ideal and supreme value. 5. Fully materialistic and mechanical attitude. 6. It is a monistic concept.	1. Pragmatism does not believe in God or spiritual values. It has full faith in man. 2. It upholds the power of man as supreme. 3. Spiritual principles are not universal. They change according to change in times, circumstances and situations. 4. Values are not pre-determined. They are in the making. 5. Fully psychological and humanistic view points. 6. It is a pluralistic concept.
Principles of education	1. Education is based on spiritualism and ethics. 2. It emphasizes mental capacities. 3. Teacher and curriculum is the center of education. 4. Emphasizes book learning. 5. Both individual and society are valued. 6. It is a definite and specific ideology.	1. Education is based on science only. 2. It emphasizes on behavior and experiment. 3. Child and his parent life are the centers of education. 4. It opposes book learning. 5. Both individual and society are valued. 6. It is liable to change according to change in a life.	1. Education is based on psychology. 2. It emphasizes basic instincts, interests and tendencies. 3. Child is the center of education. 4. It opposes book learning. 5. Individual is considered and valued. 6. It is progressive and dynamic ideology.	1. Education is based on psychology and science. 2. It emphasizes experiment and practice. 3. Child is the focal point of all educational activities. 4. It opposes book learning. 5. Sociability is emphasized. 6. It is a progressive, dynamic and changeable ideology.
Aim of education	1. Self-realization and exaltation of personality. 2. Spiritual development. 3. Realization of truth, beauty and goodness. 4. Conservation, promotion and transmission of cultural heritage. 5. Conversion of inborn nature into spiritual nature. 6. Preparation for holy life. 7. Development of intelligence and rationality.	1. Preparing the child for real life. 2. Developing the physical and mental powers of child. 3. Preparing the child for a happy life. 4. Developing and training of senses. 5. Acquainting the child with nature and social environment. 6. Imparting vocational education.	1. To perfect the human machines. 2. Attainment of present and future happiness. 3. Preparation for the struggle of existence. 4. Adaptation to environment. 5. Improvement of racial gains. 6. Natural development. 7. Autonomous development.	1. Aims of education are not pre-determined. 2. Educational aims change according to times, places and circumstances. 3. More education. 4. Creation of new values. 5. Social adjustment and harmonious development.

Contd...

Contd...

Subject	Idealism	Realism	Naturalism	Pragmatism
Curriculum	1. Idealistic curriculum is developed according to ideals and eternal values. 2. Humanistic subjects are emphasized. 3. Main subjects of idealistic curriculum are—Religious studies, Spiritual studies, Ethics, Language, Sociology, Literature, Geography, History, Music, Fine arts, etc.	1. Realistic curriculum is developed according to utility and needs. 2. Subjects concerning day to day activities are included in curriculum. 3. Main subjects of realistic Curriculum are — Natural sciences, Biological sciences, Physical sciences, Health, Culture, Physical exercises, Maths, Geography, History, Astronomy, Sports, etc.	1. Naturalistic curriculum is constructed according to basic instincts, aptitudes and tendencies of children. 2. In such curriculum, scientific subject occupy main place. Humanities occupy subsidiary position. 3. Main subjects of Naturalistic Curriculum are—Games and Sports, Physical sciences and Physiology, Health, Culture, Material sciences and Biological sciences, etc.	1. Pragmatic curriculum is based on subjects of utility, its main principle being utilitarian. 2. Social subjects form the main body and others subsidiary. 3. Main subjects of pragmatic curriculum are—Health hygiene and Science, Physical culture, History, Geography, Maths, Home-science, Science and Agriculture, etc.
Methods of Teaching	1. Idealists have not adopted any specific and definite method of teaching. 2. They advocate many methods. Thus they think themselves as creators of methods and not the slave of any particular method. 3. Idealists prescribe the following methods of teaching—Question-Answer, Conversation, Dialogue, Discussion, Lecture, Argumentation, Intersection, Book study, etc.	1. Realists emphasize scientific and objective methods of teaching. 2. It emphasizes informal methods of teaching. 3. Realists emphasize the following methods of teaching, Self-experience and Research, Experimental method, Heuristic method and Correlation method.	Naturalists, emphasizing learning by doing, learning by self-experience and learning by play, have advocated the following methods of teaching—Observation, Play, Dalton plan, Heuristic, Montessori and Kindergarten methods.	Pragmatists have emphasized the principles of purposive process of learning, learning by doing and by experience and correlation and integration. On the basis of these principles, Kilpatric has given birth to project method, a method which is widely accepted and used in the field of education.
Teacher	1. Supreme and important place of teacher. 2. The teacher as gardner knows best as to how to care and develop a child like a plant.	1. Teacher's role is supreme because he brings the child in touch with the external realities of life. 2. Keeping aside his own view, the teacher imparts scientific knowledge to the child in an easy and effective way.	1. Teacher's role is subsidiary, whereas child's position is central. 2. Nature is the supreme to the teacher. He is to set the stage for child and retire behind the curtain.	1. Teacher's role is that of a friend, philosopher and guide. 2. Teacher puts the child in such a position so that he learns to create new values for future.
Discipline	1. Idealism advocates discipline at all costs. 2. Freedom is to be restricted by ideals. 3. Emphasizes impressionistic discipline.	Realism emphasizes the systematic form of impressionistic and emancipatory discipline according to natural and social procedures.	1. The slogan of naturalism is freedom. 2. This doctrine, supporting emancipatory discipline, emphasizes discipline according to natural consequences.	Pragmatism emphasizes limited emancipatory or social discipline.
School	1. According to Idealism, school is the only place for regular and effective education. 2. School is an ideal form of pleasing and joyful activities for children.	1. According to Realism, school is a socially well planned institution. 2. It is a mirror of society.	1. According to Naturalism, nature's vast campus is the real school. 2. School should be natural and spontaneous field of free activities for children.	1. According to Pragmatism, school is a laboratory for experiments to be done by children. 2. It is a society in miniature.

Appendix 2: Lesson plan on internationally accepted rights of children.

Name of the Course : BSc (N)
Placement : III year
Name of the Subject : Child Health Nursing
Name of the Unit : Introduction to modern concepts of child care
Topic : Internationally Accepted Rights of Children
Duration : 1 hour
Date and Time : 20.11.2018; 8–9 am
Size of the class : 50
Venue : III Year BSc(N) Class room
Methods of Teaching : Lecture-cum-Discussion
Instructional Aids : Pictures, Charts, OHP
Review of Previous knowledge : Students have some knowledge on rights of human beings

Central Objective

The students will gain knowledge regarding the internationally accepted rights of children and develop desirable attitude and appreciate the importance of valuing and respecting the rights of children.

Specific Objectives

The students will be able to:
- Define the terms
- Explain the milestones in the development of rights of children
- List the characteristics of human rights
- Explain the convention on the rights of the child
- Enlist the rights of children

Introduction (5 minutes)

Every person has dignity and value. One of the ways that we recognize the fundamental worth of every person is by acknowledging and respecting their human rights. Human rights are a set of principles concerned with equality and fairness. Human rights apply to all age groups; children have the same general human rights as adults. But children are particularly vulnerable and so they also have particular rights that recognize their special need for protection. Children are neither the property of their parents nor are they helpless objects of charity. They are human beings and are the subject of their own rights. The Convention offers a vision of the child as an individual and as a member of a family and community, with rights and responsibilities appropriate to his or her age and stage of development.

Sl. No.	Specific objectives	Time	Content	Teacher activity	Learner activity	Evaluation
1.	Define the terms	5 mts	**Definition** • Right is something that a person is entitled to, which cannot be taken away from them • Human rights are those rights which are essential to live as human beings – basic standards without which people cannot survive and develop in dignity. They are inherent to the human person, inalienable and universal • Human rights are standards that recognize and protect the dignity of all human beings. Human rights govern how individual human beings live in society and with each other, as well as their relationship with governments and the obligations that governments have towards them. These human rights are applicable to both adult and children.	Explaining using black board Questioning Clarifying doubts	Taking down notes and answering	• Define rights • Define human rights

Contd...

Contd...

Sl. No.	Specific objectives	Time	Content	Teacher activity	Learner activity	Evaluation
2.	Explain the milestones in the development of the rights of children	5 mts	**Milestones in the development of the rights of children** 1948—Universal declaration of human rights was passed 1959—The Declaration of the rights of the child was announced 1989—The Convention on the rights of children was adopted 2000—UN general assembly adopted two optional protocols to the convention	• Explaining using OHP • Questioning clarifying doubts	Taking down notes and answering	• When was the universal declaration of human rights passed? • When was the convention of the rights on children adopted?
3.	List the characteristics of Human Rights	10 mts	**Characteristics of human rights** *Inherent* Human rights are *inherent*; we are simply born with them and they belong to each of us as a result of our common humanity. Human rights are not owned by select people or given as a gift. *Inalienable* They are *inalienable*; individuals cannot give them up and they cannot be taken away — even if governments do not recognize or protect them. *Universal* They are *universal*; they are held by all people, everywhere – regardless of age, sex, race, religion, nationality, income level or any other status or condition in life. Human rights belong to each and every one of us equally. *Equal* All rights are equal and no right is superior to any other; there are no 'small' rights. *Indivisible and interrelated and interdependent* Human rights are indivisible and interrelated, with a focus on the individual and the community as a whole. The enjoyment of one right usually depends on fulfilment of other rights. Different rights therefore should not be considered in isolation.	• Explaining using chart • Questioning clarifying doubts	• Discussing • Taking down notes and answering	• List any four characteristics of human rights • What is the meaning of the word 'inalienable' in the context of human rights?
4.	Explain the convention on the rights of the child	10 mts	**The convention on the rights of the child** • The convention on the rights of the child was the first instrument to incorporate the complete range of international human rights— including civil, cultural, economic, political and social rights as well as aspects of humanitarian law. The Convention sets out these rights in 54 articles and two Optional Protocols. It spells out the basic human rights that children everywhere have: the right to survival; to develop to the fullest; to protect from harmful influences, abuse and exploitation; and to participate fully in family, cultural and social life. • The four core principles of the Convention are non-discrimination; devotion to the best interests of the child; the right to life, survival and development; and respect for the views of the child. Every right spelled out in the convention is inherent to the human dignity and harmonious development of every child. The Convention protects children's rights by setting standards in health care; education; and legal, civil and social services. • By agreeing to undertake the obligations of the Convention (by ratifying or acceding to it), national governments have committed themselves to protecting and ensuring children's rights and they have agreed to hold themselves accountable for this commitment before the international community. States parties to the Convention are obliged to develop and undertake all actions and policies in the light of the best interests of the child.	• Explaining using black board • Questioning clarifying doubts	• Discussing • Taking down notes and answering	• How many articles are there in the convention on the rights of the child? • What is optional protocol?

Contd...

Contd...

Sl. No.	Specific objectives	Time	Content	Teacher activity	Learner activity	Evaluation
5.	Enlist the rights of children	10 mts	**Rights of the child** 1. Right to develop in an atmosphere of affection and security and wherever possible in the care and under responsibility of his or her parents 2. Right to enjoy the benefits of social security including nutrition, housing and medical care 3. Right to education 4. Right to full opportunity for play and recreation 5. Right to a name and nationality 6. Right to a special care if handicapped 7. Right to be among the first to receive protection and relief in times of disaster 8. Right to learn to be useful member of society and develop in a healthy and normal manner and in conditions of freedom and dignity 9. Right to be brought to a spirit of understanding tolerance, friendship among people, peace and universal brotherhood 10. Right to enjoy these rights regardless of race, color, sex, religion, national or social origin	• Explaining using OHP • Questioning clarifying doubts	• Discussing • Taking down notes and answering	List any five rights of the child?

Summary (5 mts)

Right is something that a person is entitled to, which cannot be taken away from them. Human rights are those rights which are essential to live as human beings – basic standards without which people cannot survive and develop in dignity. They are inherent to the human person, inalienable and universal. In 1989, the Convention on the rights of children was adopted. The convention on the rights of the child was the first instrument to incorporate the complete range of international human rights— including civil, cultural, economic, political and social rights as well as aspects of humanitarian law. The Convention sets out these rights in 54 articles and two Optional Protocols. Right to education, health, protection from exploitation or punishment are some of the rights of children. All children in the universe have the right to develop, enjoy social security, education, play and recreation, name and nationality, special care if handicapped, etc.

Conclusion (5 minutes)

Human rights are the same for all people everywhere – men and women, young and old, rich and poor, regardless of their background, where they live, what they think or what they believe. This is what makes human rights 'universal'. A person's ability to enjoy their human rights depends on other people respecting those rights. This means that human rights involve responsibility and duties towards other people and the community. Children have the similar rights to enjoy and it is the adult's responsibility to respect it.

Assignment

Recall your childhood and write about the rights you have enjoyed as a child.
Write an assignment on the "Promotion rights of hospitalized children".

Evaluation

I. Write short answers on the following: 5 X 2 = 10 Marks
1. Define rights.
2. Define human rights.
3. List any four characteristics of human rights.
4. What are conventions on the rights of children?
5. What is optional protocol?

II. Write short notes on the following: 2 x 5 = 10 Marks
1. Characteristics of human rights.
2. Rights of the child.

References

1. Basavanthappa BT. *Community Health Nursing*, New Delhi: Jaypee Brothers Medical Publishers; 2007.pp.1420–1.
2. Park K. *Preventive and Social Medicine* (24th ed). Jabalpur, Banarsider Bhanot Publishers; 2017.pp.473–7.
3. Parthasarathy A. *IAP Textbook of Paediatrics* (6th ed). New Delhi, Jaypee Brothers Medical publishers; 2016.pp.1225–7.
4. Datta Parul. *Pediatric Nursing* (4th ed). New Delhi, Jaypee Brothers Medical Publishers; 2018.pp.8–10.
5. Paul VK, Bagga A. *Ghai Essential Paediatrics* (8th ed). New Delhi, CBS Publishers and Distributors; 2013.pp.768–71.
6. Sharma Rimple. *Essentials of Pediatric Nursing* (2nd ed). New Delhi, Jaypee Brothers Medical Publishers; 2017.pp.7–8.
7. Sudhakar A. (2017). *Essentials of Pediatric Nursing* (1st ed). New Delhi, Jaypee Brothers Medical Publishers; 2017.pp.7–8.
8. Swan JG, Sargeant J. Assuring children's human right to freedom of opinion and expression in education. *International Journal of Speech–Language Pathology*, 20(1); https://doi.org/10.1080/17549507.2018.1385852
9. Human rights for children and women: How UNICEF helps make them a reality. Retrieved from https://www.unicef.org/publications/files/pub_humanrights_children_en.pdf

Appendix 3: Lesson plan on conceptual framework.

Name of the Course : MSc (N)
Placement : I year
Name of the Subject : Nursing Research
Name of the Unit : Developing Theoretical/Conceptual Framework
Topic : Conceptual Framework
Duration : 2 hours
Date and Time : 22.11.2018; 8–10 am
Size of the class : 18
Venue : I Year MSc(N) Class room
Methods of Teaching : Lecture-cum-Demonstration
Instructional Aids : Pictures, Charts, OHP
Review of Previous knowledge : Students do not have previous knowledge on the topic

Central Objective

The students will gain knowledge on conceptual framework and develop desirable attitude and skill in development of conceptual framework for their research project.

Specific Objectives

At the end of the class, the students will be able to:
- Define the terms
- List the purposes of conceptual framework
- Determine the relationship between conceptual model and theoretical framework
- Explain the steps in developing a conceptual framework
- Prepare a conceptual framework for a Quantitative research
- Prepare a conceptual framework for a Qualitative research
- Enumerate the inputs required for the development of conceptual framework
- Enlist the limitations of conceptual framework.

Introduction (5 minutes)

We all know that the framework of a human body is our skeletal system which gives shape and structure. The pillars and columns give the shape and structure for the building without which the building cannot exist. A framework is a structure composed of many concepts proposed to serve as a support or guide for the building of something that expands the structure into something useful and meaningful. It is a broad overview, outline, or skeleton of interlinked concepts or items which supports a major theme or overall concept. In nursing research the conceptual/theoretical framework forms an important element. Conceptual framework is used in research to outline possible courses of action or to present a preferred approach to an idea or thought. Conceptual frameworks (theoretical frameworks) are a type of intermediate theory that attempt to connect to all aspects of inquiry (e.g., problem definition, purpose, literature review, methodology, data collection and analysis). Conceptual frameworks can act like a map that explains the logic to empirical inquiry.

Sl.No.	Specific objective	Time	Content	Teacher activity	Learner activity	Evaluation
1.	Define the terms	15 mts	**Concept** It is a mental image of a phenomenon, an idea or a construct in the mind about a thing or action. **Variables** Anything which varies from person to person is a variable. There are different types of variables one may come across in a study. **Model** • A model is a simplified representation of a theory or of certain complex events, structures or systems. The example for a model of structure is model of kidney or heart. • A model is a hypothetical representation of something that exists in reality. The purpose of a model is to attempt to explain a complex reality in a systematic and organized manner. An institution's organization chart is a model that attempts to demonstrate the interrelationships of the various levels of the organization's administration. **Theory** It is a set of interrelated constructs (concepts) definitions and propositions that present a systematic view of phenomena by specifying relations among variables with the purpose of explaining and predicting the phenomena (Kerlinger, 1986). **Conceptualization** It refers to the process of developing and refining abstract ideas. It is a process of thinking and organizing ideas that grows from the learning of facts and events to concepts to theory development. **Framework** It is a structure that serves to hold parts together, e.g. skeleton forms the framework of our body. **Relational statement** It is a proposition describing a specific relationship between two or more concepts. **Conceptual model** It is a group of concepts or ideas that are related but the relationship is not explicit. Conceptual models have a "set of concepts" however, the relational statement explaining the connections between the concepts are obscure. **Conceptual Framework** A written or visual presentation that explains either graphically, or in narrative form, the main things to be studied – the key factors, concepts or variables and the presumed relationship among them. (Miles and Huberman, 1994). **Theoretical framework** A structure composed of concepts related to form a whole (Chinn & Kramer). Theoretical framework consists of a set of defined concepts and relational statements linking them.	Explaining using OHP and Sample conceptual framework.Questioning	Listening and taking down notes Answering	• What is concept? • What is a model? • Name any two physiological variables of the human being? • What is framework?
2.	List the purposes of conceptual framework	10 mts	**Purposes of conceptual framework** • It clarifies the concepts on which the study is built • It specifies the relationship among the concepts • It identifies and states the assumptions and hypothesis underlying the study • It explains why a research is conducted in a particular way • It acts as a filtering tool for selecting appropriate research questions and related data collection methods. • It can also help us to understand and use the ideas of others who have done similar things. • It is a set of coherent ideas or concepts organized in a manner that helps in communication to others. • It directs the thinking process about how and why an empirical research and about how we understand its activities. • It forms the basis for thinking about what we do and about what it means, influenced by the ideas and research of others. • It also acts as a reference point/structure for the discussion of the literature, methodology and results. • The conceptual framework is like a travel map. The investigator prepares and uses to reach a destination which also is understood by others.	Explaining using OHP Questioning	Listening and taking down notes Answering	List any two purposes of conceptual framework

Contd...

Sl.No.	Specific objective	Time	Content	Teacher activity	Learner activity	Evaluation
3.	Determine the relationship between conceptual model and theoretical framework	10 mts	**Relationship between conceptual model and theoretical framework** • Conceptual model is not a theory • Conceptual model is highly abstract • Theory contains more concrete concepts • A conceptual model embodies the world view, the paradigm of a discipline or a school of thought • Each theory derived from a model explains some or all of the paradigm's phenomena but only within a limited range • A theory is more precise and limited in scope than its parent conceptual scheme • The conceptual framework serves as a stepping stone for the formulation of the "theoretical framework" which comprises established explanations, theoretical principles and suggested theoretical relations in preparation of a more specific inquiry	Explaining using real theoretical and conceptual framework Questioning	Listening and taking down notes Answering	State any two relationship between conceptual and theoretical framework
4.	Explain the steps in developing a conceptual framework	15 mts	**Steps in developing a conceptual framework** 1. State the problem as clearly as possible 2. Identify the key words or concepts or variables of the study 3. Review the literature for theories, theoretical generalizations, empirical generalizations, and systematized facts related to the phenomenon of interest (problem) 4. Review the existing conceptual or theoretical framework already used to guide professional activities 5. Write the relational statements, and organize these into a study framework 6. Draw a visual model of concepts and known or proposed relationships Statement of problem → Identification of the major concepts → Reviewing theories and frameworks → Writing relational statements → Drawing a model using symbols (arrows etc) → Review the conceptual framework	Explaining using board and chart Clarifying doubts	Listening and taking down notes Answering	• Why should we identify key variables? • How review of literature will help in the preparation of conceptual framework?
5.	Prepare a conceptual framework for a Quantitative research	15 mts	**Conceptual Framework in Quantitative Research** Conceptual framework is formulated in a quantitative research in the beginning of the study. Formulation of conceptual framework requires the researcher to review literature and his experience on the issue(s) of interest facilitate the development of the framework. One can adopt the existing theories or model and the concepts can be fit into the model. The researcher must have the knowledge of nursing theories and the major components of those theories. By adopting existing models or theories, one can test the theories.	Helping students to prepare a conceptual framework using black board and existing theoretical frameworks. Questioning Step by step demonstration	Listening and taking down notes participating and preparing a conceptual framework Answering	Why should we refer to existing theoretical model?

Contd...

Contd...

Sl.No.	Specific objective	Time	Content	Teacher activity	Learner activity	Evaluation
6.	Prepare a conceptual framework for a Qualitative research	15 mts	**Conceptual framework in a Qualitative research** Normally, qualitative work is described as starting from an inductive position, seeking to build up theory, with the conceptual framework being 'emergent', because existing literature/theories might mislead. However, Miles and Huberman (1994) note that researchers generally have some idea of what will feature in the study, a tentative rudimentary conceptual framework, and it is better to have some idea of what we are looking for/at even if that idea changes over time. This is particularly true for inexperienced and/or time constrained researchers. Yin (1994) explained about pattern matching and explanation building. Pattern matching starts with existing theory and tests its adequacy in terms of explaining the findings. Explanation building starts with theory and then builds an explanation while collecting and analysing data. *The following are the steps/ phases in the qualitative research (Yosef Jabareen, 2009):* Phase 1: Mapping the selected data sources Phase 2: Extensive reading and categorizing of the selected data Phase 3: Identifying and naming concepts Phase 4: Deconstructing and categorizing the concepts Phase 5: Integrating concepts Phase 6: Synthesis, resynthesis, and making it all make sense Phase 7: Validating the conceptual framework Phase 8: Rethinking the conceptual framework	Helping students to prepare a conceptual framework using black board and existing theoretical frameworks and qualitative research Step by step demonstration Explaining Questioning	Listening and taking down notes participating and preparing a conceptual framework Answering	• What is pattern matching? • Why it is known as emergent conceptual framework?
7.	Enumerate the inputs required for the development of conceptual framework	10 mts	**The inputs required for the development of a conceptual framework** The following inputs are required for the novice and experienced researchers and their supervisors: • The knowledge of existing theories, models and concepts • Technical knowledge of how a conceptual model is formulated • Research experience • Critical thinking and reasoning skills • Data from the literature review- related studies can be reviewed to understand the concepts and relationships between the concepts • Data from the research study in case of qualitative study	• Explaining using white board • Questioning the students	• Observing and participating in the procedure • Taking down notes • answering	List any four inputs required for the development of conceptual framework
8.	Enlist the limitations of conceptual framework	5 mts	**Limitations of conceptual framework** • It is influenced by the experience and knowledge of the investigator. There is a chance for the subjective bias (initial bias). • Once developed will influence the researcher's thinking and may result in some things being given prominence and others being ignored (ongoing bias). • The solution is to revisit the conceptual framework, particularly at the end when evaluating one's own work	Explaining using white board Questioning	• Listening and answering • Taking down notes • answering	List any two limitations of conceptual framework

Summary (5 minutes)

Theory is a set of interrelated constructs (concepts) definitions and propositions that present a systematic view of phenomena by specifying relations among variables with the purpose of explaining and predicting the phenomena. Conceptual model is a group of concepts or ideas that are related but the relationship is not explicit. Conceptual framework clarifies the concepts on which the study is built. It acts as a filtering tool for selecting appropriate research questions and related data collection methods. The conceptual framework serves as a stepping stone for the formulation of the "theoretical framework" which comprises established explanations, theoretical principles and suggested theoretical relations in preparation of a more specific inquiry. Conceptual framework is formulated in a quantitative research in the beginning of the study. Formulation of conceptual framework requires the researcher to review literature and his experience on the issue(s) of interest facilitate the development of the framework. Normally, qualitative work is described as starting from an inductive position, seeking to build up theory, with the conceptual framework being 'emergent', because existing literature/theories might mislead. The inputs required for the novice and experienced researchers and their supervisors are the knowledge of existing theories, models and concepts, technical knowledge of how a conceptual model is formulated, research experience, critical thinking and reasoning skills, data from the literature review- related studies can be reviewed to understand the concepts and relationships between the concepts and data from the research study in case of qualitative study.

Conclusion (5 mts)

Nurse researchers must be inquisitive in nature to develop a conceptual framework. It requires critical thinking and analytical skills. As skeleton is to your body, conceptual framework is for the research. Without skeleton, body is shapeless and without conceptual framework, a research is meaningless.

Assignment

Identify a problem for your research and write the objectives. Prepare a conceptual framework for the problem identified.

Evaluation

Write short notes on the following: 5 x 5 = 25 marks
1. List the purposes of conceptual framework.
2. Explain the relationship between conceptual model and theoretical framework.
3. Explain the steps in the development of conceptual framework with suitable examples.
4. Explain the development of conceptual framework in the qualitative research.
5. Write the inputs required and limitations of the conceptual framework.

References

1. Basavanthappa BT, (2007). *Nursing Research*. (2nd ed). New Delhi, Jaypee Brothers Medical Publishers (P) Ltd.
2. Elakkuvana Bhaskara Raj, (2010). *Nursing Research and Biostatistics*, Bangalore, EMMESS Medical Publishers.
3. Kothari CR, (2011). Research Methodology–Methods and Techniques. (2nd revised ed). New Delhi, New Age International Publishers.
4. Polit DF, Beck CT, (2010). *Essentials of Nursing Research*. (7th ed). New Delhi, Wolters Kluwer (India) Pvt. Ltd.
5. Rose Marie, (2008). *Foundations of Nursing Research*, (5th ed). New Delhi, DK (India) Pvt., Ltd
6. Imenda S, Is there a Conceptual Difference between Theoretical and Conceptual Frameworks? Journal of Social Sciences, 2014;38(2):185-95
7. Sharma SK, (2011). *Nursing Research*, New Delhi, Elsevier Publishers.
8. Tripathi PC, (2010) *A Textbook of Research Methodology in Social Sciences* (6th revised and enlarged ed). New Delhi, Sultan Chand & Sons.
9. Wood GB, Haber J, (2010). *Nursing Research*, (7th ed). St Louis, Moshy Elsevier Publishers.
10. Yosef Jabareen (2009). Building a Conceptual Framework: Philosophy, Definitions, and Procedure. *International Journal of Qualitative Methods*, 8(4), 49-62 Retrieved from https://journals.sagepub.com/doi/pdf/10.1177/160940690900800406

Appendix 4: Lesson plan on surgical dressing.

Name of the Course	: BSc (N)
Placement	: I year
Name of the Subject	: Nursing Foundation
Name of the Unit	: Meeting needs of Perioperative Patients
Topic	: Surgical Dressing
Duration	: 1 hour
Date and Time	: 22.11.2018; 9–11 am
Size of the class	: 50
Venue	: Nursing Foundation Lab
Methods of Teaching	: Lecture-cum-Demonstration
Instructional Aids	: Pictures, Charts, Real objects
Review of Previous knowledge	: Students have studied Anatomy of skin and wound healing

Central Objective

At the end of the demonstration, the students will be able to gain adequate knowledge on surgical dressing and develop desirable attitude and skill in performing the procedure for patients in various health care settings.

Specific Objectives

At the end of the demonstration, the students will be able to:

- Define surgical dressing
- List the purposes of surgical dressing
- Determine the types of dressing
- List the characteristics of an ideal dressing
- Explain the general instructions to be followed during surgical dressing
- Assemble all articles needed for surgical dressing
- Perform the procedure of surgical dressing
- Perform the after care of patients
- Document the findings

Introduction (5 mts)

All human beings are interested in dress and we spend considerable time in dressing up ourselves to look confident, beautiful, and also to protect ourselves. The skin is the largest organ in the human body and all of us could have experienced at least, once in our life time, the injury to the skin. A break in the continuity of the skin surface is the first step in the formation of a wound. A wound can be as simple as a surface abrasion, or it can be an extensive, life-threatening destruction of tissue that reaches down to and includes the internal organs of the body. Surgery generally involves an incision through the skin and underlying tissues. An incision disrupts the protective skin barrier. Therefore wound healing is one of the major concerns during the postoperative period. Injury to the skin provides a unique challenge, as wound healing is a complex and intricate process. Since ancient times, many different materials have been used to treat wounds in an attempt to stop bleeding, absorb exudates, and promote healing. Some of these materials consisted of honey, animal oils or fat, cobwebs, mud, leaves or animal dung. In order to promote wound healing and protect the wound from infection, a dressing of the wound is mandatory.

Sl.No.	Specific objective	Time	Content	Teacher activity	Learner activity	Evaluation
1.	Define surgical dressing	5 mts	• Surgical dressing is cleansing a wound or incision and applying sterile protective covering using aseptic technique with or without medication • A wound is a break in the continuity of any bodily tissue caused by a cut, blow, or other impact	Explaining using black board Questioning	Listening and taking down notes Answering	What is wound? What is Surgical dressing?
2.	List the purposes of surgical dressing	5 mts	**Purposes of Surgical Dressing** • To protect the wound from contamination with the microorganisms • To promote wound granulation and healing • To support or splint the wound site • To decrease purulent wound drainage (dressing material absorbs the drainage) • To apply medication to the wound • To promote thermal insulation to the wound surface • To provide for maintenance of high humidity between the wound and dressing • To promote physical, psychological and esthetic comfort	Explaining using chart Questioning	Listening and taking down notes Answering	List any five purposes of surgical dressing
3.	Determine the type of dressing	10 mts	**Types of dressing depends upon** • The location, size and type of the wound • Type and amount of exudates • Whether the wound is infected • Frequency of changing the dressing **Types of Dressing** It is classified based on the material and purpose for which it is used. Some of the dressing are as follows: • Gauze • Gauze impregnated dressing • Wet Dressing • Non-adherent dressing • Self-adhesive dressing • Transparent film dressing • Foam dressing • Alginates • Hydrocolloid • Hydrogel dressing • Pressure dressing **Gauze:** It is inexpensive, reliable, available, and highly absorbent. Gauze comes in woven and nonwoven forms, with the latter made of synthetic fibers pressed together and having a greater absorbency. It is highly permeable and nonocclusive and can be used as a primary or secondary wound dressing. **Impregnated gauze:** Gauze dressings are also available impregnated with substances such as petroleum, iodine, bismuth, and zinc. The impregnated materials help make these dressings non-adherent and moderately occlusive. They add moisture to the wound bed and facilitate wound healing by decreasing trauma and preventing desiccation during dressing changes. **Wet Dressing:** These are preferred in treating wounds that require debridement. This moistens the dressing increasing the gauze's ability to collect exudates and wound debris. **Non-adherent dressing:** These dressing have a shiny non-adherent surface that does not stick to incision or wound opening but allows drainage to pass through the softened gauze above. Non-adherent dressings are ideal for open wounds that have light to moderate exudate. The non-adherent properties keep the fabric from sticking to the wound, even as the wound heals. This will cause little to no pain during removal. Because of its gentle nature, this gauze will not disrupt any healing that takes place, nor will it leave any residue. Non-adherent gauze often needs a secondary dressing for absorption as well as a bandage to	Explaining using real objects and picture Questioning	Listening and taking down notes Answering	• When do you apply wet dressing? • What is non adherent dressing? • Which dressing does not cause pain on removal? • What dressing is ideal for pressure ulcer and venous ulcer? • Which dressing helps in controlling bleeding? • What is transparent film dressing? • What are alginate?

Contd...

Sl.No.	Specific objective	Time	Content	Teacher activity	Learner activity	Evaluation
			keep it on the wound. There are generally two distinct types of non-adherent gauze in a gauze-based dressing. There is synthetic non-woven gauze material, which makes up the majority of non-adhesive, and there is cotton based woven gauze with a non-adherent film. The film is typically a poly skin that rests against the wound bed and allows exudate to soak through the perforation into the woven gauze padding. **Self-adhesive dressing:** It is ideal for small superficial wound that do not require debridement. **Transparent film dressings:** Transparent film dressings are thin flexible transparent sheets with adhesive backing, composed of polyurethane or co-polyester. They are permeable to water vapor, oxygen, and carbon dioxide but impermeable to bacteria and water. They provide a moist healing environment and promote autolytic debridement. They do not have any absorptive capabilities and therefore do not have a role in wounds with excessive exudates. This material should not cover infected wounds because bacteria have an ideal environment to multiply without adequate drainage. **Foam dressings:** Foam dressings are made from a polyurethane base and are permeable to both gases and water vapor. Their hydrophilic properties allow high absorptive properties while they also provide thermal insulation. These highly versatile dressings are indicated for wounds with moderate-to-heavy exudates, granulating or slough covered partial and full-thickness wounds, donor sites, ostomy sites, minor burns, and diabetic ulcers. **Alginates:** Alginates are yet another dressing to use in highly exudative wounds. Alginates are useful because they allow formation of a moist wound environment, are highly absorptive, and can prevent microbial contamination. Alginates are capable of absorbing 20 times their weight. **Hydrocolloid dressing:** Hydrocolloid dressings can be used on burns, wounds that are emitting liquid, necrotic wounds, pressure ulcers, and venous ulcers. These are non-breathable dressings that are self-adhesive and require no taping. The flexible material that they are made from makes them comfortable to wear and suitable for even the most sensitive of skin types. These dressings work by creating moist conditions which help to heal certain wounds; the surface is coated with a substance which contains polysaccharides and other polymers which absorb water and form a gel, keeping the wound clean, protecting it from infection, and helping it to heal more quickly. Hydrocolloid dressings are impermeable to bacteria and are also long-lasting, biodegradable, and easy to apply. **Hydrogel dressing:** Hydrogel dressing can be used for a range of wounds that are leaking little or no fluid, and are painful or necrotic wounds, or are pressure ulcers or donor sites. Hydrogel can also be used for second-degree burns and infected wounds. Hydrogel dressings are designed to maximize patient comfort and reduce pain while helping to heal wounds or burns and fight infection. The cooling gel in products makes them so effective at reducing pain and speeding up the healing process. **Pressure dressing:** A "pressure dressing" consists of a nonadherent bandage applied over the incision that is covered by a bulky, absorbent layer and a stretchable adhesive. Application of a pressure dressing over a wound is intended to compress dead space and prevent hematoma and seroma formation. Pressure dressing helps in promoting homeostasis. It exerts pressure over an actual bleeding site. It also helps in eliminating dead space in underlying tissues and allows the wounds to heal normally. Once pressure dressing is used, the nurse should keep a constant observation for skin colour and pulse in distant extremities.			

Contd...

Contd...

Sl.No.	Specific objective	Time	Content	Teacher activity	Learner activity	Evaluation
4.	List the characteristics of an ideal dressing	5 mts	**Characteristics of an ideal dressing** (Sood A, Granick MS and Tomaselli NL (2014)) • Creates a moist, clean, warm environment • Provides hydration if dry or desiccated • Removes excess exudates • Prevents desiccation and is non-traumatic • Provides protection to peri-wound area • Allows for gaseous exchange • Impermeable to microorganisms • Free of toxic or irritant particles • Does not release particles or fibers • Can conform to wound shape • Minimal pain during application and removal • Easy to use • Cost-effective	• Explaining using chart. • Clarifying doubts	Listening and taking down notes Answering	• What is peri-wound area? • Why should a dressing remove excess exudates? • What are the characteristic of an ideal dressing?
5.	Explain the general instructions to be followed during surgical dressing.	10 mts	**General instructions** • Maintain strict aseptic technique to prevent cross infection to and from the wound. • All materials touching the wound should be sterile • One set of instruments should be used for one dressing • Use mask, sterile gloves and gown to minimize wound contamination • Dressing should not be done immediately after sweeping and dusting, wait at least for 15–20 minutes • Use individually wrapped sterile dressing and equipment for the wound • Maintain sterile field around the wound by spreading sterile towels • Avoid talking, coughing, sneezing once the wound is opened • If dressing is adherent to the wound due to secretions or blood, wet it with sterile saline before it is removed • Observe the discharge from the wound accurately for color, odour, amount and consistency • Shortening and removal of the drainage tube is done only after doctor's order • Avoid meal timing for dressing. It should be done either half an hour before or after the meal	Explaining using black board Questioning	Listening and taking down notes Answering	Tell any five general instructions to be followed to prevent infection of the wound?
6.	Assemble all the articles needed for the type of surgical dressing.	10 mts	**Preparatory phase, Equipment needed, A clean tray containing** • Clean gloves • Sterile gloves • Readymade dressing packs • Cleaning solution (Normal saline, Hydrogen peroxide of any other antiseptic solution) • Ordered medication • Adhesive plaster • Bandage scissors • Plastic bag • Mackintosh • Culture tubes	Explaining using real objects Questioning	Listening, observing and taking down notes Answering	What are the equipment to be kept in sterile dressing tray?

Contd...

Contd...

Sl.No.	Specific objective	Time	Content	Teacher activity	Learner activity	Evaluation
7.	Perform the procedure of surgical dressing	40 mts	**A sterile dressing tray containing** • Artery forceps-1 • Thumb forceps-1 • Cotton swabs • Gauze pieces • Gallipot for cleaning solution • Surgical pads • Kidney tray • Sterile scissors **Performance phase** (see sub-table below)	Step by step demonstrating the procedure Questioning the students	Observing and participating in the procedure Taking down notes answering	• What technique will you use to clean a surgical wound? • How do you clean if drain is present?

Procedure/Task	Rationale
Identify the client	Ensures right patient receives right treatment
Explain client and parents the procedure and have client lie in the bed	Encourages client and parents co-operation
Gather equipment and arrange at the bedside	An organized approach will save time and energy
Wash hands	Reduces spread of microorganisms
Check physician's order for dressing and any specific instruction	Clarifies type of dressing
Close door or curtains and place mackintosh beneath area of dressing	Provides privacy and prevents soiling of linen
Assist patient to comfort table position that provides easy access to wound area	Promotes comfort
Don clean disposable gloves and remove soiled dressings carefully from more clean to less clean area (if dressing is adherent to the skin, moisten it by pouring small amount of normal Saline)	• Protects nurse from contamination • Moistened dressing is easier to remove
Keep soiled side of dressing away from client's view	Reduces anxiety of the client
Assess the amount color and odor of dressing	Helps for identifying the wound healing process
Discard dressing in disposable bag. Pull of the gloves inside out and discard in appropriate receptacle	Prevents spread of microorganism
Open cleaning solution and pour into the sterile galipot. Don sterile gloves	Keeps supplies within easy reach and maintains sterility

Contd...

Contd...

Sl.No.	Specific objective	Time	Content		Teacher activity	Learner activity	Evaluation
			Procedure/Task	**Rationale**			
			Use sterile technique, open sterile dressing tray and supplies on working area	Maintains asepsis			
			• For a surgical wound, clean from top to bottom or from center outward	• Moving from least to most contaminated area prevents spread of microorganisms to less infected area			
			• In contaminated wound clean from periphery to center (circular motion for cleaning circular wound)	• Moisture provides medium for growth of microorganisms and drying the wound may retard the growth of organisms and improve healing process			
			• Use one cotton swab/gauge sponge for each wipe, discarding each by dropping into the kidney tray after wiping				
			• If a drain is present, clean around it, moving from center outward in a circular motion				
			• Dry the wound using sponge in same motion				
			• Pick up soaked cotton using forceps				
			Apply medication ordered (ointment) to the wound on a dry sterile gauze. Apply a layer of sterile dressing over wound	Additional dressing serves as a wick for drainage			
			Place sterile gauze slit on side under and around the drain	Drainage is absorbed and surrounding skin area is protected			
			Apply a second layer of gauze to wound site and a surgical pad as the outer most layers	Provides for absorption of wound drainage and protection from micro organisms			
			Remove gloves from inside out and discard in plastic waste bag. Apply adhesive tape to secure the dressing	Tape is easier to apply after gloves have been removed			
			Wash reusable articles to be sent for sterilization	To keep ready for next use			
			Wash hands, remove all articles and make patient comfortable	Prevents spread of infection			
			Note dressing change, appearance of wound and describe any drainage in the chart	Provide accurate documentation of procedure			
8.	Perform the after care of patient and articles	10 mts	**After care of the patient and articles** • Remove the mackintosh and treatment towel • Take all articles to the treatment room • Discard the soiled dressing in the covered container and send it for incineration • Remove the articles and instruments from the disinfectant solution and clean them thoroughly • Dry them and reset the tray and send it for autoclaving • Replace all the articles at the proper place • Help the patient to dress up and make him comfortable • Replace the bed linen • Wash hands • Keep the unit tidy and clean		Step by step demonstrating the procedure Questioning the students	Observing and participating in the procedure Taking down notes answering	How do you discard soiled dressing?

Contd...

Contd...

Sl.No.	Specific objective	Time	Content	Teacher activity	Learner activity	Evaluation
9.	Document the findings	5 mts	• Record the procedure in nurse's record • Date and time of the procedure • Dressing material used • Condition of the wound • Type and amount of discharge • Condition of suture, etc. • Patients status during and after procedure • Report to the surgeon, if any abnormalities found	Explaining using black board	Listening	What characteristics of the wound to be documented after surgical dressing?

Summary (5 mts)

Surgical dressing is cleansing a wound or incision and applying sterile protective covering using aseptic technique. The main purpose of dressing is protection of the wound against bacterial contamination that remains a significant source of postoperative morbidity. Types of dressing depend upon the location, size and type of the wound which includes wet plain gauze or impregnated gauze dressing, non – adherent dressing, foam dressing, transparent film dressing, self – adhesive dressing, hydrocolloid and hydrogel dressing and pressure dressing. Strict aseptic technique has to be followed to prevent cross infection to and from the wound. The comfort of the patient should be ensured throughout the procedure. After procedure, keep the patient and unit tidy. Document the procedure in nurses' record with the date and time, condition of the wound, type and amount of discharge, condition of suture and the patient status during and after procedure.

Conclusion (5 mts)

Nurses have to be vigilant in identifying, assessing the wound and promote wound healing. Surgical dressing is the procedure, has to be done carefully using aseptic technique, promoting at-most comfort of the patients. If done so, promotes wound healing and aids in quick recovery of the patient.

Assignment

Write assignment on the merits and demerits of the various dressing materials available in the market, used for surgical dressing.

Evaluation

Write short answers on the following: 15 x 2 = 30 marks

1. Define surgical dressing.
2. List any four purposes of surgical dressing.
3. List the four factors influencing the decision on types of dressing.
4. Define nonadherent dressing.
5. List two indications for hydrocolloid dressing.
6. Write to purposes of pressure dressing.
7. List any four characteristics of an ideal wound dressing.
8. List two purposes of hydrogel dressing.
9. List four indications of foam dressing.
10. What are alginates?
11. Write two characteristics of transparent film dressing.
12. List any four techniques to be followed to prevent infection.
13. Write any four characteristics of the wound to be documented after procedure?
14. Write the technique to be used to clean a surgical wound?
15. Write the technique to be used to clean a contaminated wound?

OSCE Station on Surgical Dressing will be Conducted

Scenario 1
Mr A underwent appendectomy surgery and today is the third postoperative day. Changing of dressing is ordered for the patient. Perform dressing.

Scenario 2
Mr B is suffering from diabetic wound on his right foot. Dressing is ordered for the patient. Perform dressing.

Scenario 3
Ms C has burns on her right forearm. The wound has more exudates and it is painful for the patient. Perform dressing.

References

1. Berman A, Snyder SJ, Frandsen G. Kozier & Erb's *Fundamentals of Nursing; Concepts, process and practice* (10th ed). Place, Darling Kindersley publication; 2018. pp.922-8
2. Dabiri G, Damstetter E, Phillips T. Choosing a Wound Dressing Based on Common Wound Characteristics. *Advances in wound care*, 2016;5(1):32-41, doi: 10.1089/wound.2014.0586
3. Hinkle JL, Cheever KH. *Brunner & Suddarth's Textbook of Medical-Surgical Nursing* (13th ed.). Philadelphia, Lippincott Williams & Wilkins; 2014.pp.670-1.
4. Lemone PT, Burke KM, Bauldoff G, Gubrud P. *Medical-Surgical Nursing: Clinical Reasoning in Patient Care* (6th ed). Pearson Publication; 2015.pp.76-8.
5. Sood A, Granick MS, Tomaselli NL. Wound Dressings and Comparative Effectiveness Data, *Advances in wound care*. 2014;3(8):511-29, doi: 10.1089/wound.2012.0401
6. Taylor C, Lillis C, Lynn P. *Fundamentals of Nursing* (8th ed). Philadelphia, Lippincott Williams & Wilkins; 2016.pp.938-9.

Appendix 5: Unit plan.

Sample Unit Plan

Name of the Course : BSc (N)
Name of the Subject : Communication and Educational Technology
Name of the Unit : Review of Communication Process
Placement : Second Year, BSc(N)
Name of the Faculty : Mrs R Sudha
Hours Prescribed : 5 hours

General Objective

At the end of this unit, the students will be able to gain knowledge and understanding regarding communication process and develop desirable attitude and skill in establishing and maintaining effective communication.

Specific Objectives

At the end of this unit, the students will be able to:
- Define communication
- Mention the levels of communication
- Explain the communication process
- List down the forms/types of communication
- Discuss the factors influencing communication
- Describe the barriers of communication
- Explain the methods of overcoming the barriers of communication.

Introduction (10 minutes)

Communication is the basic element of human interactions that allows people to establish, maintain and improve contacts with others. Communication requires at least two people, who as a result of communicating establish a relationship with each other. Nursing is based on establishing a caring and helping relationship. Nurses must learn to communicate to be an effective caregiver. Nurses should know the techniques of communication and the barriers to effective communication. Nurses should learn to be good communicators and be able to identify the hidden messages in the communication with the people. They should be skilled enough in communicating with the people.

Sl. No.	Duration	Specific objectives	Content	Teaching-learning activities	Evaluation
1.	10 minutes	Define communication	Communication is defined as a system of sending and receiving messages that forms a connection between the sender and receiving information, a form of interaction or transaction — **Ruth F Craven** Communication is the process of sharing information or the process of generating and transmitting meanings —**Taylor**	Lecture discussion	Short answer objective type
2.	10 minutes	Mention the levels of communication	• Intrapersonal communication • Interpersonal communication • Public communication	Lecture discussion role play	Short answer objective type

Contd...

Contd...

Sl. No.	Duration	Specific objectives	Content	Teaching-learning activities	Evaluation
3.	40 minutes	Explain the communication process	<ul><li>Elements of communication process</li><li>Sender</li><li>Receiver</li><li>Channel</li><li>Feedback</li></ul>	Lecture discussion role play	Short answer objective type
4.	20 minutes	List down the forms/types of communication	<ul><li>Verbal communication</li><li>Nonverbal communication</li><li>Metacommunication</li></ul>	Lecture discussion role play	Short answer objective type
5.	1 hour	Discuss the factors influencing communication	<ul><li>Development</li><li>Perception</li><li>Values</li><li>Emotion</li><li>Sociocultural background</li><li>Gender</li><li>Knowledge</li><li>Roles and relationships</li><li>Environment</li><li>Space and territoriality</li><li>Eye contact</li></ul>	Lecture discussion role play	Short answer objective type
6.	1 hour	Describe the barriers of communication	<ul><li>Barriers to listening</li><li>Barriers to accurate perception</li><li>Barriers to effective verbal communication</li><li>Others physical, sociocultural and developmental barriers.</li></ul>	Lecture discussion role play assignment	Short answer objective type evaluation of assignment
7.	1 hour	Explain the methods of overcoming the barriers of communication	<ul><li>Listening skills</li><li>Conversational skills</li><li>Interpersonal skills</li><li>Assertive skills</li><li>Nonverbal communication</li><li>Use of humor</li><li>Use of mechanical aids</li></ul>	Lecture discussion role play	Short answer objective type

Summary (10 minutes)

Communication is the process of sharing information or the process of generating and transmitting meanings. The levels of communication are intrapersonal communication; interpersonal communication and public communication. The elements of communication process are sender, receiver, channel and feedback. The forms of communication are nonverbal communication, metacommunication and verbal communication. The factors influencing communication are development, perception, values, emotion, sociocultural background, gender, knowledge, roles and relationships, environment, space and territoriality and eye contact. The main barriers to communication are barriers to listening, barriers to accurate perception, and barriers to effective verbal communication. The others are physical, sociocultural and developmental barriers. A person can overcome the barriers by improving the skills in listening, conversation, maintaining interpersonal relationship, assertiveness and nonverbal communication. Use of humor and use of mechanical aids will also facilitate communication.

References

1. Ananthakrishnan N, Sethuraman KR, Santhosh Kumar. *Medical Education Principles and Practice* (2nd edn). Pondicherry, Alumni Association of National Teacher Training Centre, JIPMER 2000.
2. Basavanthappa BT. *Nursing Education.* (1st edn). New Delhi, Jaypee Brothers Medical Publishers Pvt Ltd 2003.
3. Constance JH, and Ruth FG. Fundamentals of Nursing. Lippincott Publication 2005.
4. Dianal LH. Leadership and Nursing care Management (3rd edn). Saunders Publication 1999.
5. Ellis H. Nursing in Today's World (8th edn.) Lippincott publications 2000.
6. Hugan TH. Fundamentals of Nursing (3rd edn). Saunders Publication 2005.

Appendix 6: Course plan.

Sample Course Plan

Name of the Course : Communication and Educational Technology
Placement : II year BSc (N)
Hours Prescribed : 90 hours

General Objective

This course will help the students acquire knowledge and understanding of principles and methods of communication and teaching and develop desirable attitude and skill in communicating effectively, maintaining effective interpersonal relations, teaching individuals and groups in clinical, community health and educational settings.

Specific Objectives

- Review communication process
- Establish effective interpersonal relations
- Explain the concepts of human relations
- Discuss guidance and counseling methods
- Explain the principles of teaching and learning
- Discuss the concepts of curriculum
- Describe the methods of teaching
- Explain the audio-visual aids used in teaching
- Describe the various methods of evaluation
- Explain health education.

Sl. No.	Time (Hours)	Specific objectives	Content	Teaching-learning activities	Evaluation
1.	5	Review communication process	**Review of communication process:** Definition, elements, facilitators of communication factors influencing communication barriers and techniques of overcoming	Lecture discussion role play exercise with audio/video taps assignment	Short answer objective type evaluation of assignment
2.	5	Discuss interpersonal relationship	**Interpersonal relations:** Definition, purpose and types, theories, barriers Johari Window and techniques of overcoming.	Lecture discussion role play exercise with audio/ video taps assignment	Short answer objective type evaluation of assignment
3.	5	Explain the concepts of human relations	**Human relations:** Understanding self-motivation, social behavior, attitude, group and group dynamics, teamwork and human relations in context of nursing	Lecture discussion role play assignment	Short answer objective type evaluation of assignment
4.	8 + 5	Discuss guidance and counseling methods	**Guidance and counseling:** Definition, principles, approaches, techniques, areas of counseling, group guidance, organization of counseling services, role of counselor, problems of the counselor and counselee, management of disciplinary problems and management of crisis and referral	Lecture discussion role play assignment	Short answer objective type assess performance in role play. Evaluation of assignment
5.	5	Explain the principles of teaching and learning	**Principles of education and teaching-learning process:** Education—Definition, forms, agencies of education. Relationship between philosophy and education. Nature and characteristics of learning, principles and maxims of teaching, formulating objectives: general and specific classroom management role of the teacher lesson plan, unit plan and course plan	• Lecture discussion prepare lesson plan • Microteaching exercise on writing objectives • Role play assignment	Short answer objective type assessing lesson plans and teaching sessions evaluation of assignment

Contd...

Contd...

Sl. No.	Time (Hours)	Specific objectives	Content	Teaching-learning activities	Evaluation
6.	4 + 2	Discuss the concepts of curriculum	**Curriculum:** Definition, nature of curriculum, factors and determinants of curriculum, phases and steps in curriculum development	Lecture discussion exercise on rotation plans assignment	Short answer objective type evaluating rotation plans
7.	10 + 10	Describe the methods of teaching	**Methods of teaching:** • Definition • Classroom methods • Clinical methods	Lecture discussion conduct teaching sessions using different methods and media	Short answer objective type assessing teaching sessions
8.	8 + 6	Explain the audio-visual aids used in teaching	**Educational media:** Definition, purposes, types, principles, graphic aids, three dimensional aids, printed aids, projected aids audio aids and computer	Lecture discussion demonstration prepare and use different teaching aids	Short answer objective type assessing the teaching aids prepared
9.	8 + 4	Describe the various methods of evaluation	**Assessment:** Definition, purpose and scope, criteria for selection of assessment techniques and methods, assessment of knowledge, attitude and skill	Lecture discussion exercise on developing different types of evaluation tools assignment	• Short answer objective type evaluation of tools prepared • Evaluation of assignment
10.	5	Explain health education	**Information, education and communication for health (IEC):** Definition, principles, health behavior and health education, health educating individuals and groups, communicating health messages, methods and media and using mass media	Lecture discussion role play plan and conduct health education sessions for individuals and groups	Short answer objective type assessment of health education session

References

1. Arulsamy S. Educational Innovations and Management (1st edn). New Delhi, Neelkamal Publishers 2010.
2. Kumar KL. Educational Technology. New Delhi, New Age International (P) Limited Publishers 1996.
3. Mukalel JC. Creative Approaches to Classroom Teaching. New Delhi, Discovery Publishing House 1998.
4. Venkataiah N. Educational Technology (1st edn). New Delhi, APH Publishing Corporation 2004.
5. Wadhwa Shalini. Teaching and Learning Methodology in Higher Education (1st edn). New Delhi, Sarup & Sons 2006.

References

Books

1. Agarwal JC. Teachers and education in a developing society. New Delhi, Vikas Publishing House Pvt Ltd., 1996.
2. Enny JW. Philosophical and theoretical perspectives for advanced nursing practice (2nd edn). Jones and Bartlett Publishers, 1999.
3. Eisner E. The art of educational evaluation. London, The Falmer Press, 1985.
4. Ganong JM, Ganong WL. Nursing Management (2nd edn). Aspin Publication, 1980.
5. Green JS, Grosswald SJ, Suter E, Walthall BD. Continuing Education for Health Professions. Washington D.C. Joss-Bass Publishes, 1984.
6. Heidgerken LE. Teaching and Learning in Schools of Nursing (1st edn). New Delhi, Konark Publishers Pvt Ltd, 1996.
7. Haladyna TM. Developing and validating multiple choice test items (2nd edn). Lawrence Erlbaum Associates,.1999.
8. Knowels M. Self Directed Learning. A guide for Learners and Teachers. New York, Association Press, 1975.
9. Kemp JE, Kayton DK. Planning and Producing Instructional Media (5th edn). New York, Harper and Row Publishers, 1985.
10. Kumar KL. Educational Technology. New Delhi, New Age International (P) Limited Publishers, 1996.
11. Mukalel JC. Creative approaches to classroom teaching. New Delhi, Discovery Publishing House, 1998.
12. Ananthakrishnan N, Sethuraman KR, Kumar Santhosh. Medical Education Principles and Practice (2nd edn). Pondicherry, Alumni Association of National Teacher Training Centre, JIPMER, 2000.
13. Mcllrath D, Huitt W. The teaching/ learning process: A discussion of models. Valdosta, Valdosta State University, 1995.
14. Mukhopadhyay, Marma. Educational Technology. New Delhi, All India Association for Educational Technology, 1991.
15. Mrunalini T. Educational Evaluation (1st edn). New Delhi, Neelkamal Publishers, 2010.
16. Mrunalini T. Curriculum Development (1st edn). New Delhi, Neelkamal Publishers, 2008.
17. Neeraja KP. Textbook of Nursing Education (1st edn). New Delhi, Jaypee Brothers Medical Publishers Pvt Ltd, 2005.
18. Slavin R. Cooperative learning and inter-group relations. Handbook of Research on Multicultural Education. New York: MacMillan, 1995.
19. Sharma SK, Tomar Monica. Teaching and Learning-Learning Process (1st edn). New Delhi, Isha Books, 2005.
20. Stanhope. Community Health Nursing Process and Practice for promoting health. Mosby Publication, 1988.
21. Schroeder Patricia S, Maibusel Regena M. Nursing quality Assurance. London, Aspen Publication, 1984.
22. Stevens J. Nursing Management. New York, Mosby Publications, 1996.
23. Arulsamy S. Educational Innovations and Management (1st edn). New Delhi, Neelkamal Publishers, 2010.
24. Sampath K, Panneerselvam A Santhanam. Introduction to Educational Technology. New Delhi, Sterling Publishers Private Limited, 1981.
25. Tay Vaughan, Multimedia. Making It Work (3rd edn). California, Osborne McGraw-Hill, 1996.
26. Venkataiah N. Educational Technology (1st edn). New Delhi, APH Publishing Corporation, 2004.
27. Wadhwa Shalini. Teaching and Learning Methodology in Higher Education (1st edn). New Delhi, Sarup & Sons, 2006.
28. Basavanthappa BT. Nursing Education (1st edn). New Delhi, Jaypee Brothers Medical Publishers Pvt Ltd., 2003.
29. Bloom B. Handbook of formative and summative evaluation of student learning. New York, McGraw-Hill, 1971.
30. Boud D. The challenge of problem based learning. London, Kogan Page, 1991.
31. Bound D, Feletti GI. The Challenge of Problem Based Learing (2nd edn). London, Kogan Page, 1998.
32. Brown JW, Lewis RB, Haroleroad FF. AV Instructional Technology, Media and Methods (5th edn). New York, McGraw Hill, Inc.,1977.
33. DeVellis RF. Scale development: Theory and applications. Newbury Park: Sage, 1991.

Journal

1. Andrades Christine. Importance of clinical audit in the prevention and control of hospital acquired infection. Asian Journal of Cardio vascular Nursing. 2000;10(2):9-13.
2. DiMaria-Ghalili RA, OstrowL, Rodney K. Web casting : A new instructional technology in distance graduate nursing education. Journal of Nursing Education. 2005;44(1).
3. Ehrenberg AC, Häggblom M. Problem-based learning in clinical nursing education: integrating theory and practice. Nurse Education Practice. 2007;7(2):67-74.
4. Goldenberg D, Andrusyszyn MA, Iwastw C. The effect of classroom simulation on nursing students' self efficacy related to health teaching. Journal of Nursing Education. 2005;44(7).
5. Jagannath Mohanty. Human rights: A global challenge racing teacher education. Education Tracks. 2004;4(2).
6. Jantzi J, Austin C. Measuring learning, student engagement and program effectiveness: A Strategic Process. Nurse Educator. 2002;30(2).
7. Karuhije HF, Ruff C. External examiners: Quality assurance in nursing education. Journal of Nursing Education. 2001;40(1).
8. Khan G. Factors affecting quality assurance in nursing care. Nursing Journal of India. 1999;Vol. LXXXX (8):173-174.
9. Kyriacos U, Heever JVD. A Non traditional curriculum for the preparation of nurse educators. Journal of Nursing Education. 1999;38(7).
10. Masters JC. Hollywood in the classroom using feature films to teach. Nurse Educator. 2005;30(3).
11. Medley CF, Horne C. Using simulation technology for undergraduate. Journal of Nursing Education. 2005;44(1).
12. Bailey PA, Carpenter DR, Harrington P. Theoretical foundations of service learning in nursing education. Journal of Nursing Education. 2002;41(10).
13. Misra PK. Making teachers' component for emerging technologies: Needed Actions. New Frontiers in Education. 2009;42(2).
14. Moree K. What nurses learn from nursing audit. Nursing out look. 1988;26(1):48.
15. Murphy JM. Distance Education in nursing: An integrated review of online nursing students' experiences with technology-delivered instruction. Journal of Nursing Education. 2007;46(6).
16. Patterson B. The nature of evidence in teaching practice. Journal of Nursing Education. 2009;48(6).
17. Rosenshine B. Advances in research on instruction. The Journal of Educational Research. 1995;88(5):262-8.
18. Ryan M, Hodson Carlton K, Ali NS. A model for faculty teaching online: Confirmation of a dimensional matrix. Journal of Nursing Education. 2005;44(8).
19. Sakrida TJ, Draus PJ. Quality handout development and use. Journal of Nursing Education, 2.
20. Samanta RK. Instructional aids for educational training. Indian Journal of Training and Development. 1988;XVIII(6).
21. Savin-Baden M. Problem-based learning: a catalyst for enabling and disabling disjunction prompting transitions in learner stances? PhD thesis, University of London, Institute of Education. 1996.
22. Siu HM, Spence Laschinger HK, Vingilis E. The effect of problem based learning on nursing students' perceptions of empowerment. The Journal of Nursing Education. 2005;44(10).
23. Baker CM, McDaniel AM, Pesut DJ, Fisher ML. Learning skills profiles of master's students in nursing administration: assessing the impact of problem-based learning. Nursing Education Perspectives. 2007;28(4):190-5.
24. Sridhar S. Quality assurance in nursing. Indian Journal of Nursing and Midwifery. 1988;2.
25. Stull A, Lantz C. An innovative model for nursing scholarship. Journal of Nursing Education. 2005;44(11).
26. Telles C. A step-by-step guide to videoconferencing. Nurse Educator. 2008;l33(4).
27. Ulloth JK. A Qualitative view of humour in nursing classrooms. Journal of Nursing Education. 2003;42(3).
28. Ulloth JK. Nursing education guidelines for developing and implementing humour in nursing classrooms. Journal of Nursing Education. 2003;42(1).
29. Webber PB. A Curriculum framework for nursing. Journal of Nursing Education. 2002;41(1).
30. Welliver MD, et al. Tips for using video teleconferencing for distance education. Nurse Educator, 33(4).
31. Barrows H, Tamblyn R. Problem-based learning: an approach to medical education. Medical Education. 1980;1.
32. Beers GW. The Effect of Teaching Method on Objective Test scores: Problem based learning vs learning. Journal of Nursing Education. 2005;44(7).
33. Blowers S, Ramsey P, Merriman C. Patterns of peer tutoring. Journal of Nursing Education. 2003;42(5).
34. Brar A. An evaluation of patient care. The Nursing Journal of India. 1989;LXXXNo.(10):268-9.
35. Campbell B. MUDD mapping an interactive teaching-learning strategy. Nurse Educator. 2005;33(4).
36. Conyers Madm. Posters: An assessment strategy to foster learning in nursing education. Journal of Nursing Education. 2003;42(1).

Index

Page numbers followed by *b* refer to box, *f* refer to figure, *fc* refer to flowchart, and *t* refer to table.

A

Ability test, pre-engineering 199
Academia, responsibilities in 295
Academic aristocracy 269
Academic audit 354, 355
　advantages of 355
　objectives of 355
　to teachers, format for 355
Academic autonomy 27
Academic freedom 4
Academic growth 298
Academic learning timer 56
Academic performance 355
Accountability 294
Accreditation
　beneficiaries of 363
　benefits of 363
Accreditation in nursing 362
　purpose 363
　types 363
Accrediting programs, stages of 363
Achievement test 194, 197
　functions of 197
Acquiescence bias 184
Action skills 307
Adapt teaching strategies 225
Administering scale 185
Administering test 190
Administration
　advantages for 300
　of institutions/departments, contribution in 356
Administrative facilities 380
Administrators, evaluation of 323
Admission
　criteria 333-335
　eligibility for 208, 335
　requirements 207, 333
Adult learning 217
　principles of 217
Adult life, preparation for 17
Advanced internet connection 387
Agencies of education, classification of 20
Agreement options 183
Ahamkara (egoism) 12
Ahimsa 14
Alexander's battery of performance test 200
Alumni employment rates and profile 324
American Association of Colleges of Nursing 290
American Federation of Teacher 150
American Society for Healthcare Education and Training 212
Anchorite 13
Andragogy 217
Anecdotal records 173, 305
　advantages of 173
　basic elements of 174
　characteristics of 173
　disadvantages of 174
Anekantavada 13
Anuprasna 12
Aparigraha 14
Aperture iris diaphragm 146
Application 189
Appraisal service 301
Aptitude 198
Aptitude test 194, 197-199, 201
　general 198
　nature of 198
　specialized 198
　types of 198
Aranyakas 12
Arm, type of 147
Army alpha test 200
Art judgment tests 198
Art of living, initiating students to 16
Arteyam 14
Artha 13
Articulation 246
Artistic skill 304
Ashrams 12
Assembling and administering test 189
Assessment skills 227
Associations, types of 367
Assumptions and needs of virtual students, relationship between 381*t*
Attitude
　principle of 50
　scale 183
　types of 183
Attract observer's attention 129
Audio aids 115
Audio and visual 348
　cassettes 223
　presentation 348
Audio medium, limitations of 137, 375
Audio presentation 348
Audio response unit 142
Audio tape 138
　recordings, making 138
Audio through tape recorder, characteristics of 138
Audio-conferencing 222, 373
Audio-teleconferencing 384
Audio-video technology 377
Audio-visual aid 114, 115, 148
　advantages of 116
　classification of 115, 115*fc*
　criteria for selection of 117
　disadvantages of 116
　in teaching, uses of 116
　requisites for effective 116
　skills 275
　use of 115, 116
　utilizing 117
Auditing, significant event 219
Auditory learners 48
Authority, delegation of 338
Auxiliary nurse and midwife 44, 206
　role of 206
Auxiliary nurse midwifery 332
　course, clinical requirements for 207
Axiology 5

B

Baccalaureate Nursing Programs 206
Bachelor of nursing course 208
Bachelor of science in nursing 202, 333
　programs 204
Bandwidth 378
Bar graph 122, 122*f*
　simple 122
　types of 122
Barrow's idea 91
Basic assumptions 303
Basic human learning 91
Basic nursing educational program 212
Basic skills, schedule of 240
Bedside clinic 109
　advantages of 110
　limitations of 110
　planning of 109
Behavior
　centered objectives 248
　effective 174
　focus on 314

inner control of 310
outer control of 310
Behavioral problems 21
Behavioral sciences 208
    applied to nursing 250
Behaviorally anchored rating scales 176
Best faculty, access to 378
Better family life 299
Bhagvad Gita 13
Biological naturalism 10
Biological pragmatism 11
Black cartridge paper 115
Blackboard 126
    effective use of 127
Blocking course content 318
Bloggers 349
Blood pressure 98
Bloom's taxonomy 63, 63f
    revised 238t
Board
    background of 129
    content of 129
    height of 129
Body natural pain killer 105
Body posture, proper 306
Body tube 146
Booklets 125
    advantages of 125
    disadvantages of 125
Bowel sounds 97
Brahmacharayam 14
Breathing difficulty 181
Brochure 348
Buddhism 14
    epistemology 14
    ethics 15
    metaphysics 14
Buddhistic philosophy 15
Budget 342
    budgeting and budgetary control, differences among 342
    capital expenditure 343
    cash 343
    classification of 343
    current 343
    enrolment 343, 344
    expense 344
    fixed 343
    flexible 343
    for college 323
    library, 359
    long-term 343
    master 343
    medium-term 343
    personnel 343
    program 343
    purchase 343
    research 343
    responsibility 343
    rolling 343
    short-term 343
    types of 343
Budgetary control
    advantages of 342
    meaning of 342
Building confidence 277
Building favorable attitude 278
Building planning 337
Bulletin board 128
    advantages of 129
    classification of 128
    disadvantages of 129
    purposes of 128
    service 377

C

Camera 142, 143f
    advantages 143
    disadvantages 143
    parts 143
    purposes of 142
Capturing students interest 76
Cardboard 115
Cardiovascular disorder 189
Care and handling 148
Career development 357
Cartoon 123, 123f
    advantages of 124
    disadvantages of 124
    to attract attention 123
Case-simulation mode 102
Catharsis 315
Celebration of International Nurses' Day 370
Central Advisory Board of Education Committee on Gnanam Committee 41
Central tendency
    bias 183
    error 152
Chalkboard 125, 126
    advantages of 127
    background 126
    disadvantages of 127
    effective use of 127
    guidelines for use of 126
    placement of 126
    types of 125
Change and innovation, guidelines for 254
Changing educational paradigm 28t
Charts 117
    advantages of 119
    classification of 118
    disadvantages of 119
    effective uses of 119
    purposes of 118
Child centeredness 231
Child psychology, knowledge of 271
Citizens, creation of good 18
Citizenship 16
    creation of good 17
    education 37
    good 299
Civil and social duties, inculcation of 19
Classical lecture 75
Classroom
    bulletin boards 129
    goes to learner 379
    instruction, web-assisted 222fc
    management 71, 268
        context, effective 71
        role of student in 73
    situations 55
Class-wide peer tutoring 102
Client-centered counseling 303
    criticisms of 303
Clients, losing oneself in 309
Climates, continuum of 254
Clinical courses and distance education 222
Clinical facilities 332, 334
Clinical learning experience 327
Clinical teacher 283
Clinical teaching methods 108
Coarse adjustment knob 146
Cognitive domain 63
Cognitive interest 217
Cognitive psychologists, group of 63
Collect data 260
Collective thinking, developing art of 81
College activities, conduct of 267
College performance standards 58
Color cardboard 115
Color chalks 126
Combined aids 115
Committee on Secondary Education 39
Common crisis 315
Common educational structure 36
Commonwealth Nurses Federation, affiliation with 369
Communicates and interacts effectively with students 51
Communication
    and educational technology 372
    skills 227, 307
    technology 372-374
        educational uses of 373
        to education, barriers of 373
        uses of 373
    two-way 75
Community
    agencies 203
    based practice experiences, increased 31
    cultural imperatives of 231
    gathering places 31
    health nurse 203, 208

relations 347
    and philanthropy 349
    role of 321
Compact disks 376
Complex drawings 127
Complex overt response 65
Component bar graph 122
Compound microscope 147
Compound optical microscope 147
Computer 141, 141f, 223
    as teacher 142
    assisted learning 101
        modes of 101
        process of 101
    based simulation programs 99
    characteristics of 141
    conferencing 222, 373
    expertise 188
    graphic table 142
    joy stick 142
    keyboard 141
    light pen 141
    managed learning 384
        advantages of 384
    mouse 141
    output microfilm 142
    parts of 141
    technology 377
    teleconferencing 384
Computing scale score values 185
Conclusion 252
Condenser 146
    focus knob 146
Conduct formative evaluation 220
Conduct item analyses 195
Conduct needs assessment 218
Conduct summative evaluation 220
Conduct task analysis 220
Conduct validity studies 195
Conference 111
    and seminars 348
    direction giving 111
    large 144
Constructing scales, steps in 194
Construction, guidelines for 158
Consumer and agency, changes in attitudes of 30
Content and skills, integration of 247
Content centered teaching 57
Content conferences 111
Content development 379
Content validity 155
Context evaluation 322
Continuing education 212, 369
    characteristics of 214
    concepts of 212
    implications of 216
    need for 213
    program 215
        forms of 213
    units 214

Continuing nursing education 213, 220
    aims of research in 221
    participated 356
Control unit 142
Control vs. freedom 234
Controlling bodies 31
Cooperative attitude 272
Copying process 136
Copyright 378
Correlation, basic principles of 326
Correspondence instruction 223
Cost effectiveness 102
Council of Educational Research and Training 36
Counseling 347
    areas of 302
    characteristics of 298
    developmental 302
    dimensions of 310
    eclectic 304
    phases of 304, 304f
    program, objectives of 301
    resistance to 308
    types of 302
Counseling individuals 308
    of different cultures 308
Counseling service 301, 323
    organization of 301
    purposes of organizing 301
    types of 301
Counseling team 305
    members, roles of 306
Counselor
    burn-out 308
    functions of 306
    qualifications of 306
    qualities of good 308
Course development 321
Course management 373
Course outline 70
    planning, principles of 70
Course planner 284
Course planning 373
    content for 70
    elements of 71
    levels of 70
    structure of 70
Course syllabus, forewarning in 313
Create empowering learning environments 57
Creative movement 66
Creative teaching, promotion of 266
Crisis
    and referral services, management of 314
    counseling 302
    intervention 310, 315
    management 350
    response 314
    types of 314
Criterion validity 155

Criterion-referenced
    and norm-referenced tests, comparison of 154t
    test 153, 154, 200
Critical incident
    criteria for using 174
    recording of 174
    review 219
Criticism 283
Cross-sectional model 131
Cruickshank's model 54
Cultural development 16
Cultural invariants 240
Cultural sensitivity, developing 270
Cultural variables 240
Culture and civilization, preservation of 17
Curative health activities 206
Current awareness services 377
Curriculum 8, 229, 230, 240
    activity-centered 233
    administration 317f
    approaches of 232
    approval, level of 261
    assessor 284
    beneficiaries of 234
    broad-field 233
    building 319
    characteristics of 231
    child centered 233
    components of 317
    concepts of 230
    content of 234, 237, 239
    coordinator, role of 319
    core 233
    cultural analysis model of 240
    decisions about 256
    designing 318
    determinants of 230
    elements of 233, 234f
    enhancement 319
    evaluation of 234
    factors influencing 234
    general plan for 247
    hidden 233
    illegitimate 233
    implementation 251, 268
    improvement 25, 324
    inquiry 325
    model 235
        basic 235f
    null 233
    official 233
    operational 233
    paradigm shift in 234
    participation in 321
    philosophical determinants of 231
    planner 284
    process model of 236, 238t
    reason for formulating 234
    renewal 37

research in nursing 325
revision, steps in 255
sequence in planning 241
sociological determinants of 231
structure, developing 318
subject centered 232
three facets of 230, 230f
transaction, resources for 252
types of 232
Curriculum change 253
phases of 255
Curriculum committee
functions of 261
membership 261
Curriculum construction
drawbacks in 241
principles of 242
steps in 243, 243f
system approach to 244
trends in 235t
Curriculum design 244
conceptual framework for 247
Curriculum development 229, 268, 318, 329
facilitators of 318
faculty role in 261
forces and issues influencing 234
phases in 242, 242f
process, collaborative 61
Curriculum evaluation 257, 259, 318
model 259
purposes of 259
Curriculum framework
characteristics of 246
guiding principles for developing 319
Curriculum organization 240, 317
patterns of 232
Curriculum planning 241, 317
stages of 242

D

Damaging institution's property 316
Defensible ideas 325
Delegate 338
far down to 338
Delegation
elements of 338
obstacles to 338
problems of 338
Deliver effective lecture, strategies to 75
Delivering lecture 76
Delivery site 380
Democracy, training for 278
Democratic attitude 272
Democratic citizenship 16
Demographic revolutions 234
Demonstration 78
advantages of 78
disadvantages of 78
purpose of 78

Demonstrator, role of 79
Demotion 345
Departmental rules and regulations, awareness of 271
Departmental workshops, participation in 321
Dependence on technologies 378
Descriptive rating scales 176
Design scale 195
Designing-learning experiences 61
Dharma 13
Diagnostic skills 307
Diaz process 136
Difficulty index 165, 166
Digital environment, pricing in 378
Digital library 376, 377
factors of change to 378
objective of 377
requirement of 377
storage and preservation, advantages of 377
technological obsolescence, problems of 378
Diploma 205
advanced 205
courses 336
programs, hospital-based 202
Direct education 2
Disadvantages and criticism 194
Disaster
management 368
man-made 234
natural 234
managing victims of 31
Discharge
and dismissal 345
simpliciter 345
Disciplinary actions 311
types of 310
Disciplinary measures, need for 344
Disciplinary probation 310
and actions 310
Disciplinary procedures 345
Disciplinary warnings 310, 313
Discipline 344
approaches to 344
aspects of 344
creating climate for 346
maintenance of effective 344
negative aspect 344
positive aspects 344
Discrepancy analysis 219
Discrimination index 165, 166
Discussion lessons 283
Discussion method
advantages of 80
disadvantages of 80
purposes of 79
Discussion techniques 80
Disorderly conduct 311

Distance education
assessment for 223
in nursing 221
issues and challenges in 223
Distance education programs
development of 223
types of 221
Distractor effectiveness 165, 166
Distractor evaluation 167
District Primary Education Program 27
Doctoral program 203, 206
in nursing 205
Doctorate in clinical nursing 203
Document camera 226
Documentation 314
Dravya 14
Drill and practice mode 101
Dristanta 12
Dyad peer tutoring 102

E

East India Company 34
Economic factors
and education 23
and nursing education 25
Economic planning 231
Editing and validating test items 189
Editorials 348
Education 1, 2, 34
activities, evaluating continuing 215
agencies of 19, 20
aim of 3, 8, 9, 15
and nursing education 1
and service, different models of collaboration between 326
assessments in outcome-based 60
basic principles of outcome-based 59
changes on 21
collective 2
commission report, secondary 230
competency-based 61
concepts of 1
cost of 23
criticism of outcome-based 60
doctor of 203
dynamic 20
environment 30
familiarizing with latest in 278
flexible 20
for all age groups 20
for increased productivity 16
for leisure 16
for living 4
for modernization 16
for social, moral and spiritual values 16
forms of 2
fulfilling compulsory 35
functions of 17, 19
funding for 23

general aims of 15
general functions of 17
goal oriented 20
goals of 41
group activity 20
in group, common difficulties in outcome-based 95
in independent, aims of 16
in national life, functions of 18
indirect 2
informal 2
investment in 23
knowledge of aims of 271
level of 4
management planning, functions of 336
meeting increased demands of 30
modification of behavior 20
multidisciplinary 21
narrower meaning of 2
online 28
outcome-based 57, 61
part of 53
pervasive 20
philosophical foundations of 231
policy 36
principles of 20
programs 21
  planning continuing 214
purposes of standards in 361
science and art 21
social process 20
sociological foundations of 231
specific 2
starts 2
system 36, 59
to individual, functions of 18
type of 318
wider meaning of 2
Educational administration 331
  roles of 320
Educational advancement 355
Educational aim 6, 236
  factors determining 17
Educational and communicational technology 372
Educational commissions 38
Educational control, mechanism of 355
Educational evaluation 149
Educational factors 374
Educational implications 3
  of *Bhagvad Gita* 13
  of *Buddhism* 15
  of *Jainism* 14
  of modern
    idealism 8
    realism 9
  of naturalism 11
  of pragmatism 12
  of vedanta philosophy 12

Educational institute 91
Educational institution
  and hospital interface 328
  case of 344
  common crisis in 315
  modern infrastructure in 23
  standards for 362
Educational objectives 62, 62f, 113, 156, 248
  taxonomy of 63
  types of 62
Educational opportunity 4
Educational organization 337
Educational plan 336
  features of 336
  operational 336
  single use 337
  standing 337
  steps in educational 337
  strategic 336
  types of 336
Educational process 45
  dimensions of 45
  elements of 46
  manager of 102
Educational program
  in nursing, evaluation of 321
  objectives of 233
Educational psychology 234
  knowledge of 271
Educational radio production process 376
Educational resolution, facts of 41
Educational sector, growth of 23
Educational spiral 45f
Educational supervisors, roles of 320
Educational systems 20
Educational technology 372, 389
  objectives of 372
Educational telecast 223
Educational teleconferencing 384
Educational television 376
Educational tool, limitations 140
Educator, type of 4
Effective and ineffective
  lecture, characteristics of 76t
  praise, guidelines for 73t
Effective delegation, prerequisites for 339
Ego supporter 267
Eisner's connoisseurship model 324
E-Learning 383
  advantages of 383
Electron microscopes 147
Electronic device 374
Electronic mail 348
  components of 387
Electronic media 375
  merits of 375
Emotional development, principle of 50

Emotional impact 138
Emotional integration 19
Emotional stability 272
Emotions, strong 308
Empathy 269
Empirical to rational, proceed from 52
Employee
  communications 349
  relations 349
  services 345
Employee/member relations 347
Employer and industry (hospital) viewpoints 256
Employer product utilization and satisfaction 324
Encouraging participation 307
Environment
  changes 234
  factors 75
    related to 243
  manipulation 315
  modification of 18
  scan 322
Epistemology 4, 14
  in pragmatism 11
  of idealism 8
  of naturalism 10
Equalizer 267
Equipment, aftercare of 136
E-self-instructional
  material
    benefits of 226
    providing 227
  module
    benefits of 226
    format of 226
Essay evaluation, characteristics of 157
Essay examinations 157
  demerits of 158
  merits of 157
Essay tests, scoring of 159
E-teaching 383
Ethical behavior 6
Ethics 270
E-tutor 383
  qualities of 384
Evaluating faculty development 323
Evaluation 150, 244, 255
  and administrators 152
  and feedback 67
  and parents 152
  and students 152
  and teacher 152
  and testing, meaning of 149
  characteristics of 259
  common errors in 152
  component 282
  concepts of 151
  consider costs of 261
  formative 152

functions of 152
judgment, unity of 324
methods for different domain 156
potency and activity 184
principles of 151
process 150, 150f, 259
purpose of 151
responses 183
skills 307
steps of 156, 157fc
tools, types of 201
types of 152
Evaluator 267
Event and press support 348
Everyday activities, incorporating humor in 105
Evidence 252, 300
Examiner, role of 182
Exercises and Yoga 183
Exhibition 84, 144
advantages of 84
disadvantages of 84
Experiential lecture 75
Experimental pragmatism 11
Explanation, consideration of 345
Exploration skills 307
Extension work 356
Extracurricular activities 267
Eye contact, maintaining 306
Eyepiece (ocular) 146
tube 146

F

Fabrication 312
Facebook 350
Facilitative counseling 302
Faculty
development 295
programs 358
evaluation 323
members 322
requirements 333, 334
rights 295
role of 190, 320, 327
teaching online, model for 379t
Family nurse practitioner 203
Family planning 23
Fetus, specimen of 130f
Field test, perform 195
Field trip 85
actual conduct of 85
advantages of 85
evaluation phase 85
limitations of 86
organization of 85
preplanning 85
File transfer and file submit 385
Films 115, 140
advantages of 140
disadvantages of 140

evaluation 140
planning 140
preparation 140
Financial input 323
Financial literacy 37
Financial pressures 256
Financial relations 347
Financing education development 39
Financing higher education 25
Flannel board 128
advantages of 128
disadvantages of 128
effective use of 128
purposes of 128
Flash cards 124
advantages of 124
disadvantages of 124
method of presenting 124
Flexibility, principle of 242
Floppy disks 142
Florence Nightingale International Foundation 229
Flowchart 119fc
Focus knob, fine 146
Focus topic 134
Food, consumption of 312
Foot (base) 146
Formal education 2
Formal feedback 353
Formal talk 74
Formative evaluation, characteristics of 153
Formulating objectives, sequence for 248
Forums 350
Four noble truths 15
Friend and philosopher 267
Full-scale simulation, advantages of 100
Functional stage 242
Fundamental movement 66
Funding 329

G

Gage and Berliner's model 55
Gastric neurosis 21
Gastrointestinal disorder 189
Gather and document information 314
Genealogy chart 118, 119f
General education 2, 207
General nursing and midwifery 44, 206
program, diploma in 207
Generic approach 315
Generic movement 66
Genitourinary disorder 189
Global economy, rise of 234
Global violence 234
Gnanakanda (knowledge) 12
Gnanam Committee 24
Goal oriented 301
Goal setting 307
principle of 50

Good counsellor, characteristics of 308
Good curriculum, characteristics of 241
Good family and community relations, developing 268
Good handout, characteristics of 134
Good lecture, learner's criteria of 77
Good lesson planning, prerequisites for 67
Good poster, features of 121
Good project, qualities of 86
Good slide, characteristics of 131
Good teacher 53
qualities of 273
Good teaching, characteristics of 53
Good textbook, characteristics of 252
Gospel of humanity 13
Government affairs 347
Government Committees and Councils, affiliation with 369
Government encourages community participation 27
Government policies 26
Grading system 190, 191
Graduate student teachers, role of 321
Grahastha period 13
Graphic
aids 117
and models 115
materials 117
rating scale 176, 176f
techniques 117
Graphics/images, selection of 117
Graphs 121
disadvantages of 122
types of 121
Greaves curriculum model for nursing 240
Ground glass board 125
Group and group talk 385
Group conference 112
principles of 112
Group discipline approach 345
Group discussion 79
forms of 80
Group guidance 307
Group instruction 307
Group leader 267
Group members, role of 94
Group process skills 307
Growth and development 301
Guidance and counseling 297
basis of 298
need for 299
place for 305
principles of 300
problems in 308
relation between 299t
tools and techniques of 305
Guidance Bureau in Colleges 305
Guidance counselor and helper 267

Guidance program, characteristics of 298
Guiding principles 280

H

Hand
  drawn transparency 136
  puppet 133
  raising 385
Handmade slides 131
Handouts 134
Harassment including ragging 311
Hard disks 142
Hardboard 115
Hardware and software requirements 385
Harmonious development 15
Hashtags 351
Health
  and living conditions 302
  effects on 105
  good 306
  issues 234
  sciences 207
Healthcare
  delivery system 31
  industry 31
  problems 31
  settings 203
  system 318
  to public 212
Hearing 13
Heart
  lung 97
  model of 130f
Higher education 4
  issues in 234
  part of 21
  privatization of 24
  quality assurance in 38
  regulation in 38
  under globalization 31
High-fidelity
  simulators 98
  units 98
Holism 300
Holistic scoring 159
Home health nurse 203
Hostel 359
  block 333
  common rooms 360
  dining hall 360
  facilities 332
  indoor games and sports 360
  kitchen premises 360
  laundry 360
  pantry 360
  physical infrastructure 359
  policies for 360
  room for housekeeping staff 360
  sanitary annexes 360
  sick room 360
  store rooms 360
  student's room 360
  visitors' room 360
  warden office 360
House holder (Grahastha) 13
Huitt's model 55
Human activity 331
Human and administrative factors 374
Human behavior, modification of 2
Human civilization, values of 8
Human condition 11
Human contact 223
Human endeavor 2
Human heart 130
Human relations 344
  approach 344
Human relationships, qualities relating to 272
Human resource 339, 344
  approach 345
  inventory 340
  planning 339
    objectives of 339
  proper utilization of 299
Human society 21
Human spirit 7
Humanistic pragmatism 11
Humanistic realism 9
Humanistic teacher, acronym of 272
Humor 104, 270
  and laughter 272
  on health and learning, effects of 105
  brain activity in 104
  central theories of 104
  components of 104
  delivered orally 106
  in classroom, tips for using 105
  in print 106
  strategies 106
    high-risk 106
Hypermedia 27
Hypochondriasis 199
Hypomania 199
Hypothetical dialog 108
Hysteria 199

I

Ideal lecture 75
Idealism
  and discipline 9
  and school 9
  and teacher 8
  basic metaphysics of 8
  fundamental principles of 8
Idealistic value theory 8
Inadequacy and anxiety, feeling of 309
Incongruity theories 104
Increments, withholding of 345
Indian Institutes of Technology 233
Indian Medical Council 36
Indian Nursing Council 251, 281, 290, 364
Indian School of Philosophy 12
Indira Gandhi National Open University 35
Individual and social transformation 21
Individual case conferences 305
Individual conference 111
  advantages of 111
  disadvantages of 112
  principles of 111
Individual education 2
Individual learning 222fc
Individual rotation plan 251
Industrial alertness 4
Industry relations 347
Information provider 283
Information service 301
Information system, management of 102
Infrastructure set-up 380
Inherent limitations 102
Innovative efforts 282
Innovative teaching techniques 356
In-service education 277
Instagram 351
Instant messaging 389
Institute of Public Relation 346
Institutional code of conduct, reviewing 313
Institutional objectives 337
Institutional planning 337
  objectives of 337
  scope of 337
Institutions
  challenges for 227
  vs. community 235
Instructional design 378
Instructional media and methods 114
Instrumental values, theory of 6
Integrate teaching with practice, strategies to 327
Integumentary disorder 189
Intellectual efficiency 21
Intelligence 198
  seven forms of 29b
  terms of 29
  tests 194, 200
  uses of 200
Intercollegiate activities, organized 356
Interdepartmental activities, oganized 356
Interest inventories 194, 196
  limitation of 197
Internal evaluation
  enables 154
  limitations of 154
  shortcomings of 154
Internal mobility
  promotions 357
  purposes 358
  types of 357

International Commission on
    Development of Education 228
International Council of Nurses,
    affiliation with 369
International Institute of Science and
    Technology Education 36
Internet 348
    advantages of 386
    connection, developing an 387
    disadvantages of 386
    in education 386
    protocol 386, 390
    services 387
Interviews 293
Intrinsic programing 90
Intrinsic values, theory of 6
Introductory stage skills 275
Issues management 347
Item analysis 165
Item banks, creation of 167
Item review 187

J

Jaina metaphysics, basic category
    of 13
Jainism 13
Jains metaphysics 14
Jamshedjee Jeejeebhoy group 34
Job description 352
John Carroll's model 54
Joint consultancy 329
Judicial approach 345

K

Kama 13
Karma 14
    law of 15
Kinesthetic learners 48
Knowledge 189, 234
    advanced 5
    approach 232
    base 258
    integrating new 94
    perceptual 14
    perfect 14
    sources of 4, 14
        authority 4
        common sense 4
        controlled experience 5
        intuition 5
        reasoning 5
Kothari Commission 41, 228
Kshana bangavada 15

L

Laughter 107
Law
    of effect, principle of 50
    of proximity, principle of 50
    of readiness, principle of 50
    of similarity, principle of 50
    of use 50
LCD projector 143f
Leadership
    approach 345
    development of 16, 205
    training for 18
Leaflet 125
    advantages of 125
    disadvantages of 125
Learner 385
    centered objectives 248
    facilities 380
    factors 75
    observable behavior 236
    possesses intelligence, dimensions of
        48
Learning 46, 113
    activities (means to ends) 237-239
    affects conduct of learner 47
    anytime-anywhere 378
    by living 12
    characteristics of 46
        problem-based 91
    creative 47
    delivery system 379
    depends upon insight 47
    disadvantages of problem-based 95
    effects on 105
    eight kinds of 47
    elements of 217
    environment 49
    facilitator of 267, 283
    factors influencing 48
    four orientations to 49t
    goals of problem-based 91
    growth 47
    history of problem-based 91
    individual 46
    integration of 244
    intelligent 47
    method, limitations of computer
        assisted 102
    modalities 48
    objectives of simulation process 98
    online 378
    organization of 244
    organizing experience 47
    pillars of 47, 113
    problem scenario, developing
        problem-based 92
    purposive 47
    self-active 46
    self-directed 95
    situation, selection of 69
    social 46
    steps of problem-based 92, 92fc
    takes place through trial and error 47
    taxonomy for 63
    theoretical orientations to 49
    to operate computers 282
    to prepare 282
    to revise one's position 82
    transferable 47
    types of 47
    unitary 46
    virtual classroom 382
Learning experiences
    appropriate 30
    criteria for selection of 249
    organization of 234, 249
    planned 212
    selection of 233, 244, 249
Learning process 47
    controlled 89
    elements of 47
Learning scenario
    characteristics of problem-based 92
    criteria for problem-based 92
Learning styles 48
    four 29b
Lecturalgia 77
Lecture
    evaluation of effectiveness of 76
    presentation 224
Lecture method 74
    advantages of 77
    disadvantages of 77
    purposes of 75
Lecturer 283
Legitimate curriculum 233
Leisure 303
Lesson plan 66
    essential elements of good 67
    steps in developing 67
    types of 67
Letters to editor 348
Library 358
    equipment 358
    furniture 358
    holdings 359
    librarian 358
    library committee 359
    location 358
    organization of books 359
    policies 359
    requisites of 358
Licensed practical nurse 202, 211
Licensed vocational nurse
    programs 202, 211
    students 204
Life
    activities 234
    centeredness 232
    preparation for 18
Likert scale 183
Limb (arm) 146
Line graph 121, 121f
Linked station 180
    type of 180

Liquid crystal display projector 143
Live broadcast 139, 376
Logical and psychological requirements 247
Lord's song 13
Low-fidelity simulators 97

M

Making man civilized 18
Management
   concept of 331
   skills 205, 227
Managerial skills 275
Manifests interest 196
Maps
   aspects of 123
   types of 123
Market monitoring 349
Marketing communications 347
Marking scheme, preparation of 160
Masculinity-femininity 199
Master programs 206
Master rotation plan 251
Mastering delivering techniques 76
Mastery test 153
Matching items 168
Material organism 4
Material phenomena, external 10
Material resources 323
Materials and one's frame of mind, coordination of 81
Matte release 349
Maturational crises 314
Mechanical aptitude tests 198
Mechanical features 252
Mechanical naturalism 10
Media relations 347, 349
Media tours 349
Medical college admission test 199
Medical services 323
Medical staff, role of 306
Medical surgical nurse 203
Medical technology 28, 207
Meditation 13
Meetings and small conferences 144
Memory
   good 272
   store 142
Mental discipline 4
Mental disorder 21
Mentor 283
   choose 270
Metaphysics 3, 13
   and pragmatism 11
Methodological teaching, maxims of 51
Microscope 146, 146f
   advantages 148
   care and handling 148
   clean-up 148
   direction to use 148
   disadvantages 148
   handling and cleaning 148
   parts of 146
   simple 147
   storage 148
   transporting 148
Microteaching 100
   advantages of 101
   characteristics of 100
   disadvantages of 101
   process 100
Mid-day meal Scheme 27
Midwifery and maternal and child health 206
Miniature Society 12
Ministry of Human Resource Development 38
Minnesota clerical aptitude test 199
Minnesota engineering analogical test 199
Minnesota mechanical aptitude test 199
Minnesota multiphasic personality inventory 199
Misconduct, procedure
   for minor 312
   for serious 313
Mobile learning 388
Mobile presentations 144
Model
   advantages of 131
   classification of 130, 130t
   disadvantages of 131
   question paper, preparation of 160
Moderate-fidelity simulators 97
Modern living, art of 12
Modern technology 32
Modified National Education Policy 36
Moksha 13
Moodle 389
Moral
   educator 267
   religion and social 303
Morality, training in 19
Most favored nation treatment 32
Mother's education 56
Motivation 217
   principle of 50
MUDD mapping 107
   for learnes 108
   for teachers 108
Multimedia 27, 385
   application of 385
   classroom environment 385
   computer, constraints in using 386
   educational tools, developing 385
Multiple aptitude test 199
Multiple bar graphs 122
Multiple choice question 162
   advantages of 162
   disadvantages of 162
   paper
      general steps of formulating 164
      validating 164
   preparation of 162
   responses, analyzing 166
   types of 162
   uses of 162
Multiple completion type 163
Musical aptitude tests 198

N

Narrative chart 118
Narrower sense 2
National and international accreditation bodies 257
National Assessment and Accreditation Council 363
National Awards 370
National Conferences 369
National Council for Teacher Education 296
National Council Licensure examination for practical nurse 202
National curriculum framework 281
National development 18
National discipline 19
National education policy 37, 206
National goals and aspirations 230
National Health and Family Welfare Programs 332
National Institute Ranking Framework 38
National integration 19
National interests, priority to 19
National League for Nursing 290
National Policy on Education 25, 27, 35, 36
National security 18
Natural interaction technology 377
Natural phenomena 10
Naturalism 10
   and school 11
   forms of 10
   metaphysics of 10
   principles of 10
   values of 10
Naturalist movement 10
Naturalistic education, characteristics of 10
Nature, laws of 10
Neurological disorder 189
New Education Policy 35
New technology adaptation 329
Newer diseases emerge 325
News releases
   audio 349
   video 349
Newsletters 223, 349
   and publications, internal 348
Nirvana 15
Nishkamya karma 13

Nonparticipant observation 169
Nonprint-based resources 252
Nonstandardized tests 193
Nonuniversity programs 206
Nonverbal communication 115
Norm-referenced
   score interpretations 194
   test 153, 154, 200
Nosepiece 147
Numerical grading 192
Numerical rating scales 176
Nurse 26
   charter 368
   educator, competencies of 296
   patient interactions, recording 112
   practitioner in critical care 291, 335
   role 346
   service condition for 368
Nursing 207, 250
   application in 54, 55
   associate degree in 202
   basic sciences applied to 250
   care
      conferences 111
      standards 361
   clinic, planning 109
   continuing education in 212
   doctor of 203
   examination board, functions of 365
   foundations 208
   journal 370
   knowledge 246
   organizations, list of 367
   post-basic diploma in 336
   postgraduate diploma in 205
   science, doctor of 203
   students, counseling of 302
   teacher, preparation of 295
   trends in development of 34
Nursing care study 108
   advantages of 109
   development of 108
   disadvantages of 109
Nursing Council on Nursing Curricula 245
Nursing curriculum
   administration of 317
   nature of 232
Nursing education 205
   advantages for 99
   aims of 16
   assessment in 221
   at global level 202
   challenges in 29
   doctor of 203
   institutions
      administration of 331
      management of 331
   issues in 203
   levels of 35, 317

   programs 202
   purposes of continuing 213
   standardization of 368
Nursing profession
   issues external to 234
   issues specific to 234
Nursing program 332
   graduates of masters of 210
   types of 30
Nursing rounds 110
   motivates 110
Nursing standards 360
   characteristics of 361
   classification of 361
   importance of 361
   process of 362
   purpose of 361
   sources of 362

O

Objective tests 162
Objective type examinations
   demerits of 168
   merits of 168
Observational method, types of 169
Observational technique
   demerits of 169
   merits of 169
Online teaching
   and learning, characteristics of 378
   tutor competencies for 227
On-the-job role model 283
Operating system 377
Operation blackboard 35
Operational level, actual 374
Optical microscope 147
   simple 147
Oral examination 179
   improving 179
Organization of discussion, general principles for 79
Organization's website 348
Organizing faculty development programs, steps in 358
Orientation service 301
Orifices, open 98
Original learning, degree of 218
Overhead projector 135, 135f
   advantages of 136
   disadvantages of 137
   parts of 135
   transparencies 135

P

Painful lecture 77
Palmer's thoughts 43
Pamphlet 125
   advantages of 125
   disadvantages of 125
Pancha mahavrata 14

Panel discussion 83
Paper presentation 356
Paranoia 199
Parent surrogate 267
Patient-centered discussion 110
Peace education 37
Pediatric nurse practitioner 203
Peer evaluation 294
   advantages of 294
   criteria of good 295
   disadvantages of 294
   goals of 294
   guiding principles of 294, 353
   process 354
Peer evaluators 353
Peer review 219
   characteristics of 354
Peer tutoring 102, 103
   benefits of 103
   cross-age 102
   incidental 102
   long-term 103
   models of 102
   reciprocal 103
   same-age 103
   short-term 103
   types of 102
Peer tutors and tutees, role of 104
Pencil tests 193
Performance appraisal 351
   alternative types of 353
   meaning and concept of 291
   principles of 352
   problems of 353
   process 352
   tool for 353
Personal counseling style, developing 309
Personal digital assistance 226
Personal growth 310
Personal skills 306
Personal social development 299
Personal values 264
Personality 324
   all-round development of 17
   development of 13, 16, 18
   inventories 194
   of student, development of 14
   tests 199
   traits 264
Pestanji Hormusji Cama Hospital 34
Philosophical implications 7
Philosophical inquiry 11
Philosophical thoughts 7
Philosophy 3, 7
   and education 3
      relationship between 5
   and objectives, formulation of 248
   branch of 5
   divisions in 3, 5f
   doctor of 203

in nursing
    doctor of 210, 335
    master of 335
main divisions in 3
major systems of 7
of continuing education 214
of education 230
    significance of 7
of life 44
of nursing education 234
program in nursing, master of 210
Photograph 115, 142, 347
Photography, steps in 143
Physical and learning resources 335
Physical environment
  and facilities 324
  arrangement of 307
  management of 71
Physical facilities 323, 332, 334, 335
Physical naturalism 10
Pictorial graphs (social graph) 122, 123f
Picture 120f
  types of 120
Pie graph 122, 122f
  method of construction of 122
Planning lecture, factors influencing 75
Planning unit, essential activities in 69
Plastics 115
Plotters 142
Podcasting 388
Policy 323
  and procedures, review of 322
  emphasizes 35
Political environment 26, 30
Political factors influencing education 26
Political ideology 230
Political neutrality 272
Population sample 187
Post-basic diploma programs 211
Post-clinical discussion 110
Post-crisis intervention procedures 316
Poster 120
  advantages of 121
  color papers 115
  disadvantages of 121
  preparation of 121
  purposes of 120
Postgraduate nursing program 205
Postgraduate selection tests 199
Post-teaching 53
Powerpoint presentation 145
  criteria for developing 145
  guidelines for preparing 145
Practical examination 177, 180
  advantages of 178
  characteristics of 178
  pattern of 180
  procedure of 177
  purposes of 177
  traditional system of 179

Practical teacher 283
Practice and continuing education, relationship between 216
Practice component 282
Practice review 219
Practicing blackboard writing 282
Practicing teaching 282
Pradhan Mantri Gramodaya Yojana 27
Pragmatism
  and school 12
  forms of 11
  principles of 11
Praise and blame, judicious use of 271
Precautionary suspension 313
Preparing transparency, method of 136
Pre-school education 37
Press kits 349
Press release 347
Preteaching 52
Prevalidation 164
Preventive counseling 302
Principal, role of 306
Print
  based resources 252
  material 373
  media 347
Printers 142
Printing and publishing technology 377
Problem design, seven principles of 92
Problem, example of 93
Problem-based learning 91
  advantages of 94
  approaching group problems in 95
  methodology 91
Problem-centered model 239
Problem-solving
  skills 91
  techniques 109
Procedure station 180
Process recording
  disadvantages of 113
  phases of 112
  preparing student for 112
  purposes of 112
Proctors model 54
Produce materials 220
Production budget 343
  cost of 343
Productive association 366
Profession and professional education 33, 286
Professional activity 301
Professional aptitude tests 198
Professional association 366
  activities 367
  benefits of 366
  serve 367
Professional competence 304

Professional development 34, 287
  activities for teacher educators 288
  plays 34
  principles of 287
  techniques of 287
Professional education 33
  fundamentals of 33, 286
  responsibilities of 33, 286
Professional ethics 271
  of teacher 265
Professional organizations, role of 321
Professional practice, competencies related to 296
Professional requirements, qualities relating to 271
Professional socialization 204
Professional teacher educator 285
Professional teaching, problem of 33
Professionalize teacher education 285
Professor-cum-Vice-Principal 334
Program content 214
Program development 102
Program duration 215
Program evaluation 259, 321
  aims of 321
  plan 322
Program format 215
Program instruction 88
  material 89
Program learning, elements in 89
Program planning 337
Program textbook 90
Program writing 90
  steps in 90
Programed instruction
  advantages of 90
  characteristics of 89
  disadvantages of 90
Programing, styles of 90
Progressive educators 6
Project
  method, stages of 86
  types of 86
Projected and nonprojected media 115
Projection surfaces 143
Pseudo-privatization 25
Psychasthenia 199
Psychological factors 75
Psychological questions and theories 240
Psychological test 193
  classification of 193, 194
Psychomotor domain 65
Psychopathic deviation 199
Public address system 139, 139f
Public affairs 347
Public relations 346, 351
  advantages of 346
  disadvantages of 347
  for nursing, role of 346

objectives of 346, 347
tools 347
trends in 350
Publications 355, 368
Publicity 347
  portrait shots, types of photographs in 347
Pulse oximetry 98
Punishment
  nature of 345
  types of 345
Punitive suspension 345
Pupil's performance, evaluating and reporting 268
Puppet 132, 133f
  advantages of 133
  disadvantages of 133
  preparation of 133
  types of 133
Purposeful group activity 12

Q

Qualities of behavior, values and 273
Quality control 329
Question
  filing and storage of 188
  large number of 185
  review of unwanted 188
  screening of 186
Question bank 185, 186, 188
  advantages 186
  blueprinting for developing 186
  computerized 188
  development of 186
  disadvantages 186
  planning 186
Question paper
  editing 161
  preparation of blueprint of 160
  refining 160
  review of 161
  setting, mechanics of 160
Quite heterogeneous 91

R

Radio 137f
  limitations of 137, 375
Radio/audio medium 375
Rapport with government 369
Rashtriya Madhyamik Shiksha Abhiyan 26
Rating scale 175
  advantages of 177
  disadvantages of 177
  items 185
  types of 176
Reading 288
  habits and journals 357
Realism
  and discipline 10
  and school 10
  forms of 9
  metaphysics of 9
Realistic education, characteristics of 9
Realistic epistemology 9
Realistic equipment 97
Realistic value theory 9
Real-life instructor 1
Recorded broadcast 139, 376
Recruitment 340
  factors affecting 340
  methods of 341
  policy 341
  process, steps of 340
  sources of 341
  techniques of 341
Re-examine philosophy 255
References, inclusion of 135
Regular teaching 355
Relief theories 104
Religious doctrinaire 230
Religious student (Brahmacharya) 13
Religious tolerance 272
Remote locations, file transfer from 390
Reporting back 93
Reporting conferences 111
Reproducing test 189
Reproductive healthcare services 23
Research 33, 323, 325, 347
  and development collaboration 329
  areas of 221
  in continuing nursing education 220
  sponsorship of 329
Resource material creator 284
Resource mobilization, strategies for 23
Restitution 311
Rich learning experience 378
Rich site summary 350
Right faith 14
Right of Children to Free and Compulsory Education Act 27
Rights of Child and Adolescent Education, Protection of 37
Road traffic accidents 23
Rod puppet 133
Role model 267, 283
Role play 87
  advantages of 88
  disadvantages of 88
  during 88
  organization of 87
  preparation phase 87
  process 87
  session 88
Room setup/equipment 225
Rural university 35

S

Sage (sanyasi) 13
Samagra shiksha 26
Samyag-darsana 14
Samyak Charita 14
Sarva Shiksha Abhiyan 26
Scale dimensions, differential 184
Scanner 377
Scheduled caste communities 35
Schizophrenia 199
Scholarship 323
  funds, affiliation with 369
  of application 295
  of discovery 295
  of integration 295
  of teaching 295
Scholastic aptitude tests 198
School
  admission test, law 199
  and community contents 55
  assessment and governance 38
  climate 54
  in society, role of 6
  nurse practitioner 203
  organization, familiarizing with 278
Science in nursing, master of 203
Scientific method, application of 325
Scientific procedures, application of 325
Scorer's personal judgment 156
Scrambled textbook 90
Scriptural knowledge 14
Search engine optimization 350
Seashore musical aptitude test 199
Secularist 267
Selection and supply type, characteristics of 189
Selection procedure, steps in 341
Self-awareness and understanding 306
Self-esteem, developing 269
Self-evaluating 96, 293, 354
  demerits of 354
  disadvantages of 293
  reasons for 354
Self-financing institutions 24, 30
Self-instructional material 226
Self-instructional module 95
  characteristics of 95
Self-learning 96
  packets 95
Self-motivating 96
Self-pacing, principle of 90
Self-sufficiency, achievement of 18
Semantic differentials 184
Seminar 80, 82
  advantages of 82
  developing paper for 81
  disadvantages of 82
  method, creative aspects of 81
  offers opportunity 81
Sense
  experience, independent of 8
  realism 9
Sensitivity, principle of 242

Shadow puppet 133
Share decision 253
Short answer questions
   types of 161
   uses of 161
Simpson's categorization 65
Simulation equipment, types of 97
Simulation process, steps of 98
Simulation units, types of 98
Situational crises 315
Skill 246, 307
   in conducting interviews 306
   in questioning 271
   manpower, supply of 19
Skype 388
Slide
   projector, effective use of 132
   types of 131
Slide and film 131
   projections
      advantages of 132
      disadvantages of 132
Small group teaching method 112
Social activities, contribution in 356
Social agreements and law 6
Social and national integration 16
Social desirability bias 184
Social efficiency, promotion of 19
Social factors
   and nursing education 22
   influencing education 21
Social feelings, inculcation of 17
Social insight, creating 278
Social introversion 199
Social realism 9
Social reform 17
Social relationships 217
Social utilitarianism 232
Social welfare 217
Society 234
   needs of 231
Sociocultural tradition, transmission of 328
Socioeconomic status scale 200
Sociograms 173
Sociological considerations 230
Sociometric criteria 170
Sociometric intervention, steps in 172
Sociometry 170
Software 374
Speaking engagements 349
Spheres of work, practical knowledge of 18
Spiritual direction 21
Spiritual in nature 3
Staff development 329
Staff issues 256
Staff resources 335
Staff welfare services 357

Standardized test 193
   design of 194
   score 194
      types of 194
Standardized tools 193
Stanford scientific aptitude test 199
Stanford-Binet scale 200
Starting programs, steps in 331
State Councils of Higher Education 38
State Implementation Society 27
State Nursing Council 365
Stations and patients, types of 180
Stock, absence of 185
Storage devices, external 142
Stream chart 118, 118f
String puppet 133
Student 29, 234
   abilities 256
   admission 208
   advantages for 299
   assessor 284
   behavior 56
   better understanding of 277
   centered teaching 57
   centeredness 300
   counseling, preparation for 283
   evaluation of teacher 292, 354
   instructions to 182
   intellectual growth of 51
   management of 72
   misconduct
      in classroom 74
      responding to 314
   performance outcomes 58
   role of 94, 321
   safety of 266
   security of 266
   support services 373
   testing, principle of 90
   training of 329
   viewpoints 256
Study
   day system 250
   guide producer 284
Subject matter 252
   centered objectives 248
   factors 75
   units 68
Subject specialists, roles of 320
Subject taught 207
Suicide threat 316
Summative evaluation 153, 354
   characteristics of 153
Support staff 322
   evaluation of 323
Survey form 293
Syadvada 14
Symposium 82
   advantages of 83
   disadvantages of 83

   purpose of 82
   technique 82

T

Tabulation chart 118
Tape recorder 138
   advantages of 138
   disadvantages of 138
Tariff boards 125
Taxonomic levels-cognitive domain 238
Taxonomy hierarchy 187
Teacher 29
   academic achievements 265
   accountability 265
   acronym of 272
   advantages for 300
   as independent variable 52
   as instructor, functions of 266
   as role model 264
   behavior 55
   centered
      objectives 248
      teaching 57
   character of 264, 272
   competency 274
   concepts of 263
   development, components of 279f
   diary, maintaining 266
   duties of 266
   efficiency, test of 158
   essential qualities of 264
   expertise 69
   factors related to 243
   in classroom management, role of 72
   major functions of 267
   mental health 264
   multifarious role 267
   multiple roles of 284
   need for evaluation of 291
   personality of 264, 272
   physical health 264
   plan 70
   properties 55
   requirements in lesson planning 68
   responsibilities of 267
   role of 268, 306
   social adjustment 264
   training, aspects of 278
   twelve roles of 283
Teacher education 278, 325
   and training 275
   concepts of 276
   environment 279f
   functions 276
      and objectives of 276
   institutions, functions of 282
   outcomes of 277f
   problems in 278
   types of 277
   values of 277f

Teacher educator 279
    selection of 278
Teacher evaluation 291
    by students, tools for 293
Teacher made tests 154
    and standardized tests, difference between 193t
Teacher preparation 22, 263
    curriculum for 280
Teacher professional
    efficiency 265
    training 265
Teacher role 291
    broad classification of 267
    in society 267
    technology and 387
Teacher-led instruction, effective 72
Teaching 49, 373
    action 56
    aids 282
    and teaching strategy evaluation 323
    aptitude test 199
    as social service 266
    biases 56
    block 250
    classification of methods of 74
    curricula 30
    effectiveness, evidence for 295
    employed, methods of 108
    evaluation model 352
    faculty 333
    general principles of 50
    good 53
    interactive phase 52
    machine 89
    materials 282
    methodology of 277
    methods of 8, 12, 74, 113
    models, availability of 100
    observation of high quality 282
    online 378
    performance, evaluation of 295
    phases of 52
    postactive phase 52
    preactive phase 52
    principles and practices, effective 50
    qualifications relating to 272
    selection of methods of 74
    stages of 52
    strategies 56
    system 250
    taxonomy for 63
    technical skills of 275
    technique of 268
    technology, use of 271
    variables of 52
Teaching and learning 6, 27
    activities, selection of 69
    dialog in 107
    method 74
    process 45, 52, 54
        models of 53
        relationship between 56
    unit 68
Teaching competencies 296
    A to Z of 275
Teaching skills 227, 274
    at planning stage 275
    desirable 275
Technical ability 304
Technical competency 1
Technical skills 227
Technological explosion 234
Technological factors 373
    influencing education 27
Technological infrastructure 224
Technological problems 378
Technological skill upgradation 30
Technology
    adoption of 374
    usage of 226
Tele nursing 33
Teleconference sessions, organization of 384
Teleconferencing 384
    advantages of 385
    benefits of 385
    broadcasting through 221
    categories of 373
    limitations of 385
    regular 373
Telemedicine 33
Telepathy 14
Television 139, 139f
    as educational tool, merits of 139, 376
    broadcasts, kinds of 139, 376
    limitations of 140
    media, limitations of 376
Temperance 269
Temporal sequence 252
Tendency toward perfectionism 309
Tension to interview, maintaining 307
Test 150, 188
    criterion-referenced 188
    items, quality of 193
    norm-referenced 188
    purposes 188
    security 182
    types of 188
Textbooks, development of 252
Third party method 341
Three language formula 35
Thurstone scale 184
    construction of 185
Thurstone's vocational interest schedule 197
Time chart 119
Trades
    commercial presence 32
    consumption abroad 32
    cross border supply 32
    distance education 32
    movement of natural persons 32
Traditional blackboard 125
Traditional education methods 60
Traditional scoring system, drawbacks of 190
Traditional teacher 114
Trained nurses' association 367
    functions of 368
    membership 368
Training program 208
Transmission control protocol 386, 390
Transmission electron microscope 147
Tree chart 118, 118f
True-false completion type, multiple 163
Tutees 104
Tutor 104
    choosing 103
    trained 103
Tutorial group functions 94
Tutorial mode 102
Tutoring, hindrances to 103
Twitter 350
Tylerian model 322

U

Unit plan 68, 71
    characteristics of 68
    selection of 69
    types of 68
United Nations Development Programme 22
Unity in diversity, knowledge of 8
University Education Commission 40
University Grants Commission 23
University programs 206
Unstructured techniques 170
Unwanted questions, removal of 188
Upanishads 12
Upasanas 13

V

Vairagya 12
Vanaprastha 13
Vedanta philosophy 12
Vedic philosophy 12
Verbal warning 312
Video cassette recorder 145, 145f
    advantages of 145
    disadvantages of 146
Video compact disk 145
    advantages of 145
    disadvantages of 145
Videoconferencing 221, 224, 373
Video-teleconference 384, 389
Virtual campus 380
    limitations of 381
Virtual classroom 381
    advantages of 381

components of 383
  learning, characteristics of 382
  unique features of 381
Virtual education 381
Virtual university 28, 381
Vision, broader 205
Visual aids 115
Visual appeal 135
Visual display unit 142
Visual learners 48
Vital signs 181
Vitamin
  A 164
  B 164
  C 164
  D 164
  deficiency diseases 164
Vitreous-coated steel surface 125
Viva voce 179
  examination, characteristics of 179
Vocal sounds 98

Vocational development 299
Vocational efficiency 16, 18
Vocational interest blank, strong 197
Voice, good 272
Voicing opinion 350
Vyakarna 12

W

Wallboards 125
Weapons 315
Webcast 223
Weblogs 388
Website 348
  press room 349
Wechsler adult intelligence scale 200
Welfare activities 370
White boards 125
Wide mental flexibility 83
Wiki 388
Wireless technologies 388, 390

Wood 115
  paint-coated pressed 125
Work scheduling 337
Workshop 96
  advantages 97
  attendants of 96
  disadvantages 97
  organization of 96
  purposes of 96
World Trade Organization 31, 32
  and education 32
Writing and scoring essay questions 159
Writing assessment 321
Writing test directions 189
Writing unit plan, steps in 69
Written speech 348
Written tests, types of 157*fc*
Written warning 345
  final 313
  first 312